ARTERY BYPASS

Edited by **Wilbert S. Aronow**

Artery Bypass
http://dx.doi.org/10.5772/50852
Edited by Wilbert S. Aronow

Contributors
Lester A.H. Critchley, Inna Kammerer, Tagreed Altaei, Imad Jamal, Diyar Dilshad, Mohammed A Balghith, Rainer G. H. Moosdorf, Maseeha Khaleel, Tracy Dorheim, Daniel Anderson, Michael Duryee, Geoffrey Thiele, Takao Kato, Benetti, Haralabos Parissis, Alan Soo, Bassel Al-Alao, Aditya M Sharma, Herbert Aronow, Oguzhan Yıldız, Melik Seyrek, Husamettin Gul, Cheng-Xiong Gu, Yang Yu, Chuan Wang, AC Zago, Eduardo K Saadi, Rui M. Almeida, Wilbert S. Aronow, Sean Maddock, Gilbert L. Tang, Ramin Malekan, Yuki Igarashi, Takeo Igarashi, Ryo Haraguchi, Kazuo Nakazawa, Jiri Mandak, Martin Šimek, Martin Kalab, Martin Molitor, Patrick Tobbia, Vladimír Lonský, Marcel A. Beijk, Ralf Harskamp, Luminita Iliuta, Faisal Latif, Muhammad A. Chaudhry, Zainab Omar, Philippe Dubois, Maximilien Gourdin, Tsuyoshi Kaneko, Sary Aranki, J D Schwalm, Michael Tsang, Andrea Székely, Zsuzsanna Cserép, Masaki Yamamoto, Kazumasa Orihashi, Takayuki Sato, Kim Houlind, Johnny Christensen

Published by InTech
Janeza Trdine 9, 51000 Rijeka, Croatia

Copyright © 2013 InTech

Notice

Publishing Process Manager Viktorija Zgela
Technical Editor InTech DTP team
Cover InTech Design team

Additional hard copies can be obtained from orders@intechopen.com

Artery Bypass, Edited by Wilbert S. Aronow
p. cm.
ISBN 978-953-51-1025-5

For EU product safety concerns:
IN TECH d.o.o., Prolaz Marije Krucifikse Kozulić 3, 51000 Rijeka, Croatia,
info@intechopen.com or visit our website at intechopen.com.

Meet the editor

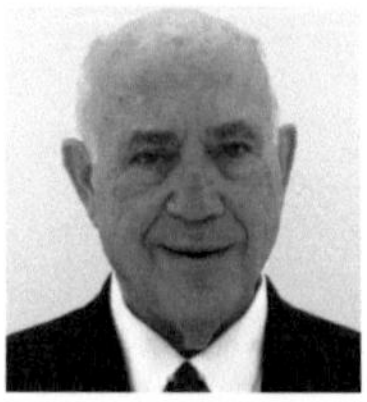

Wilbert S. Aronow, MD, FACC, FAHA, FCCP, FACP graduated from Harvard Medical School. He is Professor of Medicine at Westchester Medical Center/New York Medical College. Dr. Aronow has edited 10 books and is author or co-author of 1,272 papers (647 original research papers, 172 chapters in 96 books, 394 review papers, and 59 editorials), 190 commentaries or Letters to the Editor, and 883 abstracts. He has been a member of 75 editorial boards of medical journals, an associate editor for 9 medical journals, and a guest editor for 6 other medical journals. Dr. Aronow has been a consultant to numerous government agencies, a member of committees in numerous professional societies, and a member of guidelines committees.

Contents

Preface

The latest diagnostic and therapeutic modalities in the management of coronary artery disease by coronary artery bypass graft surgery and by percutaneous coronary intervention with stenting and in the interventional management of other atherosclerotic vascular disease have led to a reduction in cardiovascular mortality and morbidity. This book entitled Artery Bypass provides an excellent update on these advances which every physician seeing patients with atherosclerotic vascular disease should be familiar with. This book includes 27 chapters written by experts in their topics.

The first section of this book discusses basic science and physiology and includes 6 chapters. The second section of this book discusses coronary artery bypass graft surgery and includes 11 chapters. The third section of this book discusses percutaneous coronary intervention with stenting and includes 3 chapters. The fourth section of this book discusses peripheral and cerebral vascular disease intervention and includes 5 chapters. The fifth section of this book discusses miscellaneous cardiac surgical topics and includes 2 chapters. Another strength of thisbook is that unresolved issues are also discussed.

I would like to thank all of the contributors for their outstanding work. Finally, I would like to thank you, the reader, for your commitment to providing the best possible care to your patients with atherosclerotic vascular disease. I hope you will find this book a valuable resource in providing excellent care to your patients with atherosclerotic vascular disease.

Wilbert S. Aronow, MD, FACC, FAHA, FCCP, FACP
Professor of Medicine, New York Medical College
Valhalla, NY, USA

Section 1

Basic Science and Physiology

Chapter 1

Impact of Ischemia on Cellular Metabolism

Maximilien Gourdin and Philippe Dubois

Additional information is available at the end of the chapter

http://dx.doi.org/10.5772/54509

1. Introduction

As in all aerobic eukaryotic cells, oxygen is essential for homeostasis in human cells. The interruption of blood flow to tissues results in an arrested oxygen supply and disrupts the biochemical reactions that ensure the smooth functioning, integrity and survival of the cells. The limited oxygen reserves that are dissolved in the interstitial fluid and are bound to hemoglobin, myoglobin and neuroglobin do not maintain efficient, long-term metabolism.[1,2] Lack of oxygen affects all functions within the cell. Table 1 summarizes the main cellular consequences of ischemia.

(1) cellular acidosis;
(2) loss of sarcoplasmic membrane potential;
(3) cellular swelling;
(4) cytoskeleton disorganization;
(5) reduction of adenosine-5'-triphospate (ATP) and phosphocreatine is more than reduction in the energy substrates;
(6) reduction of glutathione, of a-tocopherol;
(7) increasing expression of leukocyte adhesion molecules;
(8) secretion of cytokines/chemokines
- Tumor Necrosis Factor (TNF-α)
- Interleukins (IL-) -1, 6, 8

Table 1. Major cellular consequences of ischemia

2. Adenosine triphosphate depletion

Eukaryotic cells contain mitochondria, organelles whose main function is to produce adenosine triphosphate (ATP). ATP is an essential energy substrate, as its hydrolysis provides energy for many metabolic and biochemical reactions involved in development, adaptation and cell survival. ATP production in an aerobic cell is particularly effective when the degradation of key nutrients such as glucose and fatty acids is coupled to a supramolecular complex located in the inner membrane of mitochondria to drive oxidative phosphorylation. Oxidative phosphorylation is mediated by an electron transport chain that consists of four protein complexes and establishes a transmembrane electrochemical gradient by supporting the accumulation of protons in the intermembrane space of the mitochondria. This gradient is used as an energy source by ATP synthase during the synthesis of an ATP molecule from a molecule of adenosine diphosphate (ADP) and an inorganic phosphate (Figure 1). Without oxygen, oxidative phosphorylation stops: the proton gradient between the intermembrane space and the inner mitochondria is abolished, and ATP synthesis is interrupted. The ensuing rapid fall in intracellular ATP induces a cascade of events leading to reversible cell damage. However, over time, the damage increases and gradually becomes irreversible, which may lead to cell death and destruction of the parenchymal tissue.

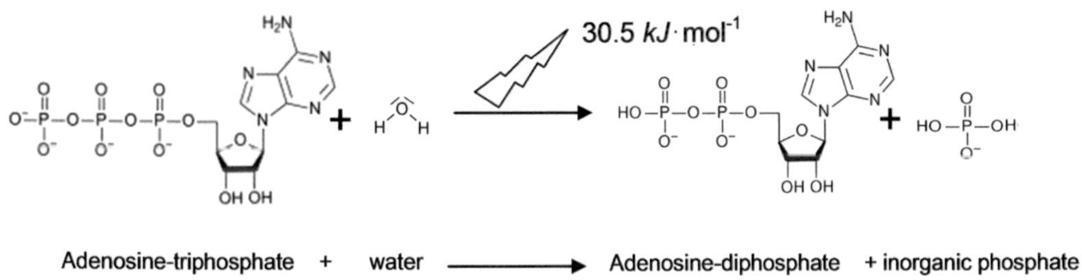

Figure 1. Hydrolysis of Adenosine-triphosphate provides energy (30.5 kJ per mole) for biochemical reactions

When devoid of ATP, the cell derives its energy from the pyrophosphate bonds of ADP as they are degraded to adenosine monophosphate (AMP) and then to adenosine. Adenosine diffuses freely out of the cell, dramatically reducing the intracellular pool of adenine nucleotides, the precursors for ATP.

3. Changes in metabolism (Figure 2)

In the presence of oxygen, human cells respire and derive their energy from the complete degradation of food (fats, carbohydrates and amino acids) by specific oxidative processes that fuel oxidative phosphorylation. A lack of oxygen completely changes these metabolic pathways, disrupting glycolysis and inhibiting the degradation pathways of lipids (beta-oxidation), amino acids and oxidative phosphorylation.

http://dx.doi.org/10.5772/54509

3.1. Glucose metabolism

During ischemia, the cell will change not only its glucose supply routes but also its glycolysis pathways and transition from aerobic glycolysis to anaerobic glycolysis. When this happens, the available cytosolic glucose is metabolized by anaerobic glycolysis and becomes the main source of ATP. The efficiency of this process is much lower than that of aerobic glycolysis coupled to oxidative phosphorylation; the anaerobic degradation of one molecule of glucose produces 2 ATP molecules compared to the 36 ATP molecules that are produced under aerobic conditions. Consumption quickly exceeds production, and the intracellular concentration of ATP decreases. For example, in the heart, the degree of glycolysis inhibition is directly proportional to the severity of coronary flow restriction.[3]-[5]

3.1.1. Glucose supply

With the complete interruption of or decrease in blood flow, the extracellular concentration of glucose drops very quickly. First, the cell optimizes the uptake of glucose from the interstitial space by improving glucose transmembrane transport by increasing the sarcoplasmic expression of the high-affinity glucose transporters GLUT-1 and GLUT-4. [6]-[8] This protective mechanism temporarily compensates for the decrease in extracellular glucose concentration. Next, the cell uses its intracellular glucose stores of glycogen. [9] The decrease in intracellular ATP and glucose-6-phosphate, the rising lactate/pyruvate ratio and the increase in intracellular AMP and the inorganic phosphate concentration activate a phosphorylase kinase, which catalyses the conversion of glycogene phosphorylase b to its active form, glycogene phosphorylase a. This cascade reaction leads to an intense and rapid consumption of glycogen. [10]-[14]

3.1.2. Glycolysis pathways

The inhibition of oxidative phosphorylation caused by lack of oxygen does not allow the pyruvate produced by glycolysis to be degraded. Under aerobic conditions, pyruvate is transported into the mitochondria and feeds into the Krebs cycle, which provides the nicotinamide adenine dinucleotide (NADH, H^+) and flavine adenine dinucleotide ($FADH_2$) cofactors for oxidative phosphorylation, significantly increasing the yield of glycolysis.

Ischemia modulates the activity of the following two key enzymes of anaerobic glycolysis: phosphofructo-1-kinase (PF1K) and glyceraldehyde-3-phosphate dehydrogenase (GAPDH).

Following the onset of ischemia, or during moderate ischemia, the activation of glycogenolysis accelerates glycolysis.[15]-[17] The decrease in both intracellular ATP and creatine phosphate, along with increases in the intracellular concentrations of AMP, inorganic phosphate and fructose-1,6-bisphosphate, intensify the activity of PF1K and GAPDH. [17]-[20]

During prolonged or sustained ischemia, the low intracellular glucose concentration, the disappearance of glycogen and severe intracellular acidosis eventually inhibit PF1K. Furthermore, high concentrations of lactate and protons in ischemic tissues also inhibit GAPDH. [21],[22]

Moreover, the lactate/pyruvate ratio, intracellular acidosis and the absence of regenerated essential cofactors, such as NADH,H^+, affect the catalytic activity of the other enzymes involved in the initial step of glycolysis and prevent the optimal performance of anaerobic glycolysis. [23]

3.2. Lipid metabolism (Figure 2)

The importance of oxygen in functional oxidative phosphorylation leads to a significant reduction in ATP production from the beta-oxidation of fatty acids that is proportional to the degree of ischemia. In mild to moderate ischemia, the rate of fatty acid oxidation decreases but still fuels oxidative phosphorylation. [4],[24] In more severe ischemia, the lack of the cofactors NADH,H^+ and FAD^+, which are normally regenerated through oxidative phosphorylation, completely inhibits acyl-CoenzymeA (acyl-CoA) dehydrogenase and 3-hydroxyacyl-CoA dehydrogenase, which are key beta-oxidation enzymes.[4],[25] The cytosolic concentrations of fatty acids, acyl-CoA and acylcarnitine rise gradually. [26]-[28] The accumulation of these amphiphilic compounds in ischemic tissues has major functional implications. They dissolve readily in cell membranes and affect the functional properties of membrane proteins. Decreased activity of Na^+/K^+-ATPase and the sarcoplasmic and endoplasmic reticulum Ca^{2+}-ATPase pumps, as well as the activation of ATP-dependent potassium channels, reduces the inwardly rectifying potassium current and prolongs the opening of Na^+ channels, delaying their inactivation.[29]-[31] The accumulation of amphiphilic compounds produces a time-dependent reversible reduction in gap-junction conductance. [31]

3.3. Metabolite detoxification pathways

Reducing the intracellular concentration of ATP inhibits the hexose phosphate cycle. This metabolic pathway regenerates glutathione, ascorbic acid and tocopherol, which are involved in the detoxification of metabolites from the cytosol and the sarcoplasmic membrane.

4. Intracellular acidosis

Intracellular acidosis is a cardinal feature of cellular ischemia. The increased production of protons due to metabolic modifications very quickly saturates the buffering capacity of the cell. Intracellular acidosis interferes directly and indirectly with the optimal functioning of the cell by increasing intracellular Na^+ through the activation of Na^+/H^+ exchangers and by Ca^{2+} activation of Na^+/Ca^{2+} exchangers, increasing the production of free radicals; changing the affinity of different proteins, such as enzymes and troponin C, to Ca^{2+}; modifying tertiary protein structures; inhibiting enzymes; and disrupting the function of sarcoplasmic pumps and carriers.[29]

http://dx.doi.org/10.5772/54509

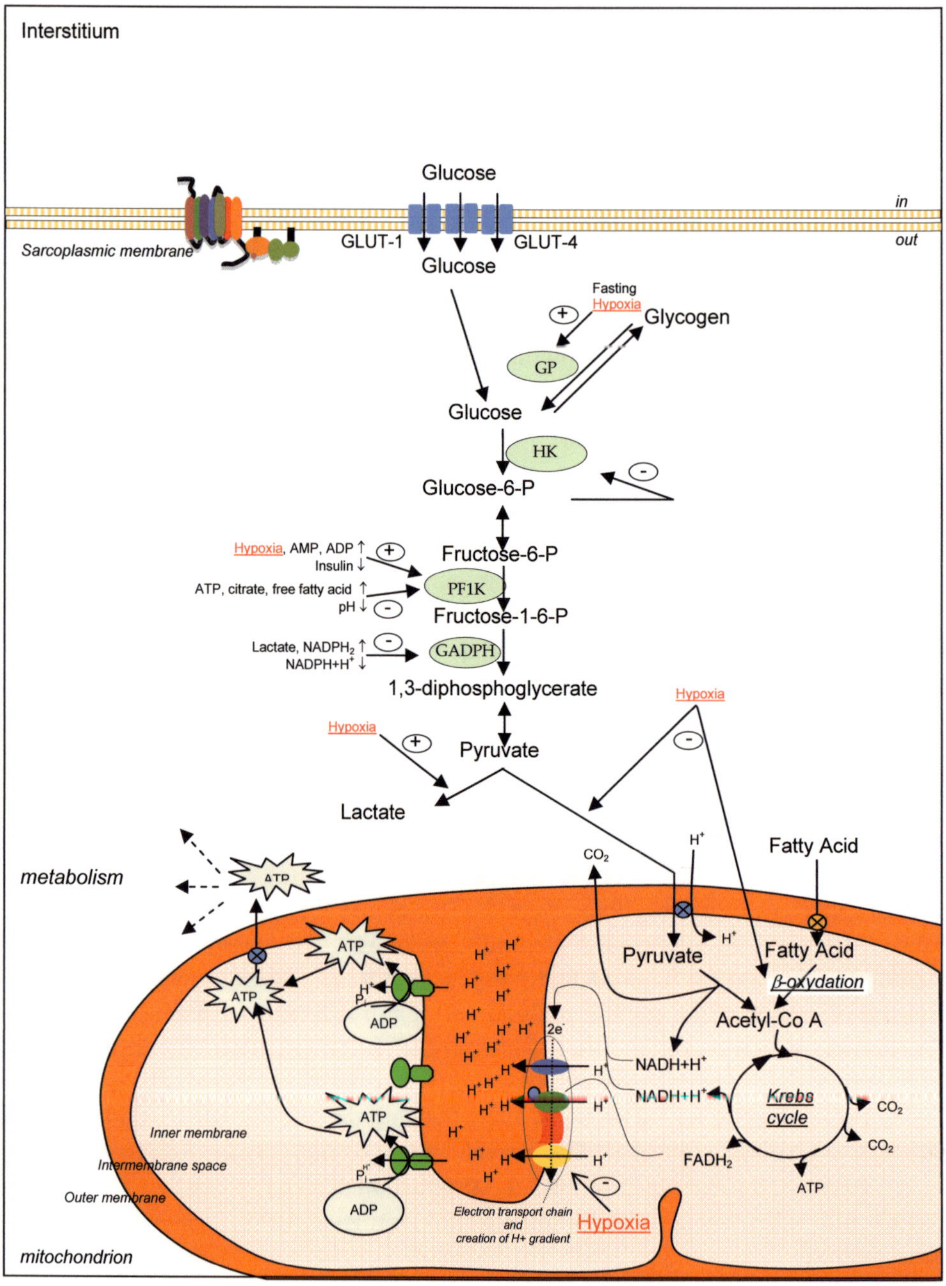

Figure 2. This figure shows schematically oxidative metabolism, ATP production and the consequences of oxygen deprivation. GLUT-1 and GLUT-4: glucose transporters; GP: Glycogene phosphorylase; HK: Hexokinase; PF1K: Phosphofructo-1-kinase; GADPH: glyceraldehyde-3-phosphate dehydrogenase; NADH, H^+: nicotinamide adenine dinucleotide; $FADH_2$: flavine adenin dinucleotide; P: phosphate;AMP, adenosine monophosphate; adenosine diphosphate;ADP: adenosine diphosphate ATP: adenosine triphosphate; CO_2 : carbon dioxide; O_2 Oxygen; - : inhibition; + activation; H^+: proton; e^-: electron.

The main source of protons during ischemia comes from the production of lactate from pyruvate by lactate dehydrogenase. The accumulation of extracellular lactate greatly reduces the effectiveness of the lactate/proton cotransporter, preventing the removal of protons. Additionally, the residual metabolic activity also contributes to acidosis, as the hydrolysis of an ATP molecule releases a proton.

5. Changes in the ionic cellular equilibrium (Figure 3)

Ischemia induces a profound disturbance of the ionic homeostasis of a cell. The two major changes are the loss of ionic transmembrane gradients, which causes membrane depolarization, and increased intracellular sodium ($[Na^+]_i$), which is responsible for inducing a rise in the intracellular calcium ($[Ca^{2+}]_i$) levels, leading to cellular edema.

Cellular depolarization occurs very rapidly after the onset of ischemia, and these mechanisms are not fully understood. However, it is recognized that both the inhibition of the Na^+/K^+-ATPase and the opening of ATP-dependent K^+ channels play a crucial role. Cellular depolarization is characterized by a negative outgoing current and a decrease in the extracellular concentrations of Na^+, Cl^- and Ca^{2+}, as well as an increase in the extracellular concentration of K^+. Progressive depolarization of the cell also promotes prolonged activation of voltage-dependent sodium channels. [29]

The accumulation of sodium in the cytosol is multifactorial. Acidosis stimulates Na^+/H^+ exchangers to purge cellular H^+, which results in increased intracellular Na^+.[32]-[34] This net movement of Na^+ is accompanied by osmotic water movement. Moreover, inhibition of the Na^+/K^+-ATPase due to a lack of ATP prevents the removal of excess intracellular Na^+. The high intracellular concentration of Na^+ affects the function of other membrane transporters, such as the Na^+/Ca^{2+} antiporter, an accelerator. This allows the extrusion of sodium from the cell at the expense of an intracellular accumulation of Ca^{2+}. The massive entry of calcium into the cell disrupts the mechanisms that regulate its intracellular concentration and induces the release of calcium from the intracellular endoplasmic reticulum stores.[35] The lack of ATP prevents calcium excretion into the interstitium and its sequestration in the endoplasmic reticulum. The accumulation of cytosolic calcium induces degradation of membrane phospholipids and cytoskeletal proteins, alters the both the calcium affinity and the efficiency of proteins involved in contractility, activates nitric oxide synthase (NOS) and proteases such as calpains and caspases, promotes the production of free radicals and alters the tertiary structure of enzymes such as xanthine dehydrogenase, which is converted to xanthine oxidase. [36]-[38]

6. Mitochondria

The mitochondrion plays a central role in ischemic injury. Not only is it the site of critical biochemical reactions in the cell, such as oxidative phosphorylation, beta-oxidation and the

citric acid cycle, but it also occupies a unique position in the cellular balance between life and death. Inhibition of the mitochondrial respiratory chain as a result of oxygen deprivation is the cornerstone of metabolic disturbances.

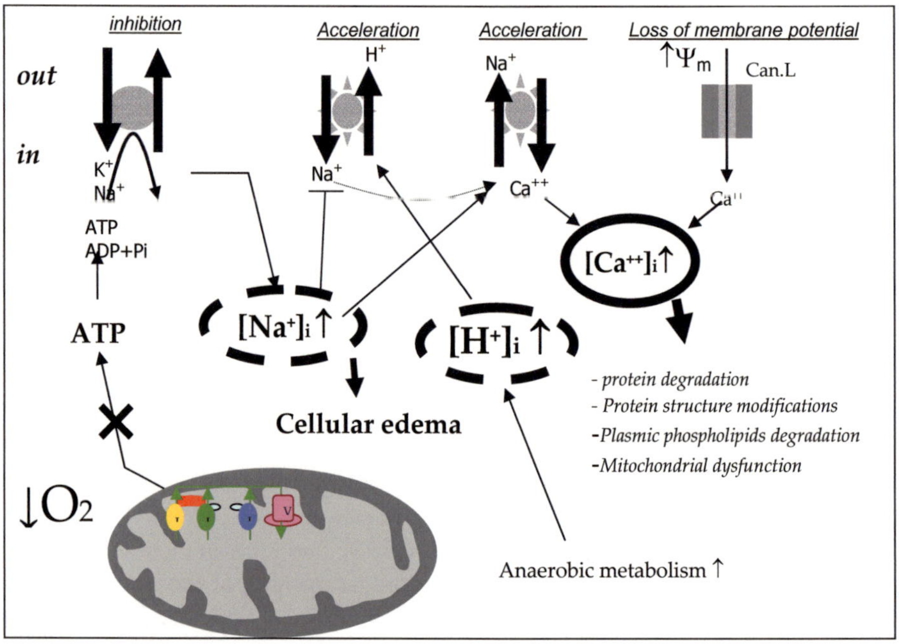

Figure 3. This figure summarizes the ionic perturbations in an ischemic cell.

6.1. Disturbance of ATP synthesis.

Without the respiratory chain oxidation-reduction reactions, proton accumulation in the mitochondrial intermembrane space is interrupted, disrupting the electrochemical gradient that allows ATP synthase to synthesize ATP. During ischemia, the proton-translocating F0F1-ATP synthase, which normally produces ATP, becomes an F0F1-ATPase and consumes ATP in order to pump protons from the matrix to the intermembrane space and maintain the mitochondrial membrane potential.[39],[40] The mitochondria therefore become a site of ATP consumption produced by anaerobic glycolysis.

6.2. An increase in free radical production

Free radical oxygen species (ROS) are highly reactive chemical compounds because they have unpaired electrons in their electron cloud. ROS are capable of oxidizing cellular constituents such as proteins, deoxyribonucleic acid (DNA), membrane phospholipids and other adjacent biological structures. In addition to their role in ischemia, ROS are constitutively generated during metabolic processes and have an important role in cell signaling. Mitochondrial respiration constitutively produces a small amount of ROS, primarily the superox-

ide anion $O_2^{-\bullet}$ at complexes I and III of the electron transport chain. The anion is rapidly converted to hydrogen peroxide (H_2O_2) by metallo-enzymes and superoxide dismutase (SOD). [41]-[43] Cellular stress, particularly oxidative stress, dramatically increases mitochondrial ROS production by disrupting and later inhibiting oxidative phosphorylation. Moreover, the rise in mitochondrial calcium increases ROS production and greatly decreases the antioxidant capacity of mitochondria by decreasing the glutathione peroxidase concentration and SOD activity.

6.3. Intramitochondrial calcium overload

The mitochondrial calcium concentration is in equilibrium between its cytosolic concentration and the proton gradient on either side of the inner membrane of mitochondria. The loss of this gradient due to the inhibition of the respiratory chain, as well as the elevated cytosolic calcium that results from ischemia, allows for the accumulation of calcium in the mitochondria and promotes mitochondrial swelling and the opening of the permeability transition pore.

6.4. Opening of the mitochondrial permeability transition pore

Ischemic disturbances within mitochondria, such as calcium overload, loss of membrane potential, oxidative stress, mass production of free radicals, low NADPH/$NADP^+$ and reduced glutathione to oxidized glutathione ratios (GSH/GSSG), low intra-mitochondrial concentration of ATP or high inorganic phosphate, will promote opening of the permeability transition pore (mPTP) upon reperfusion, a major player in I/R injury-mediated cell lethality.[42], [44] mPTP is a nonspecific channel, and its opening suddenly increases the permeability of the inner mitochondrial membrane to both water and various molecules of high molecular weight (> 1,500 kDa). The opening of mPTPs abolishes the mitochondrial membrane potential and uncouples oxidative phosphorylation, which empties the mitochondria of its matrix and induces apoptosis by releasing the intra-mitochondrial proteins cytochrome c, endonuclease G, Smac/Diablo and apoptosis-inducing factor into the cytosol. [44]-[52]

7. Structural and functional modifications

The cytoskeleton, the internal structural organization of a cell, is composed of a highly regulated complex network of organized structural proteins, including actin, microtubules and lamins. The cytoskeleton performs multiple functions. It maintains internal cellular compartmentalization and mediates the transmission of mechanical forces within the cell to adjacent cells and the extracellular matrix, the distribution of organelles, the movement of molecules or components and the docking of proteins such as membrane receptors or ion channels. Ischemia deconstructs the cytoskeleton. [53]-[56] The high intracellular concentrations of Ca^{2+} that are associated with ischemia activate multiple phosphorylases and proteases that disassemble and degrade the cytoskeleton, thereby eliminating the functions that rely on its integrity, such as phagocytosis, exocytosis, myofilament contraction, intercellular

communication and cell anchorage. Destruction of the internal architecture worsens I/R injuries and leads to apoptosis. [53],[56],[57] During ischemia, all elements of the cytoskeleton are affected, but with different kinetics.[54],[55] Moreover, the accumulation of osmotically active particles, including lactate, sodium, inorganic phosphate and creatine, induces cellular oedema.[38]

Regulatory cellular mechanisms provide intracellular homeostasis that enables optimal enzyme function in a relatively narrow range of environmental conditions. The conditions created by ischemia, such as acidosis and calcium overload, modify or inhibit the activity of many enzymes due to changes in the pH and tertiary structures, affecting cellular metabolism. For example, ischemia induces the conversion of xanthine dehydrogenase to xanthine oxidase.[36]-[38] These two enzymes catalyze the same reactions, converting hypoxanthine to xanthine and xanthine to uric acid. The first reaction uses NAD^+ as a cofactor, whereas the second uses oxygen and produces $O_2^{-\bullet}$, a free radical.

8. Protein synthesis and sarcoplasmic protein expression in an ischemic cell

Protein synthesis is a complex process that requires continuous and adequate energy intake, strict control of ionic homeostasis of the cell and the smooth functioning of many other proteins. Ischemia disrupts these necessary conditions and therefore profoundly affects protein synthesis beyond acute injury. However, the transcription of several genes is initiated at the onset of ischemia, and the mechanisms underlying this phenomenon are not fully understood. Nevertheless, it appears that the mass production of free radicals, the high concentration of calcium, acidosis and the activation of the family of mitogen-activated protein kinases (MAP kinases) play an important role. Nuclear factor heat shock transcription factor-1 (HSF-1) activates the expression of heat shock proteins (HSPs), a family of chaperone proteins, and inhibits the expression of other proteins. HSPs are synthesized in different situations of stress, including hyperthermia, ischemia, hypoxia and mechanical stress, and are intended to prevent the structural modifications of key metabolic and cytoskeletal enzymes and inhibit the activity of caspases. [58]-[60]

The low oxygen partial pressure during ischemia activates other nuclear factors, such as hypoxia-inducible factor-1alpha (HIF-1α). HIF-1α stimulates the transcription of many genes involved in cellular defense, such as those encoding NOS and GLUT-1, and other enzymes involved in glucose metabolism.[61]

In addition, ischemia activates innate immunity by stimulating sarcoplasmic receptors, such as the Toll-like receptors (TLR) TLR-2 and TLR-6, the synthesis and sarcoplasmic expression of which are increased. Receptor stimulation supports the synthesis of chemokines and cytokines and contributes to I/R injury.[61]-[66]

At the onset of ischemia, many substances are secreted by the cell. For example, ischemic cardiomyocytes secrete bradykinin, norepinephrine, angiotensin, adenosine, acetylcholine

and opioids.[67]-[69] In addition, ischemia stimulates the expression of adhesion molecules, such as P-selectins, L-selectins, intercellular adhesion molecule-1 (ICAM-1) and platelet-endothelial cell adhesion molecules (PECAM), on the surface of endothelial cells, leukocytes and other ischemic cells. [62],[63],[70],[71] Furthermore, many cytokines, such as tumor necrosis factor-α, interleukin (IL)-1, IL-6 and IL-8, and vasoactive agents, such as endothelins and thromboxane A2, are secreted by cells in response to ischemia. [62],[70],[72] Cytokines and chemokines, the production of which dramatically increases during reperfusion, initiate the local inflammatory response and prepare for the recruitment of inflammatory cells into the injured area, respectively.

Author details

Maximilien Gourdin* and Philippe Dubois

*Address all correspondence to: maximilien.gourdin@uclouvain.be

Université de Louvain (UCL), University Hospital CHU UCL Mont-Godinne – Dinant, Yvoir, Belgium

References

[1] Jennings RB, Murry CE, Steenbergen C, Jr., Reimer KA: Development of cell injury in sustained acute ischemia. Circulation 1990; 82: II2-12

[2] Kloner RA, Jennings RB: Consequences of brief ischemia: stunning, preconditioning, and their clinical implications: part 1. Circulation 2001; 104: 2981-9

[3] Neely JR, Liedtke AJ, Whitmer JT, Rovetto MJ: Relationship between coronary flow and adenosine triphosphate production from glycolysis and oxidative metabolism. Recent Adv Stud Cardiac Struct Metab 1975; 8: 301-21

[4] Neely JR, Morgan HE: Relationship between carbohydrate and lipid metabolism and the energy balance of heart muscle. Annu Rev Physiol 1974; 36: 413-59

[5] Neely JR, Whitmer JT, Rovetto MJ: Effect of coronary blood flow on glycolytic flux and intracellular pH in isolated rat hearts. Circ Res 1975; 37: 733-41

[6] Sun D, Nguyen N, DeGrado TR, Schwaiger M, Brosius FC, 3rd: Ischemia induces translocation of the insulin-responsive glucose transporter GLUT4 to the plasma membrane of cardiac myocytes. Circulation 1994; 89: 793-8

[7] Tian R, Abel ED: Responses of GLUT4-Deficient Hearts to Ischemia Underscore the Importance of Glycolysis. Circulation 2001; 103: 2961-2966

[8] Young LH, Renfu Y, Russell R, Hu X, Caplan M, Ren J, Shulman GI, Sinusas AJ: Low-flow ischemia leads to translocation of canine heart GLUT-4 and GLUT-1 glucose transporters to the sarcolemma in vivo. Circulation 1997; 95: 415-22

[9] Stanley WC, Hall JL, Stone CK, Hacker TA: Acute myocardial ischemia causes a transmural gradient in glucose extraction but not glucose uptake. Am J Physiol 1992; 262: H91-6

[10] Begum N, Graham AL, Sussman KE, Draznin B: Role of cAMP in mediating effects of fasting on dephosphorylation of insulin receptor. Am J Physiol 1992; 262: E142-9

[11] Dobson JG, Jr., Mayer SE: Mechanisms of activation of cardiac glycogen phosphorylase in ischemia and anoxia. Circ Res 1973; 33: 412-20

[12] Morgan HE, Parmeggiani A: Regulation of Glycogenolysis in Muscle. Ii. Control of Glycogen Phosphorylase Reaction in Isolated Perfused Heart. J Biol Chem 1964; 239: 2435-9

[13] Schaefer S, Ramasamy R: Glycogen utilization and ischemic injury in the isolated rat heart. Cardiovasc Res 1997; 35: 90-8

[14] Schulze W, Krause EG, Wollenberger A: On the fate of glycogen phosphorylase in the ischemic and infarcting myocardium. J Mol Cell Cardiol 1971; 2: 241-51

[15] Kubler W, Spieckermann PG: Regulation of glycolysis in the ischemic and the anoxic myocardium. J Mol Cell Cardiol 1970; 1: 351-77

[16] Rovetto MJ, Whitmer JT, Neely JR: Comparison of the effects of anoxia and whole heart ischemia on carbohydrate utilization in isolated working rat hearts. Circ Res 1973; 32: 699-711

[17] Wollenberger A, Krause EG: Metabolic control characteristics of the acutely ischemic myocardium. Am J Cardiol 1968; 22: 349-59

[18] Francis SH, Meriwether BP, Park JH: Interaction between adenine nucleotides and 3-phosphoglyceraldehyde dehydrogenase. II. A study of the mechanism of catalysis and metabolic control of the multi-functional enzyme. J Biol Chem 1971; 246: 5433-41

[19] Oguchi M, Meriwether BP, Park JH: Interaction between adenosine triphosphate and glyceraldehyde 3-phosphate dehydrogenase. 3. Mechanism of action and metabolic control of the enzyme under simulated in vivo conditions. J Biol Chem 1973; 248: 5562-70

[20] Williamson JR: Glycolytic control mechanisms. II. Kinetics of intermediate changes during the aerobic-anoxic transition in perfused rat heart. J Biol Chem 1966; 241: 5026-36

[21] Rovetto MJ, Lamberton WF, Neely JR: Mechanisms of glycolytic inhibition in ischemic rat hearts. Circ Res 1975; 37: 742-51

[22] Williamson JR: Effects of insulin and diet on the metabolism of L-lactate and glucose by the perfused rat heart. Biochem J 1962; 83: 377-83

[23] Fleet WF, Johnson TA, Graebner CA, Gettes LS: Effect of serial brief ischemic episodes on extracellular K+, pH, and activation in the pig. Circulation 1985; 72: 922-32

[24] Calvani M, Reda E, Arrigoni-Martelli E: Regulation by carnitine of myocardial fatty acid and carbohydrate metabolism under normal and pathological conditions. Basic Res Cardiol 2000; 95: 75-83

[25] Neely JR, Feuvray D: Metabolic products and myocardial ischemia. Am J Pathol 1981; 102: 282-91

[26] Ford DA, Gross RW: Differential accumulation of diacyl and plasmalogenic diglycerides during myocardial ischemia. Circ Res 1989; 64: 173-7

[27] Jaswal JS, Keung W, Wang W, Ussher JR, Lopaschuk GD: Targeting fatty acid and carbohydrate oxidation--a novel therapeutic intervention in the ischemic and failing heart. Biochim Biophys Acta; 1813: 1333-50

[28] van der Vusse GJ, Glatz JF, Stam HC, Reneman RS: Fatty acid homeostasis in the normoxic and ischemic heart. Physiol Rev 1992; 72: 881-940

[29] Martin C, Riou B, Vallet B: Physiologie humaine appliquée. 2006: First Edition, Chapter 17, pp 217-227

[30] McHowat J, Yamada KA, Wu J, Yan GX, Corr PB: Recent insights pertaining to sarcolemmal phospholipid alterations underlying arrhythmogenesis in the ischemic heart. J Cardiovasc Electrophysiol 1993; 4: 288-310

[31] Yamada KA, McHowat J, Yan GX, Donahue K, Peirick J, Kleber AG, Corr PB: Cellular uncoupling induced by accumulation of long-chain acylcarnitine during ischemia. Circ Res 1994; 74: 83-95

[32] Lazdunski M, Frelin C, Vigne P: The sodium/hydrogen exchange system in cardiac cells: its biochemical and pharmacological properties and its role in regulating internal concentrations of sodium and internal pH. J Mol Cell Cardiol 1985; 17: 1029-42

[33] Nawada R, Murakami T, Iwase T, Nagai K, Morita Y, Kouchi I, Akao M, Sasayama S: Inhibition of sarcolemmal Na+,K+-ATPase activity reduces the infarct size-limiting effect of preconditioning in rabbit hearts. Circulation 1997; 96: 599-604

[34] Tani M, Neely JR: Role of intracellular Na+ in Ca2+ overload and depressed recovery of ventricular function of reperfused ischemic rat hearts. Possible involvement of H+-Na+ and Na+-Ca2+ exchange. Circ Res 1989; 65: 1045-56

[35] Silver IA, Erecinska M: Ion homeostasis in rat brain in vivo: intra- and extracellular [Ca2+] and [H+] in the hippocampus during recovery from short-term, transient ischemia. J Cereb Blood Flow Metab 1992; 12: 759-72

[36] Chambers DE, Parks DA, Patterson G, Roy R, McCord JM, Yoshida S, Parmley LF, Downey JM: Xanthine oxidase as a source of free radical damage in myocardial ischemia. J Mol Cell Cardiol 1985; 17: 145-52

[37] Granger DN: Role of xanthine oxidase and granulocytes in ischemia-reperfusion injury. Am J Physiol 1988; 255: H1269-75

[38] Maxwell SR, Lip GY: Reperfusion injury: a review of the pathophysiology, clinical manifestations and therapeutic options. Int J Cardiol 1997; 58: 95-117

[39] Grover GJ, Atwal KS, Sleph PG, Wang FL, Monshizadegan H, Monticello T, Green DW: Excessive ATP hydrolysis in ischemic myocardium by mitochondrial F1F0-ATPase: effect of selective pharmacological inhibition of mitochondrial ATPase hydrolase activity. Am J Physiol Heart Circ Physiol 2004; 287: H1747-55

[40] Murphy E, Steenbergen C: Mechanisms underlying acute protection from cardiac ischemia-reperfusion injury. Physiol Rev 2008; 88: 581-609

[41] Balaban RS, Nemoto S, Finkel T: Mitochondria, oxidants, and aging. Cell 2005; 120: 483-95

[42] Di Lisa F, Canton M, Menabo R, Kaludercic N, Bernardi P: Mitochondria and cardioprotection. Heart Fail Rev 2007; 12: 249-60

[43] Turrens JF: Mitochondrial formation of reactive oxygen species. J Physiol 2003; 552: 335-44

[44] Hausenloy DJ, Yellon DM: Preconditioning and postconditioning: united at reperfusion. Pharmacol Ther 2007; 116: 173-91

[45] Akao M, O'Rourke B, Teshima Y, Seharaseyon J, Marban E: Mechanistically distinct steps in the mitochondrial death pathway triggered by oxidative stress in cardiac myocytes. Circ Res 2003; 92: 186-94

[46] Costantini P, Chernyak BV, Petronilli V, Bernardi P: Selective inhibition of the mitochondrial permeability transition pore at the oxidation-reduction sensitive dithiol by monobromobimane. FEBS Lett 1995; 362: 239-42

[47] Costantini P, Chernyak BV, Petronilli V, Bernardi P: Modulation of the mitochondrial permeability transition pore by pyridine nucleotides and dithiol oxidation at two separate sites. J Biol Chem 1996; 271: 6746-51

[48] Crompton M: The mitochondrial permeability transition pore and its role in cell death. Biochem J 1999; 341 (Pt 2): 233-49

[49] Danial NN, Korsmeyer SJ: Cell death: critical control points. Cell 2004; 116: 205-19

[50] Gustafsson AB, Gottlieb RA: Bcl-2 family members and apoptosis, taken to heart. Am J Physiol Cell Physiol 2007; 292: C45-51

[51] Javadov S, Karmazyn M: Mitochondrial permeability transition pore opening as an endpoint to initiate cell death and as a putative target for cardioprotection. Cell Physiol Biochem 2007; 20: 1-22

[52] Kroemer G, Galluzzi L, Brenner C: Mitochondrial membrane permeabilization in cell death. Physiol Rev 2007; 87: 99-163

[53] Cao HM, Wang Q, You HY, Li J, Yang ZY: Stabilizing microtubules decreases myocardial ischaemia-reperfusion injury. J Int Med Res 2011 39: 1713-9

[54] Hein S, Scheffold T, Schaper J: Ischemia induces early changes to cytoskeletal and contractile proteins in diseased human myocardium. J Thorac Cardiovasc Surg 1995; 110: 89-98

[55] Iwai K, Hori M, Kitabatake A, Kurihara H, Uchida K, Inoue M, Kamada T: Disruption of microtubules as an early sign of irreversible ischemic injury. Immunohistochemical study of in situ canine hearts. Circ Res 1990; 67: 694-706

[56] Nakamura Y, Miura T, Nakano A, Ichikawa Y, Yano T, Kobayashi H, Ikeda Y, Miki T, Shimamoto K: Role of microtubules in ischemic preconditioning against myocardial infarction. Cardiovasc Res 2004; 64: 322-30

[57] Ganote C, Armstrong S: Ischaemia and the myocyte cytoskeleton: review and speculation. Cardiovasc Res 1993; 27: 1387-403

[58] Chi NC, Karliner JS: Molecular determinants of responses to myocardial ischemia/reperfusion injury: focus on hypoxia-inducible and heat shock factors. Cardiovasc Res 2004; 61: 437-47

[59] Stetler RA, Gao Y, Zhang L, Weng Z, Zhang F, Hu X, Wang S, Vosler P, Cao G, Sun D, Graham SH, Chen J: Phosphorylation of HSP27 by Protein Kinase D Is Essential for Mediating Neuroprotection against Ischemic Neuronal Injury. J Neurosci 2012; 32: 2667-82

[60] Williams RS, Benjamin IJ: Protective responses in the ischemic myocardium. J Clin Invest 2000; 106: 813-8

[61] Michiels C, Minet E, Michel G, Mottet D, Piret JP, Raes M: HIF-1 and AP-1 cooperate to increase gene expression in hypoxia: role of MAP kinases. IUBMB Life 2001; 52: 49-53

[62] Eltzschig HK, Collard CD: Vascular ischaemia and reperfusion injury. Br Med Bull 2004; 70: 71-86

[63] Eltzschig HK, Eckle T: Ischemia and reperfusion--from mechanism to translation. Nat Med 2011 1391-401

[64] Into T, Kanno Y, Dohkan J, Nakashima M, Inomata M, Shibata K, Lowenstein CJ, Matsushita K: Pathogen recognition by Toll-like receptor 2 activates Weibel-Palade body exocytosis in human aortic endothelial cells. J Biol Chem 2007; 282: 8134-41

[65] Kuhlicke J, Frick JS, Morote-Garcia JC, Rosenberger P, Eltzschig HK: Hypoxia inducible factor (HIF)-1 coordinates induction of Toll-like receptors TLR2 and TLR6 during hypoxia. PLoS One 2007; 2: e1364

[66] Kuo MC, Patschan D, Patschan S, Cohen-Gould L, Park HC, Ni J, Addabbo F, Goligorsky MS: Ischemia-induced exocytosis of Weibel-Palade bodies mobilizes stem cells. J Am Soc Nephrol 2008; 19: 2321-30

[67] Arai M, Tejima K, Ikeda H, Tomiya T, Yanase M, Inoue Y, Nagashima K, Nishikawa T, Watanabe N, Omata M, Fujiwara K: Ischemic preconditioning in liver pathophysiology. J Gastroenterol Hepatol 2007; 22 Suppl 1: S65-7

[68] Kato R, Foex P: Myocardial protection by anesthetic agents against ischemia-reperfusion injury: an update for anesthesiologists. Can J Anaesth 2002; 49: 777-91

[69] Martorana PA, Kettenbach B, Breipohl G, Linz W, Scholkens BA: Reduction of infarct size by local angiotensin-converting enzyme inhibition is abolished by a bradykinin antagonist. Eur J Pharmacol 1990; 182: 395-6

[70] Briaud SA, Ding ZM, Michael LH, Entman ML, Daniel S, Ballantyne CM: Leukocyte trafficking and myocardial reperfusion injury in ICAM-1/P-selectin-knockout mice. Am J Physiol Heart Circ Physiol 2001; 280: H60-7

[71] Yadav SS, Howell DN, Gao W, Steeber DA, Harland RC, Clavien PA: L-selectin and ICAM-1 mediate reperfusion injury and neutrophil adhesion in the warm ischemic mouse liver. Am J Physiol 1998; 275: G1341-52

[72] Kakkar AK, Lefer DJ: Leukocyte and endothelial adhesion molecule studies in knockout mice. Curr Opin Pharmacol 2004; 4: 154-8

Chapter 2

Inflammation and Vasomotricity During Reperfusion

Maximilien Gourdin and Philippe Dubois

Additional information is available at the end of the chapter

http://dx.doi.org/10.5772/54508

1. Introduction

Restoration of perfusion and reoxygenation of ischemic tissues restores aerobic metabolism and supports postischemic functional recovery but also generates significant damage related to the ischemia/reperfusion (I/R) phenomenon. At the level of a blood vessel, lesions of I/R are mainly characterized by the perturbation of vasomotion and endothelial dysfunction. Moreover, despite the fact that ischemia occurs in a sterile environment, reperfusion induces a significant activation of innate and adaptive immune responses: massive reactive oxygen species (ROS) production; activation of pattern-recognition receptors or toll-like receptors (TLRs); activation of complement, coagulation, cytokine and chemokine production; and inflammatory cell trafficking into the diseased organ.[1] I/R activates different programs of cell death (necrosis, apoptosis or autophagy-associated cell death) and generates a systemic inflammatory response that lasts several days and that can lead, in some cases, to multi-organ failure and death. [2-4]

2. Posthypoxic blood vessel motricity and posthypoxic endothelial dysfunction

Blood vessels, and especially endothelium located at the blood-organ interface, are particularly susceptible to ischemia-reperfusion injuries. Endothelial stunning or the loss of endothelial functions during reperfusion contributes to IR injuries and compromises the postischemic recovery. [5-7]

The basal vascular tone is a continual balance between vasoconstrictors and vasodilators acting on the blood vessel. Vascular smooth muscle cells (VSMCs) and endothelium play pivotal roles in this control.

Posthypoxic vasoconstriction, in response to vasoconstrictors, and endothelium-independent vasodilation, induced by direct vasodilators (direct action on VSMCs), are slightly affected by I/R, demonstrating the relative resistance of VSMCs. [8]-[10] In contrast, endothelium-dependent dilatation is deeply affected. Despite the fact that endothelial cells seem relatively more resistant than other cells types (cardiomyocytes, neurons, renal tubular cell), I/R modifies their phenotype: diminution of their anticoagulant properties, increased vascular permeability, increased leukoadhesivity and establishment of a proinflammatory state in the endovascular milieu.

The production of some bioactive agents decreases (e.g., prostacyclin, nitric oxide), while that of others increases during I/R (e.g., endothelin, thromboxane A2). [1],[11]-[16] These endothelial modifications are called endothelial dysfunction and are widely described in human and animals studies.[15],[17]-[21] IR-related endothelial dysfunction is mainly characterized by the loss of NO availability and seems to be related to the reperfusion more than to ischemia. [10] In normal situations, NO acts in numerous pathways: direct vasodilation, indirect vasodilation by inhibiting the influences of vasoconstrictors (e.g., inhibiting angiotensin II and sympathetic vasoconstriction), inhibiting platelet adhesion to the vascular endothelium (anti-thrombotic effect), inhibiting leukocyte adhesion to vascular endothelium (anti-inflammatory effect), and inhibiting smooth muscle hyperplasia by scavenging superoxide anion (anti-proliferative effect). The diminution of NO concentration jeopardizes these functions.

Multiple hypotheses have been proposed to explain postischemic endothelial dysfunction: massive ROS production by mitochondria, activation of immune cells, activation of xanthine oxidase and $NADPH_2$ oxidase by the ceramide/sphingosine kinase pathway, the depletion of dihydrobiopterin (an essential cofactor of nitric oxide synthase), increased arginine consumption in other intracellular pathways, the production of chemokines and cytokines (tumor necrosis factor-alpha (TNF-α), interleukin-1, -6, and -8) or the activation of the complement system (C3a fraction, C5b-9 fraction). [21]-[31]

In normoxic conditions, the endothelium permits only restricted diffusion. During hypoxia, the modifications of the cytoskeleton of endothelial cells, induced by hypoxia and low intracellular cyclic adenosine monophosphate phosphate (cAMP) concentration, increase vascular permeability, leading to capillary leakage and perivascular interstitial edema.[1] Complement system activation, leukocyte endothelial adhesion and platelet-leukocyte aggregation increase after reperfusion.[1],[32] A clinical example is the acute respiratory failure with hypoxia and pulmonary edema observed in several surgeries. Acute respiratory distress syndrome is caused by heart failure but also by a disruption of the alveolar-capillary barrier.[33]-[36]

3. The inflammatory response

Ischemia-reperfusion induces a vigorous inflammatory reaction including activation of the complement system; activation of the innate and adaptive immune systems; increased ROS, cytokine, chemokine and other proinflammatory metabolite production; and activation of programmed cell death. If inflammation concerns mainly ischemic organs, its effects will

extend to the whole body and, particularly, the organs with a high capillary density, such as lung, brain and kidney. [1],[12],[37],[38]

3.1. Activation of the complement system

Reperfusion injury is characterized by autoimmune responses, including natural antibodies recognizing neoantigens and subsequent activation of the complement system (auto-immunity). [1] Locally produced and activated, the complement system amplifies inflammation during ischemia and reperfusion through complement-mediated recognition of damaged cells and anaphylatoxin release. The anaphylatoxins C3a, C4a and C5a lead to the recruitment and stimulation of immune cells, which promotes cell-cell interactions by increasing the expression of adhesion molecules (vascular cell adhesion molecule-1, ICAM-1, E-selectin and P-selectin) on the surface of the endothelial cells and neutrophils. [12],[39] Moreover, C5a is a chemotactic factor that directly stimulates leukocytes to synthesize and secrete cytokines such as interleukin (IL)-1, IL-6, monocyte chemoattractant protein-1 (MCP-1) and TNF-α. iC3b is implicated in neutrophil-endothelium interactions. C5b-9, known as the final cytolytic membrane attack complex complement, is a powerful chemotactic agent that causes direct lesions to the endothelial cells, stimulates the endothelial production of IL-8, MCP-1, and ROS and inhibits endothelium-dependent vasodilatation. [12],[39]

3.2. Cell-cell interactions during reperfusion

3.2.1. Neutrophil–endothelium interaction

During reperfusion, neutrophils play a central part in the inflammatory response and in the genesis of the I/R injuries. Activated neutrophils produce high amounts of cytokines, chemokines, and ROS in the vascular lumen but also in the parenchyma that directly contacts cells. These neutrophils and endothelial cells activated by cytokines (e.g., IL-6, TNF-α, IL-8, IL-1β) and other proinflammatory mediators (e.g., platelet-activating factor, ROS) promote a close interaction between these cell types that will result in a significant concentration of activated neutrophils in the interstitium. [1],[13],[15],[17],[32],[40]-[43] This complex process can be summarized in four steps: chemoattraction, weak neutrophil adhesion to the endothelium, followed by a stronger adhesion and, finally, neutrophil migration (Figure 1). Three families of sarcoplasmic adhesion molecules are implicated in the neutrophil-endothelium interaction: selectins, β2-integrins and immunoglobulins.

- Chemoattraction:

Upon reperfusion, the endothelium, parenchyma and resident immune cells (mainly macrophages and neutrophils) release cytokines such as IL-1, TNF-α and chemokines, inducing the production of selectins by endothelial and immune cells. Circulating leukocytes are concentrated towards the site of injury by the concentration gradient of chemokines.

- Rolling adhesion

Endothelial L-selectin interacts with the P-selectin and the E-selectin-specific ligand-1 (ESL-1) expressed by neutrophils. [44],[45] The activation of TLR-2, ROS production, the complement

system and thrombin and a high intracellular calcium concentration promotes the expression of endothelial P-selectin from the Weibel–Palade bodies. Its peak of expression occurs 10–20 min after the beginning of reperfusion.[40],[46] P-selectin interacts with P-selectin glycoprotein ligand-1 (PSGL-1) expressed by neutrophils. These interactions are weak and reversible, providing transitory neutrophil adherence, slowing down leukocytes and allowing them to "roll" along the endothelial surface. During this rolling motion, transitory bonds are formed and broken between selectins and their ligands. This phase prepares the neutrophils and the endothelium for the following stage.

- Tight adhesion

At the same time, chemokines released by endothelial and immune cells activate the rolling neutrophils. Stimulated by ROS, platelet-activating factor (PAF), IL-1, TNF-α and leukotriene B4 (LTB4), neutrophils present CD11a/CD18, CD11b/CD18 and CD11c/CD18 from intracellular granules. These sarcoplasmic proteins interact with the iC3a fraction of the complement system and ICAM-1, an endothelial protein whose expression is reinforced by TNF-α and IL-1.[47],[48] This interaction switches from a low-affinity link to a high-affinity state and firmly attaches the neutrophil to the surface of the endothelial cell, despite the shear forces of the blood flow.

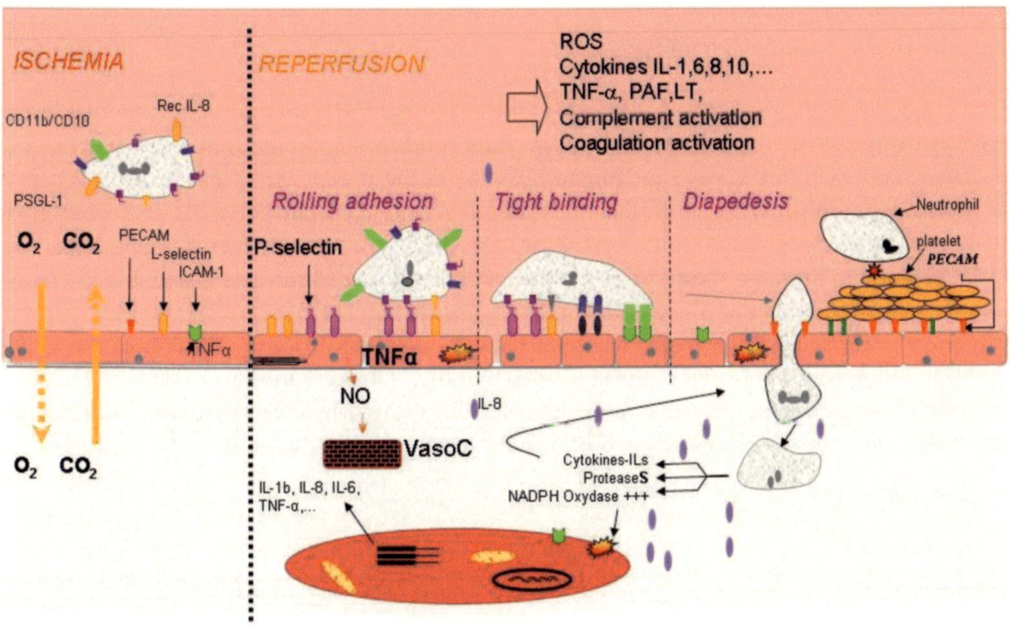

Figure 1. Ischemia–reperfusion-induced neutrophils accumulation in the interstitium is a mechanism described in three phases implicating specific complementary proteins. CD11b/CD18, sarcoplasmic neutrophil integrin; CO_2, carbon dioxide; ESL-1, E-selectin-specific ligand-1; I/R, ischemia– reperfusion; O_2, oxygen; PECAM, platelet–endothelial cell adhesion molecule-1; PSGL-1, P-selectin glycoprotein ligand-1; Rec IL-8, neutrophil IL-8 receptor; ROS, reactive oxygen species; TNF-α, tumour necrosis factor-a; WPB, Weibel–Palade body.

- Migration into the interstitium or diapedesis

Intercellular adhesion molecule-1 (ICAM-1) and platelet-endothelium adhesion molecule-1 (PECAM-1) are sarcoplasmic adhesion molecules belonging to the superfamily of the immunoglobulins. They are implicated in the transfer of neutrophils towards the interstitium, termed diapedesis. Leukocytes extravasation comprises many stages, which are not fully understood. Nevertheless, it seems that PECAM-1, found on neutrophil and endothelial cell membranes, is necessary for diapedesis. [1],[49] It interacts with several sarcoplasmic proteins of neutrophils. The cytoskeleton of the neutrophil is reorganized to allow the projection of pseudopodia between endothelial cells. This transfer is facilitated by inflammatory mediators, the CD11/CD18 ICAM 1 interaction and ROS, which combine to decrease the expression of cadherin and induce the phosphorylation vascular endothelial-cadherin and catenin, components of the intercellular junctions. [50]-[53] There is controversy concerning the mechanisms underlying this transfer through the basal membrane of the endothelium. Once into the interstitium, the neutrophil migrates along a chemotactic gradient towards the site of injury, where it causes considerable damage.

The neutrophil-related injuries in the interstitium are mainly related to the massive ROS production, proteases from the intracellular neutrophilic granules and the metabolites of arachidonic acid (PAF and LTB4). PAF and LTB4 are powerful chemoattractants that stimulate neutrophil degranulation. The neutrophil granules contain proteases, collagenases, elastases, lipoxygenases, phospholipases and myeloperoxidases that digest the protein network of the extracellular matrix. For example, elastase digests substrates such as collagen types III and IV, immunoglobulins, fibronectin and proteoglycans. Several cells, such as cardiomyocytes, stimulated by IL-6, express ICAM-1. The neutrophil binds to its receptor and empties its granules directly near the cell. [54],[55]

3.2.2. Neutrophil-platelet interaction

The role of platelets in ischemia-reperfusion injuries is unclear. However, it seems that they participate directly and indirectly in posthypoxic endothelial injury. [32],[56] Platelets affect neutrophil activation by releasing thromboxane A2, platelet-derived growth factor, serotonin, lipoxygenase products, proteases and adenosine. During reperfusion, approximately 25% of the fixed platelets are directly bound to the endothelium and the remaining 75% to neutrophils linked to the endothelium. [32],[57] This platelet-neutrophil interaction potentiates the neutrophils' capacity to produce superoxide and platelet-activating factor. [58],[59] Moreover, the neutrophil-platelet aggregates contribute to the no-reflow phenomenon and jeopardize the quality of the microcirculation. 60

3.3. Reactive oxygen species or oxygen free radicals

Reactive oxygen species, such as superoxide anion ($O_2^{-\bullet}$), hydrogen peroxide (H_2O_2) and hydroxyl radical (OH^-), are highly reactive and able to oxide all cellular constituents, includ-

ing proteins, DNA, phospholipids and other biological structures. During reperfusion, PAF, TNF-α, IL-6, IL-1β, granulocyte-macrophage colony-stimulating factor, complement fraction C5a and the ROS themselves stimulate endothelial and neutrophil ROS production. [49],[61],[62] On the other hand, ROS activate nuclear factor-κB, promote cytokine production (e.g., TNF-α, IL-6, PAF), and induce the synthesis and expression of endothelial and leukocyte adhesion molecules. [15],[41],[63]

In the reperfused tissue, the principal sources of ROS are neutrophil NADPH-oxidase, xanthine oxidase, mitochondria and the arachidonic acid pathways. [64]-[66] The massive ROS production quickly exceeds the capacity of cellular defense systems (catalase, superoxide dismutase, glutathione peroxidase and vitamins C and E). ROS directly cause much structural damage, increase the susceptibility to the opening of the mitochondrial permeability transition pore, activate immune and endothelial cells and induce apoptosis. [67]

ROS can also be produced by monoamine oxidase (MAO) of the outer mitochondrial membrane. MAO transfers electrons from amine compounds with oxygen to produce hydrogen peroxide. [68] p66Shc, a cytosolic adaptor protein for tyrosine kinase receptors that has been implicated in signal transduction, translocates to the mitochondrial matrix during reperfusion and oxidizes the reduced cytochrome *c*, which generates oxygen peroxide. [67],[69]

3.4. Ischemia-reperfusion-induced apoptosis

Reperfusion is vital for the functional recovery of an ischemic organ but also initiates the apoptosis pathways. [70],[71] Apoptosis is an active mechanism of cellular death, is genetically programmed, consumes energy, requires the expression or activation of specific enzymes, and can be induced by the oxidative stress of reperfusion. Reperfusion-induced apoptosis occurs in many organs, including heart, brain, kidney and liver. The reperfusion of an organ can induce apoptosis in other, distant organs. For example, reperfusion of a lower limb or the small bowel can induce apoptosis of cardiomyocytes or lung cells, respectively. [72],[73] The TNF-α production by the reperfused organ seems to play a crucial part in the induction of apoptosis. [70],[74]-[76] TNF-α initiates a receptor dependent death pathway by activating downstream caspases. [70],[76],[77] Other causes of reperfusion-induced apoptosis are also important: mitochondrial depolarization, high intracellular calcium, mPTP opening and the release of some mitochondrial proteins into the cytoplasm, such as cytochrome *c*. When this protein is released from mitochondria into the cytoplasm, it interacts with apoptotic protease activating factor-1 (Apaf-1) and ATP to form the apoptosome, a large oligomeric protein complex that can activate caspase 9, which activates the caspase-dependent apoptosis pathway.

Endothelial cell apoptosis precedes and influences the apoptosis of the subjacent parenchymal cells. For example, a reduction in endothelial apoptosis decreases the apoptosis of subjacent cardiomyocytes. This suggests that signals emanating from the endothelium during apoptosis can induce or reinforce that of the cardiomyocytes.

4. Integration of different aspects of ischemia-reperfusion

4.1. Blood vessel

According to the level of the vascular system considered (small arteries, capillaries and post-capillary veins), the repercussions of I/R are identical, but the clinical pictures differ.

4.1.1. At the arteriolar level

The principal manifestation of I/R in arterioles is a loss of the vasodilatation-dependent endothelium and the appearance of spasms. [78] Widespread endothelial lesions decrease the production of nitric oxide and do not counterbalance the arterioles' tendency toward vasoconstriction. This tendency is highlighted in several tissues, such as skeletal muscle, heart, lung and brain. [79]-[82] The combined effects of IR and inflammation on arteriolar vasomotricity are well documented. The increase in the contractile response of the pulmonary and mesenteric microcirculation after cardiac surgery predisposes the patient to the development of pulmonary shunt or mesenteric ischemia, particularly during the administration of vasopressive drugs in the postextracorporeal circulation. [83],[84]

4.1.2. At the capillary level

The posthypoxic recovery of an organ depends on the quality of its microcirculation and the resultant nutrient delivery and gaseous exchange. However, the microcirculation is the site of a paradoxical phenomenon called "no reflow", characterized by a major reduction in the capillary density. Despite the reestablishment of complete blood flow, an incomplete and heterogeneous perfusion of microcirculation persists. [85],[86] The capillaries are blocked by the parenchymatous and endothelial edema and the adhesion of the neutrophils and platelets to the surface of the endothelium, aided by the reduction in the production of nitric oxide. [15],[81], [85]-[87] Increased ROS and the depletion of ATP modify the cytoskeleton and the intercellular junctions, contributing to the loss of liquid from the vascular bed towards the interstitium. [88], [89] The phenomenon of no reflow persists several weeks after reperfusion. [85]

4.1.3. At the postcapillary vein level

The postcapillary veins are the sites of the inflammatory reaction. The margination and extravasation of the leukocytes are facilitated by the slower blood flow. Venous blood, arriving from the reperfused zones, is rich in proinflammatory mediators and activated neutrophils. These cause lesions both directly and indirectly through their interactions with platelets. [15],[90] Endothelial lesions prevent the intravascular oncotic pressure from recovering the excess liquid from the interstitium, thereby increasing the edema and contributing to the phenomenon of "no reflow".

4.2. Organs

In pulmonary transplantation surgery, I/R-induced lung injury is characterized by non-specific alveolar damage, lung edema and hypoxemia. The most severe form may lead to

primary graft failure and remains a significant cause of morbidity and mortality after lung transplantation.[91] Pulmonary microvascular permeability appears to have a bimodal pattern, peaking at 30 min and 4 h after reperfusion. [92] Mechanical ventilation, cardiopulmonary bypass during cardiac surgery and lung resection can also induce apoptosis and I/R-induced lung injury. [93]-[96]

Perioperative acute renal failure is associated with a high incidence of morbidity and mortality. According to the type of surgery, IR injuries in the kidney are direct or indirect. [97] For example, acute renal failure is the most important complication of remote tissue damage following abdominal aortic surgery. [98] I/R induces renal tubular injuries and contributes to the decrease of glomerular filtration. Recent data suggest that 13% of patients with acute kidney injury (AKI) evolve to end-stage renal disease within 3 years. In the case of patients with preexisting renal disease, the progression to end-stage renal disease rises to 28% within the same period. [98] These results suggest that AKI predisposes to chronic renal complication. I/R reduces blood vessel density and promotes renal fibrosis. The mechanisms mediating vascular loss are not clear but may be related to the lack of effective vascular repair responses. [99]

In cardiac surgery and in myocardial ischemia, cell death following I/R has features of apoptosis and necrosis. The loss of cardiomyocytes, which can hibernate in "no reflow" zones, and stunning, led by free radicals and calcium overload, explain the contractile posthypoxic dysfunction. The stunned cardiomyocytes can take several hours and days to recover. Intracellular ionic perturbation favors ventricular arrhythmias, such as ventricular fibrillation, ventricular tachycardia or ventricular extrasystole. [10]0 During ischemia, cardiomyocytes express ICAM-1. Neutrophils bind to this receptor and empty the contents of their granules onto the cells. [54],[55]

The mechanisms of I/R-induced brain injury have many similar aspects compared with those of I/R-induced myocardial injury. Many mediators and cytokines upregulated by I/R, such as bradykinin, purine nucleotides, nitric oxide and ROS, increase blood–brain barrier permeability and induce cerebral edema. [10]1 Although leukocyte infiltration into the ischemic brain increases cerebral damage, leukocyte accumulation in the microcirculation reduces reperfusion and increases the "no reflow" phenomenon.

The indirect repercussions of I/R on organs remote from the reperfused site are much more insidious. Neutrophils, complement activation, and massive production of cytokines and chemokines install a proinflammatory state that affects the functioning of other organs. During abdominal aortic surgery, I/R injuries are not only limited to the lower extremities but also cause damage to remote organs such as the lungs, kidneys, heart and bowel. [36],[97],[102]-[104] Lung injuries following abdominal aortic aneurysm surgery are characterized by progressive hypoxemia, pulmonary hypertension, decreased lung compliance and nonhydrostatic pulmonary edema, consistent with adult respiratory distress syndrome. [36],[103] In comparison with surgery, endovascular abdominal aortic aneurysm repair decreases I/R and I/R-induced-intestinal mucosal, renal and pulmonary dysfunction. [104]

http://dx.doi.org/10.5772/54508

Author details

Maximilien Gourdin and Philippe Dubois*

Department of Anaesthesiology, Université Catholique de Louvain, University Hospital of Mont Godinne, Belgium

References

[1] Eltzschig HK, Eckle T: Ischemia and reperfusion--from mechanism to translation. Nat Med 2011 17: 1391-401

[2] Berthonneche C, Sulpice T, Boucher F, Gouraud L, de Leiris J, O'Connor SE, Herbert JM, Janiak P: New insights into the pathological role of TNF-alpha in early cardiac dysfunction and subsequent heart failure after infarction in rats. Am J Physiol Heart Circ Physiol 2004; 287: H340-50

[3] Hotchkiss RS, Strasser A, McDunn JE, Swanson PE: Cell death. N Engl J Med 2009; 361: 1570-83

[4] Moro C, Jouan MG, Rakotovao A, Toufektsian MC, Ormezzano O, Nagy N, Tosaki A, de Leiris J, Boucher F: Delayed expression of cytokines after reperfused myocardial infarction: possible trigger for cardiac dysfunction and ventricular remodeling. Am J Physiol Heart Circ Physiol 2007; 293: H3014-9

[5] Garcia SC, Pomblum V, Gams E, Langenbach MR, Schipke JD: Independency of myocardial stunning of endothelial stunning? Basic Res Cardiol 2007; 102: 359-67

[6] Lefer AM, Tsao PS, Lefer DJ, Ma XL: Role of endothelial dysfunction in the pathogenesis of reperfusion injury after myocardial ischemia. Faseb J 1991; 5: 2029-34

[7] Qi XL, Nguyen TL, Andries L, Sys SU, Rouleau JL: Vascular endothelial dysfunction contributes to myocardial depression in ischemia-reperfusion in the rat. Can J Physiol Pharmacol 1998; 76: 35-45

[8] Besse S, Tanguy S, Boucher F, Bulteau AL, Riou B, de Leiris J, Swynghedauw B: Aortic vasoreactivity during prolonged hypoxia and hypoxia-reoxygenation in senescent rats. Mech Ageing Dev 2002; 123: 275-85

[9] Piana RN, Wang SY, Friedman M, Sellke FW: Angiotensin-converting enzyme inhibition preserves endothelium-dependent coronary microvascular responses during short-term ischemia-reperfusion. Circulation 1996; 93: 544-51

[10] Quillen JE, Sellke FW, Brooks LA, Harrison DG: Ischemia-reperfusion impairs endothelium-dependent relaxation of coronary microvessels but does not affect large arteries. Circulation 1990; 82: 586-94

[11] Deanfield JE, Halcox JP, Rabelink TJ: Endothelial function and dysfunction: testing and clinical relevance. Circulation 2007; 115: 1285-95

[12] Eltzschig HK, Collard CD: Vascular ischaemia and reperfusion injury. Br Med Bull 2004; 70: 71-86

[13] Maxwell SR, Lip GY: Reperfusion injury: a review of the pathophysiology, clinical manifestations and therapeutic options. Int J Cardiol 1997; 58: 95-117

[14] Pinsky DJ, Yan SF, Lawson C, Naka Y, Chen JX, Connolly ES, Jr., Stern DM: Hypoxia and modification of the endothelium: implications for regulation of vascular homeostatic properties. Semin Cell Biol 1995; 6: 283-94

[15] Seal JB, Gewertz BL: Vascular dysfunction in ischemia-reperfusion injury. Ann Vasc Surg 2005; 19: 572-84

[16] Zhang Y, Oliver JR, Horowitz JD: Endothelin B receptor-mediated vasoconstriction induced by endothelin A receptor antagonist. Cardiovasc Res 1998; 39: 665-73

[17] Engelman DT, Watanabe M, Engelman RM, Rousou JA, Flack JE, 3rd, Deaton DW, Das DK: Constitutive nitric oxide release is impaired after ischemia and reperfusion. J Thorac Cardiovasc Surg 1995; 110: 1047-53

[18] Loukogeorgakis SP, Panagiotidou AT, Yellon DM, Deanfield JE, MacAllister RJ: Postconditioning protects against endothelial ischemia-reperfusion injury in the human forearm. Circulation 2006; 113: 1015-9

[19] Loukogeorgakis SP, Williams R, Panagiotidou AT, Kolvekar SK, Donald A, Cole TJ, Yellon DM, Deanfield JE, MacAllister RJ: Transient limb ischemia induces remote preconditioning and remote postconditioning in humans by a K(ATP)-channel dependent mechanism. Circulation 2007; 116: 1386-95

[20] Pernow J, Bohm F, Beltran E, Gonon A: L-arginine protects from ischemia-reperfusion-induced endothelial dysfunction in humans in vivo. J Appl Physiol 2003; 95: 2218-22

[21] Weyrich AS, Ma XL, Lefer AM: The role of L-arginine in ameliorating reperfusion injury after myocardial ischemia in the cat. Circulation 1992; 86: 279-88

[22] Corda S, Laplace C, Vicaut E, Duranteau J: Rapid reactive oxygen species production by mitochondria in endothelial cells exposed to tumor necrosis factor-alpha is mediated by ceramide. Am J Respir Cell Mol Biol 2001; 24: 762-8

[23] Endres M, Laufs U: Effects of statins on endothelium and signaling mechanisms. Stroke 2004; 35: 2708-11

[24] Lefer AM, Ma XL: Cytokines and growth factors in endothelial dysfunction. Crit Care Med 1993; 21: S9-14

[25] Moens AL, Kietadisorn R, Lin JY, Kass D: Targeting endothelial and myocardial dysfunction with tetrahydrobiopterin. J Mol Cell Cardiol; 51: 559-63

[26] Salvemini D, Cuzzocrea S: Superoxide, superoxide dismutase and ischemic injury. Curr Opin Investig Drugs 2002; 3: 886-95

[27] Tiefenbacher CP, Chilian WM, Mitchell M, DeFily DV: Restoration of endothelium-dependent vasodilation after reperfusion injury by tetrahydrobiopterin. Circulation 1996; 94: 1423-9

[28] Werner ER, Blau N, Thony B: Tetrahydrobiopterin: biochemistry and pathophysiology. Biochem J; 438: 397-414

[29] Wu G, Meininger CJ: Impaired arginine metabolism and NO synthesis in coronary endothelial cells of the spontaneously diabetic BB rat. Am J Physiol 1995; 269: H1312-8

[30] Zhang C, Hein TW, Wang W, Ren Y, Shipley RD, Kuo L: Activation of JNK and xanthine oxidase by TNF-alpha impairs nitric oxide-mediated dilation of coronary arterioles. J Mol Cell Cardiol 2006; 40: 247-57

[31] Zhang C, Xu X, Potter BJ, Wang W, Kuo L, Michael L, Bagby GJ, Chilian WM: TNF-alpha contributes to endothelial dysfunction in ischemia/reperfusion injury. Arterioscler Thromb Vasc Biol 2006; 26: 475-80

[32] Rodrigues SF, Granger DN: Role of blood cells in ischaemia-reperfusion induced endothelial barrier failure. Cardiovasc Res 2010; 87: 291-9

[33] Klausner JM, Paterson IS, Mannick JA, Valeri R, Shepro D, Hechtman HB: Reperfusion pulmonary edema. Jama 1989; 261: 1030-5

[34] Ogawa S, Gerlach H, Esposito C, Pasagian-Macaulay A, Brett J, Stern D: Hypoxia modulates the barrier and coagulant function of cultured bovine endothelium. Increased monolayer permeability and induction of procoagulant properties. J Clin Invest 1990; 85: 1090-8

[35] Ogawa S, Koga S, Kuwabara K, Brett J, Morrow B, Morris SA, Bilezikian JP, Silverstein SC, Stern D: Hypoxia-induced increased permeability of endothelial monolayers occurs through lowering of cellular cAMP levels. Am J Physiol 1992; 262: C546-54

[36] Paterson IS, Klausner JM, Pugatch R, Allen P, Mannick JA, Shepro D, Hechtman HB: Noncardiogenic pulmonary edema after abdominal aortic aneurysm surgery. Ann Surg 1989; 209: 231-6

[37] Laipanov Kh I, Petrosyan EA, Sergienko VI: Morphological changes in the lungs during experimental acute ischemia and reperfusion of the limb. Bull Exp Biol Med 2006; 142: 105-7

[38] Yassin MM, Harkin DW, Barros D'Sa AA, Halliday MI, Rowlands BJ: Lower limb ischemia-reperfusion injury triggers a systemic inflammatory response and multiple organ dysfunction. World J Surg 2002; 26: 115-21

[39] Arumugam T, Magnus T, Woodruff T, Proctor L, Shiels I, Taylor S: Complement mediators in ischemia-reperfusion injury. Clin Chim Acta. 2006; 374:: 33-45

[40] Sluiter W, Pietersma A, Lamers JM, Koster JF: Leukocyte adhesion molecules on the vascular endothelium: their role in the pathogenesis of cardiovascular disease and the mechanisms underlying their expression. J Cardiovasc Pharmacol 1993; 22 Suppl 4: S37-44

[41] Vinten-Johansen J: Involvement of neutrophils in the pathogenesis of lethal myocardial reperfusion injury. Cardiovasc Res 2004; 61: 481-97

[42] Wung BS, Ni CW, Wang DL: ICAM-1 induction by TNFalpha and IL-6 is mediated by distinct pathways via Rac in endothelial cells. J Biomed Sci 2005; 12: 91-101

[43] Yadav SS, Howell DN, Gao W, Steeber DA, Harland RC, Clavien PA: L-selectin and ICAM-1 mediate reperfusion injury and neutrophil adhesion in the warm ischemic mouse liver. Am J Physiol 1998; 275: G1341-52

[44] Hidalgo A, Peired AJ, Wild MK, Vestweber D, Frenette PS: Complete identification of E-selectin ligands on neutrophils reveals distinct functions of PSGL-1, ESL-1, and CD44. Immunity 2007; 26: 477-89

[45] Steegmaier M, Levinovitz A, Isenmann S, Borges E, Lenter M, Kocher HP, Kleuser B, Vestweber D: The E-selectin-ligand ESL-1 is a variant of a receptor for fibroblast growth factor. Nature 1995; 373: 615-20

[46] Kuo MC, Patschan D, Patschan S, Cohen-Gould L, Park HC, Ni J, Addabbo F, Goligorsky MS: Ischemia-induced exocytosis of Weibel-Palade bodies mobilizes stem cells. J Am Soc Nephrol 2008; 19: 2321-30

[47] Gu Q, Yang XP, Bonde P, DiPaula A, Fox-Talbot K, Becker LC: Inhibition of TNF-alpha reduces myocardial injury and proinflammatory pathways following ischemia-reperfusion in the dog. J Cardiovasc Pharmacol 2006; 48: 320-8

[48] Ikeda U, Ikeda M, Kano S, Shimada K: Neutrophil adherence to rat cardiac myocyte by proinflammatory cytokines. J Cardiovasc Pharmacol 1994; 23: 647-52

[49] Jordan JE, Zhao ZQ, Vinten-Johansen J: The role of neutrophils in myocardial ischemia-reperfusion injury. Cardiovasc Res 1999; 43: 860-78

[50] Alexander JS, Alexander BC, Eppihimer LA, Goodyear N, Haque R, Davis CP, Kalogeris TJ, Carden DL, Zhu YN, Kevil CG: Inflammatory mediators induce sequestration of VE-cadherin in cultured human endothelial cells. Inflammation 2000; 24: 99-113

[51] Allingham MJ, van Buul JD, Burridge K: ICAM-1-mediated, Src- and Pyk2-dependent vascular endothelial cadherin tyrosine phosphorylation is required for leukocyte transendothelial migration. J Immunol 2007; 179: 4053-64

[52] Kevil CG, Ohno N, Gute DC, Okayama N, Robinson SA, Chaney E, Alexander JS: Role of cadherin internalization in hydrogen peroxide-mediated endothelial permeability. Free Radic Biol Med 1998; 24: 1015-22

[53] Wang Y, Jin G, Miao H, Li JY, Usami S, Chien S: Integrins regulate VE-cadherin and catenins: dependence of this regulation on Src, but not on Ras. Proc Natl Acad Sci U S A 2006; 103: 1774-9

[54] Davani EY, Dorscheid DR, Lee CH, van Breemen C, Walley KR: Novel regulatory mechanism of cardiomyocyte contractility involving ICAM-1 and the cytoskeleton. Am J Physiol Heart Circ Physiol 2004; 287: H1013-22

[55] Niessen HW, Lagrand WK, Visser CA, Meijer CJ, Hack CE: Upregulation of ICAM-1 on cardiomyocytes in jeopardized human myocardium during infarction. Cardiovasc Res 1999; 41: 603-10

[56] Tailor A, Cooper D, Granger DN: Platelet-vessel wall interactions in the microcirculation. Microcirculation 2005; 12: 275-85

[57] Granger DN: Role of xanthine oxidase and granulocytes in ischemia-reperfusion injury. Am J Physiol 1988; 255: H1269-75

[58] Herd CM, Page CP: Pulmonary immune cells in health and disease: platelets. Eur Respir J 1994; 7: 1145-60

[59] Suzuki K, Sugimura K, Hasegawa K, Yoshida K, Suzuki A, Ishizuka K, Ohtsuka K, Honma T, Narisawa R, Asakura H: Activated platelets in ulcerative colitis enhance the production of reactive oxygen species by polymorphonuclear leukocytes. Scand J Gastroenterol 2001; 36: 1301-6

[60] Botto N, Sbrana S, Trianni G, Andreassi MG, Ravani M, Rizza A, Al-Jabri A, Palmieri C, Berti S: An increased platelet-leukocytes interaction at the culprit site of coronary artery occlusion in acute myocardial infarction: a pathogenic role for "no-reflow" phenomenon? Int J Cardiol 2007; 117: 123-30

[61] Takahashi T, Hato F, Yamane T, Fukumasu H, Suzuki K, Ogita S, Nishizawa Y, Kitagawa S: Activation of human neutrophil by cytokine-activated endothelial cells. Circ Res 2001; 88: 422-9

[62] Takahashi T, Nishizawa Y, Hato F, Shintaku H, Maeda N, Fujiwara N, Inaba M, Kobayashi K, Kitagawa S: Neutrophil-activating activity and platelet-activating factor synthesis in cytokine-stimulated endothelial cells: reduced activity in growth-arrested cells. Microvasc Res 2007; 73: 29-34

[63] Gourdin MJ, Bree B, De Kock M: The impact of ischaemia-reperfusion on the blood vessel. Eur J Anaesthesiol 2009; 26: 537-47

[64] Abramov AY, Scorziello A, Duchen MR: Three distinct mechanisms generate oxygen free radicals in neurons and contribute to cell death during anoxia and reoxygenation. J Neurosci 2007; 27: 1129-38

[65] Kang SM, Lim S, Song H, Chang W, Lee S, Bae SM, Chung JH, Lee H, Kim HG, Yoon DH, Kim TW, Jang Y, Sung JM, Chung NS, Hwang KC: Allopurinol modulates reactive oxygen species generation and Ca2+ overload in ischemia-reperfused heart and hypoxia-reoxygenated cardiomyocytes. Eur J Pharmacol 2006; 535: 212-9

[66] Szocs K: Endothelial dysfunction and reactive oxygen species production in ischemia/reperfusion and nitrate tolerance. Gen Physiol Biophys 2004; 23: 265-95

[67] Giorgio M, Migliaccio E, Orsini F, Paolucci D, Moroni M, Contursi C, Pelliccia G, Luzi L, Minucci S, Marcaccio M, Pinton P, Rizzuto R, Bernardi P, Paolucci F, Pelicci PG: Electron transfer between cytochrome c and p66Shc generates reactive oxygen species that trigger mitochondrial apoptosis. Cell 2005; 122: 221-33

[68] Droge W: Free radicals in the physiological control of cell function. Physiol Rev 2002; 82: 47-95

[69] Pinton P, Rimessi A, Marchi S, Orsini F, Migliaccio E, Giorgio M, Contursi C, Minucci S, Mantovani F, Wieckowski MR, Del Sal G, Pelicci PG, Rizzuto R: Protein kinase C beta and prolyl isomerase 1 regulate mitochondrial effects of the life-span determinant p66Shc. Science 2007; 315: 659-63

[70] Bajaj G, Sharma RK: TNF-alpha-mediated cardiomyocyte apoptosis involves caspase-12 and calpain. Biochem Biophys Res Commun 2006; 345: 1558-64

[71] Wu D, Chen X, Ding R, Qiao X, Shi S, Xie Y, Hong Q, Feng Z: Ischemia/reperfusion induce renal tubule apoptosis by inositol 1,4,5-trisphosphate receptor and L-type Ca2+ channel opening. Am J Nephrol 2008; 28: 487-99

[72] An S, Hishikawa Y, Liu J, Koji T: Lung injury after ischemia-reperfusion of small intestine in rats involves apoptosis of type II alveolar epithelial cells mediated by TNF-alpha and activation of Bid pathway. Apoptosis 2007; 12: 1989-2001

[73] Lu X, Hamilton JA, Shen J, Pang T, Jones DL, Potter RF, Arnold JM, Feng Q: Role of tumor necrosis factor-alpha in myocardial dysfunction and apoptosis during hindlimb ischemia and reperfusion. Crit Care Med 2006; 34: 484-91

[74] Misseri R, Meldrum DR, Dinarello CA, Dagher P, Hile KL, Rink RC, Meldrum KK: TNF-alpha mediates obstruction-induced renal tubular cell apoptosis and proapoptotic signaling. Am J Physiol Renal Physiol 2005; 288: F406-11

http://dx.doi.org/10.5772/54508

[75] Sugano M, Hata T, Tsuchida K, Suematsu N, Oyama J, Satoh S, Makino N: Local delivery of soluble TNF-alpha receptor 1 gene reduces infarct size following ischemia/reperfusion injury in rats. Mol Cell Biochem 2004; 266: 127-32

[76] Sun HY, Wang NP, Halkos M, Kerendi F, Kin H, Guyton RA, Vinten-Johansen J, Zhao ZQ: Postconditioning attenuates cardiomyocyte apoptosis via inhibition of JNK and p38 mitogen-activated protein kinase signaling pathways. Apoptosis 2006; 11: 1583-93

[77] Pru JK, Lynch MP, Davis JS, Rueda BR: Signaling mechanisms in tumor necrosis factor alpha-induced death of microvascular endothelial cells of the corpus luteum. Reprod Biol Endocrinol 2003; 1: 17

[78] Ruel M, Khan TA, Voisine P, Bianchi C, Sellke FW: Vasomotor dysfunction after cardiac surgery. Eur J Cardiothorac Surg 2004; 26: 1002-14

[79] Davenpeck KL, Guo JP, Lefer AM: Pulmonary artery endothelial dysfunction following ischemia and reperfusion of the rabbit lung. J Vasc Res 1993; 30: 145-53

[80] Meredith IT, Currie KE, Anderson TJ, Roddy MA, Ganz P, Creager MA: Postischemic vasodilation in human forearm is dependent on endothelium-derived nitric oxide. Am J Physiol 1996; 270: H1435-40

[81] Nanobashvili J, Neumayer C, Fuegl A, Blumer R, Prager M, Sporn E, Polterauer P, Malinski T, Huk I: Development of 'no-reflow' phenomenon in ischemia/reperfusion injury: failure of active vasomotility and not simply passive vasoconstriction. Eur Surg Res 2003; 35: 417-24

[82] Stauton M, Drexler C, Dulitz MG, Ekbom DC, Schmeling WT, Farber NE: Effects of hypoxia-reoxygenation on microvascular endothelial function in the rat hippocampal slice. Anesthesiology 1999; 91: 1462-9

[83] Friedman M, Wang SY, Stahl GL, Johnson RG, Sellke FW: Altered beta-adrenergic and cholinergic pulmonary vascular responses after total cardiopulmonary bypass. J Appl Physiol 1995; 79: 1998-2006

[84] Sato K, Li J, Metais C, Bianchi C, Sellke F: Increased pulmonary vascular contraction to serotonin after cardiopulmonary bypass: role of cyclooxygenase. J Surg Res 2000; 90: 138-43

[85] Reffelmann T, Hale SL, Dow JS, Kloner RA: No-reflow phenomenon persists long-term after ischemia/reperfusion in the rat and predicts infarct expansion. Circulation 2003; 108: 2911-7

[86] Reffelmann T, Kloner RA: The no-reflow phenomenon: A basic mechanism of myocardial ischemia and reperfusion. Basic Res Cardiol 2006; 101: 359-72

[87] Tauber S, Menger MD, Lehr HA: Microvascular in vivo assessment of reperfusion injury: significance of prostaglandin E(1) and I(2) in postischemic "no-reflow" and "reflow-paradox". J Surg Res 2004; 120: 1-11

[88] Hinshaw DB, Burger JM, Miller MT, Adams JA, Beals TF, Omann GM: ATP depletion induces an increase in the assembly of a labile pool of polymerized actin in endothelial cells. Am J Physiol 1993; 264: C1171-9

[89] Hinshaw DB, Sklar LA, Bohl B, Schraufstatter IU, Hyslop PA, Rossi MW, Spragg RG, Cochrane CG: Cytoskeletal and morphologic impact of cellular oxidant injury. Am J Pathol 1986; 123: 454-64

[90] Han JY, Horie Y, Li D, Akiba Y, Nagata H, Miura S, Oda M, Ishii H, Hibi T: Attenuating effect of Myakuryu on mesenteric microcirculatory disorders induced by ischemia and reperfusion. Clin Hemorheol Microcirc 2006; 34: 145-50

[91] de Perrot M, Liu M, Waddell TK, Keshavjee S: Ischemia-reperfusion-induced lung injury. Am J Respir Crit Care Med 2003; 167: 490-511

[92] Eppinger MJ, Deeb GM, Bolling SF, Ward PA: Mediators of ischemia-reperfusion injury of rat lung. Am J Pathol 1997; 150: 1773-84

[93] Chang WC, Murota SI, Nakao J, Orimo H: Age-related decrease in prostacyclin biosynthetic activity in rat aortic smooth muscle cells. Biochim Biophys Acta 1980; 620: 159-66

[94] Klass O, Fischer UM, Antonyan A, Bosse M, Fischer JH, Bloch W, Mehlhorn U: Pneumocyte apoptosis induction during cardiopulmonary bypass: effective prevention by radical scavenging using N-acetylcysteine. J Invest Surg 2007; 20: 349-56

[95] Massoudy P, Zahler S, Becker BF, Braun SL, Barankay A, Meisner H: Evidence for inflammatory responses of the lungs during coronary artery bypass grafting with cardiopulmonary bypass. Chest 2001; 119: 31-6

[96] Ng CS, Wan S, Yim AP, Arifi AA: Pulmonary dysfunction after cardiac surgery. Chest 2002; 121: 1269-77

[97] O'Donnell D, Clarke G, Hurst P: Acute renal failure following surgery for abdominal aortic aneurysm. Aust N Z J Surg 1989; 59: 405-8

[98] Basile DP: The endothelial cell in ischemic acute kidney injury: implications for acute and chronic function. Kidney Int 2007; 72: 151-6

[99] Basile DP, Fredrich K, Chelladurai B, Leonard EC, Parrish AR: Renal ischemia reperfusion inhibits VEGF expression and induces ADAMTS-1, a novel VEGF inhibitor. Am J Physiol Renal Physiol 2008; 294: F928-36

[100] Ferdinandy P, Schulz R, Baxter GF: Interaction of cardiovascular risk factors with myocardial ischemia/reperfusion injury, preconditioning, and postconditioning. Pharmacol Rev 2007; 59: 418-58

http://dx.doi.org/10.5772/54508

[101] Abbott NJ: Inflammatory mediators and modulation of blood-brain barrier permeability. Cell Mol Neurobiol 2000; 20: 131-47

[102] Adembri C, Kastamoniti E, Bertolozzi I, Vanni S, Dorigo W, Coppo M, Pratesi C, De Gaudio AR, Gensini GF, Modesti PA: Pulmonary injury follows systemic inflammatory reaction in infrarenal aortic surgery. Crit Care Med 2004; 32: 1170-7

[103] Fantini GA, Conte MS: Pulmonary failure following lower torso ischemia: clinical evidence for a remote effect of reperfusion injury. Am Surg 1995; 61: 316-9

[104] Junnarkar S, Lau LL, Edrees WK, Underwood D, Smye MG, Lee B, Hannon RJ, Soong CV: Cytokine activation and intestinal mucosal and renal dysfunction are reduced in endovascular AAA repair compared to surgery. J Endovasc Ther 2003; 10: 195-202

Chapter 3

Ventricular Arrhythmias and Myocardial Revascularization

Rainer Moosdorf

Additional information is available at the end of the chapter

http://dx.doi.org/10.5772/54694

1. Introduction

Ventricular arrhythmias are closely associated with myocardial ischemia and its sequelae. Acute ischemia frequently leads to ventricular fibrillation (Vfib) and to sudden cardiac death. As well, chronic ischemia, if presented as ischemic cardiomyopathy with restricted left ventricular function, is prone to the risk of Vfib. In contrast, scar formation after myocardial infarction leads to reentry circuits as an origin of ventricular tachycardia (Vt).

2. Pathophysiology

One of the typical complications of acute myocardial ischemia respectively myocardial infarction is ventricular fibrillation. Ischemic cells loose their membrane stability and a compound of such ischemic cells may cause electrical instability. Revascularization, if in time, restores cellular function and leads to electrical restabilization. One has to be aware however, that the so called reperfusion injury in the early phase after revascularization may also cause ventricular arrhythmias.

Chronic ischemia with a significant reduction of left ventricular function, the so called ischemic cardiomyopathy, is also prone to ventricular fibrillation and also in these patients revascularization may lead to a risk reduction by an improvement of the myocardial function and left ventricular ejection fraction.

If a myocardial infarction has happened, tissue is irreversibly damaged and replaced by scar. The center of this postinfarct scar is homogenious, but the border zone to vital myocardium is not linear but shows irregular interdentations between the two tissues.Within this inhomogenious

borderzone, reentry circuits may induce ventricular tachycardia, which is not influenced by reperfusion (1).

3. Surgical treatment options

If a myocardial infarction has lead to a scar, no matter to what extent, reentry cicuits may be induced and lead to VT's. Early surgical treatments were performed in cases of major scars, so called ventricular aneurysms, which were resected (2,3) and within the same procedure, deep encircling incisions of different extent should isolate the electrically instable boarder zone from the remaining ventricle (4,5). With the introduction of electrophysiological investigations, the origin of such reentry circuits along the border zone was localized and an endocardial resection of this focus performed (6,7,8,9,10,11). However recurrent Vt's were observed frequently after these procedures, oftentimes different from the primary clinical and also electrophysiological presentation. Experimental studies could demonstrate epicardial sites as origins of these recurrencies, which could of course not be reached by endocardial resections (12).

4. Mapping guided laser photocoagulation

The search for different treatment options finally led to the introduction of laser energy into this type of cardiac surgery (13,14,15,16,17,18,19). Using a conventional Nd-Yag laser and a gas cooled fiber for energy transmission, deep photocoagulations of the diseased tissue can be performed. Tissue is not removed or ablated in the original sense, but the structural integrity of the lased area remains intact. This deep photocoagulation creates a homogenious kind of scar and stops the reentry circuit. This kind of treatment is not limited to the endocardium but can also be applied to the epicardial surface after an electrophysiological mapping.

Consequently, mapping was no longer limited to the endocardium after resection of an aneurysm, but was extended to the epicardial surface during the same procedure (18). By this combination, recurrencies could be significantly reduced.

Moreover, in cases of only small scar areas and without an aneurysm as access to the left ventricle, our group, together with the pioneering group of Svenson and Selle, performed the first cases of sole epicardial ablation, so to avoid a ventricular incision and further myocardial damage (20). Even with deep laser lesions, this limited access can of course not reach certain regions of the myocardium, especially the septum and the papillary muscles but we could still eliminate significant numbers of VT's in this special cohort of patients and avoid the implantation of an ICD.

5. Treatmentalgorithm for patients with coronary artery disease and ventricular arrhythmias

Patients with coronary artery disease and an indication for surgical revascularization, who also have experienced Vfib, receive coronary bypassgrafting alone. After surgery, the decision

for an ICD depends on the standardized criteria like reduced ejection fraction, incomplete revascularization or recurrent Vfib. In case of doubt, an electrophysiological investigation should be considered.

Patients with coronary artery disease and a status post infarct, who have experienced already a VT, are scheduled for a combined procedure of bypass grafting and VT-surgery. If the VT is documented in the charts, no further testing is necessary. If a reliable record is missing, an electrophysiological testing should be performed. The lack of major scar or an aneurysm is no exclusion criterion, in these cases a sole epicardial procedure is scheduled and the patient has to be informed about the lower cure rate because of the limited access.

Anyway, a sole revascularization with or without aneurysm resection, is an incomplete therapeutic approach. Patients, who need a surgical revascularization and/or an aneurysm resection and ventricular restoration, should also be offered a curative therapy of their ventricular arrhythmia. Without a directed ablation, a disappearance of the VT can not be expected and the implantation of an ICD is only palliative! Surgery should be curative if ever possible.

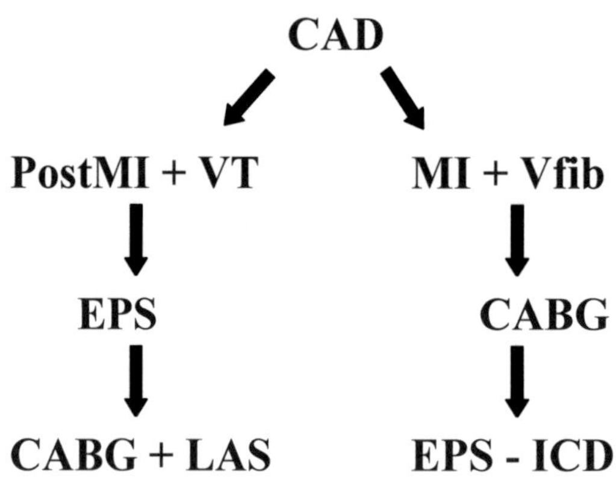

Figure 1. Treatment algorithm (CAD:coronary artery disease, MI:myocardial infarction, EPS:electrophysiological study, CABG:coronary artery bypass grafting, LAS:laser arrhythmia surgery, ICD implantable cardioverter defibrillator)

6. The surgical procedure

The procedure is performed via a median sternotomy and after establishing extracorporeal circulation and placing pacing wires on the surface of the right ventricle, the left ventricle is opened through the aneurysm and blood is evacuated by a vent, which is inserted via the right upper pulmonary vein as usual. It is important however to maintain a sufficiently high flow of the extracorporeal circulation to keep the aortic valve closed and to avoid an air embolism. After inspection of the ventricular cave and definition of the resection lines, the VT is induced with the epicardial electrodes and mapping is performed with a small finger electrode.

Whenever a typical early potential is detected by the electrophysiologist, lasing is performed with the gas cooled fiber kept at a distance of approximately 5mm away from the tissue. So a sufficiently deep lesion can be created without removal of tissue and distruction of the structural integrity of the myocardium. Laser application is terminated after the VT stops and sinus rhythm reoccures. This procedure is repeated on the endo- and afterwards on the epicardium, until no further VT is inducible. After that, surgery is continued in the normal fashion with the definitive aneurysm resection, ventricular restoration and bypass surgery.

If no aneurysm is present, the ventricle is generally not opened but mapping guided laser photocoagulation only performed epicardially. If in these cases no further epicardial focus can be mapped but a VT, mostly different to the initial clinical recording, is still inducible, the procedure must be terminated without complete cure, as already described above. According to our very strict protocol, all these patients receive an ICD in a second intervention.

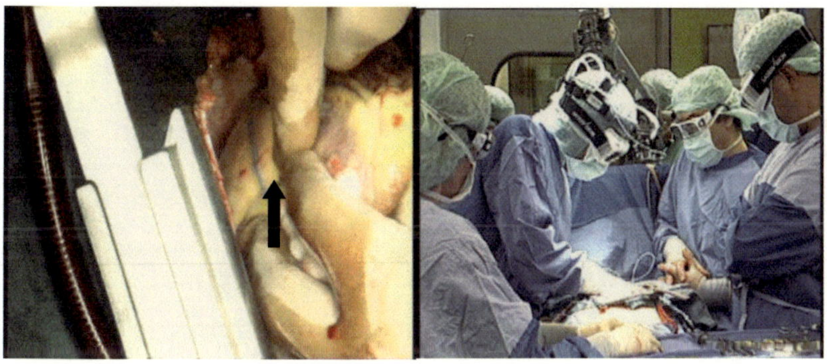

(a) (b)

Figure 2. Intraoperative mapping with a small fingerprobe (a) and laser photocoagulation with protective gogles (b)

7. Postoperative protocol

Postoperatively, no antiarrhythmic drugs are given, except the standard medication with a beta-blocker. Before discharge, every patient is submitted to a final electrophysiological investigation with an aggressive stimulation protocol to induce an arrhythmia. The photocoagulation is only considered successful, if no ventricular arrhythmia can be induced including VT´s different from the initial one or even Vfib. Patients with any type of inducible arrhythmia get an ICD before being discharged.

8. Results

Depending of course on the number of foci mapped and photocoagulated, the operative procedure is prolonged for about half an hour. The heart is not arrested during this time, so

that the arrhythmia surgery does not add to the ischemic time. In our hands, the risk of the procedure is not significantly increased. Table 2 shows the results of the initial 32 patients treated consecutively by our group at the University Hospitals Bonn and Marburg (17,20).

	Total (n=32)	Endo + Epi (n=20)	Epi (n=12)
Intraop. VT-term.	29	19	10
Postop. Ind. VT	5	1	4 (3)
Recurrent VT	5	0	5 (4)
ICD	6	0	6
Mortality (30 days)	3(9%)	2(10%)	1(8%)

Table 1. Results of 32 patients treated consecutively because of VT and severe coronary artery disease

One has to keep in mind, that all patients being treated endo- and epicardially for their VT were primarily referred because of severe coronary artery disease and large ventriclar aneurysms, resulting in a severely reduced left ventricular function prior to surgery, so that the mortality is in accordance with the predicted mortality of this high risk group alone.

Among the group with sole epicardial photocoagualation, around 40% still had inducible VT ´s during the postoperative electrophysiological examination. Most of them were not identical with the initial clinical one. However, according to our protocol, they were registered as non successful and received an ICD. Still, 60 % of those formerly not curatively treatable patients could remain without ICD and among the remaining 40% with ICD´s, shocks could be avoided or kept very rare, so that this limited access approach is also worth while being persued.

9. Summary and message

In contrast to Vfib, Vt is in the vast majority of cases associated with a clearly defined patho-anatomical substrate, an inhomogenious interdentation of scar and vital myocardium in the border zone of a postinfarct scar, which is not affected by revascularization, but has to be adressed separately.

Revascularization alone will not lead to termination of Vt´s, nor will sole resection of scar or an aneurysm be curative either, as the inhomogenious borderzone remains unaffected and may still trigger reentry circuits, which may be located subendocardially as well as subepicardially.

As a consequence, any patient with a documented VT and an indication for surgical revascularization and / or a ventricular restoration should also be submitted to an intraoperative VT ablation and be referred to specialized centers. A surgical intervention should always aim at curative result and ICD is very effective but is palliative!

Author details

Rainer Moosdorf*

Department for Cardiovascular Surgery, University Hospital Marburg, Marburg, Germany

References

[1] De Bakker, J. M, Coronel, R, Tasseron, S, Wilde, A. A, Opthof, T, Janse, M. J, Van Capelle, F. J, Becker, A. E, & Jambroes, G. Ventricular tachycardia in the infarcted, Langendorff-perfused human heart: role of the arrangement of surviving cardiac fibers. J Am Coll Cardiol, (1990). , 1594-607.

[2] Welch, T. G, Fontana, M. E, & Vasco, J. S. Aneurysmectomy for recurrent ventricular tachyarrhythmias. Am Heart J, (1973). , 685-88.

[3] Arnulf, G. Resistance and tolerance of myocardium in ischemia: experimental results. J Cardiovasc Surg (Torino), (1975). , 218-27.

[4] Guiraudon, G, Fontain, G, Frank, R, Escande, G, Etievent, P, Vignes, R, Mattei, M. F, Cabrol, C, & Cabrol, A. Circular exclusion ventriculotomy. Surgical treatment of ventricular tachycardia following myocardial infarction. Arch Mal Coeur Vaiss, (1978). , 1255-62.

[5] Schulte, H. D, Bircks, W, Ostermeyer, J, & Seipel, l. Surgery of life-threatening ventricular tachyarrhythmias associated with ventricular aneurysm. Thoarac Cardiovasc Surg, (1979). , 124-27.

[6] Josphson, ME, & Horowitz, . . Recurrent sustained ventricular tachycardia. 2. Endocardial mapping. Circulation, 1978, 57(3); 440-47

[7] Ostermeyer, J, Breithart, G, Kolvenbach, R, Borggrefe, M, Seipel, L, Schulte, H. D, & Bircks, W. The surgical treatment of ventricular tachycardias. Simple aneurysmectomy versus electrophysiologically guided procedures. J Thorac Cardiovasc Surg, (1982). , 704-15.

[8] Gallagher, J. J, Oldham, H. N, Wallace, A. G, Peter, R. H, & Kasell, J. Ventricular aneurysm with ventricular tachycardia. Report of a case with epicardial mapping and successful resection. Am J Cardiol (1975). , 696-700.

[9] Fontain, G, Guiraudon, G, Frank, R, Gerbaux, A, Cousteau, J. P, Barrillon, A, Gay, J, Cabrol, C, & Facquet, J. Epicardial cartography and surgical treatment by simple ventriculotomy of certain resistant reentry ventricular tachycardias, Arch Mal Coeur Vaiss, (1975). , 113-24.

[10] Cox, J. L, Gallagher, J. J, & Ungerleider, R. M. Encircling endocardial ventriculotomy for refractory ischemic ventricular tachycardia. IV.Clinical indication, surgical technique, mechanism of action, and results. J Thorac Cardiovasc Surg, (1982). , 865-72.

[11] Fontain, G, Guiraudon, G, Frank, R, Vedel, J, Cabrol, C, & Grosgogeat, Y. The concept of reentry in the surgical treatment of ventricular tachycardia. Ann Med Interne (Paris), (1978). , 413-17.

[12] Littmann, L, Svenson, R. H, Gallagher, J. J, Selle, J. G, Zimmern, S. H, Fedor, J. M, & Colavita, P. G. Functional role of the epicardium in postinfarction ventricular tachycardia. Observations derived from computerized epicordial activation mapping, entrainment and epicardial laser photoablation. Circulation (1991). , 1577-91.

[13] Littmann, L, Svenson, R. H, Gallagher, J. J, & Selle, J. G. High grade entrance and exit block in an area of healed myocardial infarction associated with ventricular tachycardia with successful laser photoablation of the anatomic substrate. Am J Cardiol, (1989). , 122-24.

[14] Cox, J. L. Laser photoablation for the treatment of refractory ventricular tachycardia and endocardial fibroelastosis. Ann Thorac Surg, (1985). , 199-200.

[15] Mesnildrey, P, Laborde, F, Beloucif, F, Mavolini, P, & Piwnica, A. Ventricular tachycardia of ischemic origin. Surgical treatment by encircling thermo- exclusion using the Nd-Yag laser. Presse Med, (1986). , 531-34.

[16] Svenson, R. H, Gallagher, J. J, Selle, J. G, Zimmern, S. H, Fedor, J. M, & Robicsek, F. Neodymium:Yag laser photocoagulation: a successful new map guided technique for the intraoperative ablation of ventricular tachycardia, Circulation, (1987). , 1319-28.

[17] Moosdorf, R, Pfeiffer, D, Schneider, C, & Jung, W. Intraoperative laser photocoagulation of ventricular tachycardia. Am Heart J, (1994). pt2); , 1133-38.

[18] Svenson, R. H, Littmann, L, Gallagher, J. J, Selle, J. G, Zimmern, S. H, Fedor, J. M, & Colavita, P. G. Termination of ventricular tachycardia with epicardial laser photocoagulation: a clinical comparison with patients undergoing successful endocardial photocoagulation alone. J Am Coll Cardiol, (1990). , 163-70.

[19] Isner JmEstes NA, Payne DD, Rastegar H, Clarke RH, Cleveland RJ. Laser assisted endocardiectomyfor refractory ventricular tachyarrhythmias. Clin Cardiol (1987). , 201-4.

[20] Pfeiffer, D, Moosdorf, R, Svenson, R. H, Littmann, L, Grimm, W, Kirchhoff, P. G, & Lüderitz, B. Epicardial Neodymium.Yag laser photocoagulation of ventricular tachycardia without ventriculotomy in patients after myocardial infarction. Circulation, (1996). , 3221-25.

Chapter 4

Minimally Invasive Cardiac Output Monitoring in the Year 2012

Lester Augustus Hall Critchley

Additional information is available at the end of the chapter

http://dx.doi.org/10.5772/54413

1. Introduction

"Cardiac output the "Holy Grail" of haemodynamic monitoring"

Physicians have been assessing the circulation long before the birth of Christ (BC). The Egyptian physicians used simple palpation of the pulse and the use of the pulse in Chinese medicine dates back over two thousand years. However, it was not until the 1940s that the clinical sphygmomanometer was invented, and blood pressure measurement became routinely available [1].Today pulse rate and blood pressure measurement is performed in almost every patient.

Cardiac output is the volume of blood that is pumped by the heart around the systemic circulation in a given time period, usually one minute. It is equal to the volume pumped out by the heart in one contraction, known as stroke volume, multiplied by heart rate. The need to measure cardiac output in a clinical setting arose in the 1970s because of the development of intensive care units and the increasing need to manage unstable patients during high risk surgery. In parallel with these clinical developments the technology also became available to make more sophisticated cardiac output monitors and in particular monitors that can be used continuously at the bedside.

When evaluating the circulation, and thus haemodynamics, a very simply model can be drawn of the heart pumping blood through the arteries to peripheral capillaries and then returning to the heart via the veins. The haemodynamics of the model has flow, the cardiac output, leaving the heart, and passing through a resistance, the peripheral capillaries. Blood pressure is generated in the arteries by the heart pumping against this resistance. A very simple formula exists that describes the model of Blood Pressure = Cardiac Output x Peripheral Resistance, which is often compared to Ohm's law for electricity (i.e. Voltage = Current x Resistance).

During clinical assessment pulse rate and blood pressure are very easy to measure. However, cardiac output and peripheral resistance are much less easy to obtain. Usually, the physician is only able to measure the pulse rate, and thus does not know how much blood the heart pumps each minute, nor the degree of the peripheral vasoconstriction. Knowing these variables becomes important when treating critically ill patients with low blood pressures who may be either hypovolaemic or septic, as it helps one to differentiate between the two conditions.

Cardiac output has proved very difficult to measure reliably in the clinical setting. The Fick method is considered the most accurate method and gold standard. It involves measuring oxygen uptake by the body and comparing oxygen content in arterial and venous blood samples. It is based on a very simple principle that blood flow through an organ is related to the uptake of a marker (oxygen) and the difference in concentration of that marker between blood entering (arterial) and blood leaving (venous) that organ, in the case of the Fick method, the heart and lungs. However, the method is cumbersome and time consuming, and usually performed in the laboratory. It is not suitable for bedside clinical use. The concept of using a marker is also used in other methods of cardiac output measurement, such as a dye and thermo (i.e. cold solution) dilution. Alternatively, a flow probe can be placed around the aorta, but this is highly invasive requiring surgery to access the heart or a beam aimed at the aorta that detects some property of flowing blood, such as the Doppler shift when using ultrasound. A secondary effect of blood flow or the action of the heart can also be used as a surrogate, such as bioelectrical changes in the thorax or the arterial blood pressure wave.

What makes cardiac output so difficult to measure accurately in the clinical setting, when compared to other haemodynamic variables, is its dispersion as blood travels away from the heart. Whereas the pulse rate and blood pressure can be measured from any location in the arterial tree, such as the arm, cardiac output should ideally be measured at its origin the ascending aorta, before it is split up into smaller regional blood flows.

Because of the clinical desire to known some patients' cardiac output and the inherent difficulties encountered when measuring cardiac output, developing a reliable bedside cardiac output monitoring has become the "Holy Grail" of haemodynamic monitoring.

In this chapter, I will review the main clinical methods available for measuring cardiac output and address the important issue of how they are evaluated.

2. Historical perspective

2.1. Earliest theories and methods

In the second century AD the Greek physician Galen taught his students that there were two distinct types of blood, nutritive venous blood arising from the liver and vital arterial blood arising from the heart. Galen believed that the heart acted not as pump, but sucked in blood from the veins which passed through tiny pores in the septum. Galen's explanation was believed until the beginning of the seventeenth century when an English physician William Harvey described the true nature of the circulation with the heart pumping blood around a system of arteries, capillaries and veins.

It was not until 1870 that cardiac output was first measured by the German physician and physiologist Adolf Fick using an oxygen uptake method. The Fick method was later modified in 1897 by Stewart to use a continuous saline infusion and then in 1928 by Hamilton to use a bolus injection of dye technique [2,3]

2.2. Dye dilution methods

The Stewart-Hamilton dye dilution method to measure cardiac output was one of the earliest to be used clinically. In the 1950's indocyanine green dye became available clinically and was used to measure cardiac output, as well as blood volume and liver blood flow. However, sampling of arterial blood for dye levels was messy. A photocell detector placed on a finger was developed. Today, lithium dilution is the main indicator dilution technique in clinical use [4] and it is also a popular method in veterinarian practice.

2.3. The Swan-Ganz catheter

The idea of using a cold temperature solution as an indicator, or thermodilution, dates back to the 1950's. At first fine catheter tubes were placed in the pulmonary artery, but this proved very difficult to perform clinically. The idea of using an inflated balloon to float the catheter tip into position was credited to Swan in 1970 and the triple lumen pulmonary artery catheter (PAC) with a thermistor at its tip to Ganz in 1971 [5,6]. Their PAC was produced by the Edwards Laboratory Company. The PAC became the principle method of measuring cardiac output and reached its peak usage by the end of the 1980's with sales worldwide of 1 to 2 million catheters per year. However, doubts about its clinical usefulness arose in the 1980's [7], which were later confirmed by several multicentre clinical trials [8,9]. Since the 1990's there has been a major decline in the use of the PAC catheter [10] as alternative technologies such a TOE have become available. Today, many anaesthetists and critical care doctors are unfamiliar with using PACs. Only a few companies worldwide still manufacture PACs notably Arrow International (Reading, PA, USA) and Edwards Lifesciences (Irvine, CA, USA). More sophisticated multifunction PACs are now being sold that measure continuous cardiac output using a heated wire and mixed venous oxygen saturation.

Minimally invasive cardiac out monitoring (MICOM) that measured cardiac output continuously at the bedside started to become available in the 1970's with the emergence of microprocessor and computer technology. Today they have become the main focus of clinical monitoring of cardiac output.

3. Background to main methods

3.1. Bioimpedance

In 1957 Nyboer made the observation that the cardiac cycle was associated with repetitive changes in thoracic impedance and that stroke volume could be estimated from the area under the curve of the resulting impedance waveform. In 1966 Kubicek applied this observation to

developing a method that could measure cardiac output in space by astronauts. Later he developed the first commercial impedance cardiograph, the Minnesota [11]. In the 1980's the BoMed NCCOM3 (BoMed Ltd., Irvine, CA, USA) (Figure 1) was developed by Bernstein and Sramek [12]. It used a modified Kubicek method to calculate cardiac output. It also automated the process calculating cardiac output, and provided continuous cardiac output readings in real-time. Thus, the first continuous MICOM had been developed.

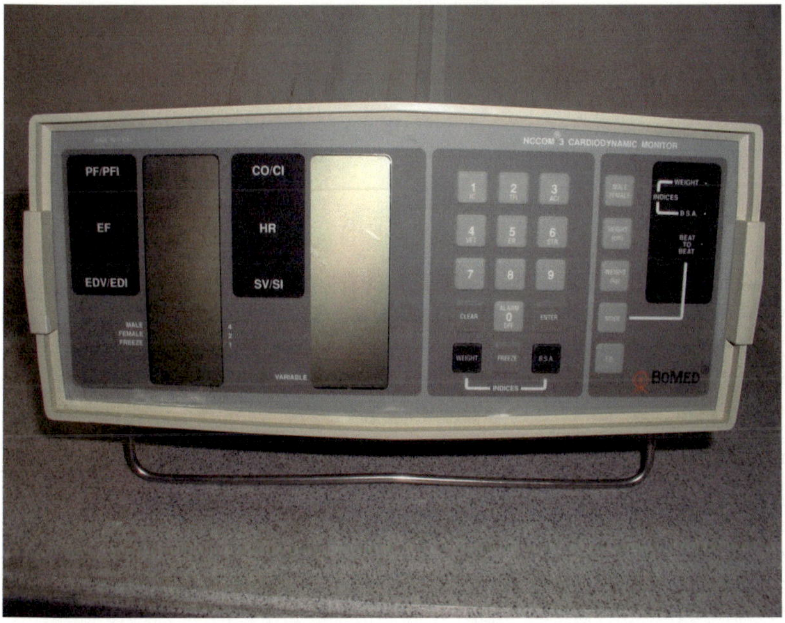

Figure 1. The BoMed NCCOM3. It connects to the patients using eight skin surface electrodes applied to the mid-neck and lower chest at the level of the diaphragm. Two additional ECG electrodes can be added. The BoMed is calibrated by inputting the patient's height and weight. Cardiac output and related bioimpedance variables are displayed as numbers. Data is averaged over 16 heart-beats.

Unfortunately, the BoMed had problems with its reliability and was never was accepted into clinical practice [13]. The presence of lung fluid corrupted impedance readings [14,15] and it was never determined with any certainty what the BoMed actually measured [16]. A digitalized version is still marketed and called the BioZ (CardioDynamics, San Diego, CA, USA). A number of companies have tried over the years to produce a more reliable version, but none have been very successful [17]. There is a haemodynamic monitoring system that incorporates bioimpedance cardiac output as one of its modalities call the Task-Force Monitor (CNSystems, Graz, Austria). It is used mainly to study autonomic responses such as syncopy and head up tilting. There is also a device on the market called the NICOM (Cheetah Medical Ltd., Tel-Aviv, Israel) that uses a principle call bioreactance, which measures shifts in alternating current phase, rather than electrical resistance. Potentially, this device may be immune to the problems that afflicted the BoMed, but good validation data are still needed.

http://dx.doi.org/10.5772/54413

3.2. Doppler ultrasound

Ultrasound was first described in 1842. It was introduced into clinical practice in the 1950s by Ian Donald, a Scotsman. Echocardiography was developed in 1960's and used pulsed ultrasound for imaging. The measurement of blood flow using Doppler ultrasound was developed later to detect aortic and peripheral blood flow using continuous wave Doppler systems. In the 1980's Singer a London critical care physician was instrumental in the clinical development of oesophageal Doppler cardiac output monitoring [18]. In the early 1990's several prototype monitor and probe systems were developed such as the Hemosonic 1000, (Arrow International, Reading, PA, USA), and the Abbott ODM II, (Abbott Laboratories, Chicago, Il, USA). The only successful model has been the CardioQ, (Deltex Medical, Chichester, England) released in the early1990's. In early 2000 an external continuous wave Doppler system was developed called the USCOM, (USCOM Ltd., Sydney, Australia). Previously one had to use echocardiography machines with limited Doppler capabilities for external monitoring. The USCOM measures cardiac output from both the ascending aorta and pulmonary artery using a hand held probe placed over the anterior neck (i.e. thoracic inlet) or left anterior chest wall (i.e. 3th to 5th intercostals spaces). Thus, the USCOM measures cardiac output intermittently.

3.3. Pulse contour analysis

Noninvasive continuous blood pressure measurement using a pneumatic finger cuff (i.e. plethysmography) was developed over 30-year ago. In 1993 Wesseling et al described a method of using the finger cuff arterial pressure wave to derive cardiac output [19]. Their method known as "Model Flow" was incorporated into the Finapres series of noninvasive continuous blood pressure monitors. Currently, the manufacturers produce the Nexfin, (BMEYE, Amsterdam, Netherlands).

Systems that used the arterial blood pressure trace to measure cardiac output were later developed. In 1997 the first commercial system, the PiCCO (Pulsion, Munich, Germany) was released. The PiCCO was calibrated using transpulmonary thermodilution and monitored cardiac output from a femoral arterial line. Since, several other systems have been developed including in 2002 the LiDCO-plus (and later rapid), (LiDCO Ltd., Cambridge, England), and in 2004 the FloTrac-Vigileo, (Edwards Lifesciences, Irvine, CA, USA). Early versions of these monitors relied on external calibration, usually by thermodilution. However, more recent versions self-calibrate using patient demographic data. Pulse contour monitoring of cardiac output has not proved all that successful and current systems are unreliable when large fluctuations in peripheral resistance occur [20]. Recently there has been a change in the marketing policy. The focus is now towards "functional haemodynamic variables", such as pulse pressure and stroke volume variation in response to fluid and postural challenges.

3.4. Other methods

Several other novel techniques of measuring cardiac output have also been developed. In the 1970's researchers explored the possibility of using the mechanical impulse produced by heart as it contracted. In the 1990's a modified Fick method based on carbon dioxide rebreathing

that used a special breathing circuit extension loop was developed call the NICO (Respironics, Philips Healthcare, USA). The NICO is still produced but its use is restricted to intubated and ventilated patients (Figure 2).

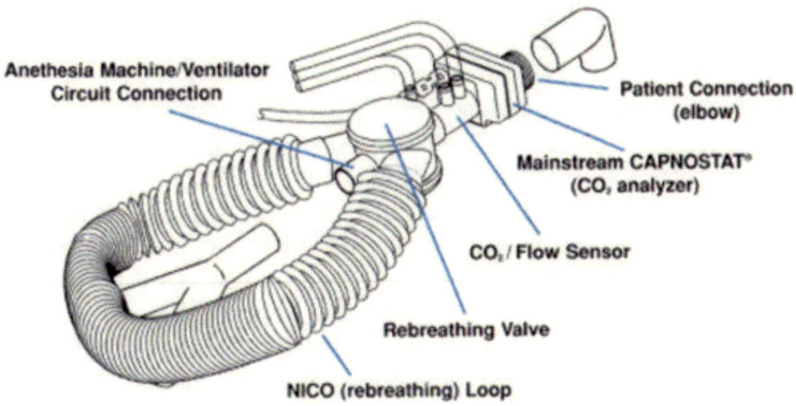

Figure 2. Elaborate NICO rebreathing loop and circuit attachment that was added to the patient's breathing circuit when performing the partial carbon dioxide rebreathing method.

In 2004 a device that used the time lags between the ECG and pulse oximetry signals was developed called the FloWave 1000, (Woolsthorpe Technologies, Brentwood, TN, USA). A Japanese group has recently developed a similar device called the esCCO monitor (Nihon Kohden, Tokyo, Japan) [21]. The esCCO also calculates pulse wave transit time from the ECG and pulse oximetry signal which it uses to calibrate the arterial pressure derived cardiac output (Figure 3).

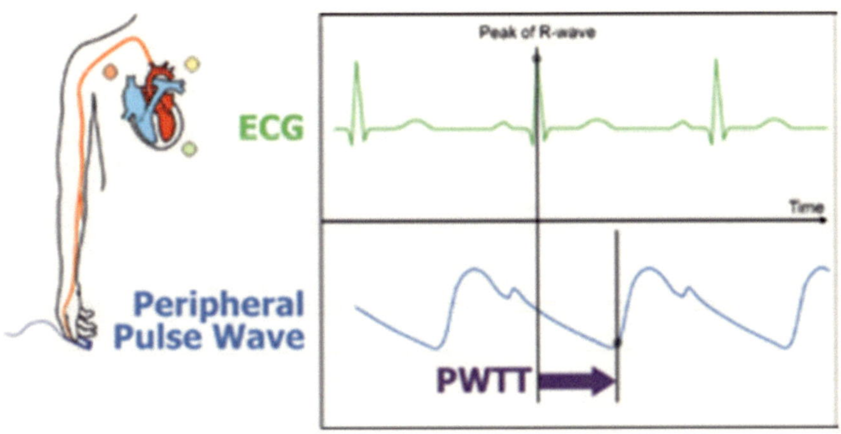

Figure 3. Illustration of the pulse wave transit time method used by the esCCO monitor. (Image from Nihon Kohden)

4. Description of the main methods

4.1. Bioreactance

To understand how the bioreactance method (NICOM, Cheetah Medical) works one first must understanding bioimpedance cardiac output. The older bioimpedance method involved detection of electrical resistance changes within the thorax. A high-frequency (50-100 kHz) low amplitude alternating current (<4mA), is passes between skin electrodes placed around the neck and upper abdomen. Inner current sensing skin electrodes detect voltage changes across the thorax and thus the impedance signal produced by the cardiac cycle (Figure 4). Originally, band electrodes were uses, but in the BoMed this was changed to eight dot electrodes. Bioimpedance is safe electrically because of the high frequency and low amperage of the current. The only report of injury with its use has been a pacemaker malfunction [22].

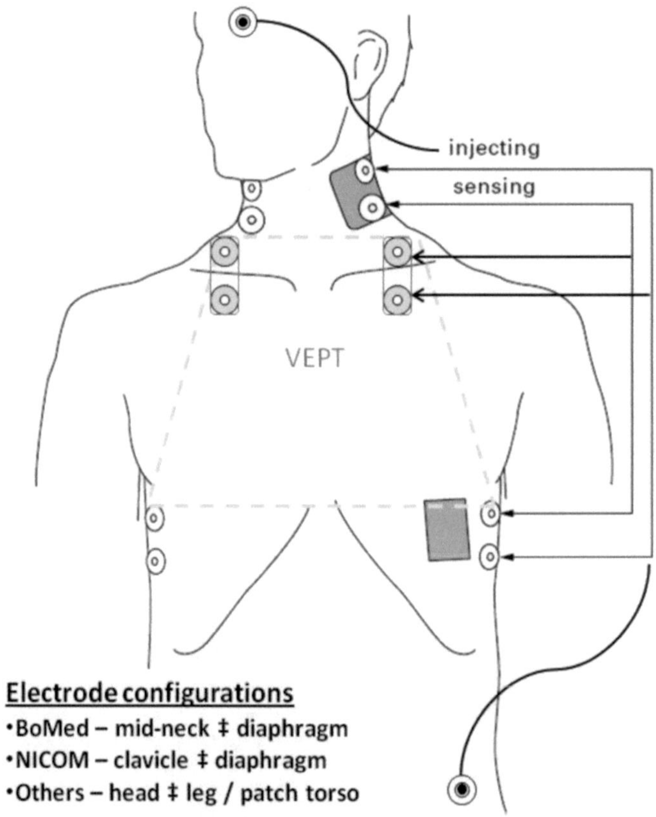

Figure 4. Electrode configurations used by different bioimpedance devices. The BoMed used an eight electrode configuration with outer current injecting and inner current sensing skin dot electrodes. Some other devices were designed with fewer but larger patch electrodes on the head and lower torso (current injecting) and neck and lower thorax (current sensing). The bioreactance system (NICOM) also uses a four dual dot electrode configuration with the neck electrodes placed slightly lower at the level of the clavicles.

In the original description of the impedance method the area under the bioimpedance signal curve during systole was used to estimate cardiac output. To simply the method Kubicek et al used the differential signal and its peak reading (dZ/dt(max)) as a surrogate for aortic blood flow [11]. The method also involves measuring the left ventricular ejection time (LVET) from the impedance signal (Figure 5). dZ/dt (max) multiplied by LVET provides stroke volume, but the reading still needs to be calibrated. Cardiac output is calculated by multiplying by heart rate. Other bioimpedance variables measured from the waveforms include: (i) the thoracic impedance which can be used as an index of lung fluid, (ii) the systolic time intervals, pre ejection period (PEP) and LVET, which can be used to calculate ejection fraction and (iii) the second differential (i.e. $d^2Z/dt^2(max)$) which can be used as an index of contractility.

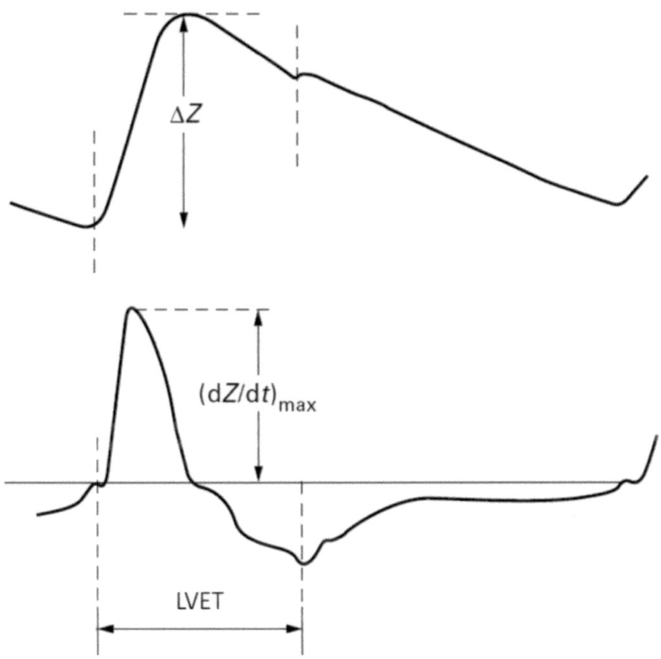

Figure 5. The bioimpedance method uses both the impedance signal (Z – upper waveform) and the differential signal (dZ/dt – lower waveform). From the differential signal the flow variable dZ/dt(max) is measured. The time variable LVET is also measured. A number of other indices that reflect lung fluid and contractility are also measured.

Bioreactance uses a different electrical signal. It detects a property of alternating current called phase. An alternating current has a sinusoidal waveform. As the current flows through different body tissues its passage is delayed by capacitive and inductive tissue effects (X) which cause a shift in its phase. As blood volume in the central thorax region varies with the cardiac cycle so does the phase shift of the current. Like resistance when measuring bioimpedance, a signal of the phase shift (bioreactance signal) can be plotted and from it variables that reflected blood flow (dX/dt(max)) and ventricular ejection time are measured (Figure 6). It is thought that the bioreactance signal is less affected by the factors that troubled the bioimpedance method, such as lung water [15].

http://dx.doi.org/10.5772/54413

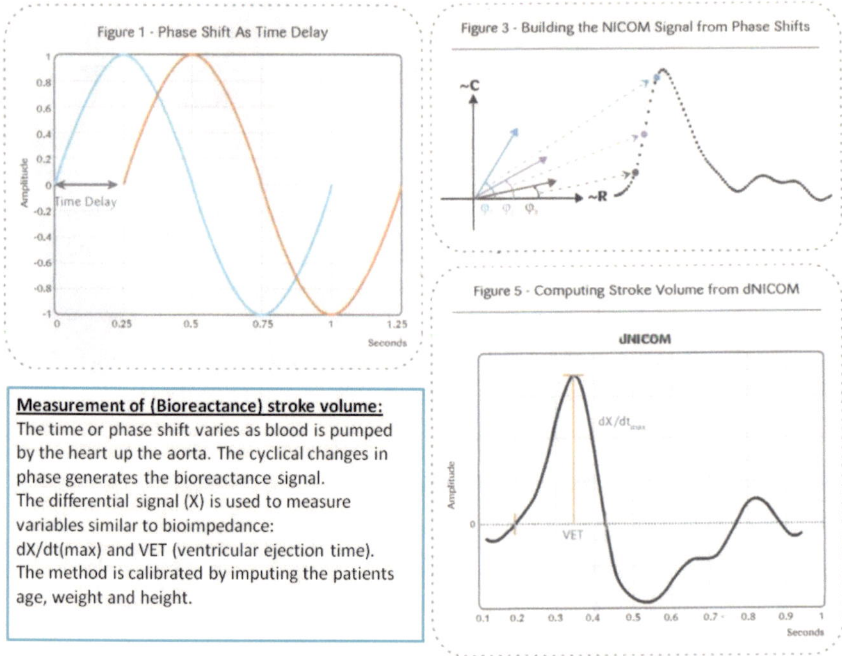

Figure 6. The steps in deriving bioreactance cardiac output (Images from Cheetah Medical).

Like all surrogate cardiac output methods the bioreactance method needs to be calibrated. When using bioimpedance this requires estimation of the volume of electrically participating tissue (VEPT) lying between the current sensing electrodes. Kubicek et al modeled the thorax on a cylinder [11]. Bernstein later modified the equation to a truncated cone [12]. In the NICOM an undisclosed algorithm based on age, weight and height is used for calibration.

Just like bioimpedance, it is not known precisely what the bioreactance signal truly represents. Rather than the flow of blood, it probably reflects blood volume expansion in the aorta as the vessel distends with the rise in blood pressure generated during systole [16]. Thus readings may also be influenced by variations in peripheral resistance.

4.2. Continuous wave Doppler

When pressure is applied to certain solid materials, notably crystals, they produce an electric charge. Equally, the same crystal will change shape when an electric charge is applied to it. This is known as the piezoelectric effect. If a high frequency current (i.e. 1-10 MHz) is applied the crystal will vibrate producing high frequency sound waves, or ultrasound. If the crystal is place in contact with the skin the ultrasound will be propagated through the underlying tissues. When the ultrasound beam hits an interface between two tissue structures part of beam is reflected back. If a short burst of ultrasound is used and a second crystal is used as a receiver, then the time delays between transmission and return of this pulse can be used to create an image of the underlying tissue structure. This is the basis of ultrasound imaging.

When a beam of continuous ultrasound encounters moving blood cells flowing In a blood vessel the ultrasound is reflected back at a slightly altered frequency. This phenomenon is known as the Doppler affect. The change or shift in frequency is related to the velocity of the blood cells. The Doppler shift signal can be separated from the ultrasound signal and a profile of the Doppler signal displayed (Figure 7). The angle (theta θ) that the ultrasound beam makes with the direction of blood flow is also important as it affects the magnitude of the Doppler shift frequency. If the direction of the ultrasound beam is parallel to the blood flow the Doppler shift will be maximal, whilst a perpendicular angle of insonation produces no Doppler shift. The angle of insonation (θ) and Doppler shift frequency are related to the cosine of theta (cos(θ)). The velocity of the blood flow is related to the Doppler frequency by the equation $velocity = c \times fD / 2 \times fT \cos\theta,$ where f_D is the Doppler shift frequency, f_T is the ultrasound probe or transmitter frequency, and c is the speed of ultrasound in the tissues, 1540 m/s. The speed of sound in air is around 340 m/s.

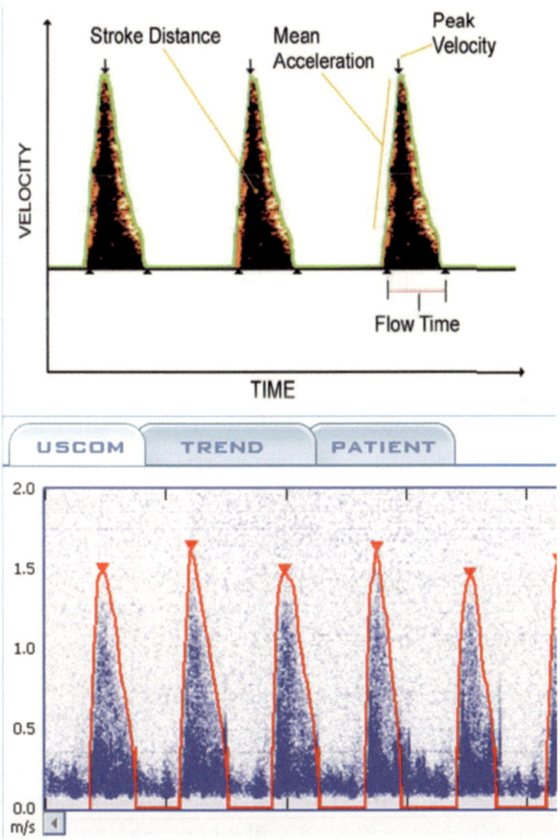

Figure 7. Doppler flow profiles from the oesophagus (upper - CardioQ) and the supra-sternal window (lower - USCOM). Velocity is shown on the y-axis (m/s) and time along x-axis. The outline of each Doppler signal is automatically detected and drawn. The area of each envelop (stroke distance) is related to stroke volume. A series of cardiac cycles are shown. (Upper image from Deltex Medical)

http://dx.doi.org/10.5772/54413

Blood flow in the aorta pulsates rather than being continuous, thus a continuous Doppler ultrasound signal needs to be recorded with sufficient sampling rate to show the details of the flow profile (Figure 7). Most ultrasound machines are imaging systems and use pulses of ultrasound to measure distance from the probe or depth like radar or sonar. Doppler is different because it detects change in velocity rather than position and requires a continuous ultrasound beam from a transmitting crystal and a separate receiving crystal. From the Doppler profile of blood flow in the aorta the peak velocity of the blood and the duration of flow can be determined. By drawing an envelope around the Doppler flow profile one can calculate the total flow during systole, which is called the stroke (or minute) distance (Figure 7).

To convert stroke distance to a volume (i.e. stroke volume) the cross-sectional area of the blood vessel is needed. In conventional echocardiography machines this is measured by ultrasound imaging using the relationship $CSA = \pi \times d^2 / 4$, where CSA = cross sectional area and d = diameter of blood vessel.

Two Doppler cardiac output systems are currently on the market, the CardioQ (Deltex Medical) (Figure 8) and the USCOM (USCOM Ltd.) (Figure 9). Neither measures the CSA of the aorta directly and both estimate it but in different ways. The CardioQ uses an empirical algorithm based on population data, where the calibration constant is based on the patient's age, gender, height and weight. As the CardioQ measures blood flow from descending aorta where about 30% of the blood flow has left the aorta for the head and arms, its algorithm corrects for this reduction in total flow. The USCOM measures blood flow across the aortic or pulmonary valve. It uses an empirical formula to calculate valve CSA [23] which also requires the patient's age, gender, weight and height.

The angle of insonation with blood flow of the probe needs to be considered. When the CardioQ is used its probe is in the oesophagus and lies parallel to the descending aorta. The ultrasound crystals at the tip are set to 45-degrees (Figure 8). Therefore, its angle of insonation is 45-degrees. The USCOM probe has a wide beam angle. It is directed at the aortic or pulmonary valves and its beam axis usually lies almost parallel to the direction of flow because of the anatomy. Thus, the angle of insonation (θ) is close to 90-degrees and the cosine of the angle approximates to 1.0. Neither device is corrected for deviations in beam angle to blood flow.

Focusing of the probe to obtain the optimal and maximum Doppler signal plays an extremely critical role in using these two Doppler devices effectively. Focusing can be performed both visually by observing the shape of Doppler profiles on the monitor screen or by listening to the quality of the audible Doppler signal. Various numbers of patient examinations are quoted to acquire competence in the focusing technique, 12 for the CardioQ and 20 for the USCOM [24,25]. However, it takes a much longer time to become sufficiently familiar with the different signal sounds and patterns to recognize when a truly reliable signal has been obtained. Significant experience and psychomotor skill is needed to be able to acquire clinically reliable data, with the CardioQ being easier to learn. Both companies provide training and support.

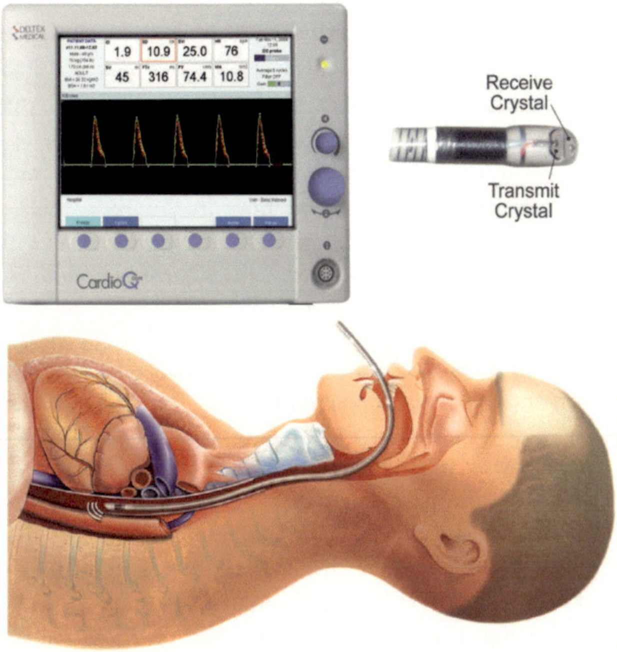

Figure 8. The CardioQ oesophageal Doppler monitor. Monitor and probe tip shown with transmitter and receiver crystals set at a 45-degree angle. Anatomical diagram shows insertion of the probe into the oesophagus via the mouth and insonation of the aorta which lies posterior. (Images from Deltex Medical)

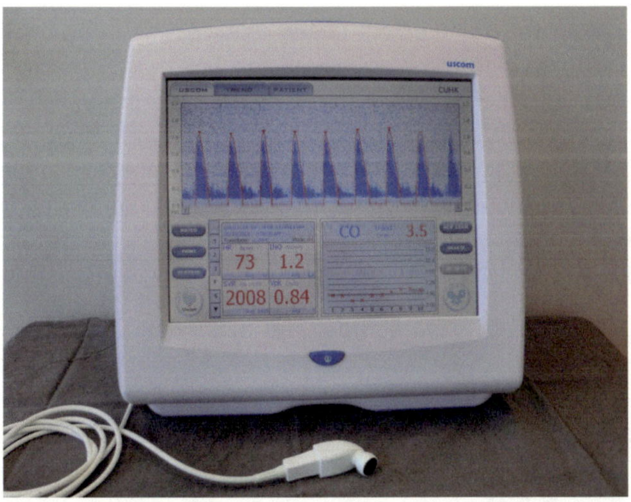

Figure 9. USCOM monitor showing Doppler signal data on its screen. The flow profiles are automatically outlined to measure stroke volumes. Below numerical readings are displayed. Lower right is a trend plot of saved cardiac output readings. The hand held USCOM probe is shown in front of the monitor. Ultrasound gel is applied to the probe to improve its acoustic contact.

In addition to measuring stroke volume and cardiac output, both Doppler devices provide internal software to (a) calculate other haemodynamic parameters, (b) display data trends and (c) store data for future reference. One particularly useful parameter measured by these Doppler systems is the flow time corrected (FTc), an index of preload or ventricular filling. It measures the duration of systole corrected for heart rate. More advanced models are sold that calculate inotropy and oxygen delivery from the blood pressure and oxygen saturation readings.

4.3. Pulse contour analysis

The arterial pulse contour method in essence is very simple. An arterial catheter is inserted into a peripheral artery, usually the radial or femoral. The catheter is connected to a pressure transducer which is zeroed and checked for under or over damping. The analog arterial pressure signal is fed into a device that calculates cardiac output from the trace. However, there are at least ten different algorithms that can be used to derive cardiac output from arterial pressure. The theoretical basis to these different algorithms is extremely complicated and involves different mathematical models that describe the circulation and adjust for changes in its impedance and compliance of the peripheral circulation. A brief outline of how these algorithms is given.

a. The simplest model that describes the circulation is the pressure = flow x resistance relationship. The area under the arterial pressure curve is directly proportional to cardiac output providing peripheral resistance remains constant. Unfortunately, peripheral resistance does not remain constant. It is constantly changing under the influence of the sympathetic nervous system which helps to maintain blood pressure and the circulation as body position changes or the person exercises.

b. Changes in peripheral resistance are reflected in diastolic pressure, so the simplest adjustment to the model is the use of pulse pressure (i.e. systolic-diastolic) rather than the arterial pressure to calculate cardiac output. This method is used in several pulse contour systems.

c. The dynamics of the circulation is not as simple as pressure = flow x resistance. The circulation is a pulsitile system and when the heart pumps the arterial system has to expand to accommodate the additional blood. Windkessel compared the arterial system to a capacitor and proposed a two element model of the circulation with both resistive and capacitive components.

d. The two element model still did not describe the circulation in its entirety. Wesseling et al added a third inductive element to compensate for time lags as blood flowed through the arterial system [19]. Their three-element model was called "Model Flow" and was first used in the Finapres, a finger blood pressure cuff technology.

e. Although, blood flow in the ascending aorta occurs during systole, as the blood travels more distally a significant proportion of blood flow also occurs in diastole and this component forms part of the peripheral arterial pressure wave. Thus, algorithms that measure cardiac output from a peripheral site such as the radial artery also should compensate for the diastolic component. One method is to identify the dichotic notch in the pulse wave and thus differentiate between the systolic and diastolic components.

f. Finally, just as arterial pressure and blood flow changes over the course of one cardiac cycle, so does the impedance and compliance of the circulation. In most Windkessel based models the impedance and compliance remains static. The Liljestrand-Zander model compensates for this non-linearity. Sun in his thesis on cardiac output estimation using arterial blood pressure waveforms found the Liljestrand-Zander algorithm to be the most robust one he tested [26].

The main pulse contour systems currently available use several of these models. The FloTrac-Vigileo (Edwards Lifesciences) uses an empirical model based of pulse pressure and vascular tone. The PiCCO (Pulsion) uses a Windkessel model measuring area under the pressure curve. The LiDCO uses a similar approach but calculates the power, or root mean square (RMS), under the pressure curve. The PRAM-MostCare (Vytech) calculates the pulsitile area under both the systolic and diastolic curves [26,27].

Pulse contour systems need to be calibrated. The early models used a reading from a second cardiac output measurement system, such as thermodilution. However, this proved inconvenient and not conducive to clinical sales. Thus, later models were designed that self calibrated using patient demographic data. The PiCCO uses transpulmonary thermodilution and the LiDCO-plus lithium dilution. Self calibration is performed by the FloTrac, LiDCO-rapid and PRAM-MostCare methods (Figure 10). Normograms have been developed based on population data and require input of the patient's age, gender, weight and height.

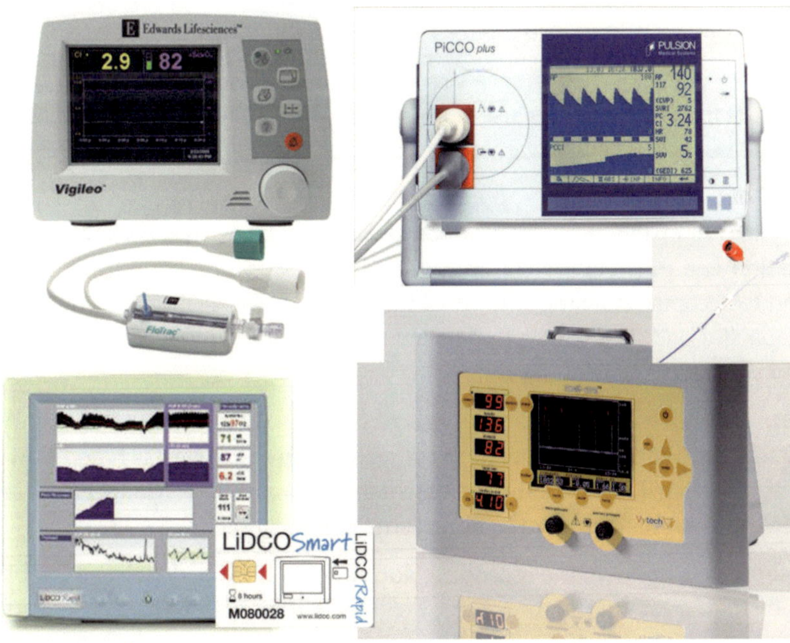

Figure 10. Four main pulse contour monitors being used. FloTrac-Vigileo (top left), PiCCO with femoral artery catheter that provides transpulmonary thermodlitation (top right), LiDCO with user card (bottom left) and PRAM-MostCare (bottom right). LiDCO system also provides lithim dilution cardiac output. (Images downloaded from manufacturers websites)

4.4. Nonivasive pulse contour

Very few pulse contour systems are available that measure arterial blood pressure using a finger cuff. The most well known system is the Nexfin (BMEYE) (Figure 11). It is able to track blood pressure from the digital artery in real time. Cardiac output is calculated from a three element Windkessel model [19].

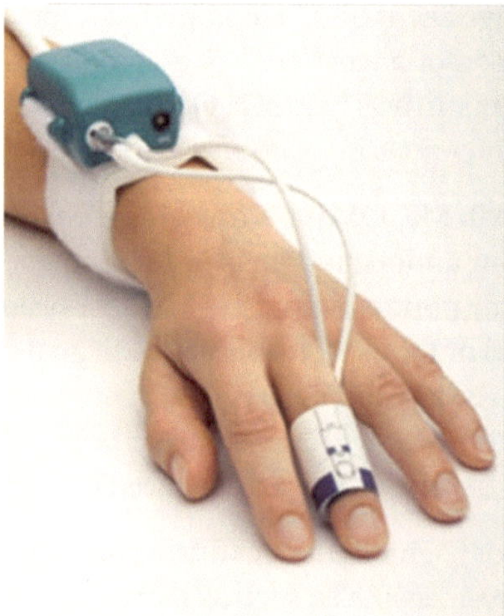

Figure 11. Finger cuff system used by the Nexfin. (Image from BMEYE)

4.5. Partial carbon dioxide rebreathing

In patients connected to a ventilator and breathing circuit it is possible to measure cardiac output using a modified Fick method based on carbon dioxide. A loop of dead-space tubing is intermittently added to the patient circuit which facilities the rebreathing of carbon dioxide (Figure 2). Based on certain assumptions and measuring carbon dioxide levels in the circuit cardiac output is derived. The NICO (Respironics) was the only system to be produced. The system was not very successful because it too sensitive to interruption of the regular breathing patterns.

5. Clinical areas & indications

5.1. Overview

MICOM has a number of desirable features: (i) It can provide continuous patient monitoring, (ii) it is relatively safe to use clinically, and (iii) it can be simple to use. The main modalities currently being used clinically are Doppler, pulse contour and bioreactance. These modalities have different attributes and thus each modality works better in different clinical areas. Bioimpedance devices are no longer in regular clinical use.

5.2. Anaesthesia

In the operating room setting a skilled operator who can interpret haemodynamic data is nearly always in attendance. Therefore, safety and reliability rather than ease of use are the main issues when selecting a MICOM for anaesthesia.

Until recently cardiac output monitoring was seldom used in anaesthesia unless the patient was having ultra-major surgery or had a significant circulatory problem. In the past a pulmonary artery catheter would have been used to monitor heart function. In more recent times the vogue has been to use transoesophageal echocardiography (TOE), though TOE does not measure cardiac output continuously. Thus, MICOM had not until very recently been widely implemented in anaesthesia.

However, anaesthetic interest in MICOM has grown in recent years and this interest has been largely driven by changes in our understanding of intra-operative fluid management [28]. Goal directed therapies have become popular with new MICOM systems being developed to drive protocols. The most successful of these protocols has been goal directed fluid therapy guided by oesophageal Doppler in high risk surgical patients. A number of low powered clinical trials attest to improved patient outcomes with its use have been published [29]. It is now being recommended in Britain and Europe as part of enhanced surgical recovery programs [30,31].

MICOM can be used to monitor haemodynamics during major high risk surgery. It has become popular in specialized areas of anaesthesia such as managing the circulation and intravenous fluids of patients undergoing oesophageal surgery and there are other examples.

I will now describe the pros and cons of the main MICOM modalities with reference to anaesthesia and operating room use.

Successful use of Doppler is very operator dependant as the probe has to be refocused regularly to assure reliability and this can prove very time consuming and distracting for the solo anaesthetist.

Oesophageal Doppler (CardioQ) provides continuous monitoring, but its placement in the oesophageal limits its use to unconscious (anaesthetized) and sedated patients. Furthermore, operations involving the head and neck or upper gastrointestinal trace may prohibit its use because of interference with the surgical field.

External precordial Doppler (USCOM) requires use of a hand held probe that is focused via the thoracic inlet and sternal notch on the aortic valve. The flow signal from the pulmonary artery via the left 3rd to 5th intercostals space can also be use but is less popular in anaesthesia because access to the anterior wall is often restricted, lung ventilation may obscure the probe beam and repositioning of the patient to improve the signal is prohibited. During anaesthesia the probe can be used more effectively to locate the Doppler signal from the aortic valve because discomfort from pressure applied to the thoracic inlet is no longer felt. Readouts are in real-time and the monitor benefits from data trending. Serial changes from up to four flow parameters can be displayed. The type of surgery may restrict use of the probe, such as head and neck operations and the prone position. The quality of the external Doppler signal and thus its reliability are very patient dependant. Age appears to have major effect with reliability

declining over the age of 50-years. A 12-point scoring system that determines the quality of the Doppler flow profile has been described by Cattermole and this score helps to determine whether readings are reliable [32].

Use of pulse contour cardiac output necessitates the placement of an arterial line which limits use to more major hospital centres and high risk surgical cases. It provides continuous monitoring and thus during anaesthesia it can be used to monitor haemodynamics and drive goal directed protocols. Also, once set up it requires very little adjustment unlike Doppler systems. There are least four pulse contour systems on the market. However, the reliability of these systems in anaesthesia and intensive care has been questioned because current algorithms do not compensate for changes in peripheral resistance, particularly when vasopressor drugs are used [33].

We do not know much about the clinical performance of bioreactance devices (NICOM, Cheetah Medical) and whether they are more reliably when compared to bioimpedance. However, bioreactance does have several features that make it theoretically the perfect monitor. It is noninvasive and safe, it provides continuous cardiac output monitoring, it does not require a great deal of skill to set up and it is inexpensive to run. It is being promoted in the anaesthesia field as a cardiac output monitor and to drive goal directed protocols.

5.3. Intensive care

MICOM is used in intensive care to manage critically ill patients with circulatory shock and to optimize ventilator settings such as when positive end expiratory pressure (PEEP) and lung recruitment strategies are used. Monitoring systems that measure cardiac output accurately are needed for bedside diagnosis, whilst reliable trending ability is needed to guide fluid and cardiovascular drug therapies. In addition to cardiac output, oxygen delivery (DO_2) and indices of contractility are also monitored. In more stable patients such as head injuries MICOM can be used for continuous surveillance to pick up sudden alterations in the patient's condition.

The use of Doppler systems is limited because the patient has to be sedated to tolerate an oesophageal probe and external Doppler does not provide continuous patient monitoring. Oesophageal Doppler was originally developed for the intensive care setting [18] and still has a role in haemodynamic optimization, lung ventilation and driving goal directed therapies. Signal quality can be an issue when using external Doppler (USCOM), particularly in elderly patients with low cardiac outputs. As Doppler MICOM requires time and skill to operate and obtain reliable signals, and an intensive care doctor trained in its use may not always be available, some intensive care units have move towards training nursing staff in its use.

The use of pulse contour methods in intensive care is attractive as most critically ill patients have an arterial line in-situ and continuous monitoring of their haemodynamic status is required. Furthermore, once it is set up pulse contour methods require very little adjustment. The main issue has been the reliability of current systems. It is a worrying fact that in response to a potent vasoconstrictor such as phenylephedrine pulse contour cardiac output increases, whereas other cardiac output modalities like thermodilution and Doppler decrease [33]. The

algorithms currently being used to convert pressure to blood flow are still in need of improvement. The most successful pulse contour system in use in the intensive care setting is the PiCCO plus (Pulsion) that integrates transpulmonary thermodilution readings with femoral artery pulse contour readings. The PiCCO system can be upgraded to measure blood volume, liver blood flow and mixed venous saturation. The FloTrac-Vigileo system (Edwards Lifesciences) also been upgraded from just monitoring cardiac output to a more global approach in their new EV1000 clinical platform monitor.

Functional haemodynamic monitoring has also become popular using arterial trace based parameters such as stroke volume (SVV) and pulse pressure (PPV) variation to guide therapy [34].

5.4. High dependency units

When MICOM is used in high dependency areas for patient monitoring continuous noninvasive systems are required. Pulse contour systems can be used providing the patient has an arterial line. The noninvasive nature of bioreactance (NICOM) makes it a potentially useful monitor in this setting.

5.5. Accident and emergency

MICOM has two potential roles in accident and emergency (i) to facilitate resuscitate and (ii) rapid bedside haemodynamic assessment of patients. Thus, systems that can be rapidly set up and used at the bedside are ideal.

For resuscitation both Doppler and pulse contour methods can be used, though for pulse contour monitoring an arterial line would need to be set up. Furthermore, a self calibrating system would be necessary. The development of noninvasive external, supra-sternal and precordial, Doppler (USCOM) has resulted in some novel application in the emergency medicine setting. Assessment of cardiac output in elderly patients admitted with general malaise can help identify early septic shock and may potentially reduce the number that need intensive care admission. Bedside cardiac output measurement in patients with hypertension helps one to differentiate between high peripheral resistance and high cardiac output as a cause and helps in determining the most appropriate drug therapy.

5.6. Medicine and cardiology

NICOM in medicine contribute to the haemodynamic assessment of patients by providing cardiac output and related measurements. They form part of multiple modality haemodynamic investigation systems, such as the Task Force Monitor (CNSystems), where they are used to assess autonomic dysfunction in diabetes and postural reflexes in patients with syncopy by head up tilting and similar tests. In cardiology they have been used to optimize pacemaker settings. MICOM devices that are noninvasive such as bioimpedance and finger plethysmography tend to be used.

5.7. Paediatrics

Most MICOM modalities have been adapted for use children. Noninvasive modalities like external Doppler (USCOM) has become increasingly popular in children because there is no need to insert lines. It works extremely well in small children and neonates as signal acquisition is good [35]. There is a growing interest in developing its use in paediatric intensive care for clinical situations such as rapid identification and treatment of shock [36].

5.8. Cost and availability

When using MICOM running costs need consideration. In addition to the monitor most systems require disposable items to operate. Oesophageal Doppler requires disposable oesophageal probes which are made for single use (Figure 8). The FloTrac-Vigileo uses a disposable pressure transducer (Figure 10). The PiCCO uses a femoral artery catheter that also acts as a thermodilution catheter. The LiDCO and PRAM systems work on a credit card system to buy user time (Figure 10). The NICOM uses purpose made skin electrodes (Figure 4). The NICO had a disposable breathing attachment to facilitate carbon dioxide rebreathing (Figure 2). Most of these disposables are priced around the same cost as thermodilution catheter. The only system that does not to require disposable items other than ultrasound gel is the USCOM. The ultrasound probe is cleaned between patient uses. Financing ones supply of these disposable items can be a problem when first introducing what is a relatively new and unproven technology into ones clinical practice and may limit use. Manufacturers will calm that it is a necessary evil to sustain the company financially and replay their investment in research and development.

6. Overview of clinical validation

6.1. Main objectives

The aim of clinical validation is to determine whether a new monitor measures cardiac output reliably, which is done by comparing its performance with that of an accepted clinical standard such as single bolus thermodilution cardiac output. If the new monitor performs as well or better than the reference method, it can be accepted into clinical practice.

However, there are two important aspects to reliable cardiac output measurement:

i. The accuracy of individual readings, and

ii. The ability to detect changes, or trends, between readings.

The type of clinical data and statistic analysis needed to evaluate these two aspects are different.

If ones objective is to diagnose a low or high cardiac output, then the accuracy of individual readings in relation to the true value is of greatest importance. However, if ones objective is to follow the change in haemodynamic response to a therapeutic intervention, then serial cardiac output readings are needed and their absolute accuracy becomes less important,

providing the readings reliably show the changes. This division into two roles may at first seem a little pedantic, but a monitor that does not measure cardiac output accurately may still be useful clinically if it detects trends reliably. As most bedside cardiac output monitors used today are now able to measure cardiac output continuously, although many are not particularly accurate, the issue of being a reliable trend monitor becomes very relevant. Unfortunately, the majority of published validation studies have only addressed accuracy [37].

6.2. Understanding errors

The error that arises when measuring cardiac output has two basic components:

i. Random error that arises from act of measuring and

ii. Systematic error that arises from the measurement system.

If I use a measuring tape to measure the heights of patients attending a clinic, my readings may vary by few millimeters from the true height of each patient. This is random error. But if the measuring tape is stretched by 2 to 3 centimeters, then every reading I take will consistently under read the height of each patient by a few centimeters. This is a systematic error. The division of measurement error into random and systematic components plays an important role in the choice of statistical techniques used for validation.

One of main sources of systematic error is imprecise calibration. Calibration is performed by (a) measuring cardiac output using a second method such as thermodilution, or (b) using population data to derive cardiac output from the patient's demographics, (i.e. age, height and weight)). Unfortunately, cardiac output, and related parameters vary between individuals. In the Nidorf nomogram used to predict aortic valve size when using suprasternal Doppler cardiac output the range of possible values about the mean for valve size at each height is ±16% [23]. This gives rise to a significant systematic error between patients and this error impacts upon accuracy when Bland-Altman comparisons are made against a reference method [38]. However, reliability during trending may still be preserved because trending involves a series of readings from one single patient. Providing the systematic error remains constant, and the random measurement errors between the series of readings are acceptably low, the monitor can still detect changes in cardiac output reliably.

The accepted method of presenting errors in validation statistics is to use (a) percentages of mean cardiac output and (b) 95% confidence intervals, which approximates to two standard deviations. The term precision error is used, and should not be confused with the percentage error which is one of the outcomes of Bland-Altman analysis.

7. Addressing statistical issues

7.1. Simple comparisons against a reference method

Validation in the clinical setting is usually performed by comparing readings from the method being tested against a reference method. Traditionally single bolus thermodilution cardiac

output performed using a PAC has been used. The average of three thermodilution readings is used, and aberrant readings that differ by more than 10% are rejected, in order to improve the precision. However, thermodilution is not a gold standard method and significant measurement errors, both random and systematic, arise when it is used. It is generally accepted that thermodilution has a precision error of ±20%. True gold standard methods such as aortic flow probes have precisions errors of less than ±5%. Thus, thermodilution is an imprecise reference method and its use greatly influences the statistical analysis. Most of the benchmarks against which the outcomes of validation studies are judged are based on this precision of ±20%.

Other more precise and gold standard reference methods could be used, such as the Fick method or a flow probe surgically placed on the aorta. However, in the clinical setting their use is inappropriate and thus the current clinical standard for cardiac output measurement thermodilution via a PAC is used. The current decline in the clinical use of PACs has left a void. Thus, some recently published validation studies have used transpulmonary thermodilution using the PiCCO system or oesophageal Doppler monitoring using the CardioQ as alternative reference methods.

7.2. The precision error of thermodilution

Recently, the precision of ±20% for thermodilution has come under scrutiny. The reason that thermodilution is said to have a precision error of ±20% can be attributed to our 1999 publication on bias and precision statistics which first proposed percentage error [39]. In the 1990's consensus of opinion was that for a monitor to be accepted into clinical use it should be able to detect at least a change in cardiac output of 1 L/min when the mean cardiac output was 5 L/min, which was a 20% change [40,41]. Furthermore, Stetz and colleagues meta-analysis of studies from the 1970's validating the thermodilution method suggested that it had a precision of 13-22% [42]. The 30% benchmark percentage error that everyone today quotes was based on a precision error of ±20% for thermodilution. However, it is now seems that the precision of thermodilution can be very variable and depends on type of patient and measurement system used [43]. Recently Peyton and Chong have suggested that the precision of thermodilution may be as large as ±30% [44].

7.3. Study design

Study design becomes significant when ability to detection trends, in addition to accuracy, is investigated. To determine accuracy one needs only a single pair of cardiac output readings, test and reference, from each patient. Test refers to the new method being validated and reference to the clinical standard thermodilution, though ideally a gold standard method should be used. Readings, test and reference, should ideally be performed simultaneously, because cardiac output is not a static parameter and fluctuates between cardiac cycles. The size of the study usually includes twenty or more pairs of readings.

Study design becomes more complicated if the ability to detect trends is being investigated. A series of paired readings from the same patient are now needed that show changes in cardiac

output. A wide range of values of cardiac output readings is also needed. A new parameter called delta cardiac output (ΔCO) is calculated for both test and reference data which uses the difference between consecutive readings. Trend analysis is performed on the ΔCOs. The data can be collected (a) at random or (b) at predetermined time points. Readings collected at random can lead to uneven data distribution. Thus, a more rigid protocol with data being collected at predetermined time points tends to be used. Commonly 6 to 10 time points are used. A typical protocol for a patient having cardiac surgery might be: (T1) - before anaesthesia, (T2) – after induction, (T3) - after sternotomy, (T4) – after by-pass, (T5) – after closure of the chest and (T6-8) - at set times on the intensive care.

8. Graphical presentation and analysis

8.1. Scatter plots

Validation data first should be plotted on a graph that shows the relationship between the test and reference cardiac output readings. The simplest approach is to plot the data on a scatter plot where the x-axis represents the reference readings and the y-axis represents the test readings (Figure 12). The data points should lie within close proximity to the line of identity x=y for there to be good agreement. A regression line can be added. However, correlation is not performed if the aim of the analysis is to assess the agreement between two methods rather than assessing trending ability. This point was highlighted by Bland and Altman when they published their well known method of showing agreement [45].

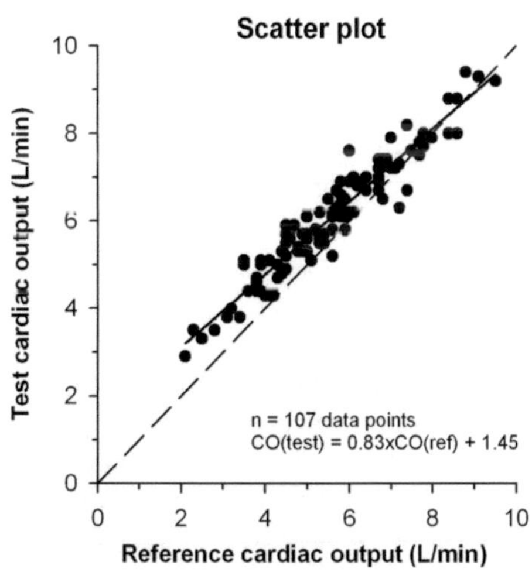

Figure 12. Scatter plot showing test and reference cardiac output (CO) data points. The regression line (solid) crosses y-axis at 1.45 L/min, indicating an offset in calibration between the two methods. A line of identity (dashed) y=x is added. There is good agreement between the test and reference methods because data points lie close to the regression line. The correlation coefficient (r) is not provided.

8.2. The Bland-Altman plot

The agreement between two measurement techniques, test and reference, is evaluated by calculating the bias, which is the difference between the each pair of readings, test minus reference. In the Bland-Altman plot the bias of each pair of readings (y-axis) is plotted against the average of the two readings (x-axis) (Figure 13). Then, three horizontal lines are added to the plot: (a) The mean bias for all the data points and (b) The two 95% confidence interval lines for the bias (1.96 x standard deviation of the bias) known as the "Limits of Agreement". Sufficient data should also be provided to allow the calculation of percentage error.

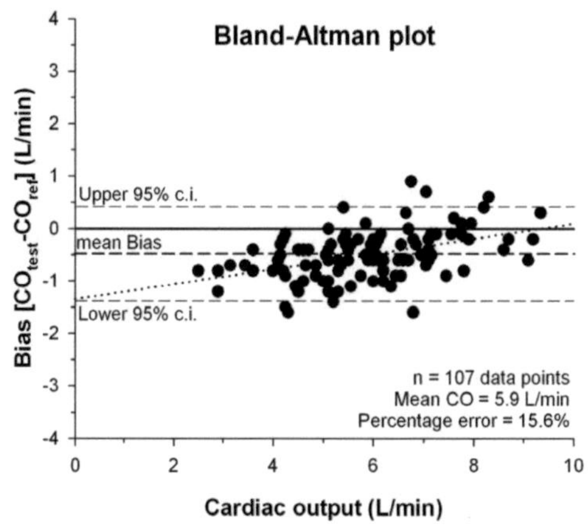

Figure 13. Bland and Altman plot showing test and reference cardiac output (CO) data points. The mean bias and limits of agreement lines (dashed) have been added to plot. 95% of the data points falls between these limits. The percentage error has been calculated from the mean CO and limits of agreement. Note the slightly skewed distribution of the data shown by the sloping regression line (dotted).

8.3. Modifications to the B-A plot

i. Some investigators argue that the best estimate of cardiac output (x-axis), or the reference value, should be used instead of the average.

ii. When the study protocol collects more than one set of data from each patient the limits of agreement should be adjusted for repeated measures. The effect of having multiple readings from the same subject is to reduce the influence of systematic errors, thus decreasing the standard deviation of the bias and narrowing the limits of agreement. As a consequence the limits become falsely small. Two recent articles describe how to perform a correction for repeated measures [46,47]. The models used in the two corrective methods are slightly different.

iii. The Bland-Altman plot assumes that both the test and reference methods have the same calibrated scales for measuring cardiac output. Otherwise, the distribution of data will be sloping and the limits of agreement falsely wide. Bland and Altman described a logarithmic transformation to deal with this scenario [45].

8.4. Which parameters should be present?

In the past many authors have not known how to present their cardiac output data from validations studies in a meaningful and useful manner. When presenting data on a scatter plot one should include the number of data points in the plot. Attention also needs to be given the scale used on the axes so that false impressions of the spread of the data are avoided. Ideally the axes should be of equal scale and range from zero to the maximum value of cardiac output. If a regression line is added, the equation of line should be shown. Correlation analysis is not required unless serial data that shows trending is being used.

Similar issues apply to the Bland-Altman plot. In particular, the range of cardiac output on the x-axis and the range of values for bias need to be appropriate. If several plots comparing data from several devices or patient groups are shown the scales on each plot should be equivalent.

The important data measured using the Bland-Altman analysis are:

i. The mean bias,

ii. The standard deviation of the bias which is presented as the 95% confidence intervals or Limits of Agreement,

iii. The mean cardiac output and

iv. A calculated parameter called the percentage error.

The study size and percentage error at least should be presented with the Bland-Altman plot.

8.5. Percentage error and the 30%

The percentage error is calculated using the formula "1.96 x standard deviation of the bias / mean cardiac output" and is expressed as a percentage. It represents a normalized version of the limits of agreement. The percentage error enables one to compare data from different studies when the ranges of cardiac outputs are different. Even today many authors still fail to present percentage error.

Following a meta-analysis of data from cardiac output studies published pre-1997 that used Bland-Altman analysis we proposed that when the percentage error was less than 28.4%, it was reasonable to accept the new test method. However, the reference method had to be thermodilution with an estimated precision was ±20% [39]. Our work lead to the 30% benchmark for percentage error quoted in many publications over the last a decade. An error-gram was published in our 1999 paper to allow for adjustment to this threshold when reference methods of different precision errors were used.

8.6. Showing reliable trending ability

To assess the trending ability of a new monitor against a reference method one uses serial cardiac output readings. The simplest way to show trending is to plotting the test and reference methods together against time (Figure 14). However, time plots only show data from a single subject, but to confirm reliable trending data from several subjects needs to

be shown. Also, time plots provide only graphical evidence and an objective measure of trending is also needed.

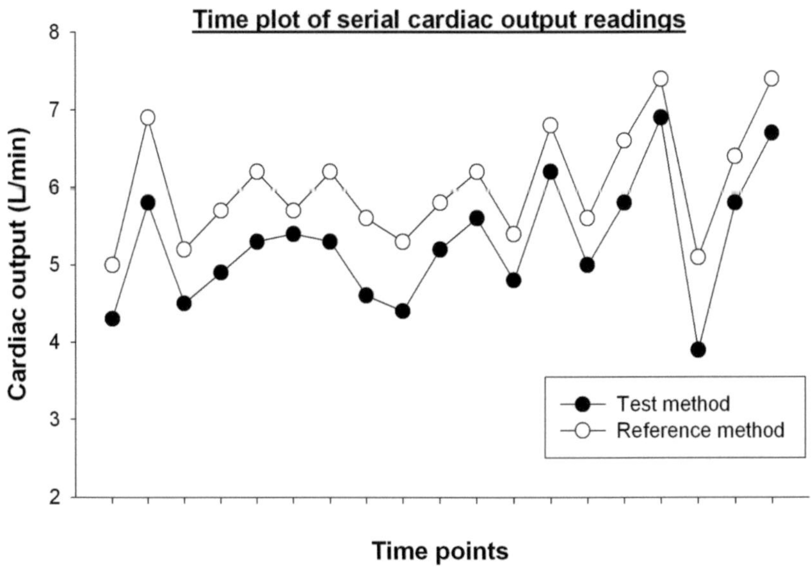

Figure 14. Time plot showing the relationship between test and reference cardiac output readings over time. Data pairs come from a single patient collected at intervals during surgery. The test method follows changes in reference cardiac output despite the test method under-reading by approximately 0.75 L/min. Thus, reliable trending ability is demonstrated in the patient.

8.7. The four-quadrant plot

The variable commonly used to assess trending in statistical analysis is delta cardiac output (ΔCO), the difference between successive readings, or the change in cardiac output (CO_b-CO_a).

Bland-Altman analysis does not show trending, so other analytical methods are used. There is limited consensus on which analytical method should be used [37]. In clinical trials concordance using a four-quadrant plot has become the standard method.

The four quadrant plot is simply a scatter plot showing delta cardiac output (ΔCO) for the test method against the reference method. Because the changes in cardiac output are used, the x and y axes pass through zero (0,0) at the centre of the plot. The delta data points should lie along the line of identity (y=x) if good trending is present (Figure 15). The earliest reference to this method appeared in the mid 1990's [48,49].

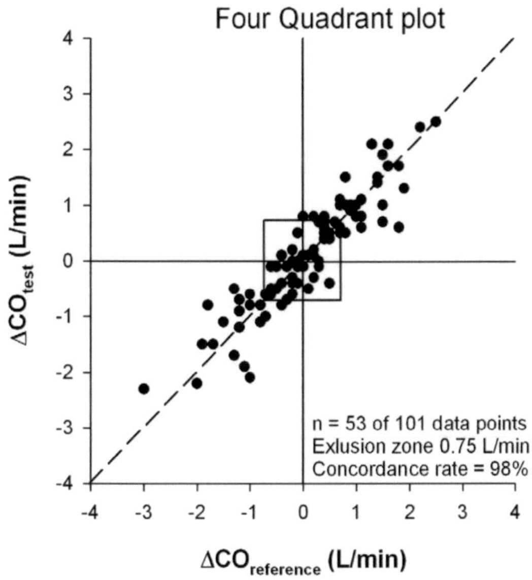

Figure 15. Four quadrant scatter plot comparing changes in test and reference cardiac output (ΔCO) readings. The plot is divided into four quadrants about the x and y axis that cross at the centre (0,0). Data points lie along the line (dashed) of identity y = x. A square exclusion zone is drawn at the centre to remove statistical noise. Concordance analysis is performed by counting the number of data points remaining after central zone exclusion that lie within the two quadrants of agreement (upper right and lower left). In the plot 98% of the data concords, thus trending ability is very good. Supra-sternal and oesophageal Doppler were being compared.

The concordance is measured as the proportion of data points in which either both methods change in a positive direction (i.e. increase and lie within the right upper quadrant) or change in a negative direction (i.e. decrease and lie within the left lower quadrant). Data points that do not concord (i.e. change in different direction) lie within the upper left or lower right quadrants. The concordance rate is the percentage of data points that are in concordance or agree regarding the direction of change of cardiac output.

8.8. The central exclusion zone

One of the main problems encountered when using the four quadrant plot is that data points close to its centre, which represent relatively small cardiac output changes, often do not concord because random error effects are of similar magnitude to the cardiac output changes. This phenomenon results in statistical noise that adversely affects the concordance rate. Perrino and colleagues introduced a central exclusion zone to reduce the level of these random error effects [49].

Receiver operator characteristic (ROC) curve analysis of Perrino and colleagues data was performed to predict the most desirable exclusion zone [48]. For a mean cardiac output of 5.0 L/min these author recommended an exclusion zone of 0.75 L/min or 15%. In the above example it can seen that after central zone exclusion of data, most of the remaining data lie

with the upper right (i.e. positive changes) and lower left (i.e. negative changes) quadrants of concordance. The concordance rate is 98% as one data point lie outside these quadrants.

When performing concordance analysis one needs to know what is an acceptable rate? In a recent publication on trend analysis, we analyzed data from nine studies that used concordance analysis. From this data we concluded that for good trending ability to be shown against thermodilution as a reference method the concordance rate should be 92% or above [37].

8.9. Polar plots

Concordance analysis and the four quadrant plot have limitations. The changes in cardiac output between the test and reference methods can be very different yet concord if both have the same direction of change and the magnitude of the change in cardiac output plays no part in the analysis other than determining what data is excluded. To address these issues we developed a method of concordance analysis based on converting the data to polar coordinates. The polar angle represented agreement whilst the radius represented the magnitude of change in cardiac output [50]. The polar data is generated from the ΔCO(test) and ΔCO(reference). Descriptions on how to draw polar plots are found in our paper.

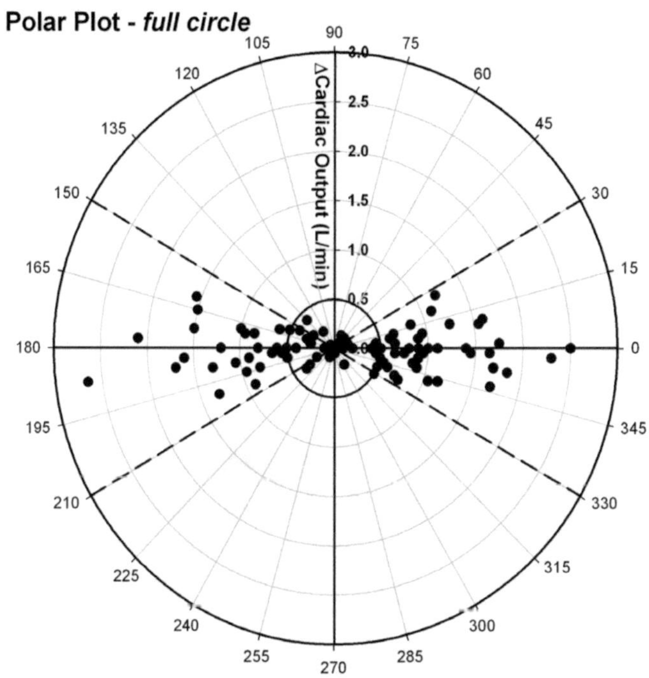

Figure 16. The polar plot displays ΔCO data. The axis of the plot lies at 0-degree (and 180-degrees). It is equivalent to the line of identity y=x on the scatter plot (figure 12), except that the plot has been rotated clockwise by 45-degrees. Concordance limits are draw at ±30-degrees. A circular exclusion zone of 0.5 L/min is draw at the centre. Data points that lies within

these limits concord. Positive changes in cardiac output (ΔCO) (right half) and negative ΔCO (left half) are presented on opposite halves of the plot. The mean polar angle and radial limits of agreement for data have been omitted.

Our earliest description of polar plots used a full 360-degree circle to show both positive and negative directional changes (Figure 16). The data points are seen to lie within narrow ±30-degree sectors about the polar axes signifying good trending ability. When 30-degree limits are used the allowable differences in size of ΔCO are limited to a ratio of 1 to 2, rather than just direction of change.

The half moon plot was later developed to show positive and negative ΔCO changes together (Figure 17).

The plot provides several parameters that describe trending:

i. The mean polar angle which shows the deviation in agreement from the polar axis zero-degrees. It is a measure of difference in scale between the test and reference methods.

ii. The radial limits of agreement which are 95% confidence intervals of the polar angles. If the angles lie within the 30-degree boundaries the original x-y ΔCO values will differ by less that 1 to 2 (i.e. half to double) in 95% of paired readings.

iii. The polar concordance rate which for comparisons against thermodilution are set at 30-degrees, but there is currently limited data to support these limits.

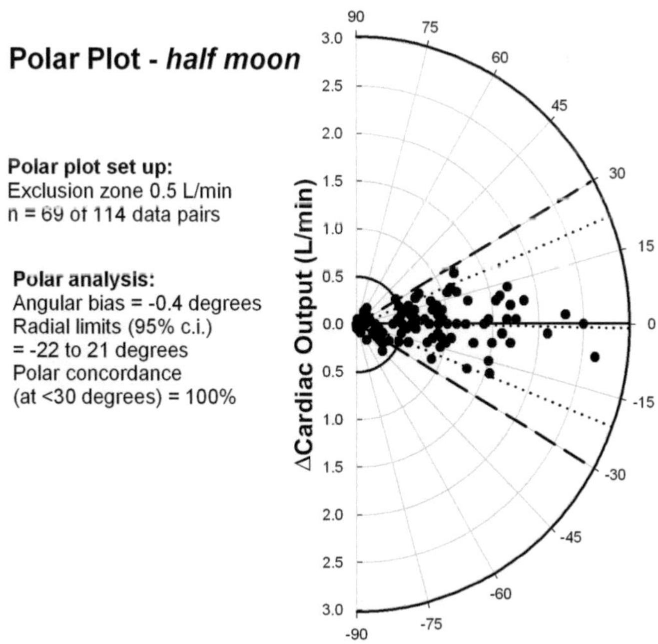

Figure 17. Half-moon polar plot showing the same data as the full-circle plot, but all within the same semi-circle. The mean polar angle and radial limits of agreement are now shown. A central exclusion zone circle removes data points where the changes in cardiac output are small. Trending of cardiac output is good because most of the data points lie within the 30-degrees of the polar axis (0-degrees). Concordance is performed by counting the percentage of data points that lie within this zone. Outcomes of the polar analysis are provided with the plots. (Graphs drawn using Sigma Plot version 7.0).

The exclusion zone is used for similar reasons as in the four quadrant plot. However, as the radial distance is mean cardiac output rather that the hypotenuse of a triangle bounded by two cardiac output readings reference and test, its 'size needs to be smaller by a ratio of 1 to 1.4. Thus, rather than using 0.75 L/min or 15% as in the four quadrant plot, we used 0.5 L/min.

8.10. Making sense of the outcomes

If evidence based approaches are to be adopted when using MICOM devices in ones clinical practice then data from clinical validation studies will need to be critically reviewed. Marketing information from most manufactures of MICOM devices provide lists of publications that they claim support their product. In reviewing such data one needs to ask the following questions:

i. Is the study design and data appropriate?

ii. Have the correct statistics been used?

iii. Have the correct criteria been applied to results?

iv. And are the conclusions correct?

Study design is critical. (a) A sufficient number of patients should have been studied, though calculating the power of validation studies is not easy. Comparison of study size with other similar validation studies may help. (b) Type of patients and clinical setting effects results. Situations where a wide range of cardiac outputs and conditions (i.e. peripheral resistance) are encountered provide a rigorous test of performance. (c) Some of the early and more favourable validation studies using pulse contour devices were performed in cardiac surgery patients in whom haemodynamics were kept relatively stable. It was only when the same devices were tested in more labile liver transplant patients with cirrhosis that the problem with these devices and peripheral resistance became apparent [51].

The different statistical methods used in validation have been systematically covered previously. (a) If a simple test versus reference method comparison has been performed then only Bland-Altman analysis is needed, but make sure the outcomes of the analysis are properly presented, including the percentage error. (b) If a sophisticated study design that allows trending to be assessed has been used, then concordance analysis using the four quadrant plot, and possibly a polar analysis should have been used to show trending. Check that central exclusions zones have been applied to the ΔCO data. (c) Animal studies are slightly different because of extent and quality of data that can be collected, and it is reasonable to use regression analysis.

When interpreting the results of Bland-Altman analysis: (a) Make sure the precision error of the reference method is correct. Normally for thermodilution it is ±20%, but other modalities

may have different precisions and criteria may need correcting, like the 30% for percentage error. (b) Make sure all the outcomes of the Bland-Altman analysis have been presented. The key to interpreting Bland-Altman is the percentage error which needs the mean cardiac output and limits of agreement to be calculated. (c) Make sure that the limits of agreement have been correct for repeated measures [46,47].

When interpreting the results of concordance analysis: (a) Make sure central exclusion zones have been used. These should be shown on the four quadrant plot. (b) Make sure the exclusion criteria used in the plot are appropriate, usually set at 15% or 0.75 L/min when mean cardiac output is 5 L/min. (c) Make sure the precision error of the reference method is known as this will affect the threshold criteria for good trending. (d) When thermodilution is the reference method a concordance rate of above 90-95% signifies good trending ability of the test method.

Polar plots are relatively new to trend analysis so their usefulness and threshold criteria for good trending still need to be set. However, they are an excellent method of showing trend data from multiple patients and for good trending data should lie within the 30-degree radial limits [50].

When reading authors conclusions regarding their validation study data, be skeptical about what is written, as the statistical analyses is often incomplete and authors tend to exaggerate their findings. In general the percentage error should be less than 30% for good agreement and the concordance rate above 90-95% for good trending ability.

9. Laboratory data

9.1. Advantages of animal models

Testing in animal models has two big advantages:

i. More invasive and precise gold standard methods of monitoring cardiac output can be used, such as flow probes surgically place on the ascending aorta. Thus, the limitations of comparing against thermodilution can be avoided. The original flow probes were electromagnetic, but today ultrasonic transit time flow probes are used.

ii. The ranges of circulatory conditions and cardiac outputs that can be studied are much greater than in humans for ethical reasons.

9.2. Showing accuracy and trending

Bland-Altman and concordance analysis can still be used to assess accuracy and trending. However, the ability to perform multiple readings over a range of cardiac output and conditions against a gold standard method allow the test method to be fully assessed. Regression analysis and correlation now are the appropriate methods for analyzing the data. Regression plots from each animal experiment are used to show how the test method behaves over a range of cardiac output. The regression line defines the relationship between test and flow probe methods. Correlation reflects the repeatability and trending ability of the test method, rather

than the agreement between methods. Either r or R^2 are quoted. R^2 is used when a relationship exists between the two methods. The correlation coefficient (R^2) ranges from 0 to 1, where a value > 0.9 signifies good correlation. Ideally, if the test and reference (i.e. flow probe) methods are correctly calibrated, their data should lie along the line of identity y=x and correlation can also be performed along this line, which is known as Lin's concordance. Alternatively, the interclass correlation coefficient (ICC) is used. These methods were used in our 2005 paper to validate the supra-sternal Doppler method in anaesthetized dogs [52].

9.3. Current status of technology in 2012

Bioimpedance is no longer used clinically. Bioreactance (NICOM, Cheetah Medical) has only recently been released and still needs further clinical evaluation. It is being promoted in a wide range of clinical areas.

Pulse contour methods have not proved universally successful because of issues with the current algorithms failing to cope with swings in peripheral resistance. The PiCCO has a role in intensive care for continuous cardiac output monitoring in combination with transpulmonary thermodilution. The other modalities seem more useful when used to measure "functional haemodynamic variables" such as stroke volume variation in response to the straight leg raise test and fluid challenge. They are now being promoted to drive fluid optimization protocols.

Oesophageal Doppler (CardioQ, Deltex Medical) appears to be a useful intra-operative and intensive care monitor of haemodynamic status. It has been used successfully to drive goal directed fluid therapy protocols in high risk surgical patients. It has recently become popular in Britain as part of enhanced surgical recovery programs. External Doppler (USCOM) is less commonly used but appears useful in a number of clinical settings including paediatrics.

Other MICOM technology does exist but none currently have a major role to play in developing patient monitoring.

Nomenclature

MICOM – Minimally invasive cardiac output monitoring

TOE – Transoesophageal Echocardiography

PAC – Pulmonary Artery Catheter

CSA – Cross sectional area

LVET – Left ventricular ejection time

PEP – Pre ejection period

VEPT – Volume of electrically participating tissue

ECG – Electrocardiogram

ΔCO – delta cardiac output

Author details

Lester Augustus Hall Critchley

Address all correspondence to: hcritchley@cuhk.edu.hk

Department of Anaesthesia and Intensive Care, The Chinese University of Hong Kong, Prince of Wales Hospital, Shatin, New Territories, Hong Kong, S.A.R.

References

[1] Booth J. A short history of blood pressure measurement. Proceedings of the Royal Society of Medicine 1977;70(11) 793-799.

[2] Stewart GN. Researches on the circulation time and on the influences which affect it: IV. The output of the heart. Journal of Physiosiology 1897;22 159–181.

[3] Hamilton WF, Moore JW, Kinsman JM, Spurling RG. Simultaneous determination of pulmonary and systemic circulation times in man and of a figure related to the cardiac output. American Journal of Physiology 1928;84 338-344.

[4] Linton R, Band D, O'Brien T, Jonas MM & Leach R. (1997) Lithium dilution cardiac output measurement: A comparison with thermodilution. Critical Care Medicine 1997;25(11) 1796-1800.

[5] Ganz W, Donoso R, Marcus HS, Forrester JS and Swan HJ. A new technique for measurement of cardiac output by thermodilution in man. American Journal of Cardiology 1971;27 392–396.

[6] Swan HJ, Ganz W, Forrester J, Marcus H, Diamond G and Chonette D. Catheterization of the heart in man with use of a flow-directed balloon-tipped catheter. New England Journal of Medicine 1970;283(9) 447–451.

[7] Robin ED. Death by pulmonary artery flow directed catheter: Time for a moratorium? Chest 1987;92(4) 727–731.

[8] Connors AF, Speroff T, Dawson NV, Thomas C, Harrell FE Jr, Wagner D, Desbiens N, Goldman L, Wu AW, Califf RM, Fulkerson WJ, Vidaillet H, Broste S, Bellamy P, Lynn J, Knaus WA. The effectiveness of right heart catheterization in the initial care of critically ill patients. Journal of the American Medical Association 1996;276(11) 889–897.

[9] Harvey S, Harrison DA, Singer M, Ashcroft J, Jones CM, Elbourne D, Brampton W, Williams D, Young D, Rowan K. PAC-Man study collaboration. Assessment of the

clinical effectiveness of pulmonary artery catheters in management of patients in intensive care (PAC-Man): A randomized controlled trial. Lancet 2005;366(9484) 472–477.

[10] Koo KK, Sun JC, Zhou Q, Guyatt G, Cook DJ, Walter SD, Meade MO. Pulmonary artery catheters: evolving rates and reasons for use. Critical Care Medicine 2011;39(7) 1613-1618.

[11] Kubicek WG, Kottke J, Ramos MU, Patterson RP, Witsoe DA, Labree JW, Remole W, Layman TE, Schoening H, Garamela JT. The Minnesota impedance cardiograph-theory and applications. Biomedical Engineering. 1974;9(9) 410-416.

[12] Bernstein DP. A new stroke volume equation for thoracic electrical bioimpedance: theory and rationale. Critical Care Medicine 1986;14(10) 904-909.

[13] Clarke DE, Raffin TA. Thoracic electrical bioimpedance measurement of cardiac output: not ready for prime time. Critical Care Medicine 1993;21(8) 1111–1112.

[14] Peng ZY, Critchley LA, Fok BS. An investigation to show the effect of lung fluid on impedance cardiac output in the anaesthetized dog. British Journal of Anaesthesia 2005;95(4) 458-464.

[15] Critchley LA, Calcroft RM, Tan PY, Kew J, Critchley JA. The effect of lung injury and excessive lung fluid, on impedance cardiac output measurements, in the critically ill. Intensive Care Medicine 2000;26(6) 679-685.

[16] Kubicek WG. On the source of peak first time derivative (dZ/dt) during impedance cardiography. Annals of Biomedical Engineering 1989;17(5) 459-462.

[17] Critchley LA. Impedance cardiography: Impact of new technology. Anaesthesia 1998;53(7) 677-685.

[18] Singer M. Oesophageal Doppler. Current Opinion in Critical Care 2009;15(3) 244-248.

[19] Wesseling KH, Jansen JR, Settels JJ, Schreuder JJ. Computation of aortic flow from pressure in humans using a nonlinear, three-element model. Journal of Applied Physiology 1993;74(5) 2566-2573.

[20] Cecconi M, Rhodes A. Pulse pressure analysis: to make a long story short. Critical Care 2010;14(4) 175.

[21] Ishihara H, Sugo Y, Tsutsui M, Yamada T, Sato T, Akazawa T, Sato N, Yamashita K, Takeda J. The ability of a new continuous cardiac output monitor to measure trends in cardiac output following implementation of a patient information calibration and an automated exclusion algorithm. Journal of Clinical Monitoring and Computing (E Pub Aug 2012:26(6) 465-471)

[22] Aldrete JA, Brown C, Daily J, Buerke V. Pacemaker malfunction due to microcurrent injection from a bioimpedance noninvasive cardiac output monitor. Journal of Clinical Monitoring 1995;11(2) 131-133.

[23] Nidorf SM, Picard MH, Triulzi MO, Thomas JD, Newell J, King ME, Weyman AE. New perspectives in the assessment of cardiac chamber dimensions during development and adulthood. Journal of the American College of Cardiology 1992;19(5) 983-988.

[24] Lefrant JY, Bruelle P, Aya AG, Saïssi G, Dauzat M, de La Coussaye JE, Eledjam JJ. Training is required to improve the reliability of esophageal Doppler to measure cardiac output in critically ill patients. Intensive Care Medicine 1998;24(4) 347-352.

[25] Dey I, Sprivulis P. Emergency physicians can reliably assess emergency department patient cardiac output using the USCOM continuous wave Doppler cardiac output monitor. Emergency Medicine Australasia. 2005;17(3) 193-199.

[26] Sun JX, Reisner AT, Saeed M, Heldt T, Mark RG. The cardiac output from blood pressure algorithms trial. Critical Care Medicine 2009;37(1): 72-80.

[27] Thiele RH, Durieux ME. Arterial waveform analysis for the anesthesiologist: past, present, and future concepts. Anesthesia and Analgesia 2011;113(4) 766-776.

[28] Chappell D, Jacob M, Hofmann-Kiefer K, Conzen P, Rehm M. A rational approach to perioperative fluid management. Anesthesiology 2008;109(4) 723-740.

[29] Hamilton MA, Cecconi M, Rhodes A. A systematic review and meta-analysis on the use of preemptive hemodynamic intervention to improve postoperative outcomes in moderate and high-risk surgical patients. Anesthesia and Analgesia 2011;112(6) 1392-1402.

[30] Kehlet H, Mythen M. Why is the surgical high-risk patient still at risk? British Journal of Anaesthesia 2011;106(3) 289–291.

[31] Mythen MG, Swart M, Acheson N, Crawford R, Jones K, Kuper M, McGrath JS, Horgan A. Perioperative fluid management: Consensus statement from the enhanced recovery partnership. Perioperative Medicine 2012;1(1) 2.

[32] Cattermole GN, Leung PYM, Tang CO, Smith BE, Graham CA, Rainer TH. A new method to score the quality of USCOM scans (Abstract 14). Hong Kong Journal of Emergency Medicine 2009;16(4) 288.

[33] Meng L, Tran NP, Alexander BS, Laning K, Chen G, Kain ZN, Cannesson M. The impact of phenylephrine, ephedrine, and increased preload on third-generation Vigileo-FloTrac and esophageal Doppler cardiac output measurements. Anesthesia and Analgesia 2011;113(4) 751-757.

[34] Marik PE, Cavallazzi R, Vasu T, Hirani A. Dynamic changes in arterial waveform derived variables and fluid responsiveness in mechanically ventilated patients: a systematic review of the literature. Critical Care Medicine 2009;37(9) 2642–2647.

[35] He SR, Zhang C, Liu YM, Sun YX, Zhuang J, Chen JM, Madigan VM, Smith BE, Sun X. Accuracy of the ultrasonic cardiac output monitor in healthy term neonates during postnatal circulatory adaptation. China Medical Journal 2011;124(15) 2284-2289.

[36] Brierley J, Peters MJ. Distinct hemodynamic patterns of septic shock at presentation to pediatric intensive care. Pediatrics 2008;122(4) 752-759.

[37] Critchley LA, Lee A, Ho AM. A critical review of the ability of continuous cardiac output monitors to measure trends in cardiac output. Anesth. Analg. 2010;111(5) 1180-1192.

[38] Chong SW, Peyton PJ. A meta-analysis of the accuracy and precision of the ultrasonic cardiac output monitor (USCOM). Anaesthesia 2012;67(11) 1266-1271.

[39] Critchley LA, Critchley JA: A meta-analysis of studies using bias and precision statistics to compare cardiac output measurement techniques. Journal of Clinical Monitoring and Computing 1999;15(2) 85–91.

[40] LaMantia KR, O'Connor T, Barash PG: Comparing methods of measurement: An alternative approach. Anesthesiology 1990;72(5) 781–783.

[41] Wong DH, Tremper KK, Stemmer EA, O'Connor D, Wilbur S, Zaccari J, Reeves C, Weidoff P, Trujillo RJ: Noninvasive cardiac output: Simultaneous comparison of two different methods with thermodilution. Anesthesiology 1990; 72(5) 784 –792.

[42] Stetz CW, Miller RG, Kelly GE, Raffin TA. Reliability of the thermodilution method in the determination of cardiac output in clinical practice. American review of respiratory disease 1982;126(6) 1001–1004.

[43] Yang XX, Critchley LA, Joynt GM. Determination of the measurement error of the pulmonary artery thermodilution catheter using in-vitro continuous flow test rig. Anesthesia and Analgesia 2011;112(1) 70-77.

[44] Peyton PJ, Chong SW. Minimally invasive measurement of cardiac output during surgery and critical care: a meta-analysis of accuracy and precision. Anesthesiology 2010;113(5) 1220-1235.

[45] Bland JM, Altman DG. Statistical methods for assessing agreement between two methods of clinical measurement. Lancet 1986;1(8476) 307-310.

[46] Bland JM, Altman DG. Agreement between methods of measurement with multiple observations per individual. Journal of Biopharmaceutical Statistics 2007;17(4) 571–582.

[47] Myles PS, Cui J. Using the Bland–Altman method to measure agreement with repeated measures. British Journal of Anaesthesia 2007;99(3) 309–311.

[48] Perrino AC, O'Connor T, Luther M. Transtracheal Doppler cardiac output monitoring: comparison to thermodilution during noncardiac surgery. Anesthesia and Analgesia 1994;78(6) 1060–1066.

[49] Perrino AC, Harris SN, Luther MA. Intraoperative determination of cardiac output using multiplane transesophageal echocardiography: a comparison to thermodilution. Anesthesiology 1998;89(2) 350–357.

[50] Critchley LA, Yang XX, Lee A: Assessment of trending ability of cardiac output monitors by polar plot methodology. Journal of Cardiothoracic and Vascular Anesthesia 2011;25(3) 536-546.

[51] Biancofiore G, Critchley LA, Lee A, Bindi L, Bisa` M, Esposito M, Meacci L, Mozzo R, DeSimone P, Urbani L, Filipponi F. Evaluation of an uncalibrated arterial pulse contour cardiac output monitoring system in cirrhotic patients undergoing liver surgery. British Journal of Anaesthesia 2009;102(1) 47–54.

[52] Critchley LAH, Peng ZY, Fok BS, Flach J, Wong SC, Lee A, Phillips RA. Testing the reliability of a new ultrasonic cardiac output monitor, the USCOM using aortic flow probes in anaesthetized dogs. Anesthesia and Analgesia 2005;100(3) 748-753.

Chapter 5

Intraoperative Indocyanine Green Imaging Technique in Cardiovascular Surgery

Masaki Yamamoto, Kazumasa Orihashi and Takayuki Sato

Additional information is available at the end of the chapter

http://dx.doi.org/10.5772/55311

1. Introduction

The number of patients with arteriosclerotic disease requiring revascularization surgery such as coronary arterial bypass grafting (CABG) is increasing [1]. In CABG, off-pump CABG (OPCAB) has reduced incidence of operative mortality, which was reported to be as low as 0.6% in the Japanese database of 2009 cases and has enabled surgical treatment for those patients who could not tolerate conventional CABG under cardiac arrest [1]. However, off-pump technique can adversely deteriorate the quality of coronary anastomosis due to technical difficulties, potentially leading to a higher rate of graft occlusion or stenosis [2]. In addition, surgery for peripheral arterial disease (PAD) has become more complicated due to an increasing number of patients with longer period of chronic renal failure [3]. They often necessitate revascularization surgery to the paramalleolar arteries.

In both groups, quality of anastomosis affects the prognosis: an inadequate graft perfusion in CABG deteriorates cardiac function while that in PAD patient may lead to an amputation of ischemic limb. Graft patency and quality of anastomosis has been evaluated postoperatively by means of fluoroscopic angiography or computed tomography angiography (CTA). However, a redo surgery for restoring an adequate perfusion based on these assessment has a higher risk compared to the primary surgery, and thus intraoperative assessment of graft is desirable. Since intraoperative coronary angiography (CAG) is not necessarily feasible unless hybrid operating room is equipped, transit time flowmeter (TTF) has been employed [4, 5]. However, it does not provide morphological information and some alternative to fluoroscopic CAG is anticipated. Indocyanine green (ICG) angiography could be an alternative.

Intestinal ischemia remains a devastating complication in vascular surgery, especially in surgical repair of abdominal aortic aneurysms (AAA) [6, 7]. The incidence of intestinal ischemia in elective surgery for AAA and emergency surgery for ruptured AAA is reported to be 6% and 42%, respectively [6, 7]. In cases of suspected intestinal ischemia, however, it is not easy to make a treatment strategy of either revascularization or intestinal resection based on the inspection and digital palpation. ICG imaging system may provide an another useful clue for decision-making [8].

In this chapter, basic principles to the clinical applications of ICG imaging in cardiovascular surgery are described [9].

2. Property of ICG

Indocyanine green is a hydrophilic tricarbocyanine dye that rapidly binds to plasma proteins in the body and is mostly incorporated to the liver and excreted in the bile [10]. As ICG in the blood is exposed to near infrared ray of 760- 780 nm wave length, it generates fluorescence of 800 - 850 nm wave length (Figure 1A, B) [10, 11]. Our preliminary study showed that the peak spectral absorption of ICG diluted in the human blood was at 760 - 780 nm (Figure 2) [12]. The amplitude of ICG fluorescent luminescence is not proportional to its concentration but is highest at the ICG concentration of 2.5×10^{-3} mg/mL.

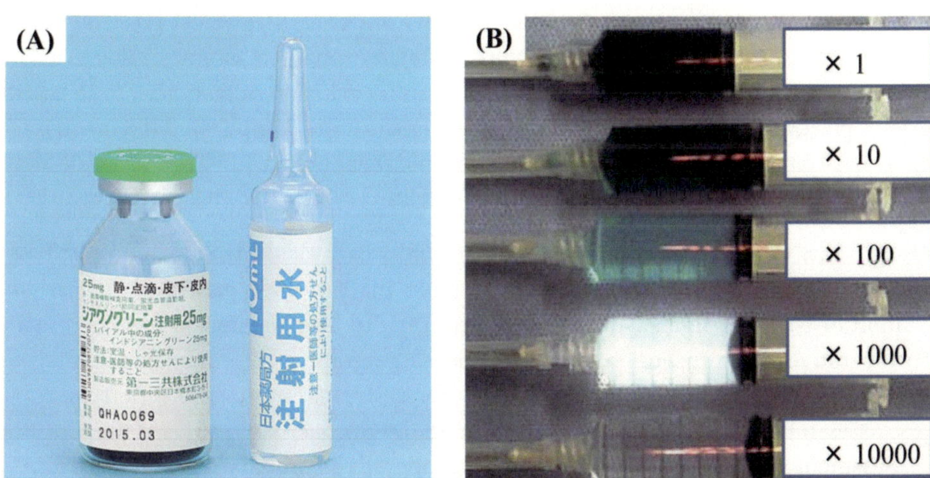

Figure 1. ICG and fluorescent luminescence in various dilution. A: drug product of ICG (Diagnogreen™; DaiichiSankyo Co., Tokyo, Japan). B: Fluorescent luminescence is not proportional to its concentration. The luminescence was highest at a concentration of 2.5×10^{-3} mg/mL.

http://dx.doi.org/10.5772/55311

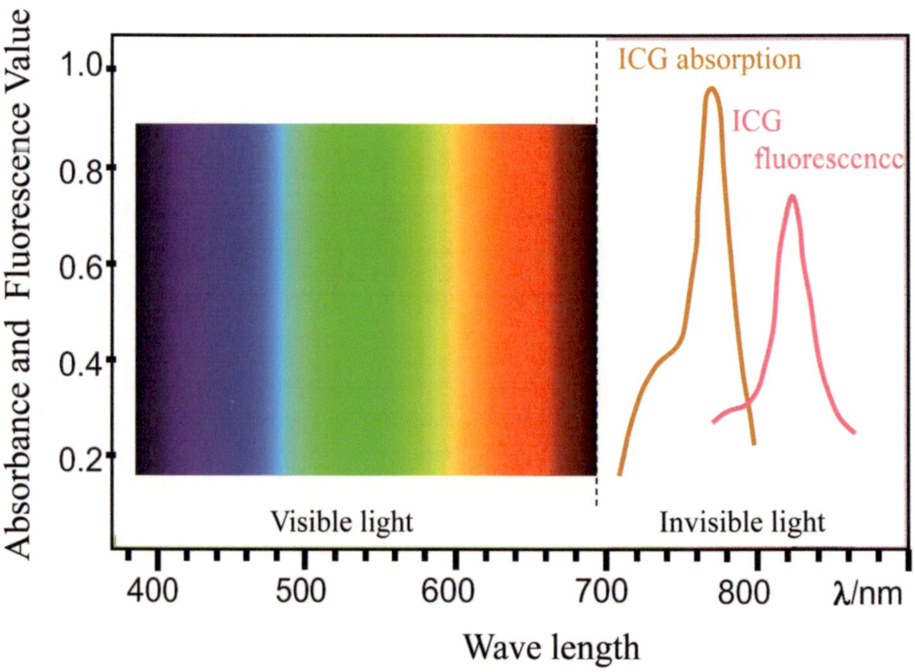

Figure 2. Absorbance and fluorescence value of ICG. ICG emits a flash of light with a wavelength of 806nm. The peak spectral absorption of ICG diluted in human blood is 760 - 780 nm.

3. ICG angiography

Fluorescence property of ICG has been used not only in ophthalmology as fluorescein fundus angiography to visualize retinal and choroidal circulation but for breast cancer surgery (sentinel node mapping), gastroenterological surgery, and cardiovascular surgery [8, 13, 14]. Following intravenous injection of ICG, fluorescence generated in the blood by near infrared light is captured by a camera and the vessels are visualized, although fluorescence is partially absorbed by the water and hemoglobin. This principle was applied to the commercially available intraoperative imaging system, SPY ™ (Novadaq Technologies Inc., Toronto, Canada) and Photodynamic Eye (PDE; Hamamatsu Photonics K.K., Shizuoka, Japan) [15, 16]. The PDE enable to image with a hand-held camera in the surgical

field. These devices visualize the blood flow clearly in monochrome imaging under irradiation of excitation light after ICG injection. The former emits a low-intensity laser (2.7 watts) and demonstrates angiographic image at a frame rate of 30 per second. They allow irradiation and recording time for up to 34 seconds but demonstrate the vessels in monochrome image. These systems have been applied to coronary and graft angiography [17] and peripheral arterial surgery [18].

4. Characteristics of ICG angiography

ICG angiography has several advantages. First, it can visualize arterial blood flow by intravenous injection of ICG without catheter manipulation or contrast agent. Second, stenotic portion can be visualized like fluoroscopic angiograms. Third, it takes only ten minutes from preparation to imaging.

However, ICG angiography systems mentioned above have several drawbacks. First, they use laser light source, and the time duration for irradiation is limited to 35 seconds because of the danger of thermal injury. Second, the angiograms are shown in monochrome, making it difficult to recognize the color of tissue. Third, penetration of fluorescence is poor and vessels in the deep layer is hardly visualized.

We have developed a new ICG imaging system, HyperEye Medical System (HEMS, Mizuho Co., Tokyo, Japan) to solve these problems (Figure 3) [9, 12]. It is composed of an imaging unit, a control unit and a monitor. The imaging unit consists of multiple light-emitting diodes (LEDs) which is allocated around an ultra-sensitive color charged-coupled device (CCD) imaging camera with non- Bayer color filter arrays (HyperEye Technology; SANYO Co., Ltd, Tokyo, Japan). This camera detects near infrared rays (380-1200 nm) and visible light at 30 frames per seconds. The control unit is composed of a personal computer and a controller for recording and adjusting the focus, iris and range of imaging.

HEMS can demonstrate the fluorescent images on the background of natural color (Figure 4), which facilitates surgeons to recognize the vessels in the surgical field [12]. Unlimited recording is another advantage of this system because it uses LEDs as the light source. The imaging head is draped by a sterile cover and is placed at 30 to 50 cm above the targets (Figure 5A). The illumination area is approximately 78.5cm^2 (5 × 5 × 3.14cm) on the surgical field. A 5mg of ICG (Diagnogreen™, DaiichiSankyo Co., Tokyo, Japan) dissolved in 2 mL of distilled water is injected via a central venous catheter and is flushed by 10 mL of saline per each imaging sequence (Figure 5B) [19]. The right atrium immediately glows white, then right ventricle and pulmonary artery, followed by ascending aorta and the coronary grafts as well as native coronary arteries. Cardiac output affects the time lag of opacification. The images are recorded using a digital image-processing system such as audio video interweave (AVI) or Smart Draw (SDR) format.

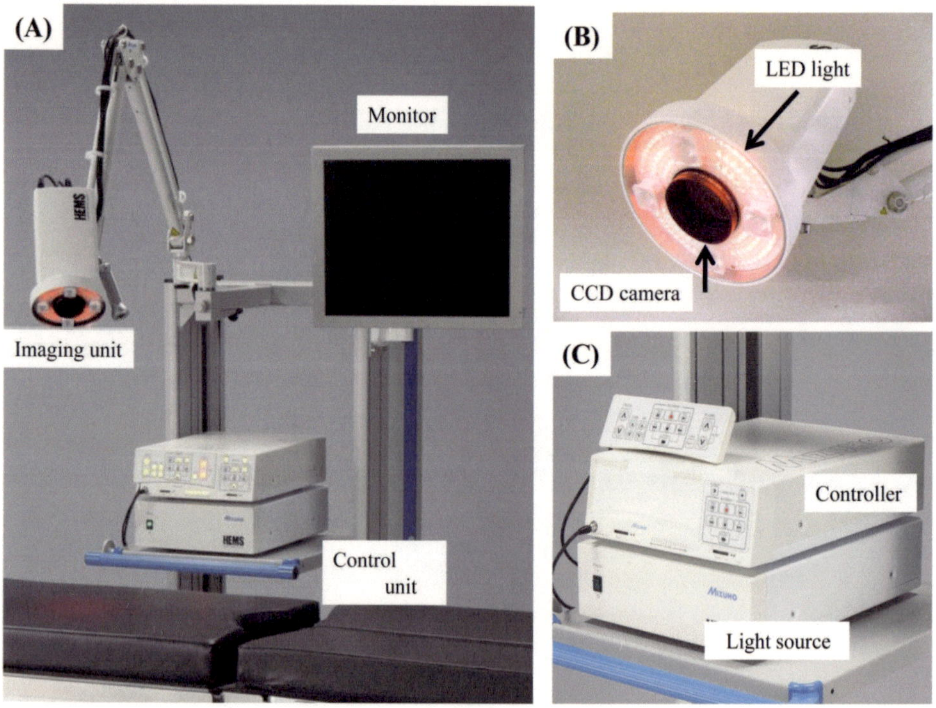

Figure 3. HyperEye Medical System (HEMS) A: Full view of HEMS, composed of imaging unit, control unit, and monitor. B: The imaging head consists of multiple light-emitting diodes (LED) and an ultrasensitive color charge-coupled device (CCD) camera. C: Control unit consists of controller and analyzing system.

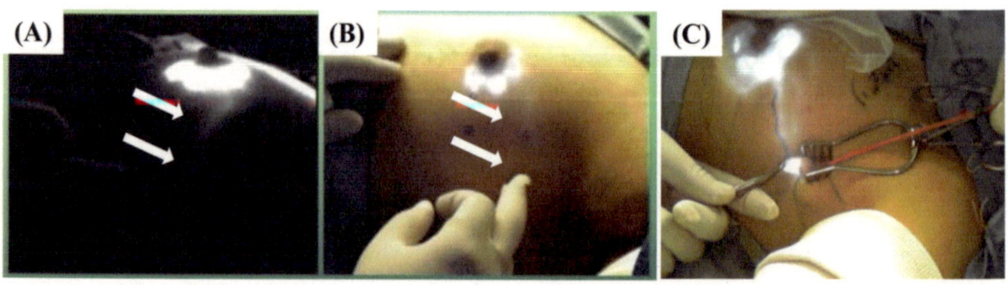

Figure 4. Sentinel node mapping in breast cancer surgery. The ICG stream in lymphatic duct is observed from subareolar to the axillar lymph nodes after ICG injection to subcutaneous of areolar. A: Fluorescence emitted from ICG injected in the breast. The lymphatic duct is identified as fluorescence line (arrow). B: The ICG stream in lymphatic duct. C: ICG in the axillar lymph nodes. The sentinel lymph node is identified as strong fluorescence leading out of lymphatic duct.

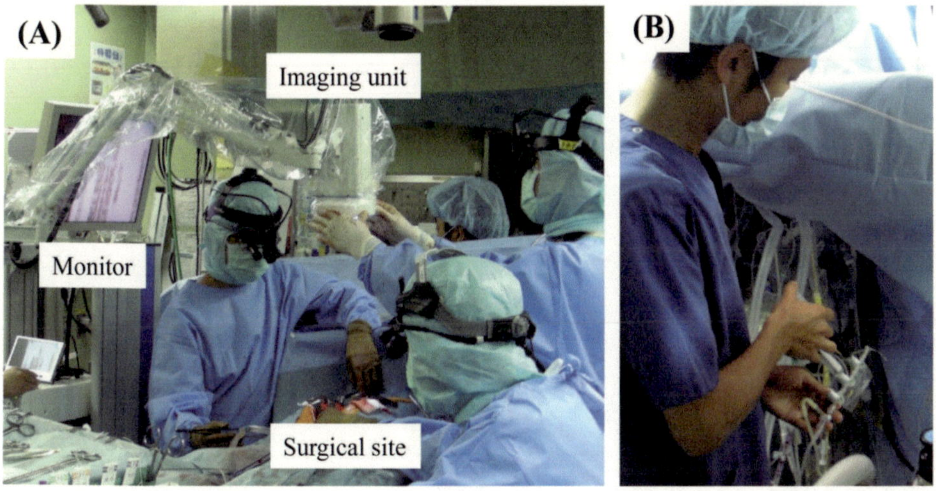

Figure 5. HEMS in use during cardiac surgery. A: The imaging head is draped by a sterile cover and placed at 30 to 50 cm above the targets. B: ICG solution is injected via a central venous catheter.

5. Application of ICG angiography in CABG

Since the first report of intraoperative ICG coronary angiography by Rubens et al. and Detter et al. in 2002, usefulness of this modality have been reported by several investigators (Table 1) [5, 12, 16, 17, 20-22]. Reuthebuch and Taggart showed the clinical utility of the SPY system for assessment of the quality of bypass grafts of usage from experience [20, 21]. Takahashi et.al. described the verification of ICG angiography with using the SPY imaging system [16].

TTF (MediStim AS, Oslo, Norway) has been used as well in CABG for intraoperative assessment of coronary graft [23]. The time for ultrasound beam to travel from one crystal across a vessel to another crystal is called as transit time. In TTF, the graft flow is assessed by three parameters: mean graft flow, pulsatility index, and diastolic filling percentage. Desai et al. researched the utility of two intraoperative assessments of graft, TTF and ICG graft angiography [24]. A total of 139 grafts were reviewed and the sensitivity and specificity of ICG angiography to detect greater than 50% stenosis or occlusion were 83.3% and 100%, respectively. When TTF shows an unusual data, however, imaging modality may be helpful for making treatment strategy.

Investigators	Year	Patients	Graft No	Sensitivity	Specificity
Rubens	2002	20	-	-	-
Reuthebuch	2003	38	124	-	-
Taggart	2003	84	213	-	-
Balacumaraswami	2004	200	533	-	-
Takahashi	2004	72	290	-	-
Desai	2006	46	139	83.3	100
Handa	2009	39	116	100	100
Handa	2010	51	129	85.7	100

- : not shown, ICG: indocyanine green, CABG: coronary artery bypass grafting

Reprinted from Surgery Today, 2011; 41:1467-1474, Yamamoto M et. al. Assessing Intraoperative Blood Flow in Cardiovascular Surgery., copyright (2011)

Table 1. Reported clinical studies on the indocyanine green imaging system in coronary artery bypass grafting

We have assessed coronary grafts by means of HEMS since 2007 and have classified the flow pattern as follows [12].

1. Normal flow: smooth opacification of the graft and then coronary artery (Fig 6A).

2. Abnormal flow:

Delay: delayed graft enhancement compared to other grafts (Fig 6B)

Occlusion: no enhancement of the graft (Fig 6C)

The results of HEMS assessment were compared with fluoroscopic CAG one year after CABG and have found that the former accurately predicted the outcomes of grafts (Figure.6D-F). [12]. Thus, visualization of graft flow is helpful for surgeons to make decisions of revision in the operating room.

Visualization of myocardial perfusion is another feature of HEMS. Figure 6C shows an obstructed anastomosis in the left internal thoracic arterial graft, causing perfusion defect in the anterior wall around the anastomosis, whereas myocardium in the diagonal region is well opacified. Detter et. al. reported that myocardial perfusion can be quantitatively assessed by ICG angiography with digital image processing system [25].

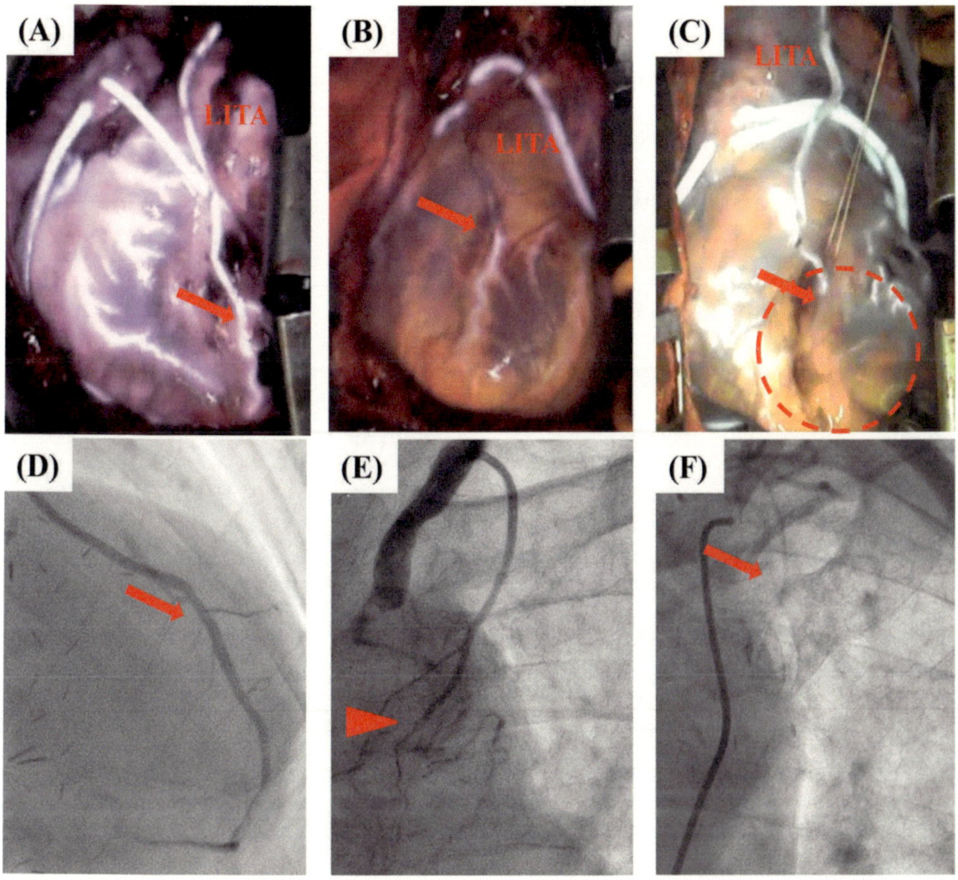

Figure 6. HEMS assessment of coronary arterial grafts. Coronary arterial bypass grafts images created by HEMS (A-C) and fluoroscopic angiography (D-F). Arrows indicate coronary anastomoses, arrow heads indicate occluded point of graft. A: Smooth opacification of graft and distal coronary artery. B: Delayed graft flow. C: Absence of fluorescence in the left anterior descending artery (LAD) despite of opacification of left internal thoracic artery (LITA) graft. There was perfusion defect in the anterior myocardial wall (circled dot line), while myocardial perfusion in the diagonal region is apparent. D-F: Fluoroscopic coronary angiography corresponding to A to C, respectively.

6. Application to peripheral arterial surgery

HEMS has been also applied to peripheral arterial surgery for assessing the blood flow in the saphenous vein graft anastomosed to the paramalleolar artery [19]. Blood flow in vascular prosthesis such as Dacron or Polytrafluoroethylene (PTFE) graft cannot be assessed due to poor penetration of fluorescence (Figure 7). Although there are varying time delay from ICG injection to opacification of graft, assessment of arterial graft via intravenous ICG injection is an advantage of HEMS. Since the target (graft) is immobile unlike coronary angiography, the image is clear despite a long distance from the injection site [18, 19].

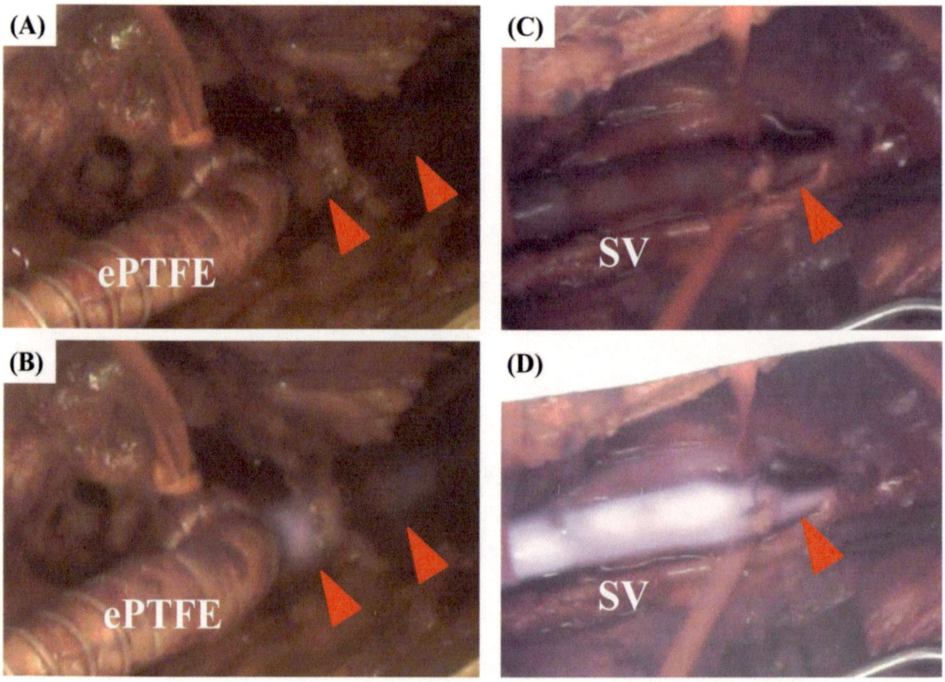

Figure 7. HEMS assessment of graft in peripheral arterial surgery. Visual image and ICG angiogram in ePTFE graft (A,B) and saphenous vein graft (C, D). Opacification is poor in PTFE graft. PTFE: polytetrafluoroethylene. SV: saphenous vein. Arrow heads show native peripheral arteries.

Figure 8 compares the intraoperative HEMS image and postoperative CT angiogram in a case of arterial revascularization. The blood flow through the anastomosis was smooth (Figure 8A) and there was no stenosis at the anastomosis by CTA (Figure 8B). Figure 9 demonstrates the data of a case who underwent bypass grafting to the posterior peroneal artery (PTA) with a saphenous vein graft [19]. HEMS revealed an inadequate blood flow in the PTA distal to the anastomosis (Figure 9A), although TTF showed fairly acceptable graft flow (7 mL/min of mean flow: Figure 9B). Based on the HEMS findings, an additional bypass to the PTA was placed with a saphenous vein graft. HEMS following additional grafting showed smooth flow in the graft as well as in the PTA distal to the anastomosis (Figure 9C). The TTF assessment showed doubled graft flow (15 mL/min, Figure 9D). Since the TTF data can be largely affected by hemodynamic condition as well as peripheral perfusion area, it is not easy to make reliable TTF criteria. HEMS may be helpful for making a decision in such instances.

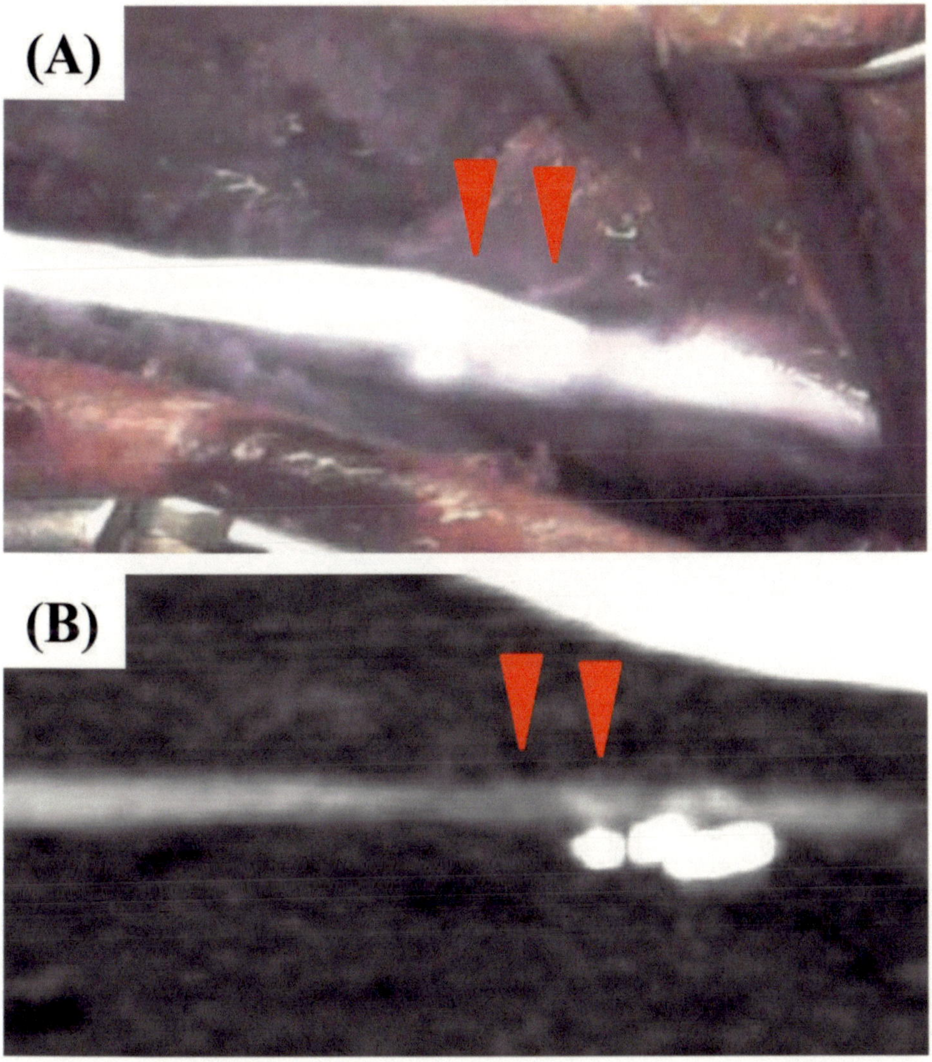

Figure 8. Intraoperative ICG angiogram compared with postoperative CT angiogram. The patient underwent femoro-tibial arterial bypass with saphenous vein graft. A: ICG angiogram of femoro- tibial arterial bypass with saphenous vein graft. Blood flow through the anastomosis is smooth. B: The CTA showed there was no anastomotic stenosis.

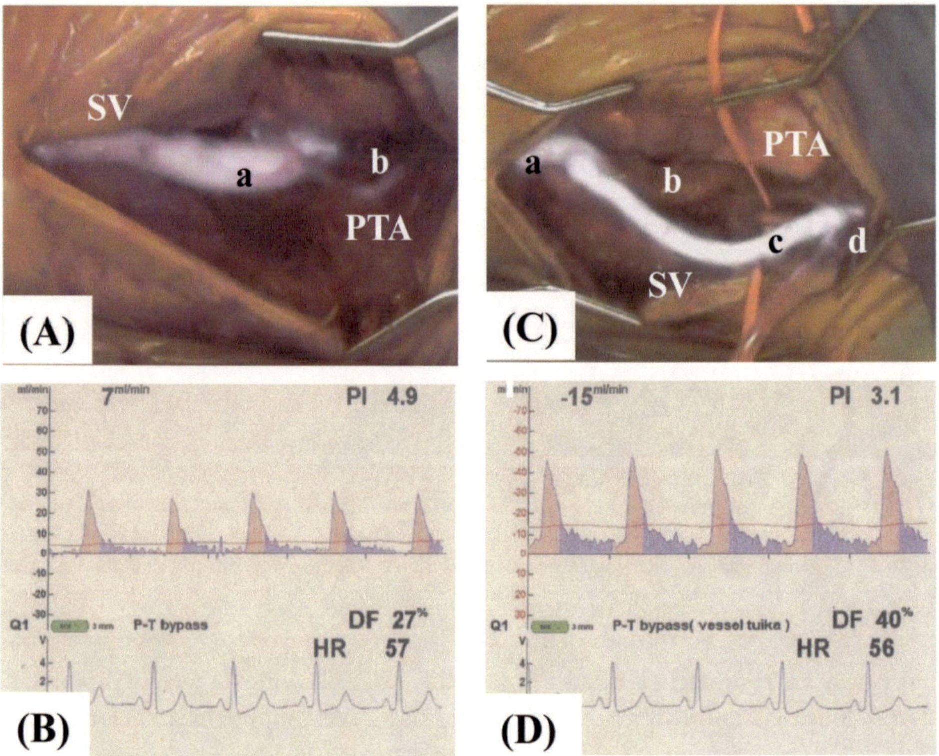

Figure 9. HEMS assessment and transit time flowmetry (TTF) data in peripheral arterial surgery. A: HEMS image of saphenous vein (SV) graft which was anastomosed to the posterior tibial artery (PTA). Fluorescence is poorly detected in the PTA (b). B: TTF data showing graft flow in the initial bypass (a). C: An improved flow in HEMS assessment in additional SV (c) as well as in the PTA (d). D: TTF data showing doubled graft flow after revised bypass (c).(Reprinted from Eur J Vasc Endovasc Surg 2012; 43:426- 432)

7. Application to AAA surgery

Intestinal ischemia is one of undesirable complications in AAA surgery. It can be well demarcated caused by embolism of mesenteric artery or poorly demarcated in diffuse malperfusion. HEMS is capable of visualizing the blood flow in the mesenteric artery as well as tissue perfusion in the intestinal wall (Figure 10) [9, 19]. The mesenteric artery is opacified first, then marginal artery, and illuminescence sequentially spreads to the entire intestines and colon, but slightly delayed in the sigmoid colon, probably because inferior mesenteric artery arises at the most distal portion of the aorta.

Bowel necrosis can develop under markedly reduced perfusion despite the presence of detectable blood flow in the mesenteric artery [19, 26]. Assessment of tissue perfusion such as intestinal wall appears to be a unique and advantageous feature of HEMS which allows a longer duration for imaging.

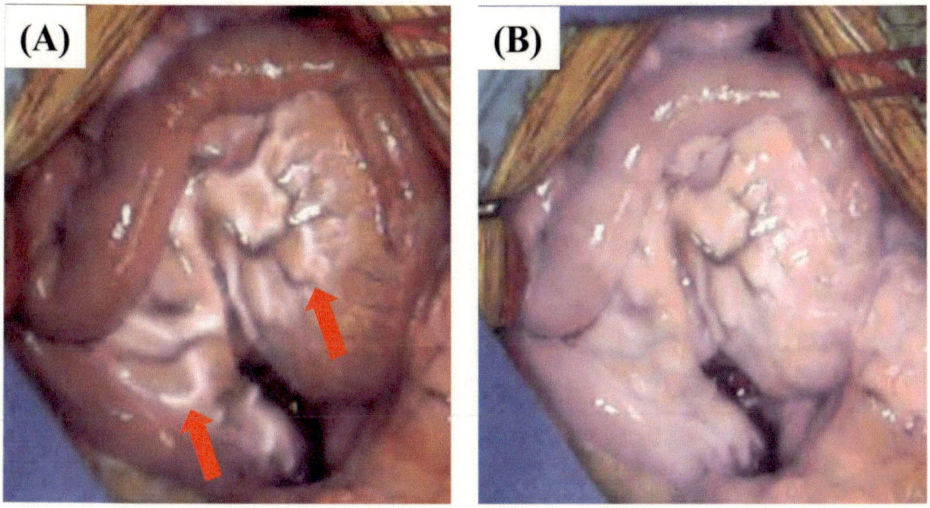

Figure 10. HEMS images showing sequential mesenteric perfusion. A: Fluorescence appears first in the mesenteric arteries (arrow). B: The entire mesenterium and intestinal wall is opacified. (Reprinted from Eur J Vasc Endovasc Surg 2012; 43:426- 432)

Champagne et al. reported the incidence of ischemic colitis following surgery for ruptured AAA as 42% [27]. Shock status in the preoperative period is the most important predictor of ischemic colitis [28]. Although resection of necrotic intestine and colon is necessary to rescue the patients, it is not easy to determine the extent of resection by visual inspection. Figure 11 shows the corresponding images of inspection and HEMS images in two cases. Figure 11A shows the appearance of intestine in an 85 year-old woman who underwent emergent surgery for ruptured AAA. HEMS revealed malperfusion in the sigmoid colon (Figure 11B). Figure 11C is the visual finding of an 80 year-old woman after transient hypotension during AAA surgery. The intestine appeared to be diffusely malperfused in spotty fashion (Figure 11C). HEMS showed spotty malperfusion of intestinal wall (Figure 11D). ICG opacification in addition to the color image of surgical field facilitates to precisely locate the ischemic region [19].

8. Limitation of ICG angiography

Despite the advantages of HEMS, quick and less invasive assessment without contrast agent as well as assessment of tissue perfusion superimposed on the color views [9, 19, 29], it also has several limitations to be noted.

First, penetration of fluorescence is less than 2 to 3 mm and visualization of blood flow is limited to the superficial portion of the vessel and tissue [25]. The coronary artery covered with adipose tissue or hemostatic stuff cannot be visualized clearly.

http://dx.doi.org/10.5772/55311

HEMS does not provide the projectional image as in fluoroscopic angiography but the en-face view of superficial layer. Therefore, densitometric analysis for assessing the severity of stenosis is not feasible.

The intensity of brightness is not absolute but rather relative. Furthermore, HEMS assessment can be affected by hemodynamic status such as blood pressure or cardiac output. Therefore, the results cannot be simply compared among individuals.

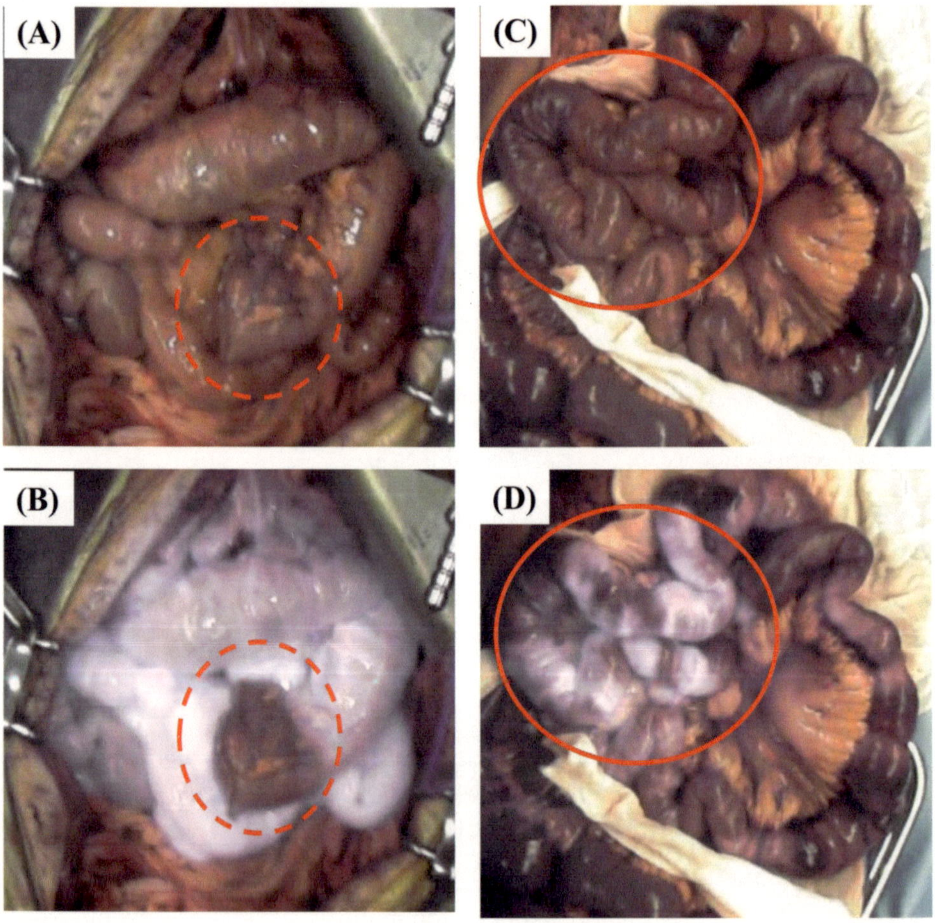

Figure 11. HEMS images showing intestinal ischemia. A,B: Segmental ischemia in the sigmoid colon in an 85 year-old female patient who underwent emergent surgery for ruptured abdominal aortic aneurysm (AAA). The sigmoid colon appears slightly ischemic in visual inspection (A) but is apparent in ICG angiograms (B). C,D: Diffuse and spotty ischemia in an 80 year-old female patient after transient hypotention during AAA surgery. (Reprinted from Eur J Vasc Endovasc Surg 2012; 43:426- 432)

9. Future prospects of HEMS

Despite the qualitative nature of HEMS assessment, we have ambitiously attempted more quantitative analysis of data obtained in peripheral arterial surgery and AAA surgery [19]. The transitional changes of intensity appear to indicate the smoothness of graft flow or tissue perfusion, although further investigation is necessary.

TTF is likely to reflect another aspect of graft function which is different from that obtained in HEMS. The combination assessment may be useful for assessing the graft with higher sensitivity and specificity compared to each single assessment.

10. Conclusion

HEMS is a simple, safe, and reliable imaging tool for intraoperative assessment of blood flow. It enables intraoperative assessment in surgical treatment for ischemic heart disease, peripheral arterial disease, or abdominal aortic aneurysm and may facilitate to optimize the surgical outcomes by detecting unexpected trouble and alerting additional revision or intervention.

Author details

Masaki Yamamoto, Kazumasa Orihashi and Takayuki Sato*

*Address all correspondence to: y-masaki@kochi-u.ac.jp

Departments of Surgery II and Cardiovascular Control, Faculty of Medicine, Kochi University, Kochi, Japan

References

[1] 95963667SakataRFujiiYKuwanoHThoracic and cardiovascular surgery in Japan during 2009: annual report by the Japanese Association for Thoracic Surgery. General thoracic and cardiovascular surgery. 2011;59963667.

[2] Khan, N. E, De Souza, A, Mister, R, Flather, M, Clague, J, Davies, S, et al. A randomized comparison of off-pump and on-pump multivessel coronary-artery bypass surgery. The New England journal of medicine. (2004). , 350(1), 21-8.

[3] Criqui, M. H, Langer, R. D, Fronek, A, Feigelson, H. S, Klauber, M. R, Mccann, T. J, et al. Mortality over a period of 10 years in patients with peripheral arterial disease. N Engl J Med. (1992). , 326(6), 381-6.

[4] Ancona, D, Karamanoukian, G, Ricci, H. L, Schmid, M, Bergsland, S, & Salerno, J. TA. Graft revision after transit time flow measurement in off-pump coronary artery bypass grafting. Eur J Cardiothorac Surg. (2000). , 17(3), 287-93.

[5] Balacumaraswami, L, & Taggart, D. P. Digital tools to facilitate intraoperative coronary artery bypass graft patency assessment. Seminars in thoracic and cardiovascular surgery. (2004). , 16(3), 266-71.

[6] Ernst, C. B, Hagihara, P. F, Daugherty, M. E, & Griffen, W. O. Jr. Inferior mesenteric artery stump pressure: a reliable index for safe IMA ligation during abdominal aortic aneurysmectomy. Annals of surgery. (1978). , 187(6), 641-6.

[7] Champagne, B. J, & Darling, R. C. rd, Daneshmand M, Kreienberg PB, Lee EC, Mehta M, et al. Outcome of aggressive surveillance colonoscopy in ruptured abdominal aortic aneurysm. J Vasc Surg. (2004). , 39(4), 792-6.

[8] Flower, R. W, & Hochheimer, B. F. A clinical technique and apparatus for simultaneous angiography of the separate retinal and choroidal circulations. Investigative ophthalmology. (1973). , 12(4), 248-61.

[9] Yamamoto, M, Sasaguri, S, & Sato, T. Assessing intraoperative blood flow in cardiovascular surgery. Surgery today. (2011). , 41(11), 1467-74.

[10] Cherrick, G. R, Stein, S. W, Leevy, C. M, & Davidson, C. S. Indocyanine green: observations on its physical properties, plasma decay, and hepatic extraction. J Clin Invest. (1960). , 39, 592-600.

[11] Benson, R. C, & Kues, H. A. Fluorescence properties of indocyanine green as related to angiography. Physics in medicine and biology. (1978). , 23(1), 159-63.

[12] Handa, T, Katare, R. G, Sasaguri, S, & Sato, T. Preliminary experience for the evaluation of the intraoperative graft patency with real color charge-coupled device camera system: an advanced device for simultaneous capturing of color and near-infrared images during coronary artery bypass graft. Interactive cardiovascular and thoracic surgery. (2009). , 9(2), 150-4.

[13] Kitai, T, Inomoto, T, Miwa, M, & Shikayama, T. Fluorescence navigation with indocyanine green for detecting sentinel lymph nodes in breast cancer. Breast Cancer. (2005). Epub 2005/08/20., 12(3), 211-5.

[14] Novotny, H. R, & Alvis, D. A method of photographing fluorescence in circulating blood of the human eye. Technical documentary report SAM-TDR USAF School of Aerospace Medicine. (1960).

[15] Balacumaraswami, L, & Taggart, D. P. Intraoperative imaging techniques to assess coronary artery bypass graft patency. The Annals of thoracic surgery. (2007). , 83(6), 2251-7.

[16] Takahashi, M, Ishikawa, T, Higashidani, K, & Katoh, H. SPY: an innovative intra-operative imaging system to evaluate graft patency during off-pump coronary artery bypass grafting. Interactive cardiovascular and thoracic surgery. (2004). , 3(3), 479-83.

[17] Rubens, F. D, Ruel, M, & Fremes, S. E. A new and simplified method for coronary and graft imaging during CABG. The heart surgery forum. (2002). , 5(2), 141-4.

[18] Unno, N, Suzuki, M, Yamamoto, N, Inuzuka, K, Sagara, D, Nishiyama, M, et al. Indocyanine green fluorescence angiography for intraoperative assessment of blood flow: a feasibility study. Eur J Vasc Endovasc Surg. (2008). , 35(2), 205-7.

[19] Yamamoto, M, Orihashi, K, Nishimori, H, Wariishi, S, Fukutomi, T, Kondo, N, et al. Indocyanine green angiography for intra-operative assessment in vascular surgery. European journal of vascular and endovascular surgery : the official journal of the European Society for Vascular Surgery. (2012). , 43(4), 426-32.

[20] Reuthebuch, O, Haussler, A, Genoni, M, Tavakoli, R, Odavic, D, Kadner, A, et al. Novadaq SPY: intraoperative quality assessment in off-pump coronary artery bypass grafting. Chest. (2004). , 125(2), 418-24.

[21] Taggart, D. P, Choudhary, B, Anastasiadis, K, Abu-omar, Y, Balacumaraswami, L, & Pigott, D. W. Preliminary experience with a novel intraoperative fluorescence imaging technique to evaluate the patency of bypass grafts in total arterial revascularization. The Annals of thoracic surgery. (2003). , 75(3), 870-3.

[22] Detter, C, Russ, D, Iffland, A, Wipper, S, Schurr, M. O, Reichenspurner, H, et al. Near-infrared fluorescence coronary angiography: a new noninvasive technology for intraoperative graft patency control. Heart Surg Forum. (2002). , 5(4), 364-9.

[23] Canver, C. C, & Dame, N. A. Ultrasonic assessment of internal thoracic artery graft flow in the revascularized heart. The Annals of thoracic surgery. (1994). , 58(1), 135-8.

[24] Desai, N. D, Miwa, S, Kodama, D, Koyama, T, Cohen, G, Pelletier, M. P, et al. A randomized comparison of intraoperative indocyanine green angiography and transit-time flow measurement to detect technical errors in coronary bypass grafts. The Journal of thoracic and cardiovascular surgery. (2006). , 132(3), 585-94.

[25] Detter, C, Wipper, S, Russ, D, Iffland, A, Burdorf, L, Thein, E, et al. Fluorescent cardiac imaging: a novel intraoperative method for quantitative assessment of myocardial perfusion during graded coronary artery stenosis. Circulation. (2007). , 116(9), 1007-14.

[26] Iwai, T, Sakurazawa, K, Sato, S, Muraoka, Y, Inoue, Y, & Endo, M. Intra-operative monitoring of the pelvic circulation using a transanal Doppler probe. European journal of vascular surgery. (1991). , 5(1), 71-4.

[27] Champagne, B. J, Lee, E. C, Valerian, B, Mulhotra, N, & Mehta, M. Incidence of colonic ischemia after repair of ruptured abdominal aortic aneurysm with endograft. Journal of the American College of Surgeons. (2007). , 204(4), 597-602.

[28] Piotrowski, J. J, Ripepi, A. J, Yuhas, J. P, Alexander, J. J, & Brandt, C. P. Colonic ischemia: the Achilles heel of ruptured aortic aneurysm repair. The American surgeon. (1996)., 62(7), 557-60.

[29] Handa, T, Katare, R. G, Nishimori, H, Wariishi, S, Fukutomi, T, Yamamoto, M, et al. New device for intraoperative graft assessment: HyperEye charge-coupled device camera system. General thoracic and cardiovascular surgery., 58(2), 68-77.

Chapter 6

Peripheral Tissue Oxygenation During Standard and Miniaturized Cardiopulmonary Bypass (Direct Oxymetric Tissue Perfusion Monitoring Study)

Jiri Mandak

Additional information is available at the end of the chapter

http://dx.doi.org/10.5772/54300

1. Introduction

Coronary artery bypass grafting (CABG) using a cardiopulmonary bypass (CPB) is a routine therapeutic method in the surgical treatment of ischemic heart disease. Although CPB is successfully used thousands of times each day worldwide it is still associated with some unanswered questions [1].

One of the basic questions that arise with the use of this technology is an adequate blood flow during surgery [1,2]. There are no standards for optimal pump flow during CPB and institutional practices are largely based on empirical experience. Optimal blood flow rate has not been definitively established by large-scale randomized trials carried out on animal models more than fifty years ago and proved by clinical experiences [1,3]. Initial flow is calculated based upon the body surface area and a temperature management strategy. The flow rate most commonly used during hypothermic CPB is 2.2 - 2.4 l.min-1.m-2 and during normothermic CPB 2.5 - 2.8 l.min-1.m-2 [3].

Despite progress, cardiopulmonary bypass predominantly used during coronary operations is still associated with profound physiological reactions and changes. In the majority of cases these reactions are caused by contact of blood with artificial material within the system and by other sources such as coronary suction, blood-air contact, non-turbulent flow, hemodilution and hypothermia.

A large number of advancements in the technology, equipment and techniques have been introduced to decrease the negative impact of CPB. One of the latest complex innovations is miniaturized CPB (mini CPB). The use of more biocompatible materials and minimization of equipment and internal surface of the system can reduce pathological reactions [4-8].

Volume constant perfusion (perfusion without a reservoir) is a major advantage of mini CPB, but it can be associated with significant problems. The calculated blood flow (pump flow) must often be reduced to compensate for the volume in case of lower venous return during perfusion. Other reasons for reduction in pump flow are an increase in arterial pressure and flooding of the operating field with blood.

Delivery of oxygen to the tissues is equally dependent on blood flow and the O2 content of blood. Reduction of blood flow can decrease optimal tissue oxygenation. Inadequate oxygenation and perfusion can be associated with severe pathological peripheral tissue changes associated with clinical complications [1,9,10].

It is difficult to assess local changes in perfusion or blood circulation in the periphery. The direct measurement of blood flow through separate organs or skeletal muscles during cardiac surgery is both technically difficult and ethically unacceptable. Evaluation of the standard biochemical and hemodynamic parameters (blood pressure, blood lactate, heart rate, O2 saturation in the capillary bed, diuresis, etc.) yields for general results but not for regional changes [1,3,9].

For this purpose, direct continuous measurement of interstitial tissue oxygen tension (ptO2) of a skeletal muscle, as a typical peripheral tissue, was used in this study. Tissue oxygen tension reflects the adequacy of regional tissue oxygenation and perfusion [11,12].

Oxygen tension was measured with a special optical multiparametric sensor inserted into the patient´s deltoid muscle. The sensor is based upon the principle of fluorescence quenching whereby the intensity of a fluorescent optical emission form, an indicator, is quenched (reduced) in the presence of oxygen. Oxygen from the surrounding blood equilibrates with the sensor materials and quenches the fluorescent light. This method was introduced into brain and liver perfusion measurement but it has not been used in connection with cardiopulmonary bypass until now.

The present study was designed to evaluate changes in peripheral tissue (skeletal muscle) oxygenation during cardiac surgery and to compare tissue perfusion in relation to blood flow during standard CPB versus mini CPB.

2. Patients, materials and methods

The study was carried out at the Department of Cardiac Surgery, University Hospital and Faculty of Medicine in Hradec Kralove, Charles University in Prague, Czech Republic. The study was approved by the university Ethics Committee. Patients were given a prior detailed explanation of the study and signed an informed consent.

2.1. Patients

The sample included 40 patients with ischemic heart disease (32 men and 8 women). All patients underwent elective cardiac surgery. The exclusion criteria were concomitant surgery,

an emergency procedure, patients with local, systemic infection or inflammation, severe left ventricular dysfunction (ejection fraction < 25%), renal failure (serum creatinine >180 μmol l^{-1} or active renal replacement therapy).

The patients were randomized to two groups. Group A, consisting of 20 patients who underwent the conventional myocardial revascularization, coronary artery bypass grafting (CABG) using standard CPB and Group B, consisting of 20 patients who underwent coronary surgery using miniaturized CPB (Figure 1).

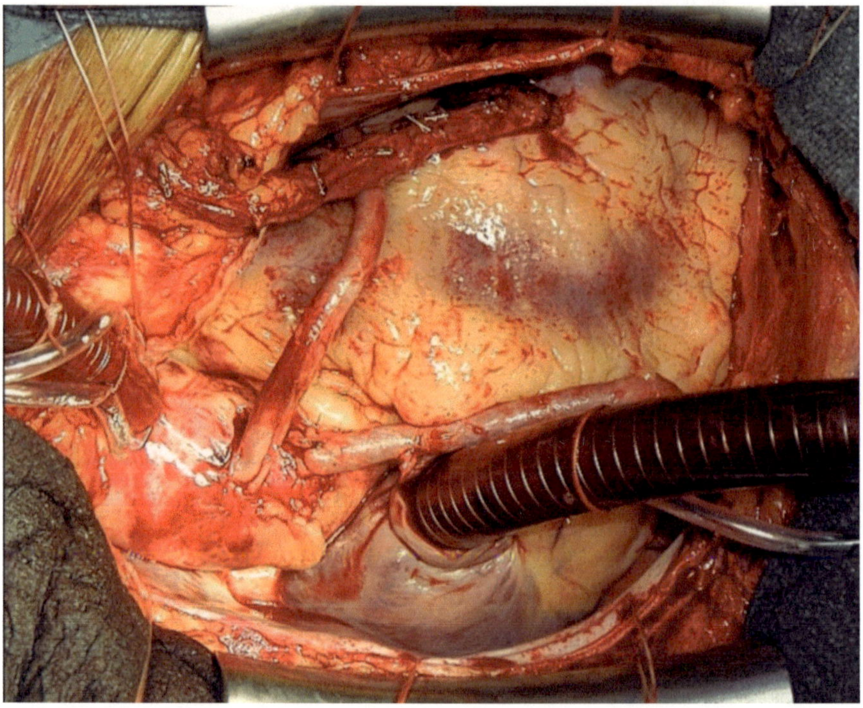

Figure 1. Coronary artery bypass grafting using cardiopulmonary bypass

Patient preoperative characteristics (Table 1), operative (Table 2) and postoperative data (Table 3) were prospectively recorded. The differences between groups (age, accompanying disease) were not statistically significant (Table 1). All routine therapeutic and monitoring steps commonly used with this diagnosis were performed. After clinical and angiographic evaluation the patients were randomly assigned to the study (n = 40).

	Group A (n=20)	Group B (n=20)	p-value
Male sex (%)	17 (85%)	15 (75%)	n.s.
Age (y)	69 ± 5.8	67 ± 6.8	n.s.
Body mass index(kg.m^{-2})	29 ± 4.9	28 ± 4.3	n.s.
Ejection fraction(%)	57.8 ± 9.8	56.2 ±12.7	n.s.
Prior myocardial infarction	12	12	n.s.
Prior PCI	4	4	n.s.
Hypertension	18	18	n.s.
Diabetes mellitus	7	6	n.s.
Chronic obstructive airway disease	3	2	n.s.
Euroscore	5.2 ± 4.7 (1.4-15.1)	4.6 ± 3.5 (0.9-15.6)	n.s.

Table 1. Preoperative characteristics of Group A (standard CPB) and Group B (mini CPB)

	Group A (n=20)	Group B (n=20)	p-value
Operation time (min)	254 ± 21.7	247 ± 58.1	n.s.
CPB time (min)	87.4 ± 21.7	75.7 ± 20.9	n.s.
Aortic crossclamp (min)	48.9 ± 14.5	45.4 ± 14.8	n.s.
No. of distal anastomoses	2.9 ± 0.8	2.7 ± 0.7	n.s.
Flow calculated (l.min^{-1})	4.7 ± 0.39	4.6 ± 0.45	n.s.
Flow real (l.min^{-1})	4.9 ± 0.41	3.5 ± 0.51	<0,001
Priming (ml)	1501 ± 44	837 ± 205	<0,001
Mean hematocrit (%)	25.3 ± 1.1	31.0 ± 2.3	<0,001
Lowest temperature (°C)	35.5 ± 0.4	35.7 ± 0.7	n.s.

Table 2. Operative characteristics of Group A (standard CPB) and Group B (mini CPB)

http://dx.doi.org/10.5772/54300

	Group A (n=20)	Group B (n=20)	p-value
IM	0	0	n.s.
Strokes	1	0	n.s.
Atrial fibrilation	6	2	<0,001
30-d mortality	0	0	n.s.
Low cardiac output	2	1	n.s.
Renal failure	0	0	n.s.
Blood loss per 24 hours (ml)	685 ± 342	861 ± 552	n.s.(0.57)
Blood transfusion (units)	2.5 ± 1.4	2.7 ± 1.2	n.s.
ICU stay (hours)	70 ± 68	112 ± 225	n.s.
Hospital lenght of stay (d)	16.4 ± 6.8	16.2 ± 5.4	n.s.

Table 3. Postoperative characteristics of Group A (standard CPB) and Group B (mini CPB)

2.2. Anesthetic technique

The anesthetic managements, CPB and surgical procedures were standardized in both groups. Anesthesia was induced with intravenous thiopenthal or midazolam and sufentanyl with muscle relaxation using cisatracurium. Anesthesia was maintained by an infusion of cisatracurium, sufentanyl and propofol at doses sufficient to keep the patient adequately anesthetized and hemodynamically stable. Isoflurane was added in the inhaled air. Antibiotic prophylaxis was given in accordance with the standard protocol (Unasyn, Pfizer, Italy; 3x1.5 g). In all cases the surgical approach was through median sternotomy.

2.3. Technique of CPB

2.3.1. Standard CPB technique (Group A)

Cardiopulmonary bypass was established by standard aortic cannulation and two-stage venous cannulation of the right atrium. Antegrade cold blood cardioplegia (blood and St. Thomas´ solution in a ratio of 4:1) and topical cooling for the arrested heart and myocardial protection were employed. Anticoagulation was induced before CBP with heparin (2.5 mg ⁺kg-1), and the activated clotting time (ACT over 480 seconds) was monitored. Heparin was neutralized with protamin in a 1:1 ratio.

The extracorporeal circuit consisted of a hollow fiber membrane oxygenator (PrimO2x, Sorin Group, Italy) and roller pump with a non-pulsatile flow (Stockert S3, Sorin Group, Germany) in an open modification with 40.0 μm arterial line filter (Dideco Micro 40R, Mirandola,

Italy). The oxygenator and tubing system were primed with a mixture of crystalloid (Hartmann´s solution), colloids (Voluven), 10% Mannitol solution, 8.4% sodium bicarbonate, magnesiumsulphur solution, 5.000 IU of heparin. The CPB involved normothermia and calculated blood flow 2.4 - 2.8 $l.m^{-2}$. Mean arterial pressure during CPB was maintained at 50 to 75 mmHg and hematocrit above 0.22%. The acid base status was maintained using the alpha-stat perfusion strategy (Figure 2).

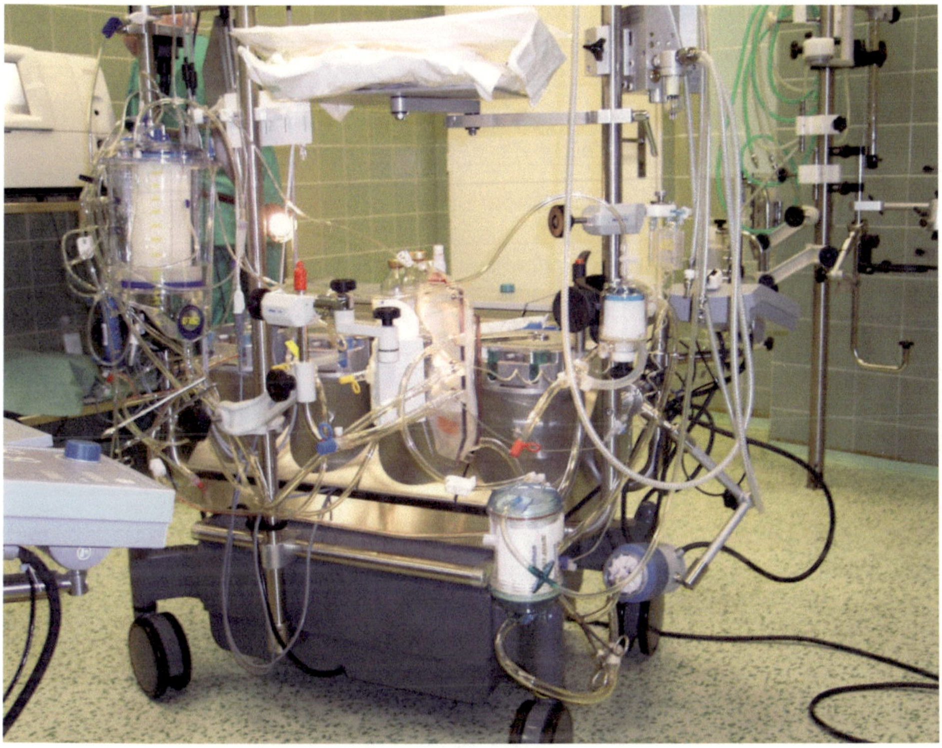

Figure 2. Standard cardiopulmonary bypass equipment

2.3.2. Miniaturized CPB technique (Group B)

Miniaturized CPB was established using aortic cannulation and a two-stage venous cannulation of the right atrium. A fully integrated minisystem (Synergy SorinR, Sorin Group, Italy) consisted of a centrifugal pump, membrane oxygenator, 40.0 μm arterial line filter and a venous bubbletrap. Cardiotomy suction and vents were not used. The whole system was a closed loop with the internal surface treated with a phosphorylcholin coat

(PH.I.S.I.O, Sorin Group, Italy) and very short tubing. The priming solution, heparinization, calculated blood flow, temperature and surgery technique were identical to the standard CPB (Group A). While initiating CPB, crystalloid priming was retrogradely flushed with blood from the arterial line to minimize hemodilution (retrograde autologus priming). Pro-

http://dx.doi.org/10.5772/54300

tection of the myocardium during surgery (blood cardioplegia and topical cooling) was the same as in Group A (Figure 3, 4).

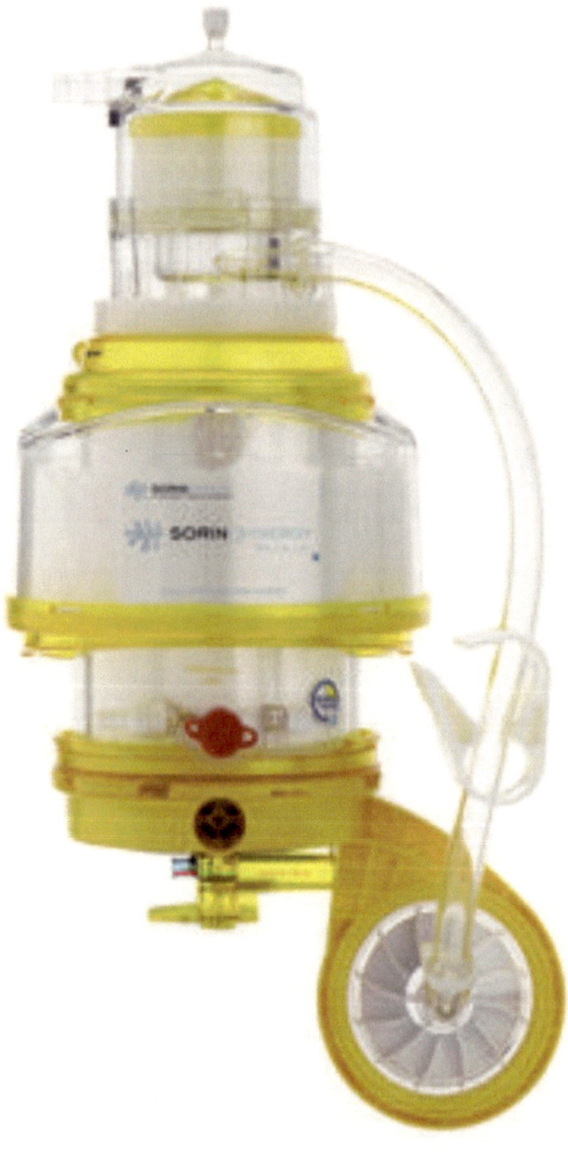

Figure 3. Miniaturized integrated CPB system (Synergy Sorin, Sorin Group, Italy)

2.4. Monitoring technique

Before the surgical procedure, at the time of anesthesia introduction, the optical multiparametric sensor (NeuroventR PTO, Raumedic AG, Germany) (Figure 5) was inserted under sterile conditions into the right deltoid muscle without the use of local anesthesia (Figure 6). Continuous measurement of interstitial tissue oxygen tension (ptO2) was made during the surgical procedure and postoperatively by a special monitoring system (DataloggerR MPR2 logO, Raumedic AG, Germany) (Figure 7,8).

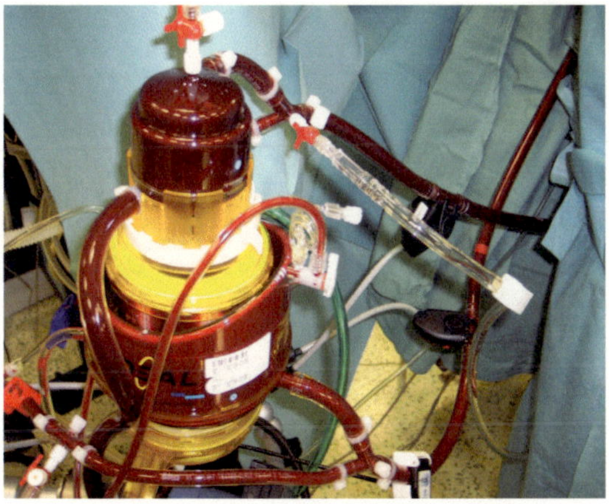

Figure 4. Miniaturized integrated CPB system (Synergy Sorin, Sorin Group, Italy) during surgery

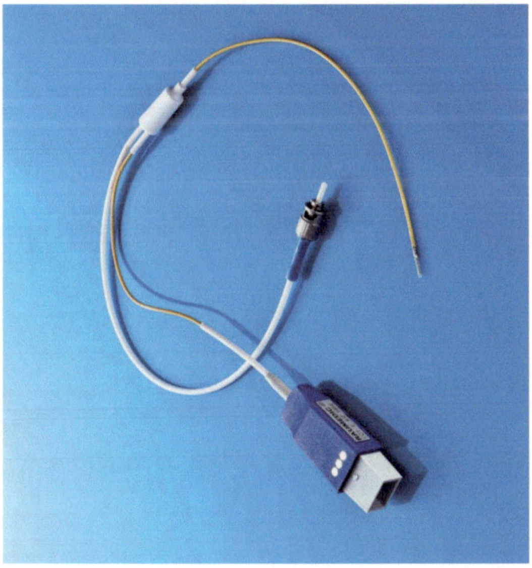

Figure 5. Multiparametric sensor Neurovent® PTO (Raumedic AG, Germany)

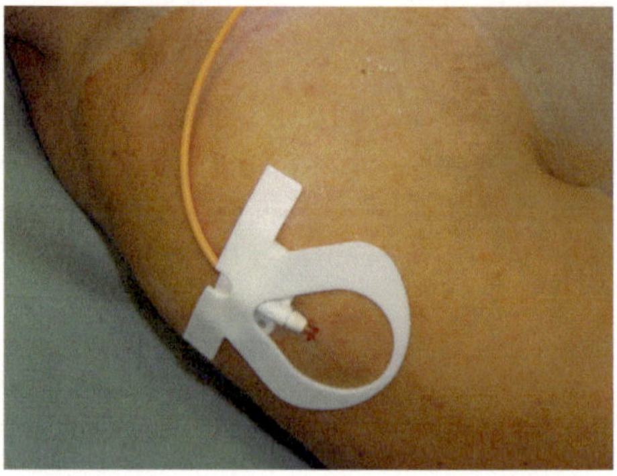

Figure 6. Sensor inserted into the right deltoid muscle

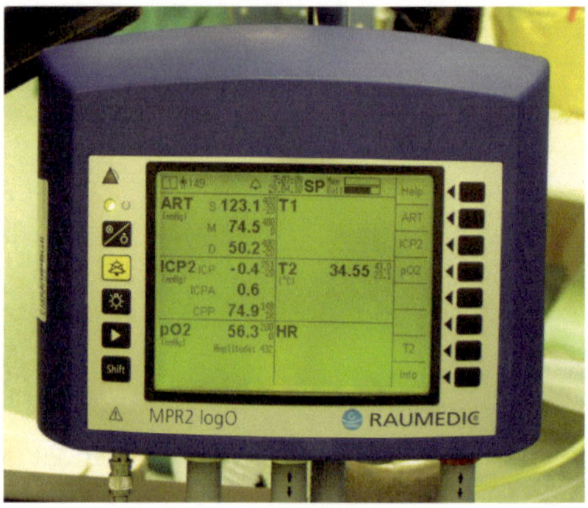

Figure 7. Analyzer Dattaloger® MPR2 logO (Raumedic AG, Germany)

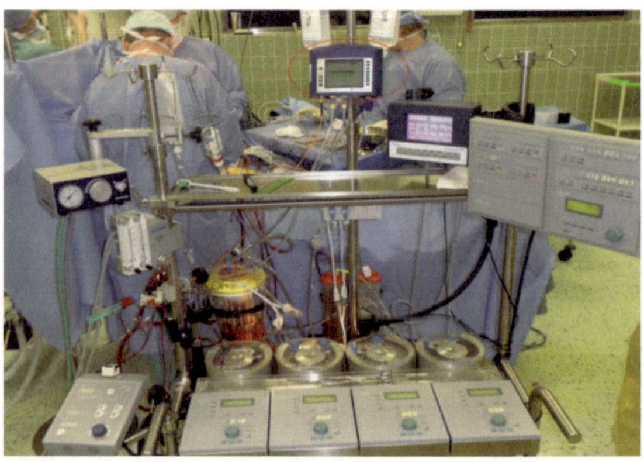

Figure 8. Analyzer Dattaloger® MPR2 logO (Raumedic AG, Germany) during CPB

Arterial blood pressure, blood flow during CPB, laboratory markers of tissue perfusion, blood gases and body temperature were recorded and analyzed as well.

Data from the oxymetric catheter in all patients were compared at the following time intervals: 1) 30 min after incision, 2) 15 min before CPB, 3) CPB, 4,5,6- at 20 min intervals during CPB, 7) end of crossclamp, 8) 15 min. after release of crossclamp, 9) end of CPB, 10) 15 min after termination of CPB, 11) end of surgery, 12,13,14- at 1 h intervals in the I.C.U.

2.5. Statistical analysis

Demographic and perioperative data are reported as number, means ± standard deviation (S.D.) or median. Comparisons between preoperative characteristics and perioperative data were made using the Student's *t* test or the Mann-Whitney U-test and Kolmogorov-Smirnov test where appropriate. Values are expressed as means ± standard error of the mean (S.E.M.). Intergroup comparisons between two variables at the same time point were performed using the Mann-Whitney U-test. Group comparison was done using the Wilcoxon test for paired data.

The data were analyzed using the programs NCSS 2004 and Statistica. Differences were considered statistically significant at the level of $P<0.05$.

3. Results

40 patients (32 men, 8 women) were included in the study. The mean age ± S.D. was 69 ± 5.8 years in Group A and 67 ± 6.8 years in Group B. Preoperative patient characteristics are presented in Table 1. There were no statistical significant differences in preoperative characteristics between the groups.

Operative data are listed in Table 2. The groups were comparable for these parameters.

Statistically significant differences were found when groups were compared in regard to the use of a lesser priming volume in mini CPB as one of its main advantages in comparison with standard CPB (1501 ± 44 ml in Group A vs. 837 ± 205 ml in Group B). It was also associated with a lower drop in hematocrit level during CPB (25.3 ± 1.1% in Group A and 31.0 ± 2.3% in Group B). The immediate postoperative values of hematocrit (ICU admission) were not significantly different.

Analysis of the data during CPB showed differences betweens groups.

The main difference was a lower real blood flow during CPB in Group B (3.5 ± 0.51 $l.min^{-1}$) vs. calculated flow (4.6 ± 0.45 $l.min^{-1}$) than real flow in Group A (4.9 ± 0.41 $l.min^{-1}$) vs. calculated flow (4.7 ± 0.39 $l.min^{-1}$) (Table 2).

There was a direct correlation between mean arterial pressure (MAP) and ptO2 in Group A during CPB (↓MAP ≈ ↓ ptO2). Pumped blood flow was continuously maintained at the same calculated level. A decrease in ptO2 levels without correlation to MAP was found during surgery after CPB (Figure 9).

On the other hand, a direct correlation between pumped blood flow and MAP (↓flow ≈↓MAP) was found during CPB in Group B. The value of ptO2 was continuously higher and independent at this time. A decrease in ptO2 levels without correlation to MAP was found during surgery after CPB as in Group A (Figure 10).

Lower levels of ptO2 without correlation to MAP were analysed postoperatively in both groups and we observed a trend towards a reduced ptO2 during the first hours after admission to the intensive care unit (Figure 9,10).

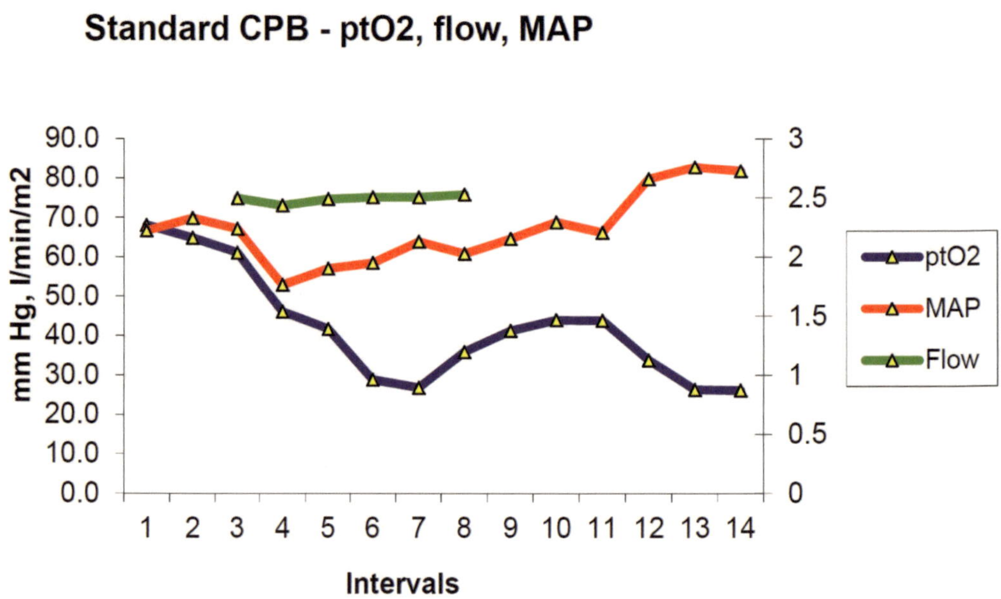

Figure 9. Levels of ptO_2, blood flow and MAP in Group A (standard CPB) in intervals (Intervals: 1- 30 min. after incision, 2- 15 min. before CPB, 3- CPB, 4,5,6- à 20 min. of CPB, 7- end of crossclamp, 8- after 15 min., 9- end of CPB, 10- after 15 min., 11- end of surgery, 12,13,14- à 1 h. I.C.U.)

Changes of ptO2 at this time compared with initial level are shown in Figure 11.

Higher levels of ptO2 during and after CPB in comparison with initial levels were observed in Group B. A decrease in ptO2 levels after surgery was found in both groups.

Changes in flow (%) in time compared to calculated flow are shown in Figure 12.

A higher blood flow during perfusion was analysed in Group A and lower than calculated blood flow was found in Group B.

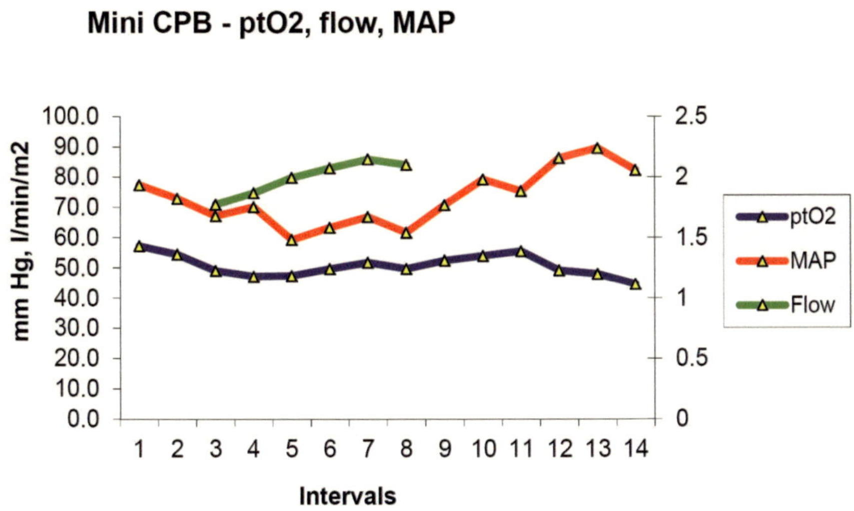

Figure 10. Levels of ptO_2, blood flow and MAP in Group B (mini CPB) in intervals (Intervals: 1- 30 min. after incision, 2- 15 min. before CPB, 3- CPB, 4,5,6- à 20 min. of CPB, 7- end of crossclamp, 8- after 15 min., 9- end of CPB, 10- after 15 min., 11- end of surgery, 12,13,14- à 1 h. I.C.U.)

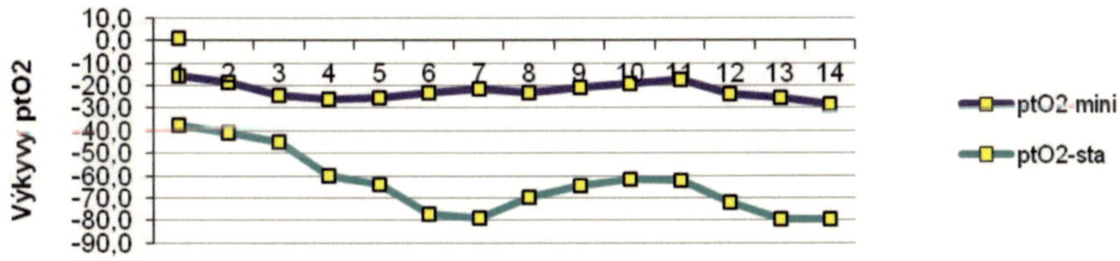

Figure 11. Changes of ptO_2 compared to initial levels (%)(Group A- green line, Group B- blue line. Intervals: 1- 30 min. after incision, 2- 15 min. before CPB, 3- CPB, 4,5,6- à 20 min. of CPB, 7- end of crossclamp, 8- after 15 min., 9- end of CPB, 10-after 15 min., 11- end of surgery, 12,13,14- à 1 h. I.C.U.)

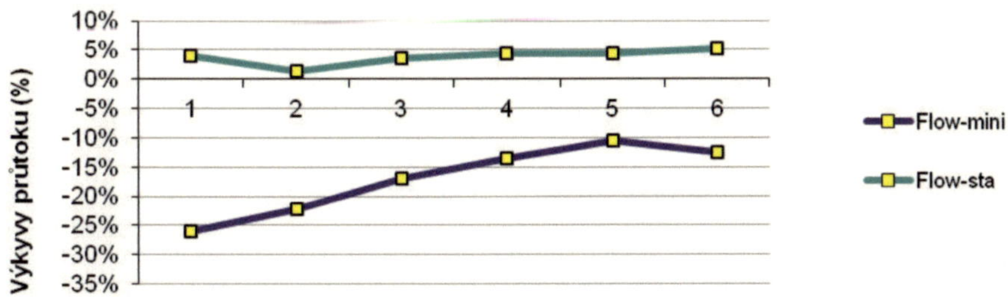

Figure 12. Changes in blood flow (%) during perfusion compared to calculated flow (Group A- green line, Group B- blue line. Intervals: 1- CPB, 2,3,4- à 20 min. of CPB, 5-end of crossclamp, 6- after 15 min.)

http://dx.doi.org/10.5772/54300

We also observed a lower muscle oxygen (ptO2) tension than in arterial blood during the whole operation in both groups.

Peri-operative biochemical parameters of perfusion (arterial blood gas variables) are shown in Table 4. There were no statistically significant differences.

	Group A (n=20)	Group B (n=20)	p-value
pH			
before CPB	7.41 ± 0,06	7.42 ± 0,04	n.s.
during CPB	7.42 ± 0,07	7.41 ± 0,03	n.s.
after CPB	7.39 ± 0,03	7.37± 0,04	n.s.
pO_2 [mm Hg]			
before CPB	142 ± 81	182 ± 72	n.s.
during CPB	171± 31	191 ± 31	n.s.
after CPB	191 ± 71	189 ± 48	n.s.
pCO_2 [mm Hg]			
before CPB	35 ± 3	37 ± 4	n.s.
during CPB	38 ± 6	39 ± 3	n.s.
after CPB	39 ± 5	37 ± 7	n.s.
BE			
before CPB	- 0.53 ± 1.72	- 0.54 ± 1.34	n.s.
during CPB	0.45 ± 1.91	0.29 ± 1.72	n.s.
after CPB	- 1.39 ± 1.8	- 0.40 ± 1.4	n.s.
DO_2 [ml.min-1.m-2]	259 ± 34	256 ± 39	n.s.

Table 4. Laboratory characteristics of perfusion (arterial blood gases)

There were no significant differences in postoperative levels of lactate and arterial blood gas variables between groups (Table 5).

	Group A (n=20)	Group B (n=20)	p-value
pH			
I.C.U. admission	7,45 ± 0,03	7,46 ± 0,06	n.s.
I.C.U after 6 h	7,37 ± 0,05	7,43 ± 0,03	n.s.

	Group A (n=20)	Group B (n=20)	p-value
1. postoper. day	7,40 ± 0,07	7,39 ± 0,05	n.s.
pO_2 [mm Hg]			
I.C.U. admission	98 ± 48	97 ± 60	n.s.
I.C.U after 6 h	171 ± 25.9	170 ± 50	n.s.
1. postoper. day	135 ± 39	141 ± 28	n.s.
pCO_2 [mm Hg]			
I.C.U. admission	30 ± 5	32 ± 4	n.s.
I.C.U after 6 h	35 ± 4	39 ± 6	n.s.
1. postoper. day	36 ± 5	35 ± 4	n.s.
BE			
I.C.U. admission	- 2.93 ± 2.34	- 3.28 ± 2.31	n.s.
I.C.U after 6 h	- 1.8 ± 1,71	- 2.16 ± 2.0	n.s.
1. postoper. day	- 2.61 ± 1.83	- 3.15± 1.91	n.s.
Lactate [mmol/l]			
I.C.U. admission	1.9 ± 0.7	2.1 ± 1.3	n.s.
I.C.U after 6 h	1.8 ± 0.5	2.4 ± 1.7	n.s.
1. postoper. day	2.1± 0.9	2.3 ± 0.8	n.s.

Table 5. Postoperative laboratory characteristics of perfusion (arterial blood gases, lactate)

No death, acute renal failure, or stroke occured during the postoperative course either group. The only differences were postoperative atrial fibrillation (6 in Group A, 2 in Group B) (Table 3).

There were no cases of local complications at the site of inserted sensors, and there were no signs of general infection or sepsis in either group.

4. Discussion

The technology of miniinvasive systems has been in development since the beginning of the 1990s.

The benefits of using miniinvasive systems have been clearly proven in many publications. Studies show that the use of miniinvasive systems result in a decrease in quantity of administered blood derivatives, a decrease in blood loss, lower incidence of postoperative neurologic complications, a shorter stay in the ICU, period of artificial ventilation and total hospital stay [4-8].

http://dx.doi.org/10.5772/54300

On the other hand some studies do not entirely confirm the positive clinical effect of using minisystems [13], even though the laboratory tests of these studies lean towards miniinvasive systems compared to standard CPB.

One discussed question while using CPB is the constant value of blood flow during the operation [1,2]. Preoperative calculated value of optimal blood flow using mini CPB is the same as standard CPB.

Nevertheless adequate and optimal blood flow during CPB is still an important question. There are no standards for optimal pump flow during CPB. Initial flow is calculated on the basis of body surface area and a temperature management strategy. The calculated blood flow often has to be decreased during perfusion using mini CPB.

The reason for the necessary decrease in pumped blood flow is the increase in arterial blood pressure during the operation most likely as a result of increased blood in the vascular bed (an absence of a CPB reservoir).

Another reason for decreased flow could be the flooding of the operating field during worsened venous return.

Decreased venous return could be another reason. The flow of a centrifugal pump during mini CPB is fully dependent upon adequate venous return with resultant filling of the venous bed of the patient.

In an effort to achieve the calculated blood flow the centrifugal rotational velocity is increased resulting in increased suction pressure within the venous part of the system and thus suction of the artifact with the venous cannulas. The ability to control flow via a cardiotomy reservoir is missed in this case. A possible solution is an increase of blood in the body (patient´s body position in space, application of vasopressors, filling of the circulatory system) or decreasing blood flow in the system. The "antitrendelenburg" position (head up), during which the filling of the lower half of the body is partly increased and consequently an increased venous flow (return), is of some advantage. Further, in this position the heart chambers are adequately emptied. The trendelenburg position described in the literature as a means to increase venous return has typically no effect when mini CPB is applied. In the case of a closed system the patient´s own body is the reservoir.

It is necessary during the procedure to have a coordinated approach between the surgeon, anesthesiologist and perfusionist.

During an acute case of a decrease in the pumped blood flow, in the presence of an impaired venous return, filling was supplemented by blood collected in a collapsible bag at the beginning of the operation. To restore satisfactory parameters usually a sufficient volume of less than 100ml was required.

The perfusion pressure in both groups was maintained at levels between 50-70 mmHg [1,3,9,10]. In the case of mini CPB this did not fall below 50 mmHg while on the other hand there was a tendency for higher levels of pressure.

Different results in comparison with both groups after analysis of ptO2, MAP and blood flow during CPB and postoperative course were found to our greatest surprise.

A direct correlation between mean arterial pressure (MAP) and ptO2 was observed in Group A during CPB. Pumped blood flow was continuously maintained at the same calculated level. On the other hand, direct correlation between pumped blood flow and MAP was found during mini CPB in Group B. The value of ptO2 was continuous, higher and independent at this time.

So far, we have no clear explanation for these differences in both groups. The main reason could most likely be due to differences in the amount of circulating blood volume, the possibility of using a cardiotomy reservoir, and the subsequent need to use catecholamines during perfusion.

A decrease in the ptO2 levels not correlated with MAP were analysed during CPB, after CPB and in the postoperative course in both groups. This is the most likely cause of decreased circulatory volume resulting in the use of vasopressors (catecholamines). A decrease in body temperature during this phase of the operation leading to peripheral vasoconstriction can also contribute equally to this phenomenon.

The lower level of acquired hemodilution (higher hematocrit) during the operation, determined by a lower filling volume and retrograde autologous priming are major advantages of using perfusion by mini CPB.

Supply of oxygen to the tissues during reduced flow of the bypass machine is therefore safe in the case of an increased hematocrit. In the mini CPB group, only 2/3 of the priming fluid was used as opposed to classical CPB and another 1/3 of this fluid was replaced by the patient's blood using retrograde autologous priming. The hematocrit provides sufficient capacity to supply oxygen in normothermia. A combination of decreased primary filling and a shortened tubing system resulted in an increased hematocrit and concentration of hemoglobin as expected in Group B (mini CPB).

In our study a closed integrated system coated with phosphorylcholine was used. The tubing system was shortened to a minimum, by placing it as close as possible to the patient, to minimalize priming. The system used allowed for partial back-flow of the patient´s own blood (retrograde autologous priming). Coronary suction was not used and neither was a venous reservoir. No cell saver device was used.

There were no technical perfusion linked complications.

In comparison to the perfusion parameters of both groups there were no differences during surgery. The monitored values of arterial blood gases were comparable and showed optimal perfusion management in both groups. Likewise, the values in both groups were comparable in the early postoperative course.

No death, acute renal failure, or stroke occurred in the postoperative course of either group. The only difference noted was in the incidence of postoperative atrial fibrillation with group B (mini CPB) showing better results. This study was limited by a small number of patients.

http://dx.doi.org/10.5772/54300

In a comparison of monitored parameters of the clinical course we can suggest that lower values of blood flow during perfusion in group B (mini CPB) were sufficient and had no negative impact in the postoperative course.

Tolerance to decreased flow in mini CPB, with maintained sufficient blood pressure, is in our opinion due to a higher hematocrit. Decrease in volume of priming fluid together with technique of RAP ensures a decreased perioperative hemodilution and thus an increase in blood oxygen carrying capacity.

Another improtant postive aspect of using mini CPB is also a decrease in microcirculatory dysfunction. The system design (closed loop, biocompatible surface area, centrifugal pump, and elimination of cardiotomy suction) and decreased contact with artificial surfaces (shortened tubing system and absence of cardiotomy reservoir) during lower flow decreases the negative impact on the organism. A lower intensity in the inflammatory reaction results in a decreased dysfunction of the endothelium and subsequent malperfusion. To verify this impact of the minisystem on the microcirulation it is necessary to perform further studies.

5. Conclusion

A miniaturized system of CPB enables perfusion with relatively low flow and in normothermic conditions. Monitoring perfusion of skeletal muscle during the operation and our experience shows that it is a safe method of perfusion.

Our work experience and the results of this pilot study suggest that a flow decrease in mini CPB is well tolerated by the organism.

The chapter was supported by PRVOUK P 37/04/440.

Author details

Jiri Mandak

Address all correspondence to: jiri.mandak@centrum.cz

Department of Cardiac Surgery, Charles University in Prague, Faculty of Medicine and University Hospital in Hradec Kralove, Hradec Kralove, Czech Republic

References

[1] Murphy GS, Hessel EA, Groom RC. Optimal perfusion during cardiopulmonary bypass: An evidence-based approach. Anesth Analg 2009; 108:1394-417.

[2] Fernandes P, MacDonald J, Cleland A, Walsh G, Mayer R. What is optimal flow using a mini-bypass system? Perfusion 2010; 25:133-9.

[3] Lonsky V. Mimotelni obeh v klinicke praxi (Cardiopulmonary bypass in clinical practice). Praha: Grada Publishing, 2004. ISBN 80-247-0653-9.

[4] Koivisto SP, Wistbacka JO, Rimpilainen R, Nissinen J, Loponen P, Teittinen K, Biancari F. Miniaturized versus conventional cardiopulmonary bypass in high-risk patiens undergoing coronary bypass surgery. Perfusion 2010; 25:65-70.

[5] Curtis N, Vohra HA, Ohri SK. Mini extracorporeal culit cardiopulmonary bypass system: a review. Perfusion 2010; 25:115-24.

[6] Dobele T. Schwirtz G, Gahl B, Eckstein F. Mini ECC vs. Conventional ECC: an examination of velus oxygen saturation, hemoglobin, haematocrit, flow, cardiac index and oxygen delivery. Perfusion 2010; 25:125-31.

[7] Mazzei V, Nasso G, Salamone G, Castorino F, Tommasini A, Anselmi A. Prospective randomized comparison of coronary bypass grafting with minimal extracorporeal circulation system (MECC) versus off-pump coronary surgery. Circulation 2007; 116:1-7.

[8] Beghi C, Nicolini F, Agostinelli A, Borrello B, Budillon AM, Bacciottini F, Friggeri M, Costa A, Belli L, Battistelli L, Gherli T. Mini-Cardiopulmonary Bypass System: Results of a Prospective Randomized Study. Ann Thorac Surg 2006; 81:1396-1400.

[9] Boston US, Slater JM, Orszulak TA, Cook DJ. Hierarchy of regional oxygen delivery during cardiopulmonary bypass. Ann Thorac Surg 2001; 71:260-4.

[10] Haugen o, Farstad M, Kvalheim M, Rynning SE, Mongstad A., Husby P. Intraoperative fluid balance during cardiopulmonary bypass: effects of different mean arterial pressures. Perfusion 2007; 22:273-8.

[11] Benaron DA, Parachikov IH, Friedland S, Soetikno R, Brock-Utne J, van der Starre PJ, Nezhat C, Terris MK, Maxim PG, Carson JJ, Razavi MK, Gladstone HB. Continuous, noninvasive and localized microvascular tissue dimetry using virble light spectroscopy. Anesthesiology 2004; 100.1469-75.

[12] Soller BR, Idwasi PO, Balauger J, Levin S, Simsir SA, Vander Salm TJ, Collette H, Heard SO et al. Noninvasive, NIRS-measured muscle pH and PO2 indicate tissue perfusion for cardiac surgical patients on cardiopulmonary bypass. Crit Care Med 2003; 31:2324-31.

[13] Svitek V, Lonsky V, Mandak J, Krejsek J, Kolackova M, Brzek V, Kubicek J, Volt M. No clear clinical bendit of using mini-invasive extracorporeal circulation in coronary artery bypass rafting in low risk patiens. Perfusion 2009; 24:389-95.

Section 2

Coronary Artery Bypass Graft Surgery

Chapter 7

Total Arterial Revascularization in Coronary Artery Bypass Grafting Surgery

Sean Maddock, Gilbert H. L. Tang, Wilbert S. Aronow and Ramin Malekan

Additional information is available at the end of the chapter

http://dx.doi.org/10.5772/54866

1. Introduction

Coronary artery bypass graft (CABG) operations are one of the most commonly performed surgical procedures, with a worldwide prevalence of over 800,000 annually and more than 350,000 operations being performed in the United States each year [1]. The use of the left internal mammary artery (LIMA) is widely considered to be the gold standard for conventional CABG operations. Its use has been shown to result in a lower incidence of reintervention, fewer myocardial infarctions, a lower incidence of angina, and lower associated mortality rates than with the use of saphenous vein grafts alone. Also when compared to saphenous vein grafts, LIMA use has been shown to have greater long-term patency results [1, 2]. For patients with multivessel coronary disease undergoing what is usually referred to as conventional CABG, the LIMA is typically grafted to the left anterior descending (LAD) artery with saphenous vein grafts often used to bypass the remaining coronary occlusions. However, arterial conduits are now being more frequently used as choices for the second and third conduits in place of saphenous vein grafts to achieve total arterial revascularization (TAR) of the myocardium due to superior patency and long-term survival results. This article provides a review of TAR using the right internal mammary artery (RIMA) and radial artery as additional arterial conduits in conjunction with the LIMA as a first choice conduit. The reported benefits of TAR when compared to conventional CABG procedures using the LIMA and saphenous vein grafts are discussed.

2. LIMA use in CABG

The LIMA is widely considered to be the best conduit for CABG procedures. In a study of the Society of Thoracic Surgeons National Cardiac Database performed by Tabata *et al.*, data from 541,368 CABG surgeries taking place between 2002 and 2005 were analyzed. Among all

procedures performed, 92.4% of patients had at least one IMA graft, and the frequency of LIMA usage by each hospital ranged from 48.0% to 100% with a median of 94% [3]. The presence of an IMA graft has also been identified as an independent predictor of survival and confers significantly better long-term survival rates than the use of saphenous vein grafts alone [2].

While anatomically identical to the LIMA, the RIMA is rarely used in CABG procedures, and is almost always used as part of bilateral internal mammary artery (BIMA) grafts when it is utilized. Despite several studies showing that BIMA use confers significantly improved clinical outcomes [4-6], between 2003 and 2005 the frequency of BIMA use was only 4% [3]. Reasons for not using the RIMA include increased operative time and perceived technical difficulty associated with the harvest, concern for perioperative morbidity and mortality, the possibility of reoperations for bleeding, sternal wound infection, and uncertainty as to whether there is a significant benefit with BIMA grafting [7, 8]

3. Outcomes of BIMA in CABG

Despite its low prevalence of use, many studies have shown that RIMA use in conjunction with the LIMA can confer significantly better clinical outcomes when compared to conventional CABG procedures with the LIMA and saphenous vein grafts.

Survival benefits of BIMA versus Single Internal Mammary Artery (SIMA)

Several observational, retrospective studies have found that there are significantly greater long-term survival benefits in patients who received BIMA grafting compared to SIMA grafting. Lytle *et al.* studied 10,124 elective CABG patients receiving either SIMA or BIMA grafts with or without any additional vein grafts in a retrospective, non-randomized study with a mean follow-up of 10 post-operative years. Hospital mortality rates were identical for the SIMA and BIMA groups (0.7%). However, over 12 years of post-operative follow up, survival rates for BIMA patients were significantly better than for SIMA patients (79.1% versus 71.6% respectively, $p < 0.001$) [9]. In a follow-up to the original study, which extended the mean post-operative follow up to 16.5 years, survival rates for BIMA and SIMA patients at 20 years were 50% versus 37% respectively ($p < 0.0001$), demonstrating a significant long-term survival advantage for patients receiving two internal mammary grafts compared to just one [10].

Nasso *et al.* aimed to determine whether or not there were significant benefits to using two arterial conduits rather than just a single arterial conduit. 815 patients were randomized to one of four revascularization strategies: *in situ* LIMA to LAD plus isolated RIMA Y graft, *in situ* RIMA to LAD plus *in situ* LIMA, *in situ* LIMA to LAD plus free radial artery, and *in situ* LIMA to LAD with saphenous vein grafts as a control. All revascularization groups received saphenous vein grafts to bypass the remaining coronary occlusions, if needed. Although the authors found no significant overall survival advantage between any of their revascularization groups over a follow-up period of two years, there was a significant difference in survival when considering cardiac event-free survival. Patients in groups receiving two arterial grafts had significantly better cardiac event-free survival rates when compared to patients who only

http://dx.doi.org/10.5772/54866

received a single internal mammary artery (LIMA) grafted to the LAD with saphenous vein grafts. These arterial revascularization strategies were also seen to convey significantly better cardiac event-free survival rates to elderly (> 75 years) patients as well. The study did not find any significant differences in survival based on the choice of either the RIMA or the radial artery as the second arterial conduit [11].

In the longest reported retrospective analysis of CABG procedures, ranging from 6 weeks to 32 years of follow up, Kurlansky *et al.* conducted a review of 4,584 isolated CABG procedures between 1972 and 1994. When patient differences were accounted for and comparisons made between 2,197 matched patients, survival was 16.5% for SIMA patients and 28.5% for BIMA patients after 25 years ($p = 0.001$). The median survival for SIMA patients was 11.8 years compared to 15.9 years for BIMA patients. There were no significant differences between the two groups in the rates of non-fatal myocardial infarction, reoperation, percutaneous coronary intervention, permanent stroke, or composite freedom from late adverse cardiac events. [12

The location of the distal anastomosis of the RIMA graft also does not appear to significantly affect clinical outcomes of patients undergoing BIMA grafting. Kurlansky *et al.* performed a propensity-matched study of 2,215 patients undergoing BIMA CABG procedures having the RIMA grafted to either the right coronary system or to the left coronary system. In both the matched and unmatched analyses, there was no significant difference in operative or late mortality between the two groups. The median survival for propensity-matched patients in both groups was 16.1 years ($p = 0.671$) [13]. In another study by Rankin *et al.* there were no significant differences in long-term outcomes based on grafting territory of BIMA grafts as long as they are anastomosed to the two largest coronary systems [14].

Not all studies have found significantly increased survival rates for BIMA use over SIMA use. In a study performed by Dewar *et al.*, there was not a significant difference in the 5 or 7-year survival rates for patients undergoing either unilateral or bilateral IMA grafting with supplemental vein grafts. 5-year survival rates for SIMA and BIMA revascularization for patients less than 60 years of age were 94.4% and 94.8%, respectively (p = not significant). There was also no significant difference in 5-year survival rates for patients over 60 years of age. However, the authors did note that there was a trend in lower rates of angina in the patient group receiving BIMA grafts less than 60 years of age [15].

4. Patency of RIMA versus LIMA

Patency is the most important determinant in long-term prognosis [7]. Due to the extremely low prevalence of use for the RIMA, there have been few studies evaluating its patency compared to the LIMA. However, the studies that have been performed suggest that the RIMA has similar early and even long-term patency rates as the LIMA, especially when grafted to similar coronary territories [17].

Fukui *et al.* reviewed the angiographic records of 705 patients undergoing BIMA CABG procedures. Early angiography and 1-year angiographic results for RIMA patency are good,

with an overall patency of 98.8% at early angiography and 94.3% at 1-year postoperative follow-up compared to 99.1% and 97.0% for the LIMA at the same follow-up times ($p = 0.7732$ and $p = 0.1288$, respectively). In terms of grafting technique, at both early and 1-year angiographic follow up, there were no significant differences in the patencies of *in situ* versus free RIMA grafts. For free RIMA grafts, there were also no significant differences in patency rates between sites of proximal anastomoses (composite versus aorta). However, for the *in situ* RIMA, patency rates were significantly better when anastomosed to the anterior coronary territory when compared to other grafting methods ($p < 0.0001$)[16].

Tatoulis *et al.* evaluated the results of 991 consecutive RIMA postoperative CABG angiograms taking place between 1986 and 2008. The main focus was graft patency, with grafts considered non-patent if they had a greater than 80% stenosis, string sign, or total occlusion. When compared to the LIMA for identical grafting territories, there was no significant difference in RIMA and LIMA patency. For the LAD, overall LIMA patency was 96.9% while overall RIMA patency was 94.6% ($p=0.74$). When grafted to the circumflex, LIMA patency was 90.7% versus RIMA patency of 91.9% ($p = 0.85$). Long-term patency results for the RIMA were favorable as well, with 92% of 352 RIMA grafts in place for greater than 10 years being patent. RIMA patencies were always better than radial artery or saphenous vein graft patencies. At 15 years, RIMA patency was 79% compared to 50.7% for saphenous vein grafts ($p<0.001$). 15-year data were not available for the radial artery; 10-year patency was 78% ($p<0.01$ when compared to RIMA 10-year patency). However, the authors noted that data for radial artery patency is limited [17].

There are a variety of grafting techniques for BIMA, such as *in situ* grafting versus Y/T-grafts that may have an impact on patency rates. In a study by Glineur *et al.*, 304 patients receiving BIMA grafts were randomized to receive either an *in situ* RIMA graft or a Y-graft with the RIMA anastomosed proximally to the *in situ* LIMA as an end-to-side graft. Follow-up angiography was performed at 6 months and the RIMA patency rate in both groups was 97% ($p = 0.99$) [18]. In a similar but slightly larger study, Calafiore *et al.* also found no significant differences in patency rates between *in situ* and Y-graft RIMA grafts at both early (13 days) and long-term (17 months) angiographic follow up [19]. A longer study by Hwang *et al.* studied 5-year angiographic patency results of BIMA grafting configurations. At 1 year of follow-up, *in situ* RIMA patency rates were not significantly different than Y-graft RIMA patency rates (92.5% versus 95.7%, respectively, $p = 0.138$). Similarly at 5 years of follow up, there were also no significant differences in patency rates (92.5% *in situ* versus 92.4% Y-graft, $p = 0.978$) [20].

5. Myocardial infarction, cerebrovascular accidents, freedom from reoperation, and quality of life

Stevens *et al.* report that patients undergoing BIMA CABG operations had significantly better long-term freedom from myocardial infarction (MI) and from coronary reoperation. After 10 post-operative years, 85% of BIMA patients were free of myocardial infarction compared to 82% of patients receiving LIMA grafts ($p = 0.001$). 99% of BIMA patients also were free from coronary reoperation compared to 98% of LIMA patients ($p = 0.01$) [4].

While Burfeind *et al.* found no significant difference in 15-year mortality rates for patients receiving single IMA grafts or multiple (bilateral) IMA grafts, they did find significant differences in the rates of MI and CABG reoperation. However, these rates differ based on the definition of what constitutes a patient receiving multiple IMA grafts. In their study 1,067 patients that had undergone isolated CABG procedures were analyzed by three different methods. In the first analysis (analysis I), patients were analyzed based on the initial surgical strategy for revascularization – SIMA or BIMA grafts. However, not all patients who were designated to receive BIMA grafts were able to be revascularized with multiple IMAs, and likewise some patients designated to receive SIMA grafts ultimately received BIMA grafts. Analyses II and III were therefore performed based on the surgery the patient ultimately received and not the initial surgical strategy. Analysis II defined "multiple IMA grafts" based on the number of distal anastomoses performed. Therefore, in analysis II, multiple coronary systems anastomosed with multiple IMA grafts were considered "multiple IMA grafts" as well as a single coronary system sequentially anastomosed with a single IMA graft. In analysis III only multiple coronary systems anastomosed with multiple IMA grafts were considered to be "multiple IMA grafts." In both analyses II and III, Burfeind *et al.* found that there were significantly reduced rates of CABG reoperation in patients receiving multiple IMA grafts when compared to patients only receiving a single IMA graft (analysis II: 9.7% reop SIMA, 4.5% BIMA $p = 0.0095$; analysis III: 9.7% reop SIMA, 3.4% BIMA, $p = 0.0026$). However, in analysis III there was also a significantly reduced rate of MI in BIMA patients when compared with SIMA patients (17.4% versus 11.6% for SIMA and BIMA patients, respectively, $p = 0.0181$) [6].

In their original retrospective study on BIMA versus SIMA grafting in elective CABG patients, Lytle *et al.* also found that patients receiving BIMA grafts had significantly greater reoperation-free survival rates after 12 post-operative years than patients receiving only SIMA grafts with or without any additional vein grafts. BIMA patients had a reoperation-free survival of 76.8% compared to the 62.4% reoperation-free survival rate of SIMA patients [9].

As previously mentioned, Nasso *et al.* found that patients receiving two arterial grafts had significantly better long-term, cardiac-event free survival outcomes than patients who just received a single arterial graft with or without additional saphenous vein grafts. As expected, adverse cardiac events occurred significantly less frequently in the groups receiving two arterial grafts versus the group receiving just one. There was no significant difference in the occurrence of adverse cardiac events between the three groups receiving two arterial grafts. Cerebrovascular complications occurred more frequently in the SIMA group, however this difference was not significant. The authors note that this increased incidence of cerebrovascular complications may be due to the more extensive manipulation of the ascending aorta needed in the SIMA group due to the greater number of proximal anastomoses [11].

Damgaard *et al.* performed a study to assess the health-related quality of life improvements in patients undergoing traditional CABG procedures versus patients undergoing TAR CABG procedures. 331 patients were randomized between the two revascularization techniques and over 90% of patients responded to the questionnaire at the specified time points. Preopera-

tively, patient scores in all areas of the questionnaire were significantly lower than that of the results of the standardized Danish population. Post-operatively, both revascularization groups showed significant improvement in all areas at 3 months and 11 months, with the TAR group showing improvement in the 'social functioning' category that was significantly higher than the conventional revascularization group. There was no significant difference in post-operative improvement in the categories 'physical component summary,' 'bodily pain,' and 'vitality' between the two revascularization groups [21].

6. Incidence of sternal wound infection, subset of patients benefiting from BIMA, IMA harvesting techniques, and operative time in BIMA CABG

One of the main concerns amongst surgeons regarding the use of BIMA in CABG procedures is the occurrence of sternal wound infections (SWI). When both internal mammary arteries are harvested, blood supply to the sternum may be more severely compromised than in single IMA procedures, thus increasing the risk for developing SWI. Various pre-operative and intra-operative techniques have been used to prevent the incidence of SWI, such as the use of prophylactic antibiotics, double gloving, and skeletonized IMA harvesting [7]. Skeletonized IMA harvesting is thought to preserve the collateral blood supply to the sternum and reduce the risk of infection [22].

Patients who are insulin-dependent diabetics, morbidly obese, or who have severe COPD are at a higher risk of developing SWI (DSWI = deep sternal wound infection, definition varies) and, in general, bilateral harvesting of the IMAs is avoided in these patients [7, 8].

In a study performed by Pevni *et al.*, 1,515 consecutive patients underwent CABG procedures with skeletonized BIMA grafting. In earlier studies, the authors state that, in their past experience, patients with chronic lung disease, diabetic females, and obese diabetics represented absolute contraindications to BIMA grafting for CABG procedures because of the risk of SWI. However in this study, the authors found that there was no evidence of a relationship between diabetes mellitus and DSWI in patients receiving skeletonized BIMA grafts, even with a prevalence of diabetes mellitus of 34% in their patient population [23].

In a meta-analysis of 13 studies regarding BIMA CABG procedures and the harvesting technique for the IMAs, Saso *et al.* found that skeletonizing the IMA as opposed to harvesting it in a pedicled manner lowered the incidence of SWI by 60%. An even greater benefit of skeletonized harvesting was noted in groups at an increased risk for SWI, such as in diabetic patients. The authors also found that these decreased rates of SWI applied to the entire spectrum of sternal infections, including mediastinitis [22].

Kurlansky *et al.* found a slightly higher incidence of SWI amongst diabetic patients receiving BIMA grafting compared to diabetic patients receiving LIMA grafting, but the difference was not significant. However, amongst patients receiving BIMA grafts, the presence of diabetes did affect the occurrence of SWI. This suggests that, while the presence of diabetes mellitus

http://dx.doi.org/10.5772/54866

could still be considered a risk factor for SWI, the risk is not increased by receiving BIMA grafting [12].

One of the probable factors contributing to the low prevalence of BIMA use is the perceived increased operative time required to harvest both IMAs [7]. However, few studies have actually included operative time in their statistical analyses, most simply report aortic cross-clamp and cardiopulmonary bypass times. Gansera *et al.* do report total operative time and found that operative time was significantly increased for patients receiving BIMA grafting compared to patients receiving SIMA grafting (189 minutes versus 164 minutes, respectively, $p = 0.00$). However, the number of anastomoses in the BIMA group was significantly higher than in the SIMA group (3.8 versus 3.1, respectively, $p = 0.00$), which could in part explain the increased operative time observed [8].

7. Radial artery grafts as a second arterial conduit

The success of the LIMA in CABG procedures has lead surgeons to search for other arterial conduits. The radial artery has become a popular choice as an additional arterial conduit in attempts to achieve total arterial revascularization of the myocardium. There are numerous advantages to using the radial artery, including its long length, exposure to systemic blood pressures, and the fact that it is seldomly affected by atherosclerosis. However, the radial artery has a thicker tunica media, which is thought to contribute to its greater vasoconstrictor response than the IMA and could possibly lead to vessel occlusion. Thus, care must be taken during operative harvesting and the use of calcium-channel blockers may ameliorate a vasospastic response [24].

Like the LIMA, the radial artery has been shown to have significantly better short and long-term patency results and outcomes than vein grafts. In the radial artery patency study (RAPS), Desai *et al.* randomized 561 patients to receive a radial artery graft to either the inferior (right) coronary territory or to the lateral (circumflex) coronary territory, with a saphenous vein graft anastomosed to the opposite territory in each group as a control. All patients also received a LIMA graft to the LAD, with the main endpoint of the study being 1-year angiographic complete occlusion of the radial artery versus saphenous vein. In this definition of occlusion, grafts displaying the string-sign would be considered patent. At the mean follow-up of 10.9 months, 13.6% of saphenous vein grafts were completely occluded and 8.6% of radial artery grafts were completely occluded ($p = 0.009$). The authors also found that the patency of radial artery grafts depends on the severity of the native vessel stenosis, with better patency results corresponding with higher grades of stenosis. Thus, the authors recommend using the radial artery for the most highly occluded coronary vessel after the LAD [25].

In a follow-up to the original RAPS study, Deb *et al.* extended the mean angiographic follow-up time to 7.7 years, with 269 patients of the original 561 undergoing late angiography. The primary endpoint was functional graft occlusion; vessels displaying narrowing or reduced flow were considered occluded as well as vessels that were completely occluded. 12.0% of radial artery grafts were determined to be functionally occluded compared with 19.7% of

saphenous vein grafts (p = 0.03). For the secondary endpoint of complete occlusion, 8.9% of radial artery grafts were completely occluded compared with 18.6% of saphenous vein grafts (p = 0.002) [26].

Zacharias *et al.* compared 6-year outcomes in propensity matched CABG patients receiving LIMA to LAD grafts who also received either radial artery grafts or vein grafts only. The authors found that mortality rates were 67% and 98% greater in vein patients than in radial artery patients after 1 and 6 years, respectively. While LIMA patencies were always significantly greater than both radial and vein patencies, 6-year radial graft patencies were systematically greater than that of vein grafts, although the results failed to reach statistical significance. Overall, the use of the radial artery as a second arterial conduit in LIMA to LAD CABG patients is associated with improved long-term survival [27].

Collins *et al.* compared 142 patients receiving either radial artery or saphenous vein grafted to the left circumflex coronary artery, with the end point being 5-year angiographic patency. 98.3% of radial artery grafts and 86.4% of saphenous vein grafts were found to be patent after the 5-year angiographic study of 103 patients (p = 0.04). The rate of graft narrowing was also significantly less in radial artery grafts compared to vein grafts, with narrowing occurring in 10% of patent radial artery grafts and 23% of patent saphenous vein grafts (p = 0.01) [28].

A smaller study by Cameron *et al.* also examined the 5-year angiographic patency results of radial artery grafts. Grafts that displayed a string sign were considered not patent. With a radial artery graft patency rate of 89%, the authors found that the radial artery had a patency rate similar to that of other grafts, although the study was too small to determine whether or not this result was statistically significant [29]. Acar *et al.* report similar results for radial artery graft patencies when compared to the LIMA [30].

Not all studies of radial artery use have been favorable. In a review of 310 patients receiving radial artery grafts between 1996 and 2001, Khot *et al.* found significantly lower patency rates for radial artery grafts when compared to IMA grafts, and similar patency rates when compared to saphenous vein grafts after a mean follow up of 565 ± 511 days. Patency rates of radial artery grafts, LIMA grafts, and saphenous vein grafts were 51.3%, 90.3%, and 64.0%, respectively. While patency rates were similar between radial artery and saphenous vein grafts, there was a significantly higher incidence of severe disease in radial artery grafts (p = 0.0003). Women were also found to have significantly lower radial artery patency rates than men [31]. However, Desai *et al.* specifically note that this study did not use randomized controls, standardized surgical methods, concurrent pharmacology, or routine angiographic follow-up that could lead to potential bias [25].

8. RIMA versus radial artery as a second choice arterial conduit

With favorable clinical results for both RIMA and radial artery use, it is then necessary to decide which is the better choice as a second arterial conduit when attempting to achieve multiple arterial revascularization.

http://dx.doi.org/10.5772/54866

Ruttman *et al.* studied 1,001 patients undergoing CABG procedures either receiving RIMA grafts or radial artery grafts as second conduits after LIMA grafts with or without concomitant saphenous vein grafts added when necessary. Propensity-score matched analysis was performed on the two patient groups to examine the short and long-term outcomes of BIMA grafting versus LIMA plus radial artery grafting. Overall, the evidence provides strong support for the use of the RIMA over the radial artery as a second choice arterial conduit. Radial artery graft occlusion and disease rates were significantly higher than both IMA and saphenous vein anastomoses, with occlusion/disease rates of 37.9%, 10.2%, and 20.9%, respectively. Survival rates for BIMA grafting were 98.9% at 1, 3, and 5 years post-operatively, compared with rates for the radial artery group of 96.8%, 96.3%, and 93.0% at the same post-operative years. The BIMA group also had significantly higher rates of major cardiac and cerebrovascular events-free survival than the radial artery group at the same yearly intervals post-operatively [32].

In a 10-year prospective, randomized trial, Hayward *et al.* examined angiographic outcomes of patients receiving either a radial artery, RIMA, or saphenous vein graft to the second largest coronary target after the LAD, which was grafted with the LIMA. Patients were randomized to two groups: those less than 70 years of age received either a radial artery or RIMA as the second arterial conduit, and those greater than 70 years of age received either a radial artery or saphenous vein. At a mean follow up of 5.5 years, a total of 350 patients between the two groups had angiography performed. In the first group, Kaplan-Meier estimates of graft patency were 89.8% for the radial artery and 83.2% for the RIMA ($p = 0.06$). In the second group, patency estimates were 90.0% for the radial artery and 87.0% for the saphenous vein ($p = 0.29$). With no significant difference in the patency rates between the conduits in each of the two groups, the results show that the choice of conduit for the second largest coronary target does not significantly affect patency, giving surgeons flexibility in their revascularization plans [33].

9. Total Arterial Revascularization (TAR)

The clinical benefits of RIMA and radial artery use have been established, and many studies have indirectly examined the results of TAR in patients receiving BIMA or radial artery grafts without the need of concomitant saphenous vein grafts. However, few studies have specifically compared the clinical outcomes of TAR to conventional CABG procedures.

In a prospective study by Muneretto *et al.*, 200 patients over 70 years of age were randomized into two groups either receiving TAR or conventional CABG (LIMA to LAD with additional saphenous vein grafts if needed). Even though 31% of patients in the TAR group received BIMA grafts, the incidence of perioperative sternal wound complications was found to be 1% in both groups. At the mean follow up of 15 months, the incidence of cardiac-related events (MI, angina, coronary angioplasty, and graft occlusion) was significantly higher in the conventional CABG group compared to patients receiving

TAR. The presence of diabetes and hyperlipidemia had a negative impact on clinical outcome, especially in patients receiving saphenous vein grafts in the conventional CABG group. Conventional CABG surgery was also found to be significantly associated with coronary graft occlusion. Overall, at follow-up, TAR resulted in improved clinical outcomes in patients undergoing CABG procedures when compared to conventional CABG [34].

In a more recent, long-term study with a mean follow-up of 6 years, Chung *et al.* examined 503 patients undergoing isolated CABG procedures for three-vessel coronary disease. Patients in the study either received TAR (117 patients) or conventional revascularization (386 patients). In both the crude analysis and propensity-score matched analysis, there was no significant difference in the rates of death, reintervention, MI, or stroke between the patients receiving TAR or conventional CABG. However, the study did not examine graft patency. The authors conclude that, since the outcomes were similar between the two groups, "the selection of conduit should be more liberal" [35].

Zacharias *et al.* conducted a long-term study of 4,743 patients undergoing multivessel CABG procedures receiving either TAR (612 patients) or conventional CABG (4,131 patients). Early, 30-day mortality was similar for both patient groups, with a 1.30% mortality rate in the TAR group and a 1.67% mortality rate in the conventional group. Due to significant differences in the patient cohort for the two groups, propensity-matched analyses were performed for the 12-year follow up. Late survival was found to be significantly better in total arterial patients with three-vessel disease compared to conventional CABG patients with three-vessel disease ($p < 0.001$). However, there was not a significant difference in late survival between the two groups for patients with two-vessel disease ($p = 0.89$). The authors also noted that the completeness of myocardial revascularization was "critical for maximizing the achievable long-term benefits of total arterial grafting" [36].

10. Summary

Poor long-term patencies of saphenous vein grafts coupled with the greater long term patency results of the LIMA as the gold standard conduit for CABG has prompted surgeons to seek out additional arterial conduits [1,2]. Achieving total arterial revascularization of the myocardium would then be a natural progression for the procedure.

Since it is anatomically identical to the LIMA, the RIMA would be the next logical choice in arterial conduits, yet is rarely used in CABG operations due to the perceived technical difficulty of harvest and increased operating times, a higher risk of developing SWIs, and previous lack of long-term studies of clinical outcomes [7,8]. However, several studies have demonstrated significantly increased long-term survival rates for patients receiving BIMA grafting compared to SIMA grafting [9-12]. BIMA patients also have significantly improved cardiac event-free survival than SIMA patients [4, 6, 9]. Patency rates for RI-

http://dx.doi.org/10.5772/54866

MA grafts have also been shown to be similar to those of the LIMA, even when considering the sites of distal anastomoses and the proximal anastomosing techniques [16, 17, 18, 19, 20]. Further studies are needed to determine if there is any significant effect on operative length in BIMA grafting versus conventional CABG.

The incidence of SWI has been a significant concern for surgeons, especially among high-risk patients such as the morbidly obese, insulin-dependent diabetics, and those with COPD. BIMA harvesting is generally avoided in these patients [7, 8], however studies have shown that BIMA harvesting in general does not significantly affect the incidence of SWIs [12, 23]. The risk of SWI can be even further reduced with the use of skeletonized BIMA harvesting rather than pedicled harvesting [22, 23].

Studies have shown that the radial artery is also a good choice for an arterial conduit after the LIMA. Studies examining clinical outcomes and patency rates of the radial artery have been mixed, with some studies showing better short-term patency rates than saphenous vein grafts [25-28], while other studies have shown that radial artery outcomes are at least similar to those for the RIMA and saphenous vein [11, 32, 33].

While not all studies have been favorable with regards to BIMA and radial artery use [11, 15, 32, 33], studies generally find patency rates and clinical outcomes of these two arterial conduits are at least as good as the currently accepted standards of care, which should give surgeons flexibility in their choice of conduits, ultimately leading to total arterial revascularization.

Studies in general have provided favorable results for TAR, with TAR at least being similar in outcomes to conventional CABG [35]. Several studies have demonstrated that TAR, and the use of arterial conduits in general, provides significantly better late survival (especially in patients with three vessel coronary disease), cardiac event-free survival, and improved health-related quality of life when compared to conventional CABG [11, 21, 36].

11. Conclusion

With favorable results for the use of arterial conduits and results that are at least as good as those seen in conventional CABG, these results should allow surgeons flexibility in their choice of conduits. Due to the significantly increased long-term survival advantages over saphenous vein grafts, BIMA use should be particularly indicated for younger patients, with special attempts to achieve TAR in patients with three vessel disease. Especially with skeletonized harvesting, BIMA may be safe to use in high-risk patients for SWI, such as insulin-dependent diabetics. BIMA use may also decrease the incidence of postoperative cerebrovascular events due to the decreased manipulation of the ascending aorta if both IMAs are used *in situ*. The radial artery is also a suitable conduit to use in conjunction with BIMA or as a second arterial conduit if either the LIMA or RIMA is not suitable for use. This ultimate flexibility provided by TAR should allow surgeons to determine their revascularization strategies not based on the availability of conduits, but by the possible co-morbidities and post-operative complications that may arise based on the patient in question.

Author details

Sean Maddock[1], Gilbert H. L. Tang[1], Wilbert S. Aronow[2] and Ramin Malekan[1]

*Address all correspondence to: TangG@wcmc.com

1 Section of Cardiothoracic Surgery, Department of Surgery, New York Medical College, Westchester Medical Center, Valhalla, NY, USA

2 Division of Cardiology, Department of Medicine, New York Medical College, Westchester Medical Center, Valhalla, NY, USA

References

[1] Goldman, S, Zadina, K, Moritz, T, Ovitt, T, Sethi, G, Copeland, J. G, Thottapurathu, L, Krasnicka, B, Ellis, N, Anderson, R. J, & Henderson, W. VA Cooperative Study Group #207/297/364. Long-term patency of saphenous vein and left internal mammary artery grafts after coronary artery bypass surgery: results from a Department of Veterans Affairs Cooperative Study. J Am Coll Cardiol. (2004). Dec 7; , 44(11), 2149-56.

[2] Cameron, A. A, Green, G. E, Brogno, D. A, & Thornton, J. Internal thoracic artery grafts: 20-year clinical follow-up. J Am Coll Cardiol. (1995). Jan; , 25(1), 188-92.

[3] Tabata, M, Grab, J. D, Khalpey, Z, Edwards, F. H, Brien, O, Cohn, S. M, Bolman, L. H, & Rd, R. M. Prevalence and variability of internal mammary artery graft use in contemporary multivessel coronary artery bypass graft surgery: analysis of the Society of Thoracic Surgeons National Cardiac Database. Circulation. (2009). Sep 15; , 120(11), 935-40.

[4] Stevens, L. M, Carrier, M, Perrault, L. P, Hébert, Y, Cartier, R, Bouchard, D, Fortier, A, Hamamsy, I, & Pellerin, M. Single versus bilateral internal thoracic artery grafts with concomitant saphenous vein grafts for multivessel coronary artery bypass grafting: effects on mortality and event-free survival. J Thorac Cardiovasc Surg. (2004). May; , 127(5), 1408-15.

[5] Rizzoli, G, Schiavon, L, & Bellini, P. Does the use of bilateral internal mammary artery (IMA) grafts provide incremental benefit relative to the use of a single IMA graft? A meta-analysis approach. Eur J Cardiothorac Surg. (2002). Nov; , 22(5), 781-6.

[6] Burfeind WR JrGlower DD, Wechsler AS, Tuttle RH, Shaw LK, Harrell FE Jr, Rankin JS. Single versus multiple internal mammary artery grafting for coronary artery bypass: year follow-up of a clinical practice trial. Circulation. (2004). Sep 14; 110 (11 Suppl 1) :II27-35., 15.

[7] Tatoulis, J, Buxton, B. F, & Fuller, J. A. The right internal thoracic artery: is it underutilized?. Curr Opin Cardiol. (2011). Nov; , 26(6), 528-35.

[8] Gansera, B, Schmidtler, F, Gillrath, G, Angelis, I, Wenke, K, Weingartner, J, Yönden, S, & Kemkes, B. M. Does bilateral ITA grafting increase perioperative complications? Outcome of 4462 patients with bilateral versus 4204 patients with single ITA bypass. Eur J Cardiothorac Surg. (2006). Aug; , 30(2), 318-23.

[9] Lytle, B. W, Blackstone, E. H, Loop, F. D, Houghtaling, P. L, Arnold, J. H, Akhrass, R, Mccarthy, P. M, & Cosgrove, D. M. Two internal thoracic artery grafts are better than one. J Thorac Cardiovasc Surg. (1999). May; , 117(5), 855-72.

[10] Lytle, B. W, Blackstone, E. H, Sabik, J. F, Houghtaling, P, Loop, F. D, & Cosgrove, D. M. The effect of bilateral internal thoracic artery grafting on survival during 20 postoperative years. Ann Thorac Surg. (2004). Dec; discussion 2012-4., 78(6), 2005-12.

[11] Nasso, G, Coppola, R, Bonifazi, R, Piancone, F, Bozzetti, G, & Speziale, G. Arterial revascularization in primary coronary artery bypass grafting: Direct comparison of 4 strategies--results of the Stand-in-Y Mammary Study. J Thorac Cardiovasc Surg. (2009). May; , 137(5), 1093-100.

[12] Kurlansky, P. A, Traad, E. A, Dorman, M. J, Galbut, D. L, Zucker, M, & Ebra, G. Thirty-year follow-up defines survival benefit for second internal mammary artery in propensity-matched groups. Ann Thorac Surg. (2010). Jul; , 90(1), 101-8.

[13] Kurlansky, P. A, Traad, E. A, Dorman, M. J, Galbut, D. L, Zucker, M, & Ebra, G. Location of the second internal mammary artery graft does not influence outcome of coronary artery bypass grafting. Ann Thorac Surg. (2011). May; discussion 1383-4., 91(5), 1378-83.

[14] Rankin, J. S, Tuttle, R. H, Wechsler, A. S, Teichmann, T. L, Glower, D. D, & Califf, R. M. Techniques and benefits of multiple internal mammary artery bypass at 20 years of follow-up. Ann Thorac Surg. (2007). Mar; discussion 1014-5., 83(3), 1008-14.

[15] Dewar, L. R, Jamieson, W. R, Janusz, M. T, Adeli-sardo, M, & Germann, E. MacNab JS, Tyers GF. Unilateral versus bilateral internal mammary revascularization Survival and event-free performance. Circulation. (1995). Nov 1; 92 (9 Suppl) :II, 8-13.

[16] Fukui, T, Tabata, M, Manabe, S, Shimokawa, T, Morita, S, & Takanashi, S. Angiographic outcomes of right internal thoracic artery grafts in situ or as free grafts in coronary artery bypass grafting. J Thorac Cardiovasc Surg. (2010). Apr; , 139(4), 868-73.

[17] Tatoulis, J, Buxton, B. F, & Fuller, J. A. The right internal thoracic artery: the forgotten conduit--5,766 patients and 991 angiograms. Ann Thorac Surg. (2011). Jul; discussion 15-7., 92(1), 9-15.

[18] Glineur, D, Hanet, C, Poncelet, A, Hoore, D, Funken, W, Rubay, J. C, Kefer, J, Astarci, J, Lacroix, P, Verhelst, V, Etienne, R, Noirhomme, P. Y, & El Khoury, P. G. Comparison of bilateral internal thoracic artery revascularization using in situ or Y graft configurations: a prospective randomized clinical, functional, and angiographic midterm evaluation. Circulation. (2008). Sep 30; 118 (14 Suppl) :S, 216-21.

[19] Calafiore, A. M, Contini, M, & Vitolla, G. Di Mauro M, Mazzei V, Teodori G, Di Giammarco G. Bilateral internal thoracic artery grafting: long-term clinical and

angiographic results of in situ versus Y grafts. J Thorac Cardiovasc Surg. (2000). Nov; , 120(5), 990-6.

[20] Hwang, H. Y, Kim, J. S, Cho, K. R, & Kim, K. B. Bilateral internal thoracic artery in situ versus y-composite graftings: five-year angiographic patency and long-term clinical outcomes. Ann Thorac Surg. (2011). Aug; discussion 585-6., 92(2), 579-85.

[21] Damgaard, S, Lund, J. T, Lilleør, N. B, Perko, M. J, Madsen, J. K, & Steinbrüchel, D. A. Comparably improved health-related quality of life after total arterial revascularization versus conventional coronary surgery--Copenhagen arterial revascularization randomized patency and outcome trial. Eur J Cardiothorac Surg. (2011). Apr; , 39(4), 478-83.

[22] Saso, S, James, D, Vecht, J. A, Kidher, E, Kokotsakis, J, Malinovski, V, Rao, C, Darzi, A, Anderson, J. R, & Athanasiou, T. Effect of skeletonization of the internal thoracic artery for coronary revascularization on the incidence of sternal wound infection. Ann Thorac Surg. (2010). Feb; , 89(2), 661-70.

[23] Pevni, D, Uretzky, G, Mohr, A, Braunstein, R, Kramer, A, Paz, Y, Shapira, I, & Mohr, R. Routine use of bilateral skeletonized internal thoracic artery grafting: long-term results. Circulation. (2008). Aug 12; , 118(7), 705-12.

[24] Conklin, L. D, Ferguson, E. R, & Reardon, M. J. The technical aspects of radial artery harvesting. Tex Heart Inst J. (2001). , 28(2), 129-31.

[25] Desai, N. D, Cohen, E. A, Naylor, C. D, & Fremes, S. E. Radial Artery Patency Study Investigators. A randomized comparison of radial-artery and saphenous-vein coronary bypass grafts. N Engl J Med. (2004). Nov 25; , 351(22), 2302-9.

[26] Deb, S, Cohen, E. A, Singh, S. K, Une, D, Laupacis, A, & Fremes, S. E. RAPS Investigators. Radial artery and saphenous vein patency more than 5 years after coronary artery bypass surgery: results from RAPS (Radial Artery Patency Study). J Am Coll Cardiol. (2012). Jul 3; , 60(1), 28-35.

[27] Zacharias, A, Habib, R. H, Schwann, T. A, Riordan, C. J, Durham, S. J, & Shah, A. Improved survival with radial artery versus vein conduits in coronary bypass surgery with left internal thoracic artery to left anterior descending artery grafting. Circulation. (2004). Mar 30; , 109(12), 1489-96.

[28] Collins, P, Webb, C. M, Chong, C. F, & Moat, N. E. Radial Artery Versus Saphenous Vein Patency (RSVP) Trial Investigators. Radial artery versus saphenous vein patency randomized trial: five-year angiographic follow-up. Circulation. (2008). Jun 3; , 117(22), 2859-64.

[29] Cameron, J, Trivedi, S, Stafford, G, & Bett, J. H. Five-year angiographic patency of radial artery bypass grafts. Circulation. (2004). Sep 14; 110 (11 Suppl 1) :II, 23-6.

[30] Acar, C, Ramsheyi, A, Pagny, J. Y, Jebara, V, Barrier, P, Fabiani, J. N, Deloche, A, Guermonprez, J. L, & Carpentier, A. The radial artery for coronary artery bypass

grafting: clinical and angiographic results at five years. J Thorac Cardiovasc Surg. (1998). Dec; , 116(6), 981-9.

[31] Khot, U. N, Friedman, D. T, Pettersson, G, Smedira, N. G, Li, J, & Ellis, S. G. Radial artery bypass grafts have an increased occurrence of angiographically severe stenosis and occlusion compared with left internal mammary arteries and saphenous vein grafts. Circulation. (2004). May 4; , 109(17), 2086-91.

[32] Ruttmann, E, Fischler, N, Sakic, A, Chevtchik, O, Alber, H, Schistek, R, Ulmer, H, & Grimm, M. Second internal thoracic artery versus radial artery in coronary artery bypass grafting: a long-term, propensity score-matched follow-up study. Circulation. (2011). Sep 20; , 124(12), 1321-9.

[33] Hayward, P. A, Gordon, I. R, Hare, D. L, Matalanis, G, Horrigan, M. L, Rosalion, A, & Buxton, B. F. Comparable patencies of the radial artery and right internal thoracic artery or saphenous vein beyond 5 years: results from the Radial Artery Patency and Clinical Outcomes trial. J Thorac Cardiovasc Surg. (2010). Jan; discussion 65-7., 139(1), 60-5.

[34] Muneretto, C, Bisleri, G, Negri, A, Manfredi, J, Metra, M, Nodari, S, & Culot, L. Dei Cas L. Total arterial myocardial revascularization with composite grafts improves results of coronary surgery in elderly: a prospective randomized comparison with conventional coronary artery bypass surgery. Circulation. (2003). Sep 9; 108 Suppl 1:II, 29-33.

[35] Chung, J. W, Kim, J. B, Jung, S. H, Choo, S. J, Song, H, Chung, C. H, & Lee, J. W. Mid-term Outcomes of Total Arterial Revascularization Versus Conventional Coronary Surgery in Isolated Three-Vessel Coronary Disease. J Korean Med Sci. (2012). Sep; , 27(9), 1051-6.

[36] Zacharias, A, Schwann, T. A, Riordan, C. J, Durham, S. J, Shah, A. S, & Habib, R. H. Late results of conventional versus all-arterial revascularization based on internal thoracic and radial artery grafting. Ann Thorac Surg. (2009). Jan; e2., 87(1), 19-26.

Chapter 8

MINI OPCABG

Federico Benetti, Natalia Scialacomo,
Jose Luis Ameriso and Bruno Benetti

Additional information is available at the end of the chapter

http://dx.doi.org/10.5772/54880

1. Introduction

The majority of the worldwide Coronary surgery typically requires exposure of the heart and its vessels through median sternotomy and cardiopulmonary bypass, making it one of the most invasive and traumatic aspects of open-chest surgery.

Trying to decrease the risks of the CABG and its costs, in 1978 we repopularized the Off Pump Coronary Artery Bypass Graft (**OPCABG**) [1-2] and expand the technique, addressing lesions of the circumflex system (Cx) and applying it to diverse clinical scenarios. We tested several surgical approaches, such as full sternotomy, including left, anterolateral, posterolateral and right anterolateral thoracotomies, as well as partial sternotomy [3].

The video – assisted techniques in the nineties allowed, for the first time, to dissect the left internal thoracic artery (LITA) without opening the pleura cavity. The LITA was anastomosed to the left anterior descending (LAD) through a small left anterior thoracotomy. [4-5-6] and a new method for coronary bypass was create [7].

From 1996, a new series of technological developments allowed, widespread application of the OPCABG and MIDCAB techniques surgeons to perform high quality reproducible anastomoses and demonstrate in the great majority of reports, a decrease in postoperative morbidity [9-16].

In 1997, we performed for the first time an ambulatory coronary bypass through a xiphoid lower sternotomy incision (MINI OPCABG) using 3D technology to assist in the operation [8], shortly after we would continue to expand the operation [17-18].

Here in this chapter we will describe the technique to perform the MINI OPCABG operation today in our institution.

2. Anatomical considerations

The work area anastomosis is generally from the fourth intercostal space down (Fig. 1).

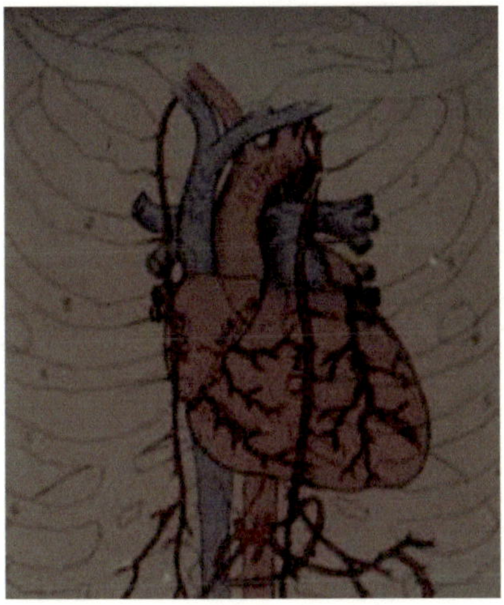

Figure 1.

The relationship between breast and distance to the coronary arteries or the anastomosis potential place can be estimated preoperatively with different imaging techniques. With a simple chest radiograph, you can also estimate the distance from the tip of heart to the midline sternum, important factor in concordance with the anatomical variations of the thorax. In the Fig. 2 you can see an ideal case where you are able to access any territory of the heart with this incision.

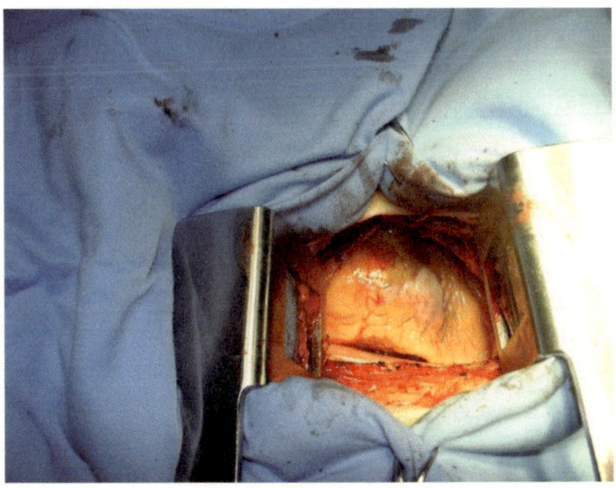

Figure 2.

http://dx.doi.org/10.5772/54880

3. Technique

The patients are prepared as for standard coronary bypass operation through medium sternotomy.

A skin incision is made from the xiphoid up to the level between the third and fourth intercostal space (Fig 3).

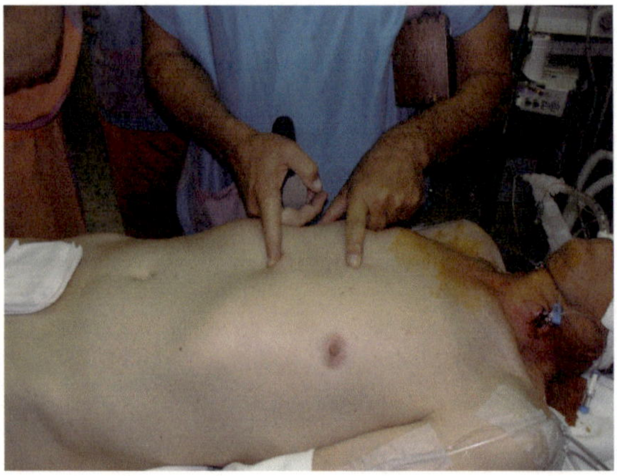

Figure 3.

The sternum is open and the left table is lifted to dissect the left mammary artery.

In the majority of the operations, we used a part of a normal Lima retractor. In the last patients **we created a new prototype retractor** that allows to potential perform a more friendly operation (Fig.4). The left mammary was dissected up to the third intercostal space, in general around 7 to 10 cm. isolated without the veins. It is important that the angle of the superior part where the mammary is attached to the sternum has to be below 20% to avoid any potential kinking. After the dissection was completed, (Fig.5), if the operation is only left internal mammary to LAD, we would heparinzed the patient with 3mg/kg to maintain ACT more than 480 sec.

When the ACT is more than 480 sec. and the patient has a normal temperature we would cut the distal part of the left internal mammary 1cm approximately from the distal bifurcation. The mammary distance is measured first with the pericardium intact, if achieved the diaphragmatic reflect of the pericardium it means that the length of the mammary is correct to perform a graft, also in the most distal segment of the LAD. After the pericardium is cleaned to identify the area of the pulmonary artery, the pericardium is open to the apex and towards the right around 5 to 6 cm., initially in that moment in most of the cases the area of the LAD is seen and the potential area of the anastomosis is defined, the distance with the heart, in normal position of the mammary, is measured to be sure there is not any potential kinking do to excess of the conduit. The retractor is changed (in the last 6 cases we used a new prototype system where you only change the angle without changing the piece) (Fig.4), the pericardium

was opened towards the right side of the aorta and a piece is taken avoiding any compression of the great vessels. 2 stitches are put around 2 cm. deep in the left border of the pericardium with a distance of 5 to 7 cm and lifted to position the LAD area. After that a Polypropylene 5-0 is put around the artery in the area we decided to perform the anastomosis, also a mechanical stabilizer is always in position in this place with the opening part towards the head of the patient to avoid any problem of damaging the graft when you need to take it. The anastomosis is performed in a running way with 7 or 8 polypropylene depending on the size of the artery. We didn't use shunt, normally except if the artery has more than 2,5 mm in size and has a very proximal occlusion.or the clinical situation require We used blower only in the moment we needed to visualized correctly the border of the artery, we tried to avoid the use of the blower directed to the mammary, also syringe with warm water is used to help and to maintain the temperature of the heart. When the bypass is finished and before we tied the suture, the stitches of 5-0 polypropylene around the artery where released as well as the clamp of the mammary, finally the anastomosis was tied.

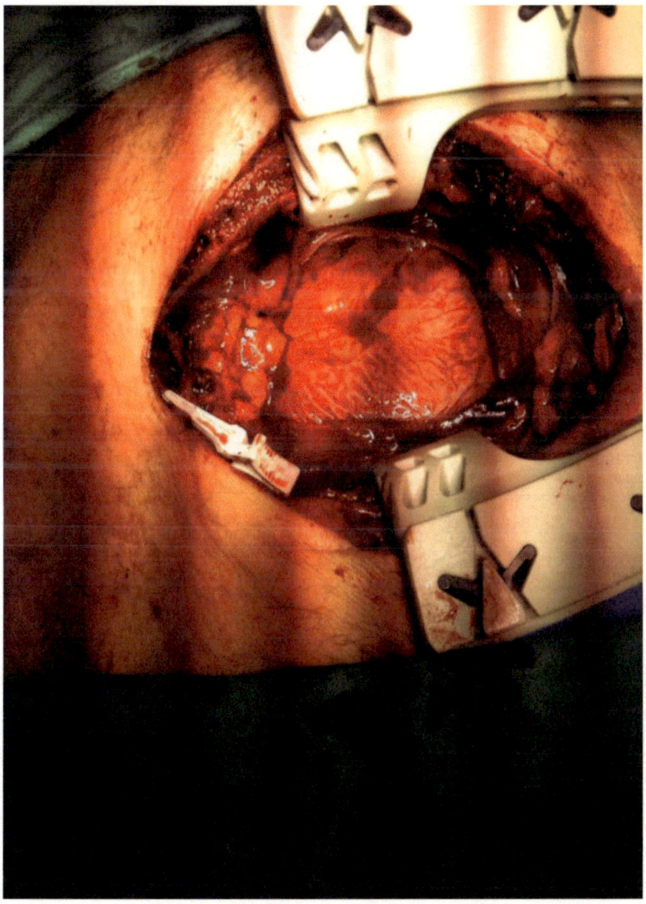

Figure 4.

http://dx.doi.org/10.5772/54880

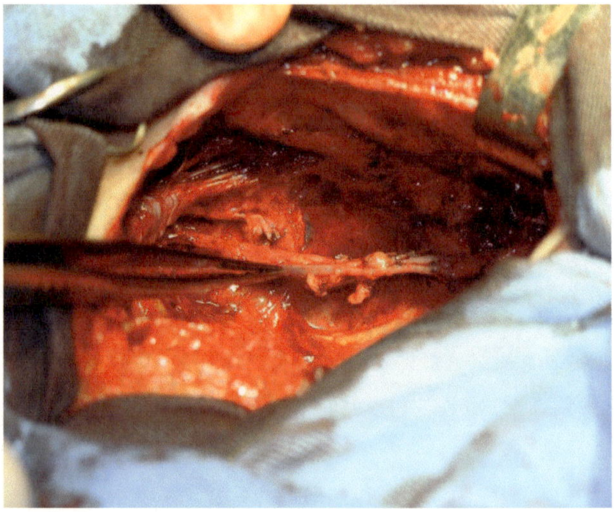

Figure 5.

The mechanical stabilizer was removed, the stitches of the pericardium where released and the Flow of the graft was measured being sure there is not any kinking, if the Flow and the PR are ok the mammary is fixed with 2 stitches of 7-0 polypropylene in both sides around 1 cm from the anastomosis.

The heparin was reverted with protamine. If the pleura was closed one drainage is positioned avoiding touching the heart and the graft. If the left pleura was opened the drainage is positioned in the left pleural space with two holes in the mediastinun area and one stitch is done between the pleura and the back of the sternum to separate the drainage from the area of the graft to avoid any damage and the sternum is closing in a normal way with less numbers of sutures.

In case we need to perform more grafts after the left internal mammary was prepared, we put the mammary retractor in the right size of the sternum and take a piece of a right mammary and perform and anastomosis (fig. 6), with a non touch vein or radial artery to perform the others grafts. In this situation after both conduits were prepared the retractor is changed and the heart is exposed opening the pericardium in the same way previously descript in the mammary to Lad graft. (fig7)

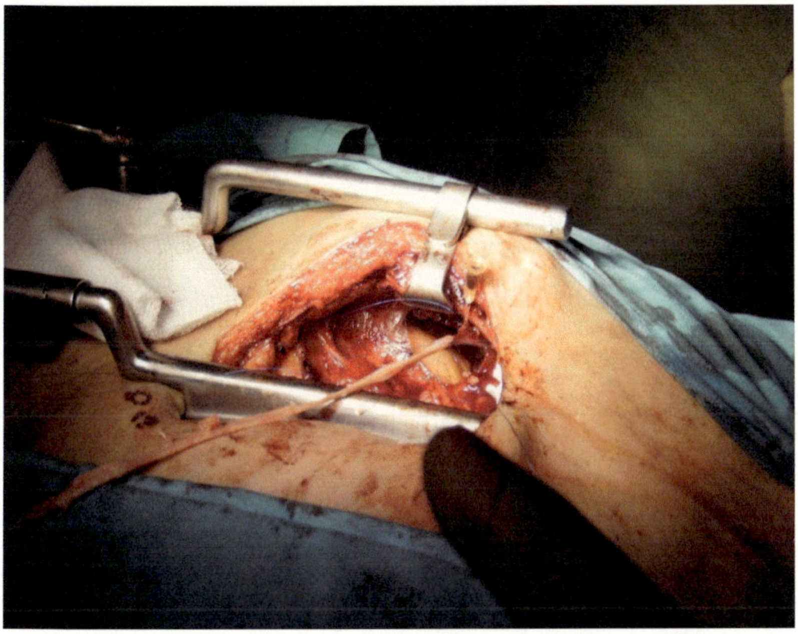

Figure 6.

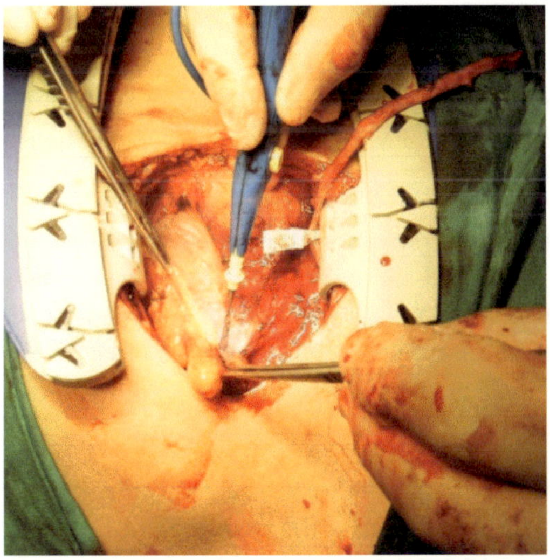

Figure 7.

http://dx.doi.org/10.5772/54880

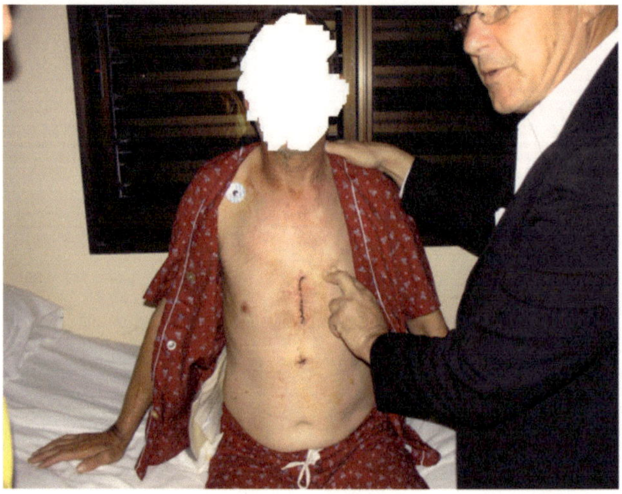

Figure 8. Patient four coronary grafts next day after operation.(ideal candidate)

If the patient is stable and need Cx graft and it is possible we put any suction cusp in the apex to expose the heart and vessels then using always mechanicals stabilizers we perform the anastomosis. After the Cx we perform the right and the LAD, last [18], if the patient because the clinical conditions require, we completed the mammary to LAD first and then the rest of the operation. Is important to notice that the heart is not touch in any moment only you require to do it when you need to put a suction cusp in the apex.

The incision is closed in the same way (Fig.8). In hybrid procedures, the operation where performed first MINI OPCABG (Mammary to LAD) and after a period of 8 hours we perform angioplasty Stent. In table 1 and 2 we see the characteristics of the patients, and in Fig 9-10-11- the different grafts we already performed in this group of patients.

Patient Characteristics	**Value**
Number of patients	55
Average age (years)	66.0 ± 8.3
Female gender	9(16.%)
One-vessel disease	24 (43%)
Two-vessel disease	12 (22.%)
Three-vessel disease	17 (31%)
Left main trunk disease	2 (4.0%)
Hypertension	35 (64%)
Lipid disorders	37 (67.0%)
Diabetes mellitus	14 (25%)
Smokers	21 (38%)
Aspirin preoperatively	17 (31%)

Table 1. MINI-OPCABG: long term results.

Previous myocardial infarction	21 (38.0%)
Previous catheter intervention	6 (11.0%)
Peripheral vascular disease	5 (9%)
Chronic obstructive pulmonary disease	8 (15%)
Previous renal disease	1 (2%)
Previous stroke	1 (2%)
Critical preoperative state	3 (5.0%)
Moderate to severe left ventricular function	7(13%)
Asymptomatic	6 (11.0%)
Stable chronic angina	17 (31.0%)
Unstable angina	32 (58.0%)
Myocardial Infarction	1 (2%)
Recent myocardial infarct	3 (5%)
Emergency operation	2 (4.0%)
Other than isolated CABG	1 (2.%)
Average Euroscore	3.4 ± 1.4
Previous CABG	2 (4%)
Preoperative Death	0.0 (0%)
Exploration for bleeding	1 (2.%)
New onset atrial fibrillation	1 (2.%)
Pleural effusion	1 (2.%)
Ventilation more than 24 hours	2 (4.0%)

Table 2.

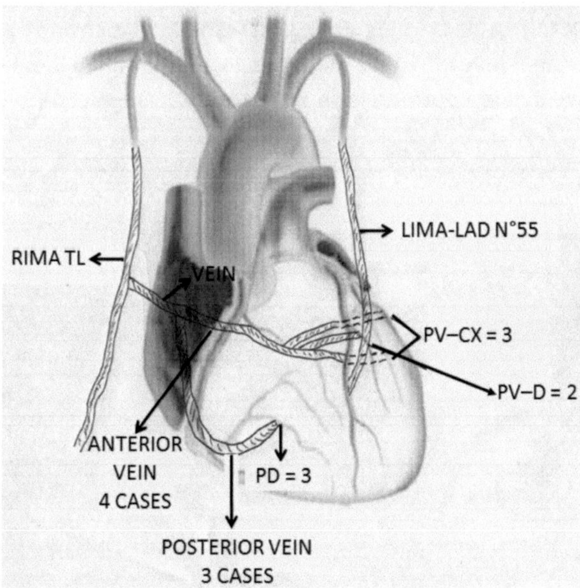

Figure 9.

http://dx.doi.org/10.5772/54880

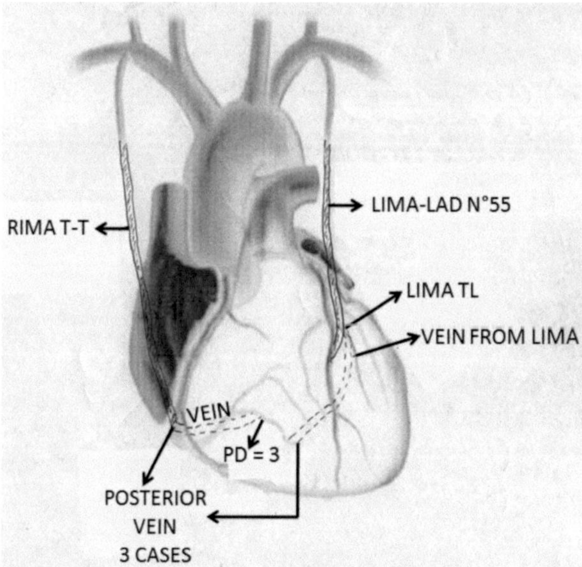

Figure 10.

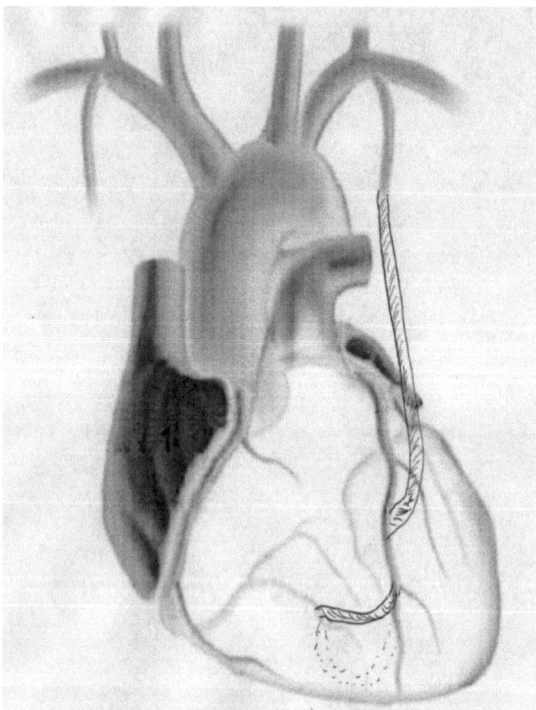

Figure 11.

4. Results

We didn't have operative mortality in this series of 55 Patients.

Two Patients in this series received plus the MINI OPCABG operation a PTCA STENT to the CX and RCA after the procedure.

We performed during the last 15 years this type of MINI OPCABG operation with the variables in 55 patients with good long term clinical results (Fig. 13-14).

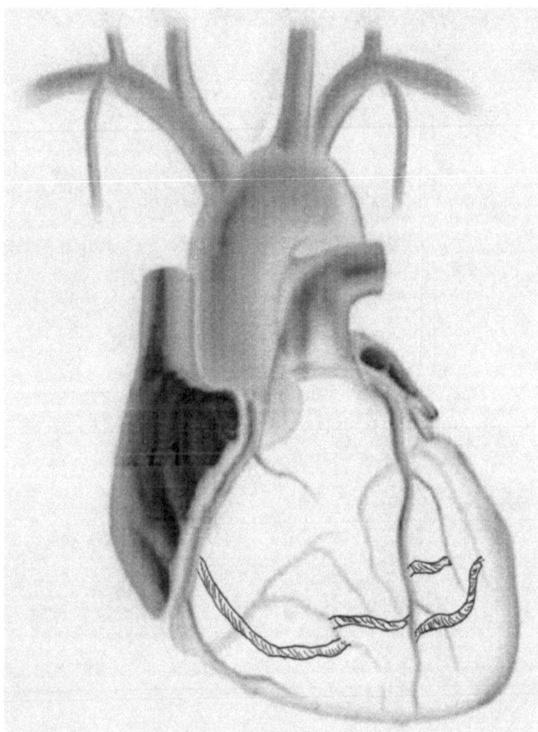

Figure 12.

http://dx.doi.org/10.5772/54880

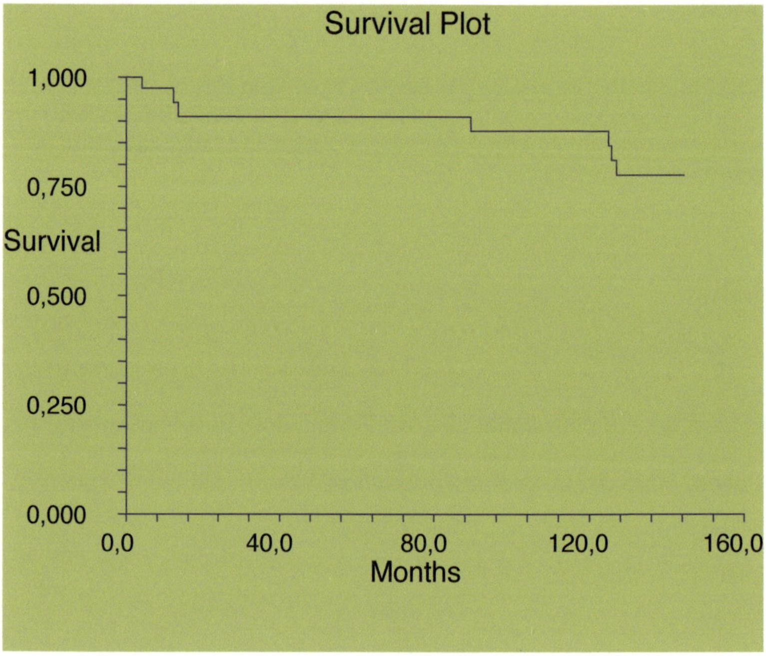

Figure 13.

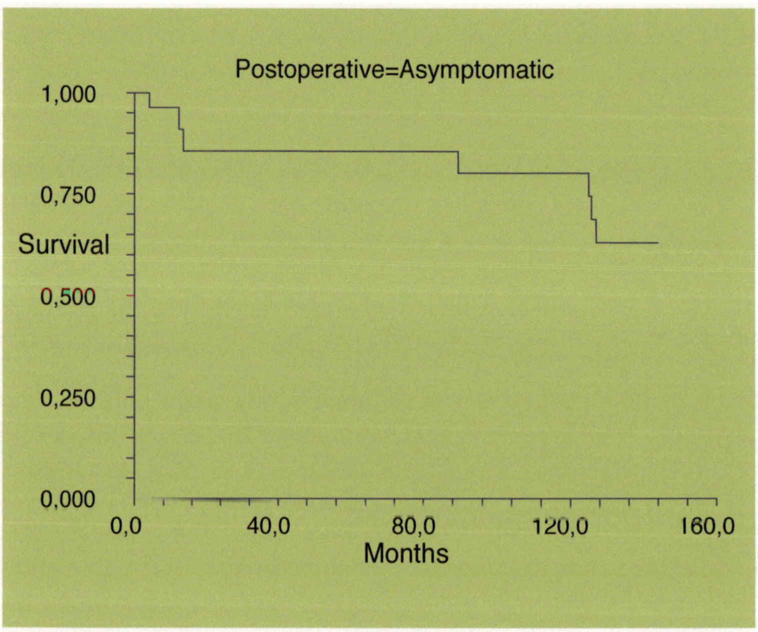

Figure 14.

5. Conclusions

More experience and better technology is needed to expand this operation in multiple vessels and also to create intracoronary connections in some situations (Fig.12). Also for the Hybrid technique is mandatory to create a more friendly retractor and others instruments that facilitate the mammary to Lad operation.

Author details

Federico Benetti[1], Natalia Scialacomo[1], Jose Luis Ameriso[1] and Bruno Benetti[2]

1 Cardiac Surgeon Benetti Foundation, Benetti Foundation, Rosario, Santa Fe, Argentina

2 Enginner Benetti Foundation, Benetti Foundation, Rosario, Santa Fe, Argentina

References

[1] Benetti, F J. "Direct coronary surgery with saphenous vein bypass without either cardiopulmonary bypass or cardiac arrest." *J Cardiovasc Surg* 26, no. 3 (May-Jun 1985): 217-222.

[2] Buffolo, E, J C Andrade, J Succi, L E Leão, and C Gallucci. "Direct myocardial revascularization without cardiopulmonary bypass." *Thorac Cardiovasc Surg* 33, no. 1 (Feb 1985): 26-29.

[3] Benetti, F J, G Naselli, M Wood, and L Geffner. "Direct myocardial revascularization without extracorporeal circulation. Experience in 700 patients." *Chest* 100, no. 2 (Aug 1991): 312-316.

[4] Benetti, F J, C Ballester, y A Barnia. «Uso de la Toracoscopía en cirugía coronaria para disección de la mamaria izquierda.» *La Prensa Médica Argentina* 9 (1994): 81-87.

[5] Benetti, F J, and C Ballester. "Use of thoracoscopy and a minimal thoracotomy, in mammary-coronary bypass to left anterior descending artery, without extracorporeal circulation. Experience in 2 cases." *J Cardiovasc Surg* 36, no. 2 (Apr 1995): 159-161.

[6] Benetti, F J, and C Ballester. "Coronary revascularization with the arterial conduits via a small thoracotomy and assisted by thoracoscopy, although without cardiopulmonary bypass." *Coronary Revasc* 4, no. 1 (1995): 22-24

[7] Federico Benetti :Method for coronary bypass United States Patent Patent Ñ 5,888,247

[8] Benetti, F J. "Minimally invasive coronary surgery (the xiphoid approach)." *Eur J Cardiothorac Surg* 16, no. Suppl 2 (Nov 1999): S10-S11.

[9] Angelini, G D, F C Taylor, B C Reeves, y R Ascione. «Early and midterm outcome after off-pump and on-pump surgery in Beating Heart Against Cardioplegic Arrest Studies (BHACAS 1 and 2): a pooled analysis of two randomised controlled trials.» *Lancet* 359, nº 9313 (Apr 2002): 1194-1199.

[10] Nathoe, H M, et al. "A comparison of on-pump and off-pump coronary bypass surgery in low-risk patients." *N Engl J Med* 348, no. 5 (Jan 2003): 394-402.

[11] Sabik, J F, et al. "Does off-pump coronary surgery reduce morbidity and mortality?" *J Thorac Cardiovasc Surg* 124, no. 4 (Oct 2002): 698-707.

[12] Mack, M J, et al. "Comparison of coronary bypass surgery with and without cardiopulmonary bypass in patients with multivessel disease." *J Thorac Cardiovasc Surg* 127, no. 1 (Jan 2004): 167-173.

[13] Calafiore, A M, et al. "Myocardial revascularization with and without cardiopulmonary bypass in multivessel disease: impact of the strategy on early outcome." *Ann Thorac Surg* 72, no. 2 (Aug 2001): 456-462.

[14] Al-Ruzzeh, S, et al. "Off-Pump Coronary Artery Bypass (OPCAB) surgery reduces risk-stratified morbidity and mortality: a United Kingdom Multi-Center Comparative Analysis of Early Clinical Outcome." *Circulation* 108, no. Suppl 1 (Sep 2003): II1-8.

[15] Plomondon, M E, et al. "Off-pump coronary artery bypass is associated with improved risk-adjusted outcomes." *Ann Thorac Surg* 72, no. 1 (Jul 2001): 114-119.

[16] Stevens, L M, et al. "Single versus bilateral internal thoracic artery grafts with concomitant saphenous vein grafts for multivessel coronary artery bypass grafting: effects on mortality and event-free survival." *J Thorac Cardiovasc Surg* 127, no. 5 (May 2004): 1408-1415.

[17] Benetti, Federico J, and Maximo Guida. "Minimally Invasive Coronary Artery Bypass Grafting." Chap. 11 in *Minimally invasive cardiac surgery*, by Daniel J Goldstein and Mehmet C Oz, edited by Daniel J Goldstein and Mehmet C Oz, 147-156. Totowa, New Jersey: Humana Press, 2004

[18] Benetti, F et al Xiphoid Lower Sternotomy Approach for multivessel revascularization of the Left internal Mammary to the left anterior descending Artery and Rigth Internnal mammary as inflow to the others vessels. The Heart Surgery Forum 2009-1131 13(1), 2010 (Epub February 2010) Doi :10.1532/ H SF 98.20091131

Chapter 9

Saphenous Vein Conduit in Coronary Artery Bypass Surgery — Patency Rates and Proposed Mechanisms for Failure

Maseeha S. Khaleel, Tracy A. Dorheim,
Michael J. Duryee, Geoffrey M. Thiele and
Daniel R. Anderson

Additional information is available at the end of the chapter

http://dx.doi.org/10.5772/55098

1. Introduction

Coronary artery disease is the single leading cause of death in the United States. Every year more than 1 million open coronary revascularization procedures are performed in the United States. Most commonly the greater saphenous veins and internal mammary and/or radial arteries are used as bypass conduits. Long term patency and avoiding repeat revascularization is every surgeon's goal following coronary artery bypass grafting. Unfortunately it is estimated that during the first year after surgery; between 10 - 15% of venous grafts occlude. The graft attrition rate is estimated to be 1 - 2 % per year during the first five years following surgery. By 10 years only 50 % of vein grafts remain free from significant stenosis [1].

The reasons for premature graft closure include; biologic, conduit quality, unsatisfactory harvest/preparation, and inappropriate operative strategy or poor surgical technique [2]. Many of these factors can be avoided with proper technique and experience of the surgical team. Currently much of the research being performed on graft failure is leading to the hypothesis of early thrombosis and neointimal hyperplasia as the physiologic basis for graft failure, although the exact mechanism is not well established.

This chapter will discuss current knowledge and ongoing research regarding the thrombosis, intimal hyperplasia and atherosclerosis of vein grafts. It will highlight harvesting techniques and preservation methods, as well as discuss proposed mechanisms that lead to intimal

hyperplasia, graft atherosclerosis, and the evolving strategies and current research for long-term prevention of graft failure.

2. How vein harvesting methods can affect patency rates

Dr. Rene Favaloro developed the first saphenous vein harvesting technique in 1967 [2]. This technique required a longitudinal incision along the length of the greater saphenous vein entering the fascial canal surrounding the vein and thus causing inadvertent damage to the adventitial layer. Following vein isolation from the surrounding tissues, ligation of side branches, as well as a transection of the vein for completion of the harvest is performed. Since that original description, many methods have evolved from Dr. Favaloro's original technique. As well, research has focused on the best method of harvesting grafts without damage. In addition to Favaloro's original technique, current and popular harvesting techniques included; "no touch", stab phlebectomy, and most recently endoscopic techniques. It is inherit that manipulation of the vein conduit causes damage to the vein itself, but the extent was unknown. Multiple studies have been done to compare; "open", "no touch", and "endoscopic vessel harvesting (EVH)" techniques [3]. The traditional open technique which is performed under direct visualization of the vein was found to preserve the endothelium of the vein quite well, but also came with the complications of leg pain i.e. wound healing, post operative cellulitis, and increased length of hospital stay [4], [5]. Initial studies performed on the long-term outcome of vein grafts harvested using the open technique did show that the vein was often stripped of the beneficial adventitial layer as well as distended to high pressures to overcome the associated vasospasm [6]. Unfortunately, the increased distention pressures caused shear stress damage to the vein intima and subsequent endothelial wall [7]. When viewed histologically the endothelial cells appeared deformed, flattened, polymorphic, and contained an abundance of cytoplasmic vesicles [8]. As a method to avoid over-handling of the vein and increased distention pressures a pedicle technique was developed and named the "no touch" technique. It was thought that veins procured in this manner would eliminate the need for conduit distention and its associated morbidities since the perivascular adipose tissue surrounding the vein was left intact [9]. It had been shown that this surrounding tissue in internal thoracic mammary arteries provided a vasodilatory effect with less arterial conduit vasospasm. Increased patency rates were demonstrated with the "no touch" technique compared to the conventional open technique [9]. 1997 began a new era in coronary artery bypass grafting with the use of EVH to harvest the saphenous vein. Endoscopic harvesting techniques were found to eliminate the need for invasive incisions, and decrease the associated risks that accrued with an open technique. Furthermore veins harvested via an EVH method were hypothesized to be promising for graft patency, since endothelial integrity was maintained following EVH harvest compared to other conventional harvesting techniques. This new technique soon became the standard of care with greater than 70% of saphenous vein conduits being retrieved in this manner [10]. Endoscopic harvesting had lower complication rates including less post-operative pain, and decreased patient length of stay. However, controversy arose about the long-term patency of the vein conduits after coronary artery

http://dx.doi.org/10.5772/55098

bypass grafting; depending upon what vein harvest method was used in surgery. It was felt veins harvested using an EVH technique failed more often and earlier than veins harvested in the traditional open technique. Studies performed by Desai et al in 2011, confirmed the relationship between the learning curve of EVH and the patency rates based on beginner and expert level of experience in harvesting vein tissue [11]. It has since been shown that when a novice is performing the procedure the vein is subjected to much more stress from trying to better visualize the vein, and 50% of the veins had discrete areas of injury [11]. It was noted that if a section of vein had more than 4 areas of injury, it had a greater than 50% risk of failure of patency [11]. Early studies, which compared the traditional open harvest method to EVH, were published in the infancy stages of EVH when all harvesters were novices to this new technique. Thus, it is now recognized that this confounding issue may have contributed to the decreased long-term patency that was noted. However, this has changed in the past years with "novice" level practitioners becoming experts. It has recently been found that when procured by expert level harvesters the physical damage to the vein is similar to that of open harvest [12], [13]. Thus, it is hypothesized that EVH and open harvest when performed by an expert will have similar patency rates if all other factors are equal.

3. The role of pressure distention and wall stress during harvest

Standard procedure in the United States is to distend the saphenous vein graft after procurement prior to myocardial implantation to ensure that all branches are ligated. The majority of the time during harvest, the vein is distended to supra-physiologic pressures [14]. While saphenous veins *in vivo* are rarely subjected to pressures greater than 60 mmHg, recorded pressure measurements during harvest easily reach 300-400 mmHg [15]. This supra-physiologic pressure severely damages the endothelium and ultimately leads to premature graft closure. This high pressure is inadvertently used to overcome vasospasm as well as to ensure ligation of all side branches [16]. The pressure causes shear wall stress that denudes the protective endothelial layer (Figure 1). As a mechanism to protect itself, the endothelium releases basic fibroblast growth factors and platelet-derived growth factors [17]. Basic fibroblast growth factor, a heparin-binding polypeptide that is present in the nucleus and cytoplasm of smooth muscle and endothelial cells and in the intracellular matrix, is normally a non-secreted cell product [18]. Platelet derived growth factor is also widely acknowledged in the process of angiogenesis and most specifically in cell migration and proliferation. The release of these 2 mitogens together initiates intimal hyperplasia [17].

4. The graft "environment" at a cellular level

The vascular endothelium has many protective functions, and it releases factors that maintain vein graft patency. The endothelium serves as the physical barrier between the blood components and the sub-endothelium, damage to this endothelium by either direct or indirect stress can disrupt this protective environment causing the formation of atheromas and subsequently

graft failure. Injury to the endothelium in addition to surgical manipulation also increases the risk for vasospasm, stenosis, and intimal hyperplasia. Studies have shown that many factors can affect the viability of endothelium; these include temperature, distention, and the composition of solution used in vein preparation. Nitric oxide controls vascular tone in addition to causing vasodilatation. Vascular endothelium contains L-arginine which when combined with nitric oxide synthase forms nitric oxide[1]. The main target of nitric oxide is to stimulate guanylate cyclase and subsequently form guanosine 3 prime 5 prime-cyclic monophosphate (cGMP). The cGMP leads to vasodilatation and inhibition of platelet aggregation [19]. Furthermore, nitric oxide also has been shown to interfere with cell migration, specifically white cells by reducing the adhesion of neutrophils to the endothelial surface. Several cytoprotective properties are conferred through nitric oxide including; scavenging of oxygen free radicals and blocking release of prostaglandin E2 and F2 alpha. These are anti-inflammatory effects, and are quite intricate in detail, but are based on regulation of transcription factors [20], [21]. Nitric oxide also has some cytotoxic effects including decreasing protein synthesis, increasing lipid peroxidation, and decreasing acute phase proteins [22]. Injury to the endothelium directly causes a decrease in nitric oxide release by the endothelial cells and destroys the integrity of the vein. Studies performed by Kown et al. showed that vein grafts treated with L-arginine (nitric oxide is a by-product created when L-arginine is converted to citrulline) can increase levels of nitric oxide and subsequently decrease hyperplasia [23].

5. Reperfusion injury

Approximately 12% of patients experience thrombosis of saphenous vein grafts within 30 days of surgery [24]. It has been shown that this acute thrombosis is likely a combination of multiple factors including ischemia and hemostasis during coronary procedures which favors thrombogenesis [25]. The ischemic period in which the vein has been harvested but not yet re-implanted into the myocardium, marks the beginning of the cascade to possible thrombosis. Upon re-establishment of blood flow through the vein it has been shown that neutrophils in the oxygenated blood are attracted to the areas of endothelial injury [26]. This ischemia-reperfusion results in a reduction in both basal and stimulated nitric oxide release, yet attenuates the vaso-relaxation responses to the agonist stimulators of endothelial nitric oxide acetylcholine and bradykinin. Together this impairs the release of nitric oxide and down regulates nitric oxide production after an ischemic event.

After the saphenous vein is harvested, the initial injury causes a decrease in nitric oxide due to the traumatic endothelial cell injury from manipulation and distention. Following the ischemic period and after implantation, nitric oxide synthesis will increase due to the reperfusion. Re-implantation causes release of multiple growth factors, and cytokines that cause the migration and proliferation of vascular smooth muscle cells and formation of extracellular matrix into the intimal compartment of the vein graft. Once neutrophils are adherent they initiate further endothelial damage and activation of the coagulation cascade which can lead to thrombosis [1]. The release of nitric oxide at this time can limit neointimal hyperplasia by inhibiting this proliferation and promoting apoptosis [27].

http://dx.doi.org/10.5772/55098

6. The role of neointimal hyperplasia in graft patency

Neointimal hyperplasia is the accumulation of smooth muscle cells and extracellular matrix that occurs in the intimal layer of vein. This thickening leads to a narrowing of the lumen and subsequent stenosis of the vein graft. Neointimal hyperplasia is the most widely accepted reason for graft failure at the present time. Many theories exist as to why this occurs but none have been completely proven. Work is currently being performed evaluating the up regulation of genes or proteins that may cause the phenomenon of intimal hyperplasia [15]. Nearly all vein grafts placed into an arterial system develop some areas of hyperplasia within the first four weeks. This acute hyperplasia can narrow the lumen of the vein conduit by as much as 25%.

Many studies have related extensive endothelial injury to neointimal hyperplasia development. Injury can be in the form of extreme venous distention, denudation of the endothelium itself, and degree of vasospasm overcome during harvest [28]. Intimal growth is stimulated by several factors including platelet derived growth factor, transforming growth factor beta, and epidermal growth factor which cause proliferation and subsequent invasion of the smooth muscle cells into the intimal layer [1]. When veins are injured, basic fibroblast growth factor is released from the endothelial cells and smooth muscle cells. This is a very potent mitogen that causes the increased production of multiple regulatory proteins, kinases, and genes that participate in DNA synthesis [29]. The sequential activation and inactivation of the cyclin dependent regulatory kinases (Cdk) leads the smooth muscle cells through the cell cycle [30]. Each cyclin exhibits a cell cycle phase specific pattern of expression with several cell cycle checkpoints at the G1/S station. At these points the kinases interact with a cyclin, specifically D and E interacting with Cdk 4/6, and 2. To progress the cell into the M phase cyclin B is activated. These Cdk proteins are inhibited by activating Cdk 1. The G1 Cdk is part of the retinoblastoma pocket proteins that when phosphorylated can sequester cell cycle regulatory transcription factors. This phosphorylation by retinoblastoma proteins as well as specific cylcin dependent kinases during late G1 leads to activation and release of genes that participate in DNA synthesis. It is this complex cascade of cellular activities that leads to proliferation of smooth muscle cells causing neointimal hyperplasia1, [30]. Further research has shown that other theories also exist as to the mechanism of neointimal hyperplasia that includes a role for perivascular fibroblasts and matrix metalloproteinases (MMP's). It is thought that fibroblasts invade through the media of the saphenous vein graft and differentiate into myofibroblasts. MMP's are the mediators of matrix deposition and degradation, which can cause neointimal hyperplasia. Theories exist that a strategy to avoid hyperplasia would be to use MMP inhibitors. MMPs compose a super family of 66 known zinc peptidases that degrade collagen, gelatin, and elastin31. MMPs are critical for cell growth and proliferation, cell migration, organ development, reproduction, and tissue remodeling. In all of these biological phenomena, matrix degradation is needed to facilitate changes in cell phenotype. For example, ligand-dependent cell-matrix associations are critical for modulating cell function, and matrix degradation. These interactions can thereby modulate responses of the cell to its microenvironment within the saphenous vein.

Vascular smooth muscle cells, monocytes/macrophages, and endothelial cells have all been shown to express MMPs. Vein graft stenosis appears to be associated with increased expression of MMP-9 and increased activation of MMP-2 [32]. Pharmacological inhibitor studies demonstrate that MMPs are, indeed, involved in the formation of the neointima. Therefore, with this data it appears that MMPs are critical for smooth muscle cell migration and proliferation, which serve as the cellular basis for neointimal proliferation *in vivo*. Tissue inhibitors of metalloprotienases (TIMPs) are four naturally occurring proteins that inactive MMP's by binding to them. Kranzhofer et al showed that three of these TIMPs are found on saphenous vein grafts [33]. Several regulatory mechanisms exist to keep a precise balance between enzymes that degrade matrix and proteins that inhibit their action. Cytokines and growth factors, specifically platelet derived growth factor BB act together through a protein kinase C dependent mechanism to increase the expression of MMP-9, whereas transforming growth factor-beta and platelet derived growth factor BB induce TIMP-3 expression in vascular smooth muscle cells [31]. However, they do not have any influence on TIMP-1, or TIMP-2 expression. Baker et al. transfected grafts with a gene for TIMP-3 and observed an 84% reduction in neointima at 14 days and 58% reduction at 28 days in porcine vein grafts [34]. This shows promise for a potential preventative treatment of neointimal hyperplasia, but problems such as weakening of pre-existing atherosclerotic plaques need to be addressed and the longer-term benefits of this therapy remain unknown.

7. Upregulation of innate inflammatory markers and graft failure

Studies have shown that patients who present with unstable angina after revascularization by previous bypass procedures do so because of an obstructive atherosclerotic lesion in the saphenous vein conduit, and graft stenosis. These plaques have been seen as early as 1 year after bypass procedures [35]. When the vein conduit plaque is viewed histologically, it is found to have an increased number of foam cells than in arterial atheromatous plaques. Recent studies support the theory that a stimulus must exist that induces the expression of inflammatory mediators and may be the inciting factor leading to intimal hyperplasia and eventual graft failure [15].

Scavenger receptor proteins play a vital early role in vascular inflammation. Scavenger receptor proteins on the surface of vascular endothelial cells and macrophage have been shown to upregulate NF-kappaB inflammatory pathways. Studies focusing on upregulation of inflammatory markers following distention compared to non distended vein segments have shown that expression of scavenger receptor-A, scavenger receptor- B, and CD36 are upregulated in the distended saphenous vein tissue [15]. This suggests that the process of distention is an inciting event that allows for the upregulation of scavenger receptors, leading to graft failure through atherosclerotic lesion progression initiated by the formation of foam cells in these saphenous vein grafts.

Pressure distention of saphenous vein conduits has been part of the standard vein preparation procedure for decades. The longer the vein is exposed to pressure distention the higher the

http://dx.doi.org/10.5772/55098

expression of biomarkers. These biomarkers include; toll like receptors (TLRs), intracellular adhesion molecules (ICAM), vascular cell adhesion molecule-1 (VCAM-1), and platelet endothelial cell adhesion molecule-1 (PECAM-1). An upregulation of ICAM, VCAM-1, and PECAM-1 was seen in veins that had undergone distention when compared with the nondistended vein [15]. The expression of these cell adhesion molecules is important because an interaction of VCAM-1 and ICAM-1 with monocytes facilitates the monocytes' recruitment to the vein [36]. Additionally, interactions of ICAM-1 and VCAM-1 with PECAM-1 mediate the process of diapedesis of the monocytes into the vessel wall. These initial cell-mediated events facilitate recruitment of more inflammatory cytokines to the area of injury caused by the damage from distention. PECAM-1 is constitutively expressed on all endothelium regardless of cytokine activation.

Toll-like receptors play a very important role in the signaling pathway of inflammation. Traditionally, TLR4 costimulates with CD14 in chronic conditions. Interestingly TLR4 has also been shown to bind directly to lipopolysaccharide without CD14 costimulation, leading to subsequent NF-kappa B activation. Studies in TLR4-deficient mice have shown that despite the presence of lipopolysaccharide, these mice do not develop neointima, suggesting that neointimal hyperplasia is a TLR4-dependent process [15], [37]. TLR4 in cooperation with interleukin-1 receptor plays a significant role in the formation of neointima. TLR4 signaling also promotes a proinflammatory phenotype and plays a role in the early response to vascular injury. Therefore, the upregulation of TLR4 may play a role in the development of graft failure in terms of neointimal hyperplasia. TLR2 activation with MYD88 leads to cytokine production through NF-kappa B pathways. Thus, these data suggest that vein graft failure is likely a multifactorial process that includes neointimal hyperplasia and inflammation. Immediate vein graft failure is most probably due to inflammatory cytokines whereas late failure (1 year after CABG) is due to neointimal hyperplasia. However, the common cause of both of these processes is quite possibly exacerbated by SV pressure distention [15].

8. The future of prevention: from the research bench to the operating room

Much interest in reducing neointimal hyperplasia by blocking gene expression is arising. The cell cycle of endothelial cells is now better understood and therefore has allowed for genetics to help play a role in preventing stenosis, thrombosis, and ischemia. If the genetic pathways that are associated with the above process can be fully identified this may ultimately influence coronary graft patency. Ex-vivo work has been promising to show that blocking of the cell cycle via gene therapy has slowed down the atherosclerosis that can lead to graft failure [1].

Repeat coronary vascular procedures will continue to be problematic until an understanding of the mechanisms of vein graft have been elucidated. Thus far, extensive research has been done on this topic, but an overall consensus exists that the saphenous vein is a very fragile and easily injured conduit. Great care must be taken while handling the vein during harvest and preparation to avoid damage or stress to either the external or internal surface of the vein. Avoiding supra-physiologic pressure, prolonged distention periods and manipulations which

result in tissue inflammation and injury should be employed to prevent graft failure. Such efforts are expected to reduce the morbidity associated with saphenous vein graft disease and repeat coronary artery bypass interventions.

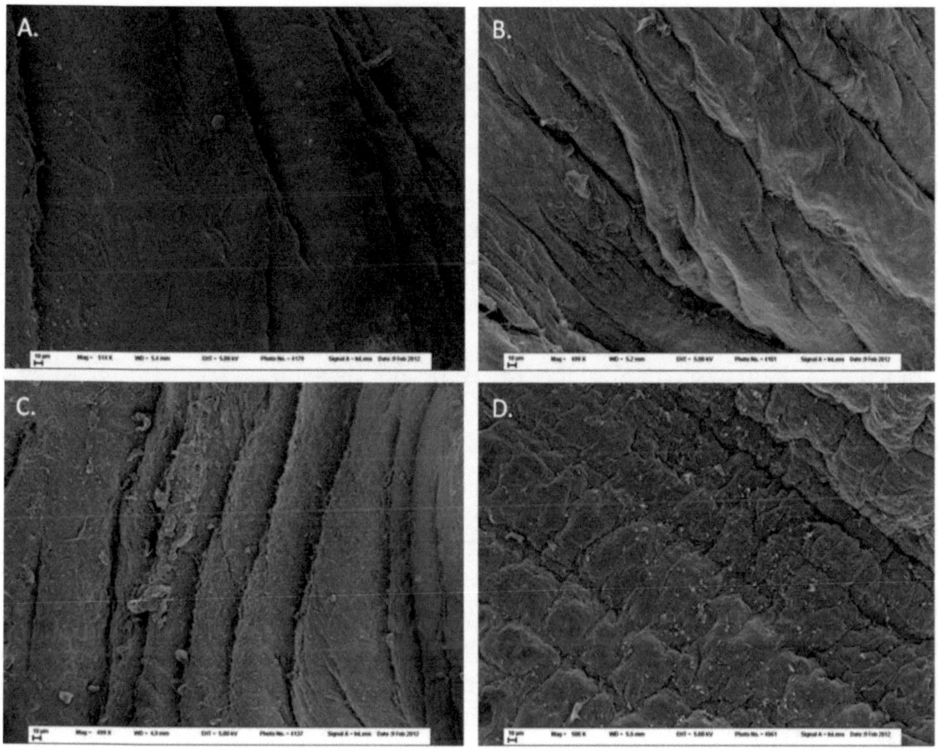

Figure 1. Scanning electron microscopy photomicrographs of vein tissue following harvest and distention. Saphenous veins underwent endoscopic harvest during bypass grafting procedures with routine pressure distention to ligate side branches. Vein distention was performed by attaching a syringe to the most anatomically distal portion of the vein. A segment of vein was obtained prior to distention and several segments along the length of the vein were harvested after distention and subjected to scanning electron microscopy. Pictures shown in the figure are (A) non-distended vein (B) most distal portion of vein from origin of distention (C) mid section of saphenous vein graft (D) vein segment closest to the syringe. Shown in the pictures are endothelial layer starting to change from a smooth flat surface to a rounded up rough surface.

Author details

Maseeha S. Khaleel[1,2*], Tracy A. Dorheim[6], Michael J. Duryee[2], Geoffrey M. Thiele[2,4,5] and Daniel R. Anderson[3,5*]

*Address all correspondence to: mkhaleel@unmc.edu or danderso@unmc.edu

1 Department of Anesthesiology, University of Nebraska Medical Center, Omaha, Nebraska, USA

2 Experimental Immunology Laboratory, Research in Autoimmune Disease, Division of Rheumatology and Immunology, Department of Internal Medicine, University of Nebraska Medical Center, Omaha, Nebraska, USA

3 Experimental Immunology Laboratory, Research in Cardiovascular Disease, Division of Cardiology, University of Nebraska Medical Center, Omaha, Nebraska, USA

4 Department of Pathology and Microbiology, University of Nebraska Medical Center, Omaha, Nebraska, USA

5 Omaha VA Medical Center, Research Services 151, Omaha, Nebraska, USA

6 Department of Surgery, Division of Cardiac Surgery, Maui Memorial Medical Center, Wailuku Hawaii, USA

References

[1] Shuhaiber, J. H, Evans, A. N, Massad, M. G, & Geha, A. S. Mechanisms and future directions for prevention of vein graft failure in coronary bypass surgery. Eur J Cardiothorac Surg. (2002). Sep;Review., 22(3), 387-96.

[2] Khaleel, M. S, Dorheim, T. A, & Duryee, M. J. High-Pressure Distention of the Saphenous Vein During Preparation Results in Increased Markers of Inflammation: A Potential Mechanism for Graft Failure. Ann Thorac Surg (2012). , 93, 552-8.

[3] Favaloro, R. Saphenous Vein Autograft Replacement of Severe Segmental Coronary Artery Occlusion: Operative Technique. Ann Thorac Surg. (1968). , 5, 334-339.

[4] Lopes, R. D, Hafley, G. E, Allen, K. B, et al. Endoscopic versus Open Vein-Graft Harvesting in Coronary-Artery Bypass Surgery. New Eng Jour Med. (2009). , 361, 235-244.

[5] Bonde, P, & Graham, A. N. MacGowan SW. Endoscopic vein harvest: advantages and limitations. Ann Thorac Surg (2004). , 77, 2076-82.

[6] Black, E. A, Campbell, R. K, Channon, K. M, Ratnatunga, C, & Pillai, R. Minimally invasive vein harvesting significantly reduces pain and wound morbidity. Eur J Cardiothorac Surg (2002). , 22, 381-6.

[7] Ramos, J. R, Berger, K, Mansfield, P. B, & Sauvage, L. R. Histologic Fate and Endothelial Changes of Distended and Nondistended Vein Grafts. Ann Surg. (1976).

[8] Souza DSRJohansson B, Bojo L, et al. Harvesting the Saphenous vein with the surrounding tissue for CABG provides Long-Term Graft Patency comparable to the Left

Internal Thoracic Artery: Results of Randomized longitudinal trial. J Thorac Cardiovasc Surg. (2006). , 132, 373-8.

[9] Dashwood, M, Savage, K, Tsui, J, et al. Retaining perivascular tissue of human saphenous vein grafts protects against surgical and distension-induced damage and preserves endothelial nitric oxide synthase and nitric oxide synthase activity. J Thorac Cardiovasc Surg (2009). , 138, 334-340.

[10] Souza, D. S, Johansson, B, Bojö, L, Karlsson, R, Geijer, H, Filbey, D, Bodin, L, Arbeus, M, & Dashwood, M. R. Harvesting the saphenous vein with surrounding tissue for CABG provides long-term graft patency comparable to the left internal thoracic artery: results of a randomized longitudinal trial. J Thorac Cardiovasc Surg. (2006). , 132(2), 373-8.

[11] STS adult cardiac surgery databaseChicago: Society of Thoracic Surgeons, (2008).

[12] Desai, P, Kiani, S, Thiruvanthan, N, et al. Impact of the Learning Curve for Endoscopic Vein Harvest on Conduit Quality and Early Graft Patency. Ann Thorac Surg (2011). , 91, 1385-92.

[13] Lancey, R. A, Cuenoud, H, & Nunnari, J. J. Scanning electron microscopic analysis of endoscopic versus open vein harvesting techniques. J Cardiovasc Surg (Torino) (2001). , 42, 297-301.

[14] Alrawi, S. J, Balaya, F, & Raju, R. Cunningham JN Jr, Acinapura AJ. A comparative study of endothelial cell injury during open and endoscopic saphenectomy: an electron microscopic evaluation. Heart Surg Forum (2001). , 4, 120-7.

[15] Thatte, H. S, & Khuri, S. F. The coronary artery bypass conduit: Intraoperative endothelial injury and its implication on graft patency. Ann Thorac Surg (2001). Sdiscussion S2267-70, 2245-52.

[16] Bonchek, L. I. Prevention of endothelial damage during preparation of saphenous veins for bypass grafting. J Thorac Cardiovasc Surg (1980). , 79, 911-5.

[17] Dashwood, M. R, & Loesch, A. Surgical damage of the saphenous vein and graft patency. J Thorac Cardiovasc Surg (2007). , 133, 274-5.

[18] Rifkin, D. B, Baumann, F. G, Colvin, S. B, et al. Mammary artery versus saphenous vein grafts: Assessment of basic fibroblast growth factors. Ann Thorac Surg (1994). , 58, 308-311.

[19] Salvemini, D, Radziszewski, W, Korbut, R, et al. The use of oxyhemoglobin to elucdate the time course of platelet inhibition induced by NO or NO-donors. Br J Pharmacol. (1990). , 101, 991-995.

[20] Feigl, E. O. EDRF- a protective factor? Nature. (1988). , 331, 490-491.

[21] Cooke, J. P, & Tsao, P. S. Is NO an endogenous antiathergenic molecule? Arterioscler Thromb. (1995). , 14(5), 653-655.

[22] Davies, M. G, Fulton, G. J, & Hagen, P. O. Clinical Biology of Nitric Oxide. Br J Surg. (1995)., 82(12), 1598-1610.

[23] Kown, M. H, Yamaguchi, A, Jahncke, C. L, et al. L-arginine polymers inhibit the development of vein graft neointimal hyperplasia. J Thorac Cardiovasc Surg (2001)., 121(5), 971-980.

[24] Fitzgibbon, G. M, Kafka, H. P, & Leach, A. J. Coronary bypass graft fate and patient outcome: angiographic follow-up of 5065 grafts related to survival and reoperation in 1388 patients during 25 years. J am Coll Cardiology(1996)., 28, 616-626.

[25] Moor, E, Hamsten, A, Blomback, M, et al. Hemostatic factors and inhibitors and coronary artery bypass grafting: preoperative alteration and relations to graft occlusion. Thromb Haemost (1994)., 72, 335-342.

[26] Verrier, E. D, & Boyle, J. R. Endothelial Cell Injury in cardiovascular surgery. Ann Thorac Surg (1996)., 62, 915-922.

[27] Sarkar, R, Meinberg, E. G, Stanley, J. C, et al. Nitric Oxide reversibly inhibits the migration of cultured vascular muscle cells. Circ Res (1996)., 78, 225-230.

[28] LoGerfo FWQuist WC, Cantelmo NL et al. Integrity of vein grafts as a function of initial intimal and medial preservation. Circulation (1983). II I II I 24., 17.

[29] Linder, V, Reidy, M. A, Baird, A, et al. Role of basic fibroblast growth factor in vascular lesion formation. Circ Res (1991)., 68, 106-113.

[30] Morgan, D. O. Cyclin-dependent kinases: engines, clocks, and microprocessors. Annu Rev Cell Div Biol (1997)., 13, 261-291.

[31] Loscalzo, J. Matrix and Vein Graft Failure: Is the Message in the Medium? Circ. (2000)., 101, 221-223.

[32] George, S. J, Zaltsman, A. B, & Newby, A. C. Surgical preparative injury and neointima formation increase MMP-9 expression and MMP-2 activation in human saphenous vein. Cardiovasc Res. (1997)., 33, 447-459.

[33] Kranzhofer, A, Baker, A. H, George, S. J, & Newby, A. C. Expression of tissue inhibitor of metalloproteinase-1,-2, and-3 during neointima formation in organ cultures of human saphenous vein. Arterioscler Thromb Vasc Biol. (1999)., 19, 255-265.

[34] Divergent effects of tissue inhibitor of metalloproteinase-1or-3 overexpression on rat vascular smooth muscle cell invasion, proliferation, and death in vitro: TIMP-3 promotes apoptosis. J Clin Invest. (1998)., 101, 1478-1487.

[35] Motwani, J. G, & Topol, E. J. Aortocoronary Saphenous Vein Graft Disease: Pathogenesis, Predisposition, and Prevention. Circulation.(1998)., 97, 916-931.

[36] Crook, M. F, Newby, A. C, & Southgate, K. M. Expression of intercellular adhesion molecules in human saphenous veins effects of inflammatory cytokines and neointima formation in culture. Atherosclerosis (2000). , 150, 33-41.

[37] Saxena, A, Rauch, U, Berg, K. E, et al. The vascular repair process after injury of the carotid artery is regulated by IL-1RI and MyD88 signalling. Cardiovasc Res (2011). , 91, 350-7.

Chapter 10

The Impact of Arterial Grafts in Patients Undergoing GABG

Haralabos Parissis, Alan Soo and Bassel Al-Alao

Additional information is available at the end of the chapter

http://dx.doi.org/10.5772/54621

1. Introduction

General population suffers at 2-3% by angina. Incidence of angina in men and women aged 55 to 75 is 9% and 5% respectively. [1]

The prevalence of angina is 24,000 people per million. Almost 1 in 1000 undergoes CABG in the USA. This means that half a million people undergo CABG around the world per year and 1.5 million patients undergo Angioplasty/ stenting (1 to 3).

Without revscularization (angioplasty or bypass) four-year survival of patients one, two or three vessels disease is 92%, 84% and 68% respectively. [2] Moreover, in patients with reduced ejection fraction and heart failure (e.g. stroke) the respective survival rates are 67%, 61% and 42%. [3]

Clearly 5-yearsurvival increases with every form of revascularization treatment. Coronary artery bypass grafting (CABG) remains the gold standard revascularisation strategy for complex 3 vessel coronary artery disease and left mainstem disease.

Recent trials such as the SYNTAX have shown that CABG is superior to PCI in most circumstances of coronary artery disease. Although there are certain anatomical lesions such as isolated left main disease treatment options to be elucidated, CABG remains the gold standard treatment for severe coronary artery disease. Data from studies such as SYNTAX and ART confirmed by the National Cardiothoracic Surgery Database have also shown the low mortality risk of CABG.

These recent evidence has prompted a rewrite of the european guidelines with regards to revascularisation. It is now recommended that no ad hoc PCI to be performed and all cases of severe coronary disease should be discussed in a multidisplinary setting involving the "Heart team".

Indicatively, with the coronary artery bypass, survival is related to the ejection fraction, according the Cardiothoracic surgeries database of Emory University, where 23960 patients are registered as follows:

	5 years	10 years	15 years
EF "/> 50%	95	80	65
EF 30-50%	78	60	50
EF <30%	58	38	15

Table 1. Mortality as per Ejection Fraction

So, the main benefit from the bypass (CABG) is not only the symptomatic improvement and avoidance of the risk of a stroke, but also the evident prolongation of the patient's survival. On the other hand, it is obvious that even with CABG, long-term survival is decreasing. Even when reviewing the sudden death risk as a result of CABG, there are three (3) stages.

Years after CABG	Loss (×1000)
½	3.4
1	0.87
5	1.2
10	3.5
15	9.0

Table 2. Risk of death following CABG

There is an early, high-risk period, a period with rapid decrease of the risk and a period after 5 years, with an ascending risk rate. This late phenomenon is related to the atheromatosis of the saphenous vein graft.

2. IMAS versus BIMAS

Arterial and vein grafts are used to perform the CABG surgery. Most patients receive three grafts in a combination of an arterial (LIMA) and vein grafts. [4]

Unfortunately, in the course of time, the atherosclerotic graft disease obstructs vein grafts. It has been shown that approximately 3 months after surgery is developed hyperplasia of the inner lining of the vascular grafts. The atherosclerotic disease of the grafts is characterized by adipose infiltration at the sites of intimal hyperplasia. Indicatively 12% of the vein grafts are occluded within 1 year, 25% within 5 years and 50% within 12 years following surgery. [5], [6] This contributes to the fact that 3% of the patients after undergoing a by-pass surgery require re-surgery in 5 years, 10% in 10 years and 25% in 20 years after the surgery. [7]

http://dx.doi.org/10.5772/54621

Arterial grafts started being systematically used in the 70's. The focus was on the internal mammary artery, which presents great biological properties:

1. Endothelial cells release of nitric oxide (NO), which has vasodilator action and also prevents the accumulation of platelets, the adhesion of neurophils and chemotaxis. NO prevents directly the development of smooth muscle fibers related to the intimal hyperplasia. [8]

2. The protective action of "vasa vasorum"

3. Increased prostacyclin production.

4. Maintenance of the inner elastic layer, which prevents the migration of the smooth muscle cells.

5. The internal mammary artery has a thin middle layer with a few smooth muscle cells, which seem to reduce infiltration in response to the growth factor produced by platelets.

For all these reasons, the internal mammary artery, contrary to other vascular grafts, is not affected by intimal hyperplasia.

IMA's attrition rate compared to the saphenous vein is given in the following table:

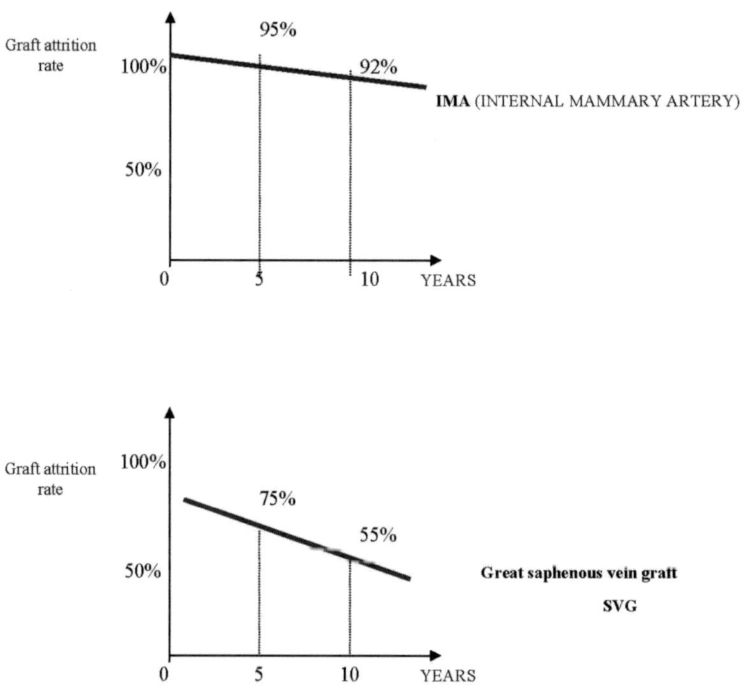

Table 3. IMA and SVG attrition rate over 10 year period

It was only a decade after the systematic use of the internal mammary artery and specifically in 1986 that a benchmark publication came from the Cleveland Clinic [9]: In an extensive retrospective study they compared the clinical outcomes and angiography findings of 2306 patients who received single internal mammary artery (IMA) graft on the left anteriordescending artery (LAD) with additional vein grafts and 3265 patients who received only vein grafts. The mean follow-up time was 8.7 years. It was found that patients on whom the internal mammary artery had been used as a graft had lower perioperative mortality rates, less re-surgery rates, smaller chances of recurrent angina or infraction and higher 10-year survival.

A second study followed, by Acinapura et al [10] in which 2100 patients were followed-up for 5 years. The study showed that:

	Patency	Recurrent angina	Re-syrgery
Internal mammary artery	96%	18%	0.5%
Vein graft	67%	31	6.3

Table 4.

Ten-year mortality rate was 10% for the IMA group and 22% for the vein grafts group.

On the same grounds, Cameron and colleagues [11] compared 479 patients with single internal mammary artery graft to 4888 patients with solely vein grafts over a period of more than 15 years. They showed that the use of a single internal mammary artery graft was an independent prognosis factor that promoted survival, especially in older patient, with a reduced LV function.

Conclusively, the use of the internal mammary artery on the anterior descending branch is indicated irrespectively to the age and to the ejection fraction. Moreover, the use of the IMA in patients with a low ejection fraction improves long-term survival.

Because of the ostensible biological similarity of the left and right internal mammary artery, many were those who believed that the use of the two internal mammary arteries as grafts could yield additional benefits.

The patency of the 2 internal mammary (left & right) artery grafts is over 90% in 10 years. The reasonable question posed is: "Why don't we use more arterial grafts during a by-pass surgery?"

Let's answer through a short review of the recent literature:

1. Calafiore [12] from Italy showed 99% patency of the 2 internal mammary arteries as shown in angiographies, at 18 months.

2. Accola et al [13] showed that in young patients, BIMAS could be safely used without putting them at higher risk of perioperative morbidity or mortality.

3. A Belgian study [14] showed 97% patency of the 2 internal mammary arteries as shown in angiographies in 161 patients at 7.5 years after by-pass.

4. Buxton [15] analyzed 962 patients and found that the patency of the right internal mammary artery is better when used for left coronary by-pass. Moroever, he underlined that arterial grafts shall by-pass a coronary artery with stenosis over 90% (to avoid the risk of competitive flow). Passing the RITA to the left, either anterior to the aorta or through the transverse sinus, did not influence patency

5. The same conclusions, meaning the use of the BIMAS on the left coronary system, were reached in a study by Schmidt [16].

6. B. Lytle [17] from Cleveland showed that the use of 2 internal mammary grafts is better than the use of a single mammary artery, regarding longer survival and lower re-surgery & recurrent angina or infraction rates. In addition, the study mentions that the benefit of the second internal mammary artery is evident 12 years after by-pass and offers a cumulative benefit. In patients with diabetes and those with a low LV ejection fraction the study showed even greater benefit regarding survival.

7. The BIMA shows no benefits in the first 4 years, however after 15 years occurrence of recurrent angina is decreased from 36% to 27%. [18]

8. Finally, the statistically strongest study comes from Oxford [19]. It is an extensive meta-analysis of seven studies. Taggard et al compared 11,200 patients with a single internal mammary artery graft versus 4,700 patients with BIMA. This study as well reached the same conclusions and showed prolonged survival when BIMA grafts were used.

Finally, it shall be underlined that all the above studies are retrospective and no prospective control studies exist till now for the single internal mammary VS the bilateral internal mammary grafting.

3. The radial artery

The fact that radial artery grafts were patent for over 18 years after surgery [20] has been the basis to re-recruit the RA (radial artery) as a graft for CABG. There is low in situ atherosclerosis incidence for this artery, however the thickened middle lining, with the abundant cells of smooth muscle fibers (contrary to the internal mammary artery) increased intimal hyperplasia of this vessel.

Angiography studies of middle time duration showed 90% patency rate in 1 year [21], 83% in 5 years [22] and over 80% in 8 years.

Although these results are encouraging, the databases should be interpreted with caution. The majority of the studies are retrospective analyses and the rate of the grafts used for follow-up via angiography varies in these studies. The recent study by Possati [23] with 92% angiographic follow-up for over 8 years, contains the most well-documented database to this day.

Two prospective randomized control studies comparing the radial artery (RA) to other grafts by means of a full angiographic follow-up are the RAPS [24] (Radial Artery Patency Study) and RSVP (Radial artery versus Saphenous Vein Patency Study) and are still in progress.

The RAPCO (Radial Artery Patency and Clinical Outcome) [25] is a prospective randomized study that compares the radial artery (RA) to grafts from the great saphenous vein and the free grafts from the right internal mammary artery. All patients received grafts from the LIMA to the LAD and then they were randomized and received either the radial artery or the right internal mammary artery on a second target in patients less than 70 years old and either the radial artery or the great saphenous vein (again within a second target) in patients aged over 70.

The 5year angiographic patency of the radial artery and the right internal mammary artery was 95 and 100% respectively, and of the saphenous vein and the radial artery it was 87% and 94% respectively.

4. Problems related to the radial artery

The tendency for vasospasm is due to the thick muscle wall of the vessel. Prevention is achieved by fine handling and the use of focal agents during denudation (papaverine / phenoxybenzamine solutions) followed by amlodipine 5mgr x 1 for one year after surgery.

5. The disadvantages of arterial grafts

The sternum infection rates when using BIMA grafts is vastly variable. Lytle reports 2.5% incidence of inflammation of the sternotomy incision when using bilateral internal mammary arteries compared to 1.4% in the group of single internal mammary artery graft. [26] Grossi and colleagues [27] published an increase of the incidence of inflammation of the sternal incision when factor 2 exists and a lot higher rate of chances, increased by 13.9% when there is concurrent diabetes. Kouchoukos [28] published that other risk factors showing an increase of the inflammation are obesity, severe chronic obstructive pulmonary disease and prolonged mechanical ventilation.

Arterial grafts shall be avoided in patients with chronic renal dysfunction and those undergoing dialysis (Steal syndrome from the AV fistula, limited survival due to dialysis.

Matsa [29] suggests the use of a skeletonized internal mammary artery (as this technique protects the collateral sternal blood flow). He argues that the complication rate of the sternal incision was the same in diabetic patients and in non-diabetic patients.

The competitive flow is the causal factor for the "string sign" which is rarely observed in arterial grafts. It had been reported when the vessel to be by-passed had not high grade stenosis. Thus, in order to avoid the competitive flow, arterial grafts are usually used only when stenosis is over 90%.

http://dx.doi.org/10.5772/54621

ARTERIAL GRAFTS PATENCY	5 year patency	10 year patency
LITA →LAD	95%	90%
LITA→ other than LAD	90%	80%
RITA→RCA	90%	80%
RITA ›LAD	95%	"/>90%
Free ITA grafts	90%,	"/>80%
Radial artery	80%	70-80%
Right gastroepiploic artery	80%	63%

Table 5. Patency of various arterial grafts over time

6. Studies on total arterial revascularization (tar)

Tavilla et al [30] reported on the 10 year follow-up of 201 CABGs in three-vessel disease using exclusively pedicled bilateral internal thoracic and right gastroepiploic arteries.Ten-year actuarial survival was 87%. The actuarial freedom from angina was 97% and 86% at 5 and 10 years respectively. None of the patients needed a repeat surgical revascularization after leaving the hospital, whereas 9 (5%) patients underwent a percutaneous transluminal coronary angioplasty. At 5 years 86% and at 10 years 69% of the patients remained free of any cardiac-related event.

Nishida [31] reported on total arterial revascularization on 239 patients with the only use of BIMAs and the right gastroepiploic artery (RGEA). ITA grafts were harvested by using the skeletonization technique. Sequential grafting was performed in 64 patients; One patient (0.4%) died of mediastinitis. Graft patency was confirmed angiographically in 230 patients (96%) 2 to 3 weeks after surgery. The patency rate was 97.1% for the left ITA, 99.6% for the right ITA, and 95.5% for the RGEA. Five-year actuarial survival rate was 92.9%, and the cardiac death-free rate was 97.8%.

Finally in a prospective randomized trial on total arterial revascularization, Muneretto et al [32] conducted a TAR study with the use of LIMA in patients over 70 years old. Follow-up was performed at 15 months, and it showed higher arterial patency and freedom from ischemic attacks in the TAR group.

Recommendation for the use of BIMA
In young patients (less than 65 years old)
- not obese and diabetic at the same time
- angiography has shown proper coronary disease (stenosis "/> 90%)
Bilateral IMAs shall go to he left system
Contraindications
- Emergencies
- Chronic renal dysfunction requiring dialysis
- Peripheral vascular disease and carotid stenosis
- Chronic obstructive pulmonary disease

Table 6. Indications and Contraindications for the use of BIMA

7. Conclusion

Experience regarding the preference of use of bilateral internal mammary arteries as grafts is growing big. However, despite the fact that the evidences are compelling, the absence of prospective randomization makes them vulnerable to ctriticism.

The use of bilateral internal mammary arteries can be conducted safely. It can offer long-term symptomatic improvement and also improve survival. Surprisingly, multiple arterial conduits are used in <15% of patients undergoing a CABG, and the radial artery is the most common choice for the second arterial conduit.

The lack of robust protocols for using BITA grafting, contributes to the variations in practises amongst surgeons. Quidelines for BIMA usage, including variables such as age, the type of diabetes, obesity, LV function and the suitability of the coronary anatomy would emergence in the future. More specifically a possible scoring system taking into consideration Syntax score and EuroSCORE maybe able to become a quide for BIMA utilization and that may overcome the difficulty for surgeons to extend the use of BIMA.

Author details

Haralabos Parissis*, Alan Soo and Bassel Al-Alao

*Address all correspondence to: hparissis@yahoo.co.uk, drsoo@hotmail.com

Cardiothoracic Department, Royal Victoria Hospital, Belfast, UK

References

[1] Pepine, C. J, Cohn, P. F, Deedwania, P. C, Gibson, R. S, Handberg, E, Hill, J. A, et al. effects of treatment on outcome in mildly symptomatic patients with ischemia during daily life. The Atenolol Silent Ischemia Study (ASIST). Circulation (1994). , 90(2), 762-8.

[2] Rogers, W. J, Coggin, C. J, Gersh, B. J, Fisher, L. D, Myers, W. O, Oberman, A, et al. Ten-year follow-up of quality of life in patients randomized to receive medical therapy or coronary artery bypass graft surgery. The Coronary Artery Surgery Study (CASS). Circulation (1990). , 82(5), 1647-58.

[3] Mock, M. B, et al. Survival of medically treated patients in the coronary artery surgery study (CASS) registry. Circulation (1982). , 66(3), 562-8.

[4] Keogh, B. E, & Kinsman, R. National Adult Cardiac Surgical Database Report (2002). The Society of Cardiothoracic Surgeons of Great Britain and Ireland; , 164-6.

[5] Fitrgibbon et alAttrition rate of saphenous vein conduit.Canadian study. Ann Thorac Surg (1996).

[6] Bourassa et alPatency rate of saphenous vein grafts. Ann Thorac Surg (1991).

[7] Lytle, B. Cleveland clinic Data from : Cardiac Surgery in the Adult, H. Edmunds, Jr).

[8] Moncada, S. Palmer RMJ, Higgs EA : Nitric Oxide : Physiology, Pathophysiology and pharmacology. Pharmacol Rev (1991).

[9] Loop, F. D, et al. Influence of the internal-mammary-artery graft on 10-year survival and other cardiac events. New Engl J Med (1986). , 314(1), 1-6.

[10] Acinapura, AJ, Rose, DM, Jacobwitz, IJ, Kramer, MD, & Robertazzi, . , Cunningham JN: Internal mammary artery bypass grafting: influence on recurrent angina and survival in 2100 patients. Ann Thorac Surg 1989, 48:186-191.

[11] Cameron, A, Davis, K. B, Green, G, et al. Coronary bypass surgery with internal-thoracic-artery grafts- effects on survival over a 15-year period. N Engl J Med (1996). , 334(4), 216-9.

[12] Calafiore, A. M, et al. Bilateral internal thoracic artery grafting: long-term clinical and angiographic results of in situ versus Y grafts. J Thorac Cardiovasc Surg (2000). , 120(5), 990 6.

[13] Accola, K. D, Jones, E. L, Craver, J. M, et al. Bilateral mammary artery grafting: Avoidance of complications with extended use. Ann Thorac Surg (1993).

[14] Dion, R, et al. Long-term clinical and angiographic follow-up of sequential internal thoracic artery grafting. Eur J Cardiothorac Surg (2000). , 17(4), 407-14.

[15] Buxton, B. F, et al. The right internal thoracic artery graft- benefits of grafting the left coronary system and native vessels with a high-grade stenosis. Eur J Cardiothorac Surg (2000). , 18(3), 255-61.

[16] Sheila, E. Schmidt, James W. Jones, John I. Thornby, Charles C. Miller, Arthur C. Beall. Improved Survival with multiple left-sided bilateral internal thoracic artery grafts. Ann Thorac Surg (1997). , 64, 9-15.

[17] Lytle, B. W, et al. Two internal thoracic artery grafts are better than one. J Thorac Cardiovasc Surg (1999). , 117(5), 855-72.

[18] Naunheim et alLong term outcome with the use of BIMAs. Annals Thorac Surgery (1992).

[19] Taggart, D. P, et al. Effect of arterial revascularisation on survival: a systematic review of studies comparing bilateral and single internal mammary arteries. Lancet (2001). , 358(9285), 870-5.

[20] Acar, C, Jebara, V. A, Portoghese, M, et al. Revival of the radial artery for coronary artery bypass grafting. Ann Thorac Surg (1992). discussion 659-60., 54(4), 652-9.

[21] Tatoulis, J, Royse, A. G, Buxton, B. F, et al. The radial artery in coronary surgery: a 5-year experience- clinical and angiographic results. Ann Thorac Surg (2002). discussion 147-8., 73(1), 143-7.

[22] Acar, C, Ramsheyi, A, Pagny, J. Y, et al. The radial artery for coronary artery bypass grafting: clinical and angiographic results at five years. J Thorac Cardiovasc Surg (1998). , 116(6), 981-9.

[23] Possati, G, Gaudino, M, Prati, F, et al. Long-term results of the radial artery used for myocardial revascularization. Circulation (2003). , 108(11), 1350-4.

[24] Fremes, S. E. Multicenter radial artery patency study (RAPS). Study design. Control Clin Trials (2000). , 21(4), 397-413.

[25] Buxton, B. F, Raman, J. S, Ruengsakulrach, P, et al. Radial artery patency and clinical outsomes: five-year interim results of a randomized trial. J Thorac Cardiovasc Surg (2003). , 125(6), 1363-71.

[26] Lytle, B. W, Blackstone, E. H, Loop, F. D, et al. Two internal thoracic artery grafts are better than one. J Thorac Cardiovasc Surg (1999). , 117(5), 855-72.

[27] Grossi, E. A, Esposito, R, Harris, L. J, et al. Sternal wound infections and use of internal mammary artery grafts (see comments). J Thorac Cardiovasc Surg (1991).

[28] Kouchoukos, N. T, Wareing, T. H, Murphy, S. F, et al. Risks of bilateral internal mammary artery bypass grafting. Ann Thorac Surg (1990).

[29] Matsa, M, Paz, Y, Gurevitch, J, et al. Bilateral skeletonized internal thoracic artery grafts in patients with diabetes mellitus. J Thorac Cardiovasc Surg (2001). , 121(4), 668-74.

[30] Tavilla, G, Kappetein, A. P, Braun, J, Gopie, J, Tjien, A. T, & Dion, R. A. Long-term follow-up of coronary artery bypass grafting in three-vessel disease using exclusively pedicled bilateral internal thoracic and right gastroepiploic arteries. Ann Thorac Surg (2004). discussion 799., 77, 794-799.

[31] Nishida, H, Tomizawa, Y, Endo, M, Koyanagi, H, & Kasanuki, H. Coronary artery bypass with only in situ bilateral internal thoracic arteries and right gastroepiploic artery. Circulation (2001). I, 76-80.

[32] Muneretto, C, Bisleri, G, Negri, A, et al. Total myocardial revascularization with composite grafts improves results of coronary surgery in the elderly: a prospective randomized comparison with conventional coronary artery bypass surgery. Circulation (2003). Suppl 1): II, 29-33.

Chapter 11

Complex Coronary Artery Disease

Tsuyoshi Kaneko and Sary Aranki

Additional information is available at the end of the chapter

http://dx.doi.org/10.5772/55251

1. Introduction

With recent increase in percutaneous cardiac intervention (PCI) the patients undergoing coronary artery bypass (CABG) are getting more complex with other medical problem. [1] In some patients standard surgical or percutaneous intervention is no longer available due to its complexity.

We define complex coronary artery disease (CAD) as condition not amenable to percutaneous coronary intervention and standard surgical intervention. Conditions for complex CAD include necessity of reoperative CABG, coronary endarterectomy, calcified aorta and trans-myocardial laser revascularization (TMR).

We will discuss each topic with preoperative workup including history and physical, tests and images. Operative steps will be discussed as well as outcomes and evidence that support the treatment.

Complex CAD is a challenge for the cardiac surgeons and advanced technique and strategies are required to treat this difficult condition surgically. Reoperative CABG can be performed with proper preoperative assessment and surgical planning. Diffusely calcified CAD can be treated with coronary endarterectomy or TMR. In case of porcelain aorta, circulatory arrest, off-pump bypass or bilateral internal thoracic artery graft may be used.

A combination of these modalities is likely necessary for cardiac surgeons in the future to treat patients with complex CAD.

2. Reoperative CABG

Data suggests that fewer patients are undergoing reoperative CABG. [2] From 1990 through 1994, 7.2% of CABG was reoperations which decreased to 2.2% from 2005 through 2009. On

the other hand, PCI before redo CABG increased from 14.5% (1990 through 1994) to 26.6% (2005 through 2009). The likely explanation for this is increased use of PCI for patients with previous CABG and more effective risk factor control. Also, use of internal thoracic artery (ITA) grafts to left anterior descending (LAD) coronary artery graft decreases the risk of reoperation and this had become standard graft choice for CABG. The patients who underwent reoperative CABG had more diabetes, dyslipidemia, hypertension, peripheral vascular disease and left main disease. In another words, we are seeing less reoperative CABG in a higher risk patients. Because ITA grafts rarely develop atherosclerosis, reoperation is primarily based on the patency of the saphenous venous grafts or other arterial grafts. Atherosclerosis occurs in majority of vein grafts explanted more than 10 years after surgery and this account for almost all the late graft stenosis. The friability of vein graft atherosclerosis is a substantial risk of distal coronary artery embolization during PCI and reoperation CABG.

Current recommendations for reoperation CABG include late stenotic vein grafts perfusing large area of myocardium mainly LAD or new distal CAD which is not perfused by the previous grafts. [3, 4, 5] Avoidance of graft injury during reentry is the key since perioperative myocardial infarction is the most significant predictor of mortality in patients undergoing reoperation. [6, 7]

2.1. Work up

Previous History Detailed specifics of the previous surgery must be obtained. Date of the surgery, operating surgeon, technical aspects of surgery including number of the grafts performed, which target was bypassed, presence of ITA grafts and what kind of grafts were harvested. Also presence of any complication during the last surgery can be obtained from medical record or directly from the patient. Information regarding aspirin, clopidogrel, warfarin and dabigatran is important that may dispose to intraoperative and postoperative bleeding.

Physical Examination Physical examination should include assessment of grafts such as Allen's test for radial arterial graft and previous scars to show saphenous vein harvest. Presence of peripheral artery disease should be assessed in case axillary or femoral cannulation is used for establishment of cardiopulmonary bypass. Venous Doppler study can be used for presence of greater and lesser saphenous vein and arterial Doppler studies can be used to assess the patency of radial and inferior epigastric arteries.

Cardiac Catheterization Cardiac Catheterization is the golden standard test to identify the new CAD. This will show native vessel anatomy, location of the lesion, patency of the previous graft including the LITA and size of the conduit. Non patency generally suggests presence of graft occlusion, but one must realize there is a chance that this may be incomplete study.

CT Angiography Another test that is being used in evaluation of the conduit is Computed tomography (CT) angiography. [8, 9] They are useful because they are able to precisely define the course of the previously placed conduits especially the LITA grafts. The condition of the Aorta, stenosis in the subclavian artery can also be assessed. Information gained from these methods will help guide the surgeons where the previous conduit will be during sternal entry.

http://dx.doi.org/10.5772/55251

Other images Chest X-ray will provide the information regarding the sternal wires and aortic calcification and lateral view will provide proximity of the heart to the sternum. If the patient does not have a sternal wire after previous CABG, it may indicate patient had sternal wound dehiscence with flap closure. Echocardiogram will provide any wall motion abnormality as well as any valve abnormality which may change operative strategy. Nuclear stress tests such as thallium scanning and positron emission tomography and/or stress (exercise or dobutamine) echocardiogram can be used to assess the viability of the myocardium. If there is no viability, surgical revascularization may not be indicated.

2.2. Operation

The reoperation CABG is more complex surgery compared to primary CABG. Technical challenges include sternal reentry, identification of old grafts, presence of graft stenosis and lack of bypass conduits.

Cardiopulmonary bypass strategy Typically, due to risk of graft injury, axillary or femoral artery cannulation is performed prior to sternotomy. Venous cannulation is obtained using femoral vein cannulation. For high risk cases, such as LITA lying underneath the sternum, Aorta underneath the sternum or right ventricle severly adhered to the sternum, CPB may be established prior to sternotomy. This allows lung deflation which retracts the heart away from the sternum.

Operating Room Setup External defibrillators must be attached to the patient prior to incision in case patient develops nonsustained ventricular arrhythmia during entry and dissection. For specific cases, thoracotomy can be performed for left sided graft to enable safe and efficient approach to the targets. [10]

Sternal Reentry Sternal wires are cut and midline of the sternum is marked for sternal reentry. Oscillating saw is used to divide the anterior table of the sternum. The sternal wires are left in place to protect the saw from cutting through the posterior table and possibly injuring the heart. When the anterior table has been divided, ventilation is stopped. And assistant elevate each side of sternum and posterior table is then sharply divided. Sternal wires are removed as posterior table is divided.

Dissection Once the sternum is divided, dissection of the mediastinum is performed. Traction superiorly not laterally is important, since lateral traction can tear the right ventricle and other important structures. Typically, dissection is performed from inferior to superior direction to minimize the chance of injuring critical structures. Identification of the diaphragm and pericardial edge is a marker for correct plane. Right pericardial edge is dissected from pericardiophrenic angle to the superior vena cava/right atrium junction and aorta is identified. Innominate vein is identified and dissected to avoid stretch injury. Anticipation of proximal anastomosis and graft is the key using the preoperative images and operative report. If there is an injury to the graft, CPB should be initiated and further dissection can be carried out. CPB can also be initiated on high risk patients to empty the heart and allow it to fall away from the sternum. Downside of this technique is the need to dissect while on heparin which results in more bleeding.

Cardiopulmonary Bypass Once Aorta and right atrium is dissected, the heart can be arrested. Effective myocardial protection is essential in previously revascularized heart. Both antegrade and retrograde coronary perfusion are critical. Antegrade cardioplegia may not be effective for areas supplied by ITA, and may dislodge emboli from the atherosclerotic debris from the disease vein grafts. On the other hand, retrograde cardioplegia protects from embolization and removes debris from the retrograde flow. 11 Epiaortic ultrasound is performed to prior to aortic crossclamp to identify any aortic plaques. [12] Mild hypothermia is induced after patient is placed on CPB. When there is patent LITA, it is standard practice to dissect and clamp. However, if the dissection is difficult, moderate hypothermia with either fibrillatory arrest or systemic hyperkalemia can be used to arrest the heart. Manipulation of the graft should be avoided until the heart is arrested since this can dislodge the debris.

Revascularization If LITA or RITA was not used, this will be the first choice for conduit. When ITA is used to replace a vein graft, the old vein graft should be left in place and arterial vessel should be anastomosed to the same coronary vessel. [13] If the vein graft is ligated this may induce ischemia to the target vessel. If saphenous vein is used for conduit, distal anastomosis can be performed directedly to the native coronary artery or to the cuff of 0.5mm of old vein graft if no distal stenosis is present. Proximal anastomosis is performed in similar fashion; however, if there are minimal aorta that can be used for anastomosis, graft can be connected to the previous proximal graft.

If there is associated procedure such as aortic procedure or valve procedure, distal anastomosis is performed prior to valve procedure to avoid manipulation of the heart after the prosthesis is in place. When adding ITA graft to stenotic LAD vein graft, it is advised to leave the stenotic vein graft to avoid hypoperfusion, although there is a risk of distal embolization from the old vein and competitive flow to the new graft.

2.3. Outcomes

From Society of Thoracic Surgeon database, surgical coronary revascularization has evolved over the last decade, with reoperative CABG now uncommonly performed in contemporary practice. reoperative CABG dropped from 6.0% in 2000 to 3.4% in 2009. [14] Reoperative mortality is high in reoperative group, operative mortality declined from 6.1% in 2000 to 4.6% in 2009 despite the fact that patients now more frequently present with left main disease, myocardial infarction, and heart failure. In centers with large operative experience, reports have demonstrated consistently lower mortality. There is increasing evidence that the preemptive strategies discussed here may minimize technical and postoperative complication. [15] Patients also now present more frequently for urgent or emergent surgery and following previous PCI. They also now have a higher incidence of other comorbidities such as increased weight, diabetes, hypertension, hypercholesterolemia, renal failure, and cerebrovascular disease.

Despite operating in patients with more complex coronary artery disease and greater medical comorbidities, there have been significant improvements in operative morbidity and mortality in this challenging population. The primary reason for increased mortality appears to be related to perioperative myocardial infarction (MI), due to graft injury, graft failure, inade-

quate myocardial protection and postoperative graft failure. Other significant predictors of mortality after reoperative coronary revascularization include age, female gender and emergency operations. [16] Long-term outcome is successful after a high risk surgery. 10-year survival is reported to be 55-69% and negative predictors of long term survival is preoperative left ventricular dysfunction, increasing age and diabetes mellitus. [17]

3. Coronary endarterectomy

Coronary endarterectomy is performed when the target has severe atherosclerosis and is not a suitable target. This procedure removes the atherosclerotic plaques with the intima and allows the conduit be anastomosed to the target. Often, decision of coronary endarterectomy is made intraoperatively and conduit is anastomosed to the endarterectomized vessel. This requires precise technique and experience since inadequate procedure leads to occlusion of the native artery and the bypass conduit. Main perioperative challenge is maintainance of patency because removal of the endothelial surface of the coronary artery disposed to platelet aggregation and subsequent thrombus formation. Therefore, anticoagulation method including usage of postoperative heparin and clopidogrel is encouraged.

3.1. Operation

Right coronary artery (RCA) is the most common vessel which coronary endarterectomy is performed. LAD endarterectomy is a technically complex procedure when compared to RCA endarterectomy due to the location and configuration of the septal and diagonal branches. LAD atherosclerotic core is narrow and delicate which increases the risk of disruption under tension. Unidirectional traction on the plaque can cause shearing off the branches. It is quite common that an extended arteriotomy or multiple arteriotomies are performed to achieve adequate plaque extraction. In cases where an extended arteriotomy is performed, the proximal third is used as the site of LITA anastomosis while the distal aspect of the vessel is reconstructed with a vein patch. In cases where 2 or more distinct arteriotomies are created, the LITA may be used for both sites as a separate graft; however, it is common practice that the LITA be used for 1 arteriotomy site and vein graft(s) used for the remainder. [18]

Endarterectomy Endarterectomy for a diffusely diseased coronary artery is used when 1-mm probe is not passed. It is often necessary to create long arteriotomy. After the coronary arteriotomy, an endarterectomy spatula was used to identify the plane of dissection and then to mobilize the plaque proximally and distally. A 1-mm probe was advanced gently through the plane of dissection to break away resistant adhesions. A combination of gentle traction on the plaque and countertraction on the adventitia is useful to extract the plaque. When proper distal tapering of the specimen was not achieved, the arteriotomy was extended distally for complete extraction of the plaque. The proximal end of the endarterectomy should be distal to the most proximal lesion, to avoid competitive flow through the native coronary artery, to the level of the first diagonal branch at most. The atherosclerotic plaque varies from soft to extremely calcified and adherent. This characteristic dictates the length of the arteriotomy

inasmuch as adherent plaques cannot be removed easily through a limited arteriotomy to at least the distal two thirds of the length of the target. If this was the case, the arteriotomy was extended to allow for complete extraction of the atherosclerotic core.

Cardioplegia Flush After complete extraction, retrograde cardioplegic solution was given to flush out any debris that may have embolized distally. A visible flow of retrograde cardioplegic solution through the diagonal and septal branches is indicative of successful endarterectomy.

Vein Patch The saphenous vein patch was applied to the endarterectomized vessel with a long arteriotomy and the LITA was then applied to either the middle of the vein patch or the proximal end of the arteriotomy or LITA onlay patch grafting was used for a relatively short arteriotomy after confirming that there was no tension on the graft.

Myocardial Protection Myocardial protection is achieved with combination of antegrade and retrograde blood cardioplegia. Retrograde cardioplegia is essential during endarterectomy as it allows for flushing of debris proximally, thereby minimizing the risk of myocardial infarction secondary to plaque emboli. Furthermore, retrograde cardioplegia serves a diagnostic purpose; brisk flow through the entire artery indicates complete plaque extraction.

Postoperative Drug Regimen Prevention of platelet aggregation and thrombus formation is crucial to prevent graft and native vessel occlusion. An aggressive protocol is generally required and includes intravenous heparin in the immediate postoperative phase as well as lifetime treatment with clopidogrel (with loading dose) and aspirin.

3.2. Outcome

The risk of endarterectomy patients are higher compared to CABG alone. In some reports, long term patency is inferior to CABG, but in experienced hands operative mortality of 3.0% and 5-year survival of 87% can be achieved. [19] The most significant complication is periooperative MI after endarterectomy. It is significant higher compared to CABG alone including MI occurrence which occurs in 5-10%. [20] Multiterritory endarterectomy is associated with worse long term survival (64% 5-year survival and 36% 10-year survival), but this could be due to higher risk patient population. [21]

LAD endarterectomy was intially reported with increased incidence of morbidity and mortality. [22 23] With technical modifications including LITA grafting with saphenous vein patch and LITA onlay patch grafting, the outcomes in this high risk group has significantly improved. [24] Endarterectomy provides good results and mainstay of the treatments for patients with severe diffuse coronary artery disease not amenable to PCI and traditional surgical intervention.

4. Calcified aorta

The atherosclerotic involvement of the ascending aorta presents technical challenge in patients undergoing CABG. The degree of calcification ranges from isolated plaques to total calcifica-

tion which is known as porcelain aorta. The danger of applying cross clamp is associated with markedly increased incidence of cerebral or systemic embolism. The avoidance of multiple aortic manipulations is the key and strategy must be designed based on this principle.

Atherosclerotic disease of the ascending aorta is becoming an increasing problem and is important to understand the prevalence of this disease entity. Mills and Everson reported 2.0% of unclampable aorta in their CABG population of 1735 patients. [25] Other reports have indicated its occurrence between 2-5% [26, 27]. Goto et al reported in their 463 patients undergoing CABG reported stroke rate of 10.5% in patients with severe atherosclerosis compared with 1.8% in normal or near-normal control patients. [28] The challenges in such situation are to make the accurate diagnosis and operative strategy.

4.1. Work up

Due to its potential to modify surgical strategy, preoperative or intraoperative diagnosis of unclampable aorta is the key. Accurate diagnosis of aortic atherosclerotic disease is of paramount importance. No diagnostic criteria have been established to date, and often unclampable aorta is diagnosed intraoperatively by manual palpation or epiaortic ultrasonography. Disease of the carotid artery and abdominal aorta, stenosis of LAD and age has been reported to be associated with unclampable aorta. [29] Given the predictors of atheromatous aortic disease are age, hypertension, diabetes, dyslipidemia, peripheral vasculopathy and diabetes [30], screening for calcified aorta is recommended in these patient groups.

Images- CXR, Cath, CT scan, TEE Chest X-ray and cardiac catheterization images may demonstrate the presence of atherosclerosis but is not always sensitive. Routine use of screening CT scan in this high risk group is useful to prevent incidence of stroke. [31] CT scan without contrast will delineate the white calcium in clear contrast to the non-calcified aorta which will appear dark. Intraoperatively, epiaortic ultrasound is superior to manual palpation of the ascending aorta and to Transthoracic echocardiography (TEE) for detection of atherosclerosis. [32]

Epiaortic Ultrasound Epiaortic ultrasound may reduce the frequency of neurological injury after surgery due to cerebral embolism by allowing for the identification and avoid atheroma at the site of cannulation and further manipulation. Introduction of epiaortic ultrasound was associated with reduction in prevalence of stroke from 1.2% to 0.7% in retrospective review of 8547 patients undergoing CABG surgery. [33] With this, epiaortic scanning now appears to be the gold standard in diagnosis of atherosclerosis in ascending aorta.

4.2. Operation

Management of this complex disease remains a major dilemma. Several techniques including aortic graft replacement, aortic endarterectomy, no touch technique and off-pump bypass has been described to cope with this difficult problem.

Techniques Using Hypothermic Circulatory Arrest Both Aortic graft replacement and endarterectomy are performed using period of hypothermic circulatory arrest.

- Deep Hypothermia Deep hypothermia (18-20°C) should be attained on CPB. Following fibrillation of the heart, a left ventricular vent is placed.
- Distal Anastomosis During the cooling phase of CPB, the distal anastomoses are performed in the following order: LAD, RCA/posterior descending artery, and marginal branches. Of note, when the heart is lifted during construction of distal anastomoses, bypass flow should be reduced to allow for decompression, thereby optimizing exposure and minimizing damage to the heart. Frequently, at least 1 proximal anastomosis is performed under a brief period of circulatory arrest.
- Endarterectomy When calcification is localized, endarterectomy can be performed under circulatory arrest to created portion of aorta which is decalcified to place a crossclamp.
- Ascending Aorta Replacement In extreme case, the ascending aorta should be replaced under deep hypothermic circulatory arrest. Proximal anastomosis is performed directly to the graft.

No touch Technique No touch technique described by Suma et al can be used [34]. In this instance, CPB is established between right atrium and aortic arch or femoral artery. Left ventricular vent is placed. Aortic cross clamping and cardioplegia delivery was avoided. Ventricular fibrillation was induced while target was occluded using elastic stitches. Pedicled artery graft is used for anastomosis. In case the saphenous vein is used, it is anastomosed to the artery graft or to the ascending aorta where calcification is spared.

Off-pump bypass Off-pump bypass can be used in case arch and femoral artery is calcified as well. In this case, all arterial revascularization is performed using in situ internal thoracic and radial artery. Y grafts are created to internal thoracic artery if radial artery is used.

4.3. Outcome

Aortic endarterectomy and aortic graft replacement provides opportunity to revascularize the coronary artery and eliminate danger of systemic emboli. It is reported to be performed safely, [35, 36] but these procedures do add complexity and risk due to the circulatory arrest.

No touch technique and off pump technique provides theoretical benefit to the procedure, but has not been able to provide definite superiority. Off pump technique offers inferior possibility of complete revascularization especially to the lateral branches of circumflex artery. On the other hand, no touch technique still requires insertion of the arterial cannula which can predispose to systemic and cerebral emboli. Gaudino et al compared these two techniques in 211 unclampable aorta cases and reported no touch technique had greater incidence of neurological complications, renal insufficiency, and stay in the intensive care unit and hospital. However, at midterm follow-up, more patients of the off pump group had ischemia recurrence. [37] Stroke rate was 2.3% and in-hospital mortality was 2.8% in this study.

5. Transmyocardial laser revascularization

Transmyocardial laser revascularization (TMR) is one of the first described surgical procedures intended to treat severe diffuse CAD not amenable to CABG or PTCA in patients who have had previous percutaneous coronary interventions and/or CABG procedures. This severe coronary artery disease can lead to incomplete revascularization following CABG and is powerful independent perioperative adverse events. Indications for TMR include NYHA class III/IV symptoms refractory to medical treatment with coronary disease that is not amenable to revascularization. [38, 39, 40]TMR is generally contraindicated in patients who are candidates for revascularization or those who are not candidates but have an ejection fraction below 20%.

By inducing angiogenesis with a laser (carbon dioxide, holminumyttrium– aluminum-garnett), TMR has been shown to decrease the severity of angina symptoms compared to medical therapy. [41, 42] As such, the primary indication for TMR is persistent and disabling angina refractory to medical therapy. Owing to its success as sole therapy, TMR is used in conjunction with CABG. The safety and efficacy of TMR in this subset of patients has been well described; operative mortality and morbidity may be significantly less than CABG alone. [43]

Since Food and Drug Administration (FDA) approval in 1998, over 20,000 TMR procedures have been performed in the United States. [44]

5.1. Operation

Left thoracotomy and Heart Exposure A left anterolateral thoracotomy is the incision of choice in patients undergoing TMR as the sole surgical procedure. The heart is exposed, allowing for the access to the anterior, apical, and posterolateral planes of the left ventricle. Careful attention must be paid to not injure the previous bypass grafts. LAD is identified and used as a landmark for the location of the septum. TMR is provided through a hand piece that delivers energy through hollow tubes to the epicardium.

Choose type of laser Type of Laser Only CO2 and Holmium-chromium: YAG lasers (Ho:YAG) are clinically approved for TMR. The result of any laser-tissue interaction is dependent on both laser and tissue variables. CO2 laser has wavelength of 10,600nm, whereas Ho:YAG laser has wavelength of 2,120nm. The laser is synchronized to occur on the R-wave of the electrocardiogram to avoid induction of arrhythmias.

Application of laser Pulse energy of 20-30 J over 4 pulses per second creates 1-mm channels in the myocardium that can be visualized with a transesophageal echocardiogram. Using the CO2 laser, channels are first created at the base of the heart and are separated from each other by 1 cm to the apex of the heart starting inferiorly and working superiorly to the anterior surface of the heart. As there is some bleeding from the channels, gravity will keep the field clean by starting inferiorly.

It should be noted that TMR does not provide any added benefit to areas of myocardium that are scarred and have no viability. TMR on the transmural scar will not only be non-beneficial,

it will cause bleeding which may be problematic. Detection of transmural penetration is primarily by tactile and auditory feedback.

5.2. Outcome

Mortality following TMR ranges from 1% to 5%; however, this low rate of mortality is primarily generalized to patients who are electively taken to the operating room and are hemodynamically stable. When these patients are taken to the operating room emergently, mortality is reported to be 10-20%. One-year survival following TMR ranges from 79% to 96% and is not significantly different from patients who undergo medical therapy. The primary advantage of TMR over medical therapy and the principal indication for intervention is the reduction in symptomatology; studies have found that 25%-76% of patients will achieve a decrease of 2 or more angina classes following intervention, which is not the case of patients undergoing medical intervention. Review of the randomized controlled study suggests improvement in perfusion for CO2 TMR treated patients. [45 46] Long term results suggest improved angina symptoms and decreased hospitalization in five years. [47]

However, the benefit of TMR is controversial. Cochrane review published it data after reviewing seven studies (1137 participants of which 559 randomized to TMR). Overall, 43.8 % of patients in the treatment group decreased two angina classes as compared with 14.8 % in the control group. Mortality at both 30 days (4.0 % in the TMR group and 3.5 % in the control group) and 1 year (12.2 % in the TMR group and 11.9 % in the control group) was similar in both groups. The 30-days mortality as treated was 6.8% in TMLR group and 0.8% in the control group, showing a statistically significant difference. Their conclusion was there is insufficient evidence to conclude that the clinical benefits of TMLR outweigh the potential risks and the procedure is associated with a significant early mortality. [48]

TMR is used in conjunction with CABG as well. One randomized controlled study have found that TMR combined with CABG may confer excellent perioperative and survival rates, including decreased opeartive mortality, inotropic support, and intensive care unit stay, while prolonging 1-year survival compared to those patients undergoing CABG alone. [49] Furthermore, patients who undergo both procedures appear to be less symptomatic at follow-up.

In conclusion application of TMR in selected group for the treatment with severe angina due to diffuse disease can be used achieves a more complete revascularization.

6. Conclusion

Complex CAD remains a challenge for cardiac surgeons; however, evolving techniques and strategies can be used to overcome this challenge. Although reoperative CABG is a high-risk procedure, proper preoperative assessment and surgical planning has yielded excellent results. Patients who are not candidates for CABG or percutaneous coronary interventions due to diffusely diseased vessels can be offered coronary endarterectomy. Calcified aorta encountered during surgery can be managed by aortic replacement, endarterectomy, using no touch

http://dx.doi.org/10.5772/55251

technique or off-pump CABG. TMR may be indicated for patients who have exhausted non surgical options. The outcomes in this complex coronary artery surgery are improving and the results have validated the safety, effectiveness and health outcomes. However, it is crucial to make good patient selection as well as intraoperative decision. Cardiac surgeons must familiarize themselves to these procedures as coronary artery disease patients will be more complex in the future.

Author details

Tsuyoshi Kaneko and Sary Aranki*

Brigham and Women's Hospital, Harvard Medical School, USA

References

[1] ElBardissi AW, Aranki SF, Sheng S, O'Brien SM, Greenberg CC, Gammie JS. Trends in isolated coronary artery bypass grafting: an analysis of the Society of Thoracic Surgeons adult cardiac surgery database. J ThoracCardiovascSurg Feb;143(2):273-81.

[2] Spiliotopoulos K, Maganti M, Brister S, RaoVivek. Changing Pattern of Reoperative Coronary Artery Bypass Grafting: A 20-Year Study. Ann ThoracSurg 2011;92:40-7.

[3] Cohn L: Cardiac Surgery in the adult, vol. 4. New York, NY, McGraw-Hill, 2011

[4] Lytle BW, Loop FD, Taylor PC, et al: Vein graft disease: The clinical impact of stenoses in saphenous vein bypass grafts to coronary arteries. J ThoracCardiovascSurg 103:831-840, 1992

[5] Lytle BW, Loop FD, Taylor PC, et al: The effect of coronary reoperation on the survival of patients with stenoses in saphenous vein bypass grafts to coronary arteries. J ThoracCardiovascSurg 105:605-612, 1993, discussion, 612-614

[6] Lytle BW, McElroy D, McCarthy P, et al: Influence of arterial coronary bypass grafts on the mortality in coronary reoperations. J ThoracCardiovascSurg 107:675-682, 1994

[7] Jones EL, Lattouf OM, Weintraub WS: Catastrophic consequences of internal mammary artery hypoperfusion. J ThoracCardiovascSurg 98:902-907, 1989

[8] Von Kiedrowski H, Wiemer M, Franzke K, et al: Non-invasive coronary angiography: The clinical value of multi-slice computed tomography in the assessment of patients with prior coronary bypass surgery. Evaluating grafts and native vessels. Int J Cardiovasc Imaging 25:161-170, 2009

[9] Yamamoto M, Kimura F, Niinami H, et al: Noninvasive assessment of off-pump coronary artery bypass surgery by 16-channel multidetectorrow computed tomography. Ann ThoracSurg 81:820-827, 2006

[10] Byrne JG, Aklog L, Adams DH, et al: Reoperative CABG using left thoracotomy: A tailored strategy. Ann ThoracSurg 71:196-200, 2001

[11] Gundry SR, Razzouk AJ, Vigesaa RE, et al: Optimal delivery of Cardioplegic solution for "redo" operations. J ThoracCardiovascSurg 103: 896-901, 1992

[12] Rosenberger P, Shernan SK, Loffler M, et al: The influence of epiaortic ultrasonography on intraoperative surgical management in 6051 cardiac surgical patients. Ann ThoracSurg 85:548-553, 2008

[13] Navia D, CosgroveDMIII, Lytle BW, et al: Is the internal thoracic artery the conduit of choice to replace a stenotic vein graft? Ann ThoracSurg 57:40-43, 1994

[14] Ghanta RK, Kaneko T, Gammie JS, Sheng S, Aranki SF. Evolving Trends of Reoperative CABG: An Analysis of the STS Adult Cardiac Surgery Database. . J ThoracCardiovasc Surg. In press.

[15] Loop FD, Lytle BW, Cosgrove DM, et al: Reoperation for coronary atherosclerosis. Changing practice in 2509 consecutive patients. Ann Surg 212:378-385, 1990

[16] He GW, Acuff TE, Ryan WH, et al: Determinants of operative mortality in reoperative coronary artery bypass grafting. J ThoracCardiovascSurg 110:971-978, 1995

[17] Weintraub WS, Jones EL, Craver JM, et al: In-hospital and long-term outcome after reoperative coronary artery bypass graft surgery. Circulation 92:II50-II57

[18] Byrne JG, Karavas AN, Gudbjartson T, et al: Left anterior descending coronary endarterectomy: Early and late results in 196 consecutive patients. Ann ThoracSurg 78:867-873, 2004

[19] Myers PO, Tabata M, Shekar PS et al. Extensive endarterectomy and reconstruction of the left anterior descending artery: Early and late outcomes. . J ThoracCardiovascSurg 143:1336-40;2012.

[20] Brenowitz JB, Kayser KL, Johnson WD: Results of coronary artery endarterectomy and reconstruction. J ThoracCardiovascSurg 95:1-10, 1988

[21] Tabata M, Shekar PS, Couper GS, et al: Early and late outcomes of multiple coronary endarterectomy. J CardiovascSurg 23:697-700, 2008

[22] Brenowitz JB, Kayser KL, Johnson WD. Results of coronary artery endarterectomyand reconstruction. J ThoracCardiovasc Surg. 1988;95:1-10.

[23] Livesay JJ, Cooley DA, Hallman GL, Reul GJ, Ott DA, Duncan JM, et al. Early and late results of coronary endarterectomy: analysis of 3,369 patients. J ThoracCardiovasc Surg. 1986;92:649-60.

[24] Myers PO, Tabata M, Shekar PS et al. Extensive endarterectomy and reconstruction of the left anteriordescending artery: Early and late outcomes. J ThoracCardiovascSurg 2012;143:1336-40

[25] Mills NL, Everson CT. Atherosclerosis of the ascending aorta and coronary artery bypass. J ThoracCardiovasc Surg. 1991;102:546 –553.

[26] Bar-El Y, Goor DA. Clamping of the atherosclerotic ascending aorta during coronary artery bypass operations: its cost in strokes. J ThoracCardiovasc Surg. 1992;104:469–474.

[27] Culliford AT, Colvin SB, Rohrer K, et al. The atherosclerotic ascending aorta and transverse arch: a new technique to prevent cerebral injury during bypass: experience with 13 patients. Ann Thorac Surg. 1986;41: 27–35.

[28] Okita Y, Ando M, Minatoya K, Kitamura S, Takamoto S, Nakajima N. Predictive factors for mortality and cerebral complications in arteriosclerotic aneurysm of the aortic arch. Ann ThoracSurg 1999;67:72-8.

[29] Razi DM. The challenge of calcific aortitis. J Card Surg. 1993;8: 102–107.

[30] Davila-Roman VG, Barzilai B, Wareing TH, et al. Intraoperative ultrasonographicevaluation of the ascending aorta in 100 consecutive patients undergoing cardiac surgery. Circulation. 1991;84(suppl III):III- 47–III-53.

[31] Nishi H, Mitsuno M, Tanaka H et al. Who needs preoperative routine chest computed tomography for prevention of stroke in cardiac surgery?Interact CardiovascThorac Surg. 2010 Jul;11(1):30-3.

[32] Das S, Dunning J. Can epiaortic ultrasound reduce the incidence of intraoperative stroke during cardiac surgery? Interact CardiovascThoracSurg 2004;3:71–5

[33] Ozatik MA, Gol MK, Fansa I, Uncu H, Kucuker SA, Kucukaksu S, Bayazit M, Sener E, Tasdemir O. Risk factors for stroke following coronary artery bypass operations. J Card Surg 2005;20:52–7

[34] Suma H. Coronary artery bypass grafting in patients with calcified ascending aorta: the no touch technique. Ann Thorac Surg. 1989;48: 728–730.

[35] Vogt PR, Hauser M, Schwarz U, et al. Complete thromboendoarterectomyof the calcified ascending aorta and aortic arch. Ann Thorac Surg. 1999;67:457– 461.

[36] Kouchoukos NT, Wareing TH, Daily BB, et al. Management of the severely atherosclerotic aorta during cardiac operations. J Card Surg. 1994;9:490–494.

[37] Gaudino M, Glieca F, Alessandrini F, et al. The Unclampable Ascending Aorta in Coronary Artery Bypass Patients A Surgical Challenge of Increasing Frequency. Circulation. 2000;102:1497-1502.

[38] Frazier OH, March RJ, Horvath KA: Transmyocardial revascularization with a carbon dioxide laser in patients with end-stage coronary artery disease. N Engl J Med 341:1021-1028, 1999

[39] Horvath KA, Aranki SF, Cohn LH, et al: Sustained angina relief 5 years after transmyocardial laser revascularization with a CO(2) laser. Circulation 104:I81-I84, 2001

[40] Aranki SF, Nathan M, Cohn LH: Has laser revascularization found its place yet? CurrOpinCardiol 14:510-514, 1999

[41] Allen KB, Dowling RD, Fudge TL, et al: Comparison of transmyocardial revascularization with medical therapy in patients with refractory angina. N Engl J Med 341:1029-1036, 1999

[42] Aaberge L, Rootwelt K, Blomhoff S, et al: Continued symptomatic improvement three to five years after transmyocardial revascularization with CO(2) laser: A late clinical follow-up of the Norwegian randomized trial with transmyocardial revascularization. J Am CollCardiol 39:1588-1593, 2002

[43] Schofield PM, Sharples LD, Caine N, et al: Transmyocardial laser revascularization in patients with refractory angina: A randomised controlled trial. Lancet 353:519-524, 1999

[44] Horvath KA. Transmyocardial Laser Revascularization. J Card Surg 2008;23:266-276

[45] Frazier OH, March RJ, Horvath KA: Transmyocardialrevascularization with a carbon dioxide laser in patientswith end-stage coronary artery disease. N Engl J Med 1999;341:1021-1028.

[46] Burkhoff D, Schmidt S, Schulman SP, et al: Transmyocardiallaser revascularization compared with continuedmedical therapy for treatment of refractory angina pectoris: A prospective randomized trial. Lancet1999;354:885-890..

[47] Aaberge L, Rootwelt K, Blomhoff S, et al: Continuedsymptomatic improvement three to five years aftertransmyocardial revascularization with CO2 laser: A late clinical follow-up of the Norwegian randomized trialwith transmyocardial revascularization. J Am CollCardiol2002;39:1588-1593.

[48] Briones E, Lacalle JR, Marin I: Transmyocardial laser revascularization versus medical therapy for refractory angina. Cochrane Database Syst Rev. 2009 Jan 21;(1).

[49] Allen KB, Dowling R, DelRossi A, et al: Transmyocardialrevascularization combined with coronary arterybypass grafting: A multicenter, blinded, prospective, randomized, controlled trial. J ThoracCardiovascSurg2000;119:540-549.

Chapter 12

Aspirin Therapy Resistance in Coronary Artery Bypass Grafting

Inna Kammerer

Additional information is available at the end of the chapter

http://dx.doi.org/10.5772/54414

1. Introduction

The success of coronary artery bypass grafting (CABG) surgery mainly depends on the patency of graft vessels. The predominant mechanism of early graft failure after coronary surgery is associated with antiplatelet treatment using drungs such as acetylsalicylic acid (ASA). Prevention using oral ASA in the early postoperative phase in patients with vascular disease is associated with a 25% to 44% reduction in adverse cardiovascular events (1; 2). Daily ASA doses ranging between 75-1200mg can similarly reduce fatal and nonfatal events (2; 3), although studies directly comparing lower and higher doses with regard to clinical outcomes in the CABG setting have been lacking [4].

2. Clinical ASA resistance

The antithrombotic effect of ASA has been primarily attributed to the irreversible blockade of the cyclooxygenase- 1 (COX-1) enzyme in platelets that leads to attenuation in the production of an important platelet agonist, thromboxane A2 TXA_2 (1; 2). ASA irreversibly inhibits cycloxygenase-1 by acetylating a serine residue at position 529, thereby preventing the conversion of arachidonic acid to unstable prostaglandine intermediate PGH_2, which is converted to thromboxane TxA_2, a potent vasoconstrictor and platelet agonist [22]. The finding that a considerable number of patients show an impaired antiplatelet effect of ASA in CAD patients, eminently after CABG threw new light into the discussion concerning poor patency rates of bypass grafts: the early period after CABG shows a coincidence of an increased risk for bypass thrombosis (amongst others, due to platelet activation and endothelial cell disruption of the graft) and an increased prevalence of ASA resistance [5]. In recent years,

an increasing number of reports about ASA resistance have led to a growing concern among clinicians and patients about the efficacy of ASA treatment (6; 7; 8; 9), although one study group could not reveal any ASA resistance after CABG [10]. ASA resistance can be defined clinically as an ischemic event while on ASA therapy. Various studies have evaluated the antiplatelet effect of ASA therapy and have reported the prevalence of ASA resistance 0.4% - 35% of cardiovascular [11, 18] and 5 - 65% of stroke patients [19, 20].

ASA failure has been attributed to many causes, including insufficient dosage, reduced absorption or increased metabolism, diabetes mellitus, genes polymorphisms, cell-cell and drug-drug interactions and poor compliance [12]. Recent findings have suggested that the pyrazolinone analgesic metamizol, ibuprofen and other nonsteroidal analgesic anti-inflammatory drugs, but not diclofenac, may prevent the irreversible inhibition of platelet thromboxane formation by ASA [15]. The variation suggests about many more treatment failures with ASA therapy (including incompliance of patients) can be explained by a reduced antiplatelet effect for pharmacological reasons Table 1.

Drug-related ASA / Clopidogrel resistance
• Incompliance (23)
• Pharmacokinetics / Pharmacodynamics
• Insufficient bioavailability (low dose-effect relationship)
• Prevention of binding to the Ser529 by other NSAID (Ibuprofen, Indomethacin, Naproxen)
• Exogenous toxins (diabetes mellitus, smoking)
• Impaired sensitivity of platelet COX-1 (CABG)
• Gene polymorphism(s) (COX-1, COX-2, Thromboxan-A2-synthase, Glycoprotein Ia / IIb-, -Ib / V / IX and IIb / IIIa receptor, Collagen, v.-Willebrand factor and factor VIII)
• Alternative metabolism of thromboxan-A2-biosynthesis (ASA resistance)
• Changing of enteral resoption and biotransformation (Clopidogrel resistance)
Disease-relatedASA / Clopidogrel *resistance*
• Platelet hyperreactivity due to ASA-insensitive mechanisms
• Changes in the collagen receptor
• Platelet "sensitizing" by Isoprostanes

Table 1. Mechanisms of ASA / Clopidogrel resistance

3. ASA response tests

The common using tests platelet function analyzer (PFA-100_{TM}) closure times (CT); turbidimetric platelet aggregation (TPA) and impedance platelet aggregation (IPA) depending of platelet and leukocyte counts, Hb, fibrinogen and von Willebrand factor collagen binding assay (VWF:CBA), the best valid laboratory procedure was not been determinate to screen for ASA or clopidogrel resistance. One of the studies on on-pump CABG patients agrees with previous findings suggesting that different platelet function assays that are suitable for

http://dx.doi.org/10.5772/54414

detecting ASA resistance can not be used interchangeably. Simple linear regression analysis revealed significant association among CEPI-CT, AA TPA and AA IPA and collagen IPA Table 2 [14]. In the majority of cases AA IPA (impedance platelet aggregation induced by arachidonic acid) [16, 17] and ADP-induced platelet aggregation [4] were utilized.

	AATPA	Collagen TPA	AAIPA	Collagen IPA
CEPI-CT	*r=0,49** / ***p<0,0001***	NS	*r=0,35* / ***p<0,0001***	*r=0,31* / ***p=0001***
AATPA		*r=0,38** / ***p<0,0001***	*r=0,43** / ***p<0,0001***	*r=0,28* / ***p=0,0006***
Collagen TPA			NS	***r=0,22*** / ***p=0,006***
AAIPA				*r=0,52* / ***p<0,0001***

*confirmed by multiple regression analysis

CEPI-CT, collagen/epinephrine closure times; TPA, turbidimetric platelet aggregation; AATPA, turbidimetric platelet aggregation induced by arachidonic acid; collagen TPA, turbidimetric platelet aggregation induced by collagen; IPA, impedance platelet aggregation; AAIPA, impedance platelet aggregation induced by arachidonic acid; collagen IPA, impedance platelet aggregation induced by collagen.

Table 2. Linear regression analysis (Spearman rank correlation coefficients, levels of significance (*P<0.01*)) determined in 42 CABG patients before, 1h and 24 h after 300 mg of aspirin intravenously (n=126)

The clean comparison between both different procedures of CABG: on- and off-pump surgery is unperformed, the role of using extracorporeal circulation as potential destroyer of cell components for ASA Response uncertain. ASA resistence is a transient phenomenon during the early postoperatively period in approximately 30% of OPCAB patients, whereby the ASA response was revered by 6 months [16, 17].

The new age antiplatelet therapy with clopidogrel, prasugrel or ticagrelor seems be effective in most cardiology diseases (Platelet Inhibition and Patient Outcomes = PLATO Study) like acute coronary syndrome (ACS), unstable angina pectoris, myocardial infarction (non-STEMI or STEMI) with non- and invasive procedures [13], however is not standard medication for patients after CABG procedure like ASA. Clopidogrel (75mg/day) is a prodrug, which needs to be metabolized in the liver to active metabolites catalysed by Cytochrom-P450-Oxygenase CYP 3A4 and 3A5, which irreversibly inactivate the platelet ADP receptor $P2Y_{12}$. Different to ASA clopidogrel does to influent the thienopyridins not cyclooxygenase and thromboxan formation. Platelet inhibition in patients group with response to clopidogrel was enhanced by switching to ticagrelol therapy and all clopidogrel. A few studies have revealed important individual heterogeneity in platelet response to clopidogrel in patients

with stable coronary disease, but the clinical significance of this phenomenon has not yet been investigated. Matetzky showed in his study that in 15 out of 60 consecutive patients STEMI (25%) were resistant to clopidogrel and subsequently were at increased risk of recurrent cardiovascular events in a 6-month follow-up [24].

Non-Responders and Responders treated with ticagrelor will have platelet reactivity below the cut points associated with ischemic risk in the RESPOND Study [4]. Their resistance in cardiac surgery after using of extracorporeal circulation (on-pump) or without (off pump) is unidentified.

Regarding the PLATO trials (Platelet Inhibition and Patient Outcome by ticagrelol) underwent CABG endpoints were a non-significant reduction of the primary endpoint like total major bleeding [HR: 0.84 (95% CI = 0.60–1.16), p = 0.29], significant reduction of CV death [HR: 0.52 (95% CI = 0.32–0.85)] and all-cause death [HR: 0.49 (95%CI = 0.32– 0.77)] [13]. CABG-related major bleedings according to PLATO or TIMI bleeding definitions were observed very commonly during CABG.

4. Conclusion

Antiplatelet therapy with ASA is the cornerstone of treatment in coronary artery disease patients especiallity after CABG surgery. The question of ASA resistence can be defined clinically as an ischaemic even while on ASA treatment daily. Laboratory assays of ASA response are surrogate measures as platelet aggregation inhibitor in *vitro* does not coincidentally translate into prevention of thrombosis in *vivo*, however the tests are not comparibale among themself. Clinical studies are needed to discover the optimal dosing and the clinical significance of laboratory aspirin resistance for sufficiency of graft function.

Abbreviations

CABG=coronary artery bypass grafting, **ASA**=acetylsalicylic acid, **CAD** = coronary artery disease,**mg**=milligram, **COX-1**=cyclooxygenase-1, **OPCAB**=off-pump coronary artery bypass, **TXA_2** = thromboxane A2, **STEMI**=ST segment elevation myocardial infarction

Author details

Inna Kammerer

Address all correspondence to: kammerei@klilu.de

Department of Cardiac Surgery, Academic City Hospital Ludwigshafen, Ludwigshafen, Germany

References

[1] Patrono C, Coller B, FitzGerald GA, Hirsh J, Roth G. 2004 Platelet-active drugs: the relationships among dose, effectiveness, and side effects: the Seventh ACCP Conference on Antithrombotic and Thrombolytic Therapy. *Chest*; 126: 234–64

[2] Antithrombotic Trialists' Collaboration. 2002 Collaborative meta-analysis of randomized trials of antiplatelet therapy for prevention of death, myocardial infarction, and stroke in high-risk patients. *BMJ*. 324:71– 86

[3] Zimmermann N, Kienzle P, Weber AA, Winter J, Gams E, Schroder K, Hohlfeld T. 2001 Aspirin resistance after coronary artery bypass grafting. J Thorac Cardiovasc Surg; 212:982–4

[4] Gurbel PA, Bliden KP, DiChiara J, Newcomer J, Weng W, Neerchal NK, Gesheff T, Chaganti SK, Etherington A, Tantry US 2007 Evaluation of dose-related effects of Aspirin on platelet function: results from the Aspirin-induced platelet effect (ASPECT) Study *Circulation*; 115;3156-64

[5] Stein PD, Schunemann HJ, Dalen JE, Gutterman D. 2004 Antithrombotic therapy in patients with saphenous vein and internal mammary artery bypass grafts: The seventh ACCP conference on Antithrombotic and Thrombolytic therapy Chest; 126(Suppl 3):600-8S

[6] Golanski J, Chlopicki S, Golan′ ski R, Gresner P, Iwaszkiewicz, A, Watala C. 2005 Resistance to aspirin in patients after coronary artery bypass graftings is transient. Ther Drug Monit;27 :484–90

[7] Yilmaz MB, Balbay Y, Caldir V, Ayez S, Guray Y, Guray U, Korkmaz S. 2005 Late saphenous vein graft occlusion in patients with coronary bypass: Possible role of aspirin resistance. Thromb Res;115: 25–9

[8] Zimmermann N, Kienzle P, Weber AA, Winter J, Gams E, Schröder K, Hohlfeld T. 2001 Aspirin resistance after coronary artery bypass grafting. J Thorac Cardiovasc Surg; 212:982–4

[9] Zimmermann N, Wenk A, Kim U, Kienzle P, Weber AA, Gams E, Schröder K, Hohlfeld T. 2003 Functional and biochemical evaluation of platelet aspirin resistance after coronary artery bypass surgery. Circulation;108: 542–7

[10] Mengistu AM, Wolf MW, Boldt J, Röhm KD, Lang J, Piper SN. 2008 Evaluation of a new platelet function analyzer in cardiac surgery: a comparison of modified thromboelastography and whole-blood aggregometry. J Cardiothorac Vasc Anesth.; 22 (1): 40-6

[11] Cox D, Maree AO, Dooley R, Byrne MF, Fitzgerald DJ. 2006 Effect of enteritic coating on antiplatelet activity of low-dose aspirin in healthy volunteers. Stroke; 37: 3153–58

[12] Tantry US, Bliden KP, Gurbel PA. 2005 Resistance to antiplatelet drugs: current status and future research. Expert Opin Pharmacother.;6: 2027–45

[13] Giannitsis E, Katus HA Antiplatelet therapy - ticagrelor. Hamostaseologie. 2012 Jun 28;32(3)

[14] Kammerer I, Bach J, Saggau W, Isgro F. Functional evaluation of platelet aspirin resistance after on-pump coronary bypass grafting using multiple aggregation tests. Thorac Cardiovasc Surg. 2011 Oct;59(7):425-9

[15] MacDonald TM, Wei L. Effect of ibuprofen on cardioprotective effect of aspirin. Lancet 2003;361:573–4

[16] Wang Z, Gao F, Men J, Ren J, Modi P, Wei M Aspirin resistance in off-pump coronary artery bypass grafting. Eur J Cardiothorac Surg. 2012 Jan;41(1):108-12

[17] Kempfert J, Anger K, Rastan A, Krabbes S, Lehmann S, Garbade J, Sauer M, Walther T, Dhein S, Mohr FW Postoperative development of aspirin resistance following coronary artery bypass. Eur J Clin Invest. 2009 Sep; 39(9):769-74

[18] Schrör K, Hohlfeld T, Weber AA Aspirin resistance - does it clinically matter? Clin Res Cardiol. 2006 Oct;95(10):505-10

[19] Mason PJ, Jacobs AK, Freedman JE (2005) Aspirin resistence and atherothrombotic disease. J Am Coll Cardiol 46:986-93

[20] Hennekens CH, Schrör K, Weisman S, Fitz GA (2004) Terms and Conditions. Semantic complexicity and aspirin resistence. Circulation 110:1706-8

[21] Mani H., E. Lindhoff-Last Resistenz gegen Azetylsalizylsäure und Clopidogrel Hämostaseologie 2006 26 3: 229-238

[22] Mani H, Linnemann B, Luxembourg B, Kirchmayr K, Lindhoff-Last E Response to aspirin and clopidogrel monitored with different platelet function methods Platelets. 2006 Aug;17(5):303-10

[23] Cotter G, Shemesh E, Zehavi M, Dinur I, Rudnick A, Milo O, Vered Z, Krakover R, Kaluski E, Kornberg A Lack of aspirin effect: aspirin resistance or resistance to taking aspirin? Am Heart J. 2004 Feb;147(2):293-300.

[24] Matetzky S, Shenkman B, Guetta V, Shechter M, Beinart R, Goldenberg I, Novikov I, Pres H, Savion N, Varon D, Hod H Clopidogrel resistance is associated with increased risk of recurrent atherothrombotic events in patients with acute myocardial infarction.Circulation. 2004 Jun 29;109(25):3171-5

Chapter 13

Treatment of Coronary Artery Bypass Graft Failure

M.A. Beijk and R.E. Harskamp

Additional information is available at the end of the chapter

http://dx.doi.org/10.5772/54928

1. Introduction

1.1. History of surgical revascularization

The concept of surgical revascularization for coronary artery disease (CAD) originated in the early 20th century. A pioneer in this field is Beck, a surgeon who in 1935 developed an indirect technique of myocardial revascularization by grafting a flap of the pectoralis muscle over the exposed epicardium to create new blood supply. [1] Later, Beck also developed another revascularization technique by anastomosis between the aorta and the coronary sinus. [2] In 1946, the Vineberg procedure was introduced in which the internal mammary artery (IMA) was used to implant directly into the left ventricular and is hence considered the forerunner of coronary artery bypass grafting (CABG). This technique was the first intervention documented to increase myocardial perfusion and was successfully performed in over 5,000 patients between 1950 till 1970. [3-5] The major breakthrough in surgery, however, was the invention of the heart-lung machine in 1953, which allowed surgeons to perform open-heart procedures on a non-beating heart and controlled operating field while protecting other vital organs. [6] Still it was not until 1960 when the first successful human coronary artery bypass surgery was performed by Goetz and Rohman, who used the IMA as the donor vessel for anastomosis to the right coronary artery. [7] The bypass graft technique as we know today was developed by Favaloro in 1967. [8] In his physiologic approach in the surgical management of coronary artery disease, Favaloro and his team initially used a saphenous vein autograft to bypass a stenosis of the right coronary artery. Shortly hereafter, Favaloro began to use the saphenous vein as a bypassing conduit. After the saphenous vein bypass procedure was extended to include the left arterial system by Johnson [9], the use of the IMA for bypass grafting was performed by Bailey and Hirose in 1968. [10] Arguably, the first successful IMA – coronary artery anastomosis was already performed 4 years earlier by the Russian surgeon Vasilii Kolesov. [11] Use of the radial artery (RA) as a bypass conduit was introduced by

Carpentier in 1971 and fell into disrepute shortly after its introduction because of high failure rates but was revisited as many of these original grafts appeared widely patent at 6 years. [12, 13] Initially used as a free graft in a fashion similar to that of the saphenous vein graft, more recently the RA has been used as a T or Y graft from the left IMA (LIMA) or an extension graft from the distal right IMA (RIMA). On the basis of superior long-term outcomes of arterial conduits compared with vein grafts, other arteries have been used in CABG such as the gastroepiploic artery (GEA), the inferior epigastric artery (IEA), the splenic artery, the subscapular artery, the inferior mesenteric artery, the descending branch of the lateral femoral circumflex artery, and the ulnar artery. However none of these arteries have shown similar patency rates as the internal mammary artery.

Surgical revascularization in the current era - A number of studies and trials have consistently shown the benefit of CABG in select patient populations. Indisputable, surgical revascularization which in most cases is performed utilizing the saphenous vein for bypassing non LAD-lesions and arterial bypass grafts for LAD lesions, has dramatically changed the management of patients with ischemic heart disease. Currently, over 300,000 patients undergo CABG in the United States each year. [14] Although the short-term outcomes of CABG are generally excellent, patients remain at risk for future cardiac events due to progression of native coronary disease and/or coronary bypass graft failure. [15-18] To illustrate, over half of saphenous vein grafts (SVG) are occluded at 10 years post CABG and an additional 25% show significant stenosis at angiographic follow-up. [19] Additionally, diseased grafts represent an increasing proportion of culprit lesions and acute graft occlusion may cause acute coronary syndromes (ACS). [20] In the next paragraphs we will describe in further detail the pathophysiologic mechanisms that lead to coronary artery bypass graft failure, and elude to management strategies.

2. Pathophysiology of coronary artery bypass graft failure

The use of the SVG, arterial grafts or both during CABG is largely depending on the site of anatomic obstruction, the availability of good quality conduits, patient preferences, and the clinical condition of the patient. Adequate arterial conduits are not always available, in contrast SVG are usually of good quality and calibre and are easily harvested, and are thus commonly used as conduits. However, there is an increasing interest for the use of arterial conduits as coronary artery bypass grafts, especially for bypassing the left coronary artery. Although, the choice to use arterial conduits partly depends on the coronary run-off, the long-term patency of arterial grafts is superior for CABG compared to SVG. As more than half of SVG are occluded at 10 years post CABG and an additional 25% show significant stenosis at angiographic follow-up. [19] SVG failure is the main cause of repeat intervention either by redo CABG or PCI and is even more common than the progression of native coronary artery disease in patients whom underwent CABG. In spite the fact that SVG failure remains a significant clinical and economic burden, the majority of CABG procedures continue to use SVG. [21]

The concept of the 'failing graft' is one of a patent graft whose patency is threatened by a hemodynamically significant lesion in the inflow or outflow tracts or within the body of the graft. Salvage of the failing and failed bypass graft remains an important clinical and technical challenge. The high incidence of graft failure has led to the evolution of graft surveillance programs to detect 'failing' grafts and research has focussed on means to control the development of intimal hyperplasia. [22]

3. Histology of saphenous vein

The saphenous vein consists of three layers: the intima, media, and adventitia. The intima is composed of a continuous layer of endothelial cells on the luminal surface of the vessel. Beneath lies the fenestrated basement membrane embedded with a fragmented internal elastic lamina. The media comprises of smooth muscle cells (SMC) arranged in an inner longitudinal and an outer circumferential pattern with loose connective tissue and elastic fibers interlaced. The middle muscle layer is most extensive at the insertion points of the valves and leaflets. The adventitia forms the outer layer and consists of longitudinally arranged SMC, collagen fibers and a network of elastin fibers, in addition to vascular and nerve supplies to the vessel.The great saphenous vein is the most frequently used conduit for myocardial revascularization but other venous conduits such the short saphenous vein or upper extremity veins (cephalic and basilica) can be used as well.

4. Saphenous vein graft failure

Studies of saphenous veins harvested for bypass procedures have shown that many have abnormal histological and physical attributes. [23,24] Moreover, the quality of the saphenous vein can have significant clinical consequences. Therefore, vein grafts in the arterial circulation must be considered as a viable, constantly adapting and evolving conduit.

Several intrinsic and extrinsic factors may play a role in the mechanism of SVG failure. At the time of harvest, the quality of the saphenous veins may be poor, demonstrating a spectrum of pre-existing pathological conditions ranging from significantly thickened walls to post phlebitic changes and varicosities. Between 2% and 5% of saphenous veins are unusable and up to 12% can be considered diseased which reduce the patency rate by one half compared to non-diseased veins. [25] In addition, the inevitable vascular trauma that occurs during SVG harvesting itself can also lead to damage to the endothelium and SMC and thereby contribute to graft failure. Surgical manipulation and high-pressure distension to reverse spasm during harvesting leads to loss of endothelial integrity and the antithrombogenic attributes of the endothelium, rendering the SVG prone to subsequent occlusive intimal hyperplasia and/or thrombus formation. [26] During harvesting the vasa vasorum and nervous network of the SVG are devided, making the graft dependent on diffusion for weeks until adequate circulation is esthablished.

[27-32] Ischemic insult and decreased production of nitric oxide and adenosine may cause SMC proliferation. [33] As it has been demonstrated that intimal hyperplasia does not occur in vein-to-vein isografts, it can be stated that pathologic changes seen in SVG in the arterial circulation are predominantly caused by hemodynamic and physiochemical changes. [34]

SVG failure can be divided into three temporal categories: early (0 to 30 days), midterm (30 days to 1 year) or late (after 1 year). Early SVG failure due to thrombotic complications is mainly attributable to technical errors during harvesting, anastomosis or comprised anatomic runoff. [19,35-37] It occurs in 15% to 18% of VG during the 1st month. [38-40] Early thrombotic complications in SVG in the arterial circulation are caused by a reduction of tissue plasminogen activator, attenuation of thrombomudulin and reduced expression of heparin sulphate. [41]

Midterm SVG failure is mainly caused by fibrointimal hyperplasia as it serves as the foundation for subsequent graft atheroma leading to occlusive stenosis. The release of a variety of mediators, growth factors, and cytokines by the injured endothelium, platelets and activated macrophages will cause migration and proliferation of SMC. Diminished production of endothelial nitric oxide (NO), prostaglandin 12 and adenosine will further contribute to and enhanced SMC proliferation, leading to development of neointimal hyperplasia. [19,33,37,42-44] Changes in the flow pattern within the vessel (shear stress) an ischemic insults may contribute to changes in the SVG at this stage. SVG are exposed to much higher mechanical pressure that they were adapted to (arterial versus venous blood pressure) which can potentially stimulate SMC proliferation. Moreover, after encountering arterial flow patterns increased levels of intracellular adhesion molecule-1, vascular cell adhesion molecule-1, and monocyte chemotactic protein-1 will facilitate leukocyte-endothelial interactions so that leukocyte infiltration of the lesions will ensue. [34] Finally, the adaptive response to hemodynamic factors, i.e. wall shear stress, may affect the distal site of the anastomosis leading to SVG failure. [45,46] Midterm SVG failure accounts for an additional 15% to 30%. [47,48] In the course of vessel remodelling, late SVG failure is characterized by progression of intimal fibrosis at the cost of a reduction in cellularity which may contribute to progression of SMC apoptosis. [19,34,41,44] In addition, perivascular fibroblasts may also be involved in neointimal formation and matrix deposition as these cells may exhibit contractile elements while migrating from the adventitia towards the media. [49] After 1 year most SVG stenosis is due to atherosclerosis but although vein graft atherosclerosis is accelerated compared to arteries, evidence show that a fully evolved plaque appear after 3 to 5 years of implantation. [35,47,50] In SVG there is no focal compensatory enlargement in the stenotic segments which is in contrast to native atherosclerotic arteries in which the development of an atherosclerotic plaque is associated with enlargement of the vessel and preservation of the lumen area until plaque progression exceeds the compensatory mechanism of the vessel. [51] Several studies show that SVG patency at 10 years is no more than 50% to 60%. [19,41,52,53] Finally, several studies have suggested a role of immune cells in neointimal formation as macrophages are found in the intima, while T-lymphocytes are present in the adventitia of neointimal lesions wit a predominance of CD4+ cells. [54-56]

In a later stage atherosclerotic lesions may be complicated by aneurysmal dilatation which is found to correlate with thrombosed SVG. (66) The occurrence of atheroembolism form the diseased graft or plaque rupture may cause late thrombosis necessitating revascularization therapy. [57,58] In general, SVG thrombosis is the major cause of morbidity and mortality. [19,41]

Predictors of graft patency 3 years after CABG were evaluated by Veterans Affairs Cooperative Study Group. [59] Multivariable analysis showed that the only factors that were predictive were vein preservation solution temperature ≤5ºC, serum cholesterol, the number of proximal anastomoses ≤2, and recipient artery diameter >5 mm. Thus, predictors of 3-year graft patency are most closely related to operative techniques and the underlying disease. In another study, factors that predict the late progression of SVG atherosclerosis were evaluated in 1248 patients in the Post-CABG trial. [47] Factors independently associated with the progression of disease were maximum stenosis of the graft at baseline angiography, years after CABG, moderate therapy to lower LDL cholesterol, prior MI, high triglyceride levels, small minimum graft diameter, low HDL concentration, high LDL concentration, high mean arterial pressure, low left ventricular ejection fraction, male gender, and current cigarette smoking. Finally, concerns have been raised about the possibility of worse outcomes when a SVG is used for multiple distal anastomosis compared to single anastomosis. In a substudy of the PREVENT IV trial, the use of SVG conduits with multiple distal anastomoses was associated with a significantly higher rate of ≥75 percent stenosis of the SVG on angiography at one year. [60] Moreover, clinical follow-up showed a trend towards a higher rate of the adjusted composite of death, MI, or revascularization at five years.

Noteworthy, the clinical impact of SVG failure is still debated. Not all grafts that have angiographic stenosis or occlusion will cause symptoms, and probably a substantial of SVG that fail do not impact outcomes.

5. Histology of arterial grafts

Several arterial conduits are suitable for myocardial revascularization and the arterial conduits can be divided into 3 types according to functional class (Table 1). Type I arterial grafts are the somatic arteries including the IMA, IEA, and subscapular artery. Type II arterial grafts are the splanchnic arteries including the GEA, splenic artery, and inferior mesenteric artery. Type III arterial grafts are the limb arteries including the RA, ulnar artery, and lateral femoral circumflex artery. Compared to functional class type II and III, type I is less spastic. [61] Although the full length of arterial grafts is reactive, the major muscular components are located at the two ends of the artery (muscular regulator). [62] Therefore, in terms of preventing vasospasm of arterial grafts, trimming off the small and highly reactive distal end of the grafts (IMA, GEA, IEA, or other grafts) may be important and clinically feasible.

Studies have demonstrated that there are differences between arterial and venous grafts: 1) arterial grafts are less susceptible to vasoactive substances then veins [63]; 2) the arterial wall

Type I - Somatic arteries	Less spastic	Internal mammary artery
		Inferior epigastric artery
		Subscapular artery
Type II - Splanchnic arteries	Spastic	Gastroepiploic artery
		Splenic artery
		Inferior mesenteric artery
Type III - Limb arteries	Spastic	Radial artery
		Ulnar artery
		Lateral femoral circumflex artery

Table 1. Functional classification of arterial grafts according to physiological and pharmacological contractility, anatomical, and embryological characteristic

is supplied by the vaso vasorum and in addition through the lumen, whereas the veins are only supplied by the vaso vasorum [64]; 3) the endothelium of the arteries may secrete more endothelium-derived relaxing factor [65]; 4) the structure of the artery is subject to high pressure, whereas the vein is subjected to low pressure. While the SVG have to adapt to the high pressure, the arterial grafts do not which may partly explain the difference in the long-term outcome.

Similar like SVG, the arterial grafts can also be divided into three layers: the intima, media, and adventitia. As a result of location at different parts of the body and supply to different organs, differences in gross anatomy among arterial grafts have been observed. Divergent anatomic structures of the arteries have been observed. One of the most obvious differences is that arteries such as the GEA, IEA, and RA contain more smooth muscle cells in their walls and are therefore less elastic compared to other arteries such as the IMA which may be more elastic because they contain more elastic laminae. [64] Such structure divergence may also explain the difference in phsysiologic and pharmacologic reactivity.

6. Arterial graft failure

The need for repeat revascularization is substantially reduced with the use of arterial conduits, since long-term patency is much higher compared to SVG. [66-68] In contrast to SVG, arterial grafts appear to be more resistant to the influence of atherogenic factors and incur only minor traumatic and ischemic lesions, since they are not removed from the blood circulation but are prepared locally, with few ligations and preservation of blood flow. [69] Since 1986, the LIMA has been used in more than 90% of CABG procedures. Less frequently, the RIMA is used. The early patency of a LIMA anastomosed to the left anterior descending (LAD) is reported to be almost 99%. [70] The mean patency of LIMA to coronary conduit at 5 years is reported 98%, at 10 years it is 95%, and at 15 years it is 88%. [71] Differences are observed between territory

grafted, the 10 year LIMA patency to the LAD is reported to be 96% and to the circumflex (Cx) 89%. [72] The early patency of the RIMA anastomosed to major branches of the left circumflex artery is approximately 94%. [70] The mean RIMA patency at 5 years is reported to be 96%, at 10 years it is 81% and at 15 years it is 65%. [71] Again differences are observed, the RIMA graft patency to the LAD artery is 95% at 10 years and 90% at 15 years. Ten-year RIMA patency to the Cx marginal is 91%, right coronary artery is 84%, and posterior descending artery is 86%. [72] In situ RITA and free RITA had similar ten-year patency, 89% vs 91% respectively. RA patency is reported to range between 83% to 98% at 1 to 20 years but lower rates have been reported. [73] The patency rate estimated by the Kaplan-Meier method for the GEA conduit was 96.6% at 1 month, 91.4% at 1 year, 80.5% at 5 years, and 62.5% at 10 years. [74] Arterial grafts are not uniform in their biological characteristics and difference in the perioperative behaviour and in the long-term patency may be related to different characteristics. It should be taken into account in the use of arterial grafts that some grafts need more active pharmacological intervention during and after operation to obtain satisfactory results.

Although, the IMA is the most used conduit to restore the blood flow to the LAD, it is less easy to use because of its complicated preparation and postoperative complications. Specific reasons for not to use the RIMA may include additional time to harvest, concerns over deep sternal wound infection, myocardial hypoperfusion, and unfamiliarity. Besides the potentially deleterious effect on the vascular supply of the forearm and hand, potential spasm and size matching to target coronary artery are the main drawback for the use of RA in CABG. [75,76]

Although all arterial grafts may develop vasospasm, it develops more frequently in the GEA and RA, than the IMA and IEA. [13,77] Two types of vasoconstrictors are found to be important spasmogens in arterial grafts. [78] Type I vasoconstrictors are the most potent and they strongly contracts arterial grafts even when the endothelium is intact. The constrictors are endothelin, prostanoids such as thromboxane A_2 and prostaglandin $F_{2\alpha}$, and alpha1-adrenoceptor agonists. Type II vasoconstrictors induce only weak vasoconstriction when the endothelium is intact, but play an important role in the spasm of arterial grafts when the endothelium is destroyed by surgical manipulation. Type II vasoconstrictor is 5-hydroxytryptamine.

Early IMA graft failure is attributed to technical errors and distal anastomosis. [79,80] Non-technical factors that may affect the patency of the arterial graft are high levels of LDL cholesterol and triglycerides, and high levels of lipoprotein(a), a thrombogenic molecule that is related to the hypercoagulable state. Other classical risk factors for coronary artery disease, such as diabetes mellitus, smoking and hypertension may also affect the patency of the arterial graft. Age may be of influence the quality of the arterial graft.

Furthermore, competitive flow and low-flow profoundly affect graft patency. Low-grade graft stenoses in the target artery proximally are a major cause of competitive flow which may lead to a decrease in antegrade flow in the arterial graft causing early failure ('disuse athrophy'). The SVG and IMA are more tolerant than the RA and GEA conduits. This is likely to be related to biological differences as the RA and GEA have a thick layer of smooth muscle or poor endothelial function in these muscular conduits. Therefore, it is recommended to avoid grafting target arteries with a stenosis less than 90% with RA grafts. [81]

Atherosclerosis in arterial grafts can develop before coronary grafting when the graft is in the in situ native position, or after. The incidence of atherosclerosis in native arteries in the in situ position in the four major arterial grafts is low, especially in the IMA. [64] The incidence of atherosclerosis in bypass grafts is also low, in IMA grafts even as late 15 to 21 years after CABG. [67,82] However, the degree of stenosis in the native vessel is a major predictor of IMA graft patency. The observed association between non-significant stenosis of the native artery and high occlusion rate of the arterial bypass conduit raises concerns about the use of IMA in the treatment of native vessels with only mild or moderate stenosis. [83] In addition, the target vessel for the IEA must be one that is completely occluded or severely stenotic, with low coronary resistance, and in territories not totally infarcted to avoid "string sign" (conduit <1 mm diameter). Although the incidence of atherosclerosis is low in arterial grafts, 2 other morphologic changes may be present in arterial graft, fibrointimal proliferation and fibrosis representing organized thrombus. [84] The presence of fibrointimal proliferation is associated with long-term IMA graft narrowing and may be an important factor for late graft failure. Despite hypertension was associated with increased fibrointimal proliferation in SVG, this correlation could not be found in IMA grafts. [84]

7. Treatment of coronary artery bypass graft failure

Following graft revascularization, patients remain at very high risk for subsequent clinical events. In a large study from the Duke Cardiovascular Databank, patients who underwent catheterization 1 to 18 months after their first CABG were evaluated. [85] Patients were classified on the basis of their worst SVG stenosis as having no (<25%), noncritical (25% to 74%), critical (75% to 99%), or occlusive (100%) SVG disease and the primary outcome measure was the composite of death, MI or repeat revascularization. At 10-years, the corresponding adjusted composite event rates were 41.2%, 56.2%, 81.2%, and 67.1%, respectively ($p<0.0001$) and most events occurred immediately after catheterization in patients with critical and occlusive SVG disease. Multivariate analysis revealed critical, non-occlusive SVG disease as the strongest predictor of composite outcome (hazard ratio 2.36, 95% CI [2.00-2.79], $p<0.0001$).

Many patients with recurrent stable angina following CABG can be treated medically for their symptoms and risk factor reduction. Evaluation for ischemia is as in other patients with stable angina without prior CABG. However, early diagnostic angiography is suggested as the different anatomic possibilities, i.e. graft stenosis or progression of native vessel disease in nonbypassed vessels can lead to recurrent ischemia. In patients with recurrent angina, ACS, change in exercise tolerance, positive exercise test after CABG, an increased risk for coronary events is observed. [86-88]

8. Medical therapy

In all patients with coronary heart disease aggressive risk factor reduction is recommended which includes aspirin, treatment for hypertension and serum lipids, avoidance of smoking,

http://dx.doi.org/10.5772/54928

and controlling serum glucose in diabetic patients. The bypass angioplasty revascularization investigation (BARI) trial illustrated that intensive risk-factor modification and hypolipid medication use slows atherosclerosis progression within native coronary arteries of CABG-treated patients and may to a lesser extent improve long-term patency of surgical conduits. [89]

Antiplatelet therapy - Antiplatelet therapy is recommended following CABG since it improves SVG patency and clinical outcomes. The 2008 EACTS guideline on antiplatelet and anticoagulation management in cardiac surgery [90] recommends that aspirin should be given postoperatively to all patients without contra-indications after CABG in order to improve the long-term patency of SVG. The recommended dose given is 150—325 mg. Several studies have shown a trend towards maximal benefit with 325 mg/day in the first year. [91-95] In contrast, there is no evidence that the use of aspirin after coronary artery bypass grafting improved the patency of arterial grafts. However, aspirin may be recommended on the basis of improved survival of patients in general who have atherosclerotic disease.

The optimal timing of the first dose of aspirin for patients after CABG was investigated in a meta-analysis of 12 studies and found that the benefit of aspirin was optimal if started at 6 h after surgery. [96] Although, the largest risk reduction was observed when aspirin was given at 1 h after operation, there was a non-significant increase in the rate of re-operation in this group. [91] In contrast, there was no benefit found in giving aspirin if starting more than 48 h postoperatively. [97] Practically, Aspirin should be commenced within 24 h of CABG.

Whether clopidogrel given in addition of aspirin to high-risk patients after CABG would reduce thrombotic complications was evaluated in several studies. Registry data showed that adding clopidogrel to aspirin was independently associated with a decrease in recurrence of anginal complaints and adverse cardiac events following off-pump CABG. Nonetheless, clopidogrel use beyond 30 days did not show a significant effect on adverse cardiac events. [98] In the randomized CASCADE (Clopidogrel After Surgery for Coronary Artery Disease) study, aspirin monotherapy was compared with aspirin plus clopidogrel in 113 patients undergoing CABG and SVG intimal hyperplasia was determined by intravascular ultrasound at 1 year. [99] Compared with aspirin monotherapy, the combination of aspirin plus clopidogrel did not significantly reduce SVG intimal hyperplasia 1 year after CABG. Although the study was not powered for clinical outcomes, there was no significant difference in SVG patency or cardiovascular events, neither was there a difference in the incidence of major bleeding between the 2 treatment groups at 1 year. Moreover, the superiority of clopidogrel over aspirin for optimising graft patency after CABG has not been established and thus aspirin should be regarded as the drug of first choice, however, clopidogrel is an acceptable alternative to aspirin. [90]

In patients whom underwent CABG for ACS subgroup analyses of the CAPRIE (Clopidogrel versus Aspirin in Patients at Risk of Ischemic Events) and CURE (Clopidogrel in Unstable angina to prevent Recurrent Events) study provides supportive evidence to prescribe clopidogrel for 9 to 12 months in addition to aspirin. [100,101] In patients undergoing coronary bypass surgery with a coronary stent in situ implanted within 1 year, clopidogrel should be continued if the stented vessel has not been grafted. Finally, in patients with SVG failure treated

with PCI, prehospital use of antiplatelet therapy compared with patients not using antiplatelets was associated with lower occurrence of major adverse cardiac events after SVG intervention. [102] Also, DAPT did not improved outcomes when compared to single antiplatelet therapy.

Warfarin – Conflicting evidence is reported whether warfarin in addition to aspirin is beneficial in patients post CABG. In an extended follow-up of 7.5 years of the post CABG trial, low-dose anticoagulation compared with placebo reduced the rate of death by 35%, deaths or myocardial infarction (MI) by 31%, and the composite clinical endpoint of death, MI, stroke, CABG, or angioplasty by 17%. [103] However, in a smaller randomized trial, moderate-intensity oral anticoagulation alone or combined with low-dose aspirin was not superior to low-dose aspirin in the prevention of recurrent ischemic events in patients with non-ST-elevation ACS and previous CABG. [104] Currently, the American College of Chest Physicians (ACCP) Evidence-Based Clinical Practice Guidelines recommended that oral anticoagulation in addition to aspirin can be considered only when it is indicated for other reasons. [105]

Lipid lowering therapy – Clinical trials have shown that lipid lowering therapy (in particular statins) is beneficial in patients who have undergone CABG. [103,106-110] Besides the lipid lowering effect, statins also exert a number of pleiotropic effects on the vascular wall which may effect SVG in a similar way. In SVG, statins have shown to reduce vascular oxidative stress, improve NO bioavailability and reduce vascular inflammation, all critical components of SVG failure. [111] Subsequently, statins have systemic antithrombotic and anti-inflammatory effects and their administration may prevent acute SVG failure post CABG. [112] Aggressive lipid lowering therapy may be beneficial for long-term patency of grafts. In the randomized Post CABG trial, patients who had undergone bypass surgery 1 to 11 years before base line with elevated serum LDL-cholesterol concentrations (130 to 175 mg/dL / 3.4 to 4.5 mmol/L) were assigned to receive either aggressive lipid lowering therapy with lovastatin and, if needed, cholestyramine (target LDL-cholesterol <100 mg/dL / 2.6 mmol/L) or to moderate therapy (target LDL-cholesterol of approximately 134 mg/dL / 3.5 mmol/L). [106] Compared to a moderate strategy, aggressive lipid lowering therapy was associated with a delay in the progression of graft disease at an average of 4.3 years as assessed by angiography. Moreover, after clinical follow-up of 7.5 years, a 30% reduction in revascularization procedures and a 24% reduction in the composite endpoint of cardiovascular death, MI, stroke, CABG, or angioplasty were seen. [103] Similar findings were observed in a post hoc analysis from the TNT trial. In patients with previous CABG, simvastatine 80 mg compared to simvastatine 10 mg, was significantly more effective in reducing the rate of a combined cardiovascular endpoint at a median follow-up of 4.9 years (9.7% versus 13.0%). [110] Repeat revascularization with either CABG or PCI was also significantly reduced in patients assigned to the higher dose (11.3% versus 15.9%).

Antiplatelet agents and statin therapy are the only modalities with proven efficacy for the prevention of SVG stenosis. The routine use of beta blockers, calcium channel blockers, angiotensin converting enzyme (ACE) inhibitors, or nitrates post CABG is not supported by data, however, many of these patients require beta blockers and ACE inhibitors for preexistent heart failure or MI according to the ACC/AHA guideline recommendations. [113,114]

The PREVENT IV trial, including almost 3,000 patients that underwent CABG, demonstrated that rates of use of secondary prevention medications in patients with ideal indications for these therapies are high for antiplatelet agents and lipid-lowering therapy, but suboptimal for beta-blockers and ACE inhibitors or ARBs. [115] The study demonstrated that the use of multiple secondary prevention medications after CABG was associated with significant improve in clinical outcome death or MI at 2 years (4.2% in patients taking all indicated medications versus 9.0% in patients taking half or fewer of the indicated medications). No association was found between the use of most individual medications and subsequent outcomes, thus underscoring the importance of ensuring appropriate secondary prevention measures after CABG.

9. Guidelines on revascularization in patients with prior CABG

In the European Society of Cardiology (ESC)/ European Association for Cardio-Thoracic Surgery (EACTS) guidelines on myocardial revascularization [116] published in 2010 states that in acute post-operative graft failure PCI may be an alternative to re-operation with acceptable results and fewer complications. [117] The target for PCI is the body of the coronary artery of the arterial graft while freshly occluded SVG or the anastomosis itself should be targeted due to the risk of embolization or perforation. When multiple grafts are occluded or the graft or native coronary artery appears unsuitable for PCI, surgery should be favoured. In asymptomatic patients, redo CABG or PCI should only be considered if the graft or coronary artery is of good size, severely narrowed and supplies a large territory of myocardium. Redo CABG or PCI should be decided by the Heart Team.

Repeat revascularization in patients with late graft failure is indicated in the presence of severe anginal symptoms despite anti-anginal medication. In patients with mild or no symptoms repeat revascularization is dependent on risk stratification by non-invasive testing. [118,119] In patients with previous CABG, PCI has worse acute and long-term outcomes than in patients without prior CABG. Redo CABG has a two- to four-fold higher mortality than the first procedure which is mainly driven by comorbidity and less by the re-operation itself. [120,121] There is limited data comparing the efficacy of PCI with redo CABG in patients with previous CABG. In a propensity analysis of long-term survival after redo CABG or PCI in patients with multivessel disease and high-risk features, short-term outcome was very favourable, with nearly identical survival at 1 and 5 years. [118] However, in the AWESOME RCT and registry the overall in-hospital mortality was higher in the redo CABG group compared to the PCI group. [17,122] Because of the initial higher mortality of redo CABG and comparable long-term mortality, the guidelines state that PCI is the preferred revascularization strategy in patients with LIMA or amenable anatomy. Redo CABG is preferred in patients with more diseased or occluded grafts, reduced systolic function, total occlusions of native coronary arteries or in the absence of a patent arterial graft. [118] If possible, the IMA is the conduit of choice when performing redo CABG. [123]

In the 2012 appropriateness criteria for coronary revascularization focussed update of the American College of Cardiology Foundation Appropriateness Criteria Task Force (ACCF),

Society for Cardiovascular Angiography and Interventions (SCAI), Society of Thoracic Surgeons (STS), American Association for Thoracic Surgery (AATS), American Heart Association (AHA), and the American Society of Nuclear Cardiology (ASNC) it is stated that in patients with prior CABG, the presence of high-risk findings on noninvasive testing, higher severity of symptoms, or an increasing burden of disease in either the bypass grafts or native coronaries tended to increase the likelihood of an appropriate rating. [119] In patients with prior CABG receiving no or minimal anti-ischemic therapy or having low-risk findings on non-invasive testing revascularization was considered inappropriate. No specific recommendations are provided on the strategy for revascularization, performing redo CABG or PCI.

Both the ESC/EACTS guidelines on myocardial revascularization and the ACCF/SCAI/STS/AATS/AHA/ASNC/HFSA/SCCT 2012 appropriate use criteria for coronary revascularization focused update do not provide recommendations for patients with prior CABG presenting with (non) ST segment elevation myocardial infarction (STEMI) or ACS.

10. Percutaneous coronary intervention

Implantation of coronary stents has become the preferred revascularization strategy for treatment of graft lesions, because redo CABG is associated with an increased morbidity and mortality. [17,124-129] Compared to native vessel stenting, stenting of graft lesions is associated with higher rates of periprocedural events as well as cardiac events at follow-up, due to distal embolization and subsequent no-reflow and higher percentages of restenosis. [124,125, 130,131] This increased risk is mainly attributed to the friable, degenerated atheromatous and thrombotic debris that develop when SVGs deteriorate. [132] Moreover, patients with graft intervention often have a higher generalized atherosclerotic burden and more comorbidities. [130,131] To date, SVG graft intervention accounts approximately for 5% to 10% of all PCI.

Early graft failure - The incidence of early graft failure within 24 h after CABG is about 1% to 3%. [133] Perioperative graft failure following CABG may result in acute myocardial ischemia which may necessitate acute secondary revascularization procedure to salvage myocardium, preserve left ventricular function and improve patient outcome. Perioperative MI and rise in cardiac markers after CABG is associated with a substantially increased in-hospital morbidity and mortality. [134-136] The most common graft-related causes of myocardial ischemia after CABG are graft occlusion due to acute graft thrombosis, graft kinking or overstretching, postoperative graft spasm and subtotal or hemodynamic relevant anastomotic stenosis. [137,138] Nongraft-related causes for myocardial ischemia after CABG are surgery-related possibly due to surgical manipulation on pre-existing microembolizing and disintegrating unstable plaque and include inadequate cardioplegic perfusion and myocardial protection, incomplete revascularization, or distal coronary microembolization. [139-141] Rapid identification of early graft failure after CABG and diagnostic discrimination from other causes enables an adequate reintervention strategy for re-revascularization, i.e. redo CABG or PCI, and may prevent irreversible myocardial ischemia. Thus far, limited non-randomized data is available showing that in patients with acute perioperative myocardial ischemia due to early

graft failure following CABG, emergency PCI may limit the extent of myocardial cellular damage compared with redo CABG. [133] A nonsignifiant numerical difference was observed in in-hospital and 1-year mortality between the PCI group or redo CABG (12.0% and 20.0% in PCI group versus 20.0% and 27% in redo CABG group). Moreover, compared to acute redo-CABG, emergency PCI is quicker and less invasive. Importantly, in this study patent grafts were observed in 25% to 34% of the patients, therefore repeat coronary angiography should be applied when myocardial ischemia due to acute graft failure is suspected. Regarding the type of bypass graft, LIMA graft failure may be responsible for acute ischemic complications after CABG in at least a third up to half of the cases. [133,138,142]

Recurrent angina during the early postoperative period is usually due to a technical problem with a graft or with early graft closure and there is an indication for prompt coronary angiography with percutaneous revascularization. The feasibility of PCI in patients presenting with clinical evidence of ischemia within 90 days of CABG was evaluated in 2 registries. Most patients presented with ACS and the most common cause of graft failure was occlusion or thrombosis. Both registries showed that patients with graft failure can undergo PCI with a relatively low risk for in-hospital mortality or nonfatal major complications. [143,144]

SVG failure - Recurrent angina after the first few months after CABG is caused by both graft disease and by progression of atherosclerosis in non-bypassed vessels. Percutaneous intervention in SVG lesions was evaluated in several randomized studies. The SAVED (Saphenous Vein de Novo) study randomized 200 patients with SVG lesions to placement of Palmaz-Schatz bare metal stent (BMS) or standard balloon angioplasty (BA) and demonstrated that compared to BA, bare metal stents (BMS) were associated with a higher procedural success (92% vs. 69%, p<0.001) but they had more frequent hemorrhagic complications (17% vs. 5 %, p<0.01). [145] At 6 months, a non-significant reduction in angiographic restenosis was observed (36% vs. 47%, p=0.11) and clinical follow-up at 9 months showed that freedom from death, MI, repeated bypass surgery, or revascularization of the target lesion was significantly better in the stent group (73% vs. 58 %, P = 0.03). Based on the results of the SAVED study, the majority of patients with SVG stenosis are treated with stenting. To prevent distal embolization form friable atheroemboli, and in addition may serve as a smooth-muscle cell barrier to decrease restenosis, stents covered with a mesh, most commonly polytetrafluorethylene (PTFE), were evaluated. However, 3 prospective randomized trails have not shown benefit with covered stents with respect to major adverse cardiac events nor in preventing restenosis. [146-148]

In native coronary arteries, drug-eluting stents (DES) have demonstrated a marked reduction in in-stent restenosis compared to BMS in the treatment of coronary artery disease. Several DES with different stent platforms, polymers or drugs are available. In the RRISC (Reduction of Restenosis in Saphenous Vein Grafts With Cypher Sirolimus-Eluting Stent) trial, 75 patients were randomized to sirolimus-eluting stent (SES) or BMS. [149] At 6 months follow-up, in-stent late loss was significantly reduced in SES (0.38 ± 0.51 mm vs. 0.79 ± 0.66 mm in BMS). Target lesion revascularization rate was also significantly reduced (5.3% vs. 21.6%) but no difference in death and MI was observed. Howbeit, a post hoc analysis of RRISC trial at 3 years reported similar rates of target vessel revascularization and while statistically underpowered for clinical outcomes, significantly higher all-cause mortality was reported with SES compared

with BMS. [150] The SOS (Stenting of Saphenous Vein Grafts) trial randomized 80 patients to either paclitaxel-eluting stent (PES) or BMS and showed significant reduction in primary end point, binary angiographic restenosis at 12 months (9% vs. 51%). [151] At 1.5 years clinical follow-up the PES patients had a significant reduction in target lesion revascularization (5% vs. 28%), target vessel failure (22% vs. 46%) and a trend towards less MI (15% vs. 31%) but increased mortality (12% vs. 5%). In contrast to the long-term results of the RRISC study, at a median follow-up of 35 months PES treated-patients had a significantly lower incidence of MI (17% vs. 46%), target lesion revascularization (10% vs. 41%), and target vessel failure (34% vs. 72%) as well as a trend toward less definite or probable stent thrombosis (2% vs. 15%). All-cause mortality (24% vs. 13%) and cardiac mortality (7% vs. 13%) did not differ between groups. [152] More evidence was provided in the ISAR-CABG (Prospective, Randomized Trial of Drug-Eluting Stents Versus Bare Metal Stents for the Reduction of Restenosis in Bypass Grafts). In this study, 610 patients with diseased SVGs were randomized to DES and BMS and the combined incidence of death, MI, and target lesion revascularisation at 1 year was significantly lower in the DES group than in the BMS group (15.4% vs. 22.1%) which was mainly driven by a nearly 50% relative reduction in the risk of target lesion revascularization (7.2% vs. 13.1%), with non-significant differences in mortality. [153] Consistent results of improved efficacy with DES and no significant safety hazard were reported in different meta-analyses which also included non randomized trails. [154-157] The RRISC, SOS and ISAR CABG all compared first-generation DES to BMS. The SOS-Xience V (Stenting of Saphenous Grafts-Xience V) prospectively examined the frequency of angiographic in-stent restenosis in SVG lesions 12 months after implantation of everolimus-eluting stent (EES), a second generation DES. Use of EES in SVGs is associated with high rates of stent strut coverage and high malapposition rates at 12 months post implantation as assessed by optical coherence tomography, however, clinical results are to be waited. [158] Finally, in a multicenter analysis no difference was observed in real-world patients comparing first-generation DES to BMS. [159] In a meta-analysis including 29 studies (3 randomized controlled trials (RCT)) involving over 7500 patients, the authors stated that DES may decrease TVR rate in treatment of SVG stenoses but no differences in reinfarction rate, stent thrombosis or mortality was found between the DES and BMS groups in the RCT's. [160] In contrast, the observational data showed lower risk for MI, stent thrombosis and death in the DES group. This may be a result of patient selection bias in the observational studies or represent a true finding that was not detected in the RCT analysis due to limited statistical power.

Stents are effective as treatment for focal lesions, however, the optimal treatment strategy for a diffusely degenerated SVG is uncertain. Endoluminal reconstruction with stent omplantation has been suggested as a treatment for diffuse lesions. This was evaluated in a study including 126 patients with diffusely degenerated stenosed or occluded SVG treated with stents. [161] At 3 year follow-up, survival free of death, infarction, or revascularization was only 43%.

Regarding stenting technique in SVG lesions, it has been suggested that direct stenting, compared to predilatation with balloon angioplasty, may be beneficial as trapping of debris could decrease distal embolization that may occur from repeated balloon inflations. Registry data showed that in unselected patients who underwent SVG intervention direct stenting was

associated with a lower CK-MB release and fewer non-Q-wave MI. [162] These results needs to be confirmed in a prospective randomized trial.

After PCI of SVG, progression of disease outside the stented segment can lead to high rates of restenosis. Therefore, treatment of native coronary artery lesions is preferred to treatment of degenerated SVG if feasible. In addition, in patients with prior CABG, early diagnostic angiography can be important as there is a high success rate of percutaneous coronary intervention (PCI) at the time of subtotal occlusion; and the substantial consequences of the loss of a bypass graft through total occlusion (e.g, low success and high complication rates of PCI for totally occluded SVG, and difficult to control angina).

A numerous of predictors for worse outcome after percutaneous SVG intervention have been identified. Multivariate analysis revealed that major CK-MB release after SVG intervention and renal insufficiency are powerful independent predictor of all-cause mortality. [163-165] Lesion length, greater angiographic degeneration of SVG, and larger estimated plaque volume which may result in a greater likelihood of distal embolization and myocardial necrosis after intervention, have been identified as predictors of 30-day major adverse cardiac events after SVG intervention. [166,167] Sexe also appeared to be a predictor as women have a significantly higher 30-day cumulative mortality rate compared with men (4.4% vs. 1.9%), a higher incidence of vascular complications (12% vs. 7.3%), and postprocedural acute renal failure (8.1% vs. 4%). [168] Whether specific stent platforms, polymers or drugs are more appropriate in SVG and arterial graft lesions has not been addressed at this time.

Arterial graft failure - Due to the superior long-term patency of arterial grafts, in specific the IMA, they are the vascular conduit of choice for patients undergoing CABG and the increasing frequency of their use has resulted in a small but increasing need for revascularization. In arterial graft failure, ostial stenoses are the least common and the pathogenesis of ostial stenoses may be affected by its proximity to the aorta and potential extension of atherosclerosis from that vessel.

Anastomosis of IMA to the native coronary is the most frequent site of a target lesion. The particular anatomical feature of the IMA-to-LAD anastomosis is subjected to continuous mechanical stress, owing to the asynchronous motion of heart, lungs and bypass. Moreover, it has been suggested that this predilection reflects scar tissue induced by injury during surgical manipulation. [169]

Published reports have demonstrated that BA of the IMA can be performed safely with high procedural success and a low incidence of clinical restenosis. [170-175] The use of BMS compared to BA alone for percutaneous revascularization of the IMA graft was investigated in several studies. In a large cohort of 174 patients who underwent BA or BMS placement, anastomotic lesions were more evident, 63% of al cases. [169] These lesions were more commonly treated with BA (91%), whereas lesions located at the ostium (8%) were more frequently treated with stents (69%). Patients who underwent stenting had a target lesion revascularization rate of 15.4% and those who underwent BA had a rate of 5.4%. In a retrospective analysis patients undergoing BMS implantation for the treatment of IMA graft stenosis were compared to patients treated with BA. [176] The minority of patients were treated

with BMS (26.4%) and received at least either ticlopidine or clopidogrel for 4 weeks post PCI. Angiographic success after stenting was high, 92%. At 1 year follow-up, target lesion revascularization rates were significantly higher in the stented lesions than lesions treated with BA alone (19.2% vs. 4.9%) and the higher rate in stented lesions was most apparent at the anastomotic site (25.0% vs. 4.2%). Moreover, a significant difference was observed between 1-year all-cause mortality between stented lesions and lesions treated with BA alone (13.6% vs. 4.4%), no difference was observed for MI. In a multivariate analysis including all available baseline factors contributing to target lesion revascularization, indicated that stent use was an independent predictor. In this observational study selection bias may have resulted in more lesions at high risk of restenosis being chosen for stenting, as stenting was at the discretion of the operator.

Comparison of BMS and DES for percutaneous revascularization of IMA Grafts, have reported conflicting results. In a retrospective study, outomes after BMS and DES treatment in IMA grafts were evaluated. [177] Baseline characteristics were comparable between the 2 groups, except for a trend toward longer stent lengths in the DES group (DES 20.2±7.7 mm vs. BMS 14.8±3.5 mm). No significant differences were present in in-hospital and 1- or 6-month outcomes between the 2 groups, including target lesion revascularization with DES (DES 3.33% vs. BMS 10%). Contrastingly, 2 small studies did not show improved clinical impact of DES compared to BMS. At 1-year clinical follow-up, no differences were detected in target lesion revascularization rates after treatment with BMS and PES (26.6% vs. 25%). [178] In the PES group, 2 late stent thromboses were observed. In addition, in a small study the long-term outcomes of 41 patients undergoing PCI of the IMA anastomosis BMS or SES were compared. [179] At a median follow-up of 29.2 months (interquartile range, 11.1-77.7 months) target lesion revascularization was 47.8% with SES and 7.1% with BMS. Patients who underwent repeat revascularization were more likely to have longer stents than those who did not (18.2 mm vs 14.2 mm).

The favourable results of BA compared to stenting in IMA graft intervention is in contrast with native coronary artery intervention. This might be explained by the fact that: 1) the proliferative response to BA in IMA may be less aggressive than that in native coronary arteries; 2) in native coronary arteries as compared to BA, stenting leads to more pronounced arterial injury, greater inflammatory response, and enhanced neointimal formation; 3) in small native coronary arteries, the high stent-to-wall ratio might predispose restenosis more frequently; and 4) stents are known to be thrombogenic and lead to neointimal formation and restenosis. [180-183]

Percutaneous treatment of ostial stenosis, presents technical challenges for the interventionalist whereas lesions in the shaft are most similar to routine intervention in a native coronary arteries. Stenting of the anastomotic site takes carefully positioning of the stent to achieve apposition to the arterial wall given the acute angle at which IMA meets the native coronary artery. In one observational study a difference in 1-year target lesion revascularization rates was present at the ostial, shaft, and anastomotic sites (30.8%, 5.0%, and 7.2%, respectively). [176] The anastomosis experiences a bending of the stent with strut shrinkage and might cause stent fracture or in DES might limit elution of drug to vessel wall.

Failure of the RA graft is most frequently a complete occlusion and less often a string-like appearance. However, on rare occasions, focal stenoses of the RA graft can occur.

RA graft stenosis treated by percutaneous intervention was evaluated in a small study including 18 patients. [184] The location of the RA stenosis was proximal (n = 2), shaft (n = 11) or distal anastomosis (n = 5). BA alone was performed on nine RA grafts at 1.7 years after surgery and stenting (3 BMS, 6 DES) of nine RA grafts was achieved at 9.2 years after surgery. At 5.8 years, clinical follow-up showed heart failure (n = 2) and recurrent angina (n = 3), all after balloon dilatation. At 4.5 years, 1 RA graft was occluded due to competitive flow from the native coronary vessel and 2 RA restenoses following BA were treated by stenting. Intrastent RA stenosis was noted in 1 patient. PCI with BA should be restricted to the early postoperative period during which spasm is difficult to exclude. Stenting showed excellent and durable results and is preferred in most cases. There are no large studies on other arterial grafts to draw definite conclusions for the treatment with PCI by BA, BMS or DES.

Antithrombotic therapy during graft intervention - The preferred parenteral antithrombotic therapy during graft intervention remains to be explored. The role of glycoprotein IIb/IIIa antagonists in graft intervention is limited as they failed to demonstrate a reduction in periprocedural MI. [185-187] Similarly, no reduction in MACE at 30 days was observed in a post hoc analysis when glycoprotein IIb/IIIa antagonists were used in conjunction with filter-based embolic protection, although there was a trend toward improved procedural success. [188] In contrast, bivalirudin as compared with unfractionated heparin may have beneficial effects on biochemical and clinical outcomes as it was associated with a significant reduction in CK-MB elevation and a trend toward lower in-hospital non–Q-wave MI, repeat revascularization, and vascular complications. [189] Moreover, bivalirudin may offer a safety advantage over heparin plus a glycoprotein IIb/IIIa anatagonist as minor bleeding complications were lower with bivalirudin alone (26% vs. 38%) with equal or greater suppression of adverse ischemic events. [190] Pharmacological treatment of slow or no-reflow is targeted at microvascular flow with intragraft administration of vasodilators and delivery of pharmaceutical agents to the distal microvasculature and can be maximized with a microcatheter like an aspiration thrombectomy catheter. Adenosine is an endogenous purine nucleoside, a vasodilator of arteries and arterioles, and inhibits platelet activation and aggregation. A high dose of intragraft adenosine (≥5 boluses of 24 μg each) can result in reversal of slow or no-reflow and improve final Thrombolysis In Myocardial Infarction (TIMI) flow grade. However, the use of adenosine is limited because severe bradycardia may occur due to its effect on sinoatrial and atrioventricular nodal conduction and the half-life of adenosine is very short. Intracoronary administration of nitroprusside, a direct donor of NO, results in a rapid improvement in both angiographic flow and blood flow velocity. Caution is warranted in patients who are volume depleted or hypotensive at baseline because profound hypotension may occur. Prophylactic intragraft administration of verapamil (100 to 500 μg) can reduce the occurrence of no-reflow and improve TIMI myocardial perfusion grade. Prophylactic intragraft administration of nicardipine, a potent arteriolar vasodilator, may reduce CK-MB elevation. Independent predictors for slow flow or no-reflow are probable patients treated for ACS, stent thrombosis, diseased SVG, and lesion ulceration.

Embolic protection Devices - Graft intervention, in particular SVG, can be complicated by distal embolization of atheroembolic debris leading to decreased epicardial and microvascular perfusion due to capillary plugging and vasospasm from the release of neurohumoral factors. Distal embolization may result in the slow or no-reflow and is associated with periprocedural myocardial necrosis and increased in-hospital mortality. However, distal embolization remains difficult to predict. Several embolic protection devices are available to prevent distal embolization and in SVG intervention it is recommended a class I according to the ACC/AHA guideline. [191] Distal balloon systems provide occlusion beyond the lesion securing the blood and may prevent plaque embolization into the myocardial bed. Hereafter, the blood with contained debris can be aspirated before occlusive balloon deflation. Advantages are the low crossing profile and entrapment of debris of all sizes as well as neurohumoral mediators such as serotonin and thromboxane that may have an adverse effect on the distal microvasculature. However, disadvantages are: 1) the need to cross the lesion before adequate protection, possibly liberating friable material before balloon occlusion; 2) temporary cessation of blood flow leading to ischemia and possible hemodynamic instability, as well as limiting visualization making accurate stent placement difficult; 3) inability to obtain full evacuation, especially near the occlusion balloon; 4) possible traumatic injury to the SVG during balloon occlusion, and 5) the need for a relatively disease-free landing zone of approximately 3 cm distal to the lesion for placement of the occlusion balloon. [192] The PercuSurge GuardWire (Medtronic, Minneapolis, Minnesota) and the TriActiv embolic protection system (Kensey Nash Corporation, Exton, Pennsylvania) both demonstrated a significant decrease the incidence of no-reflow and improved 30-day clinical outcome but the latter was associated with more vascular complications and the need for blood transfusion. [193,194]

Distal filter systems, composed of a tightly wrapped filter attached to a guidewire and sheathed within a delivery catheter for placement distal to the target lesion, can trap debris that embolize while the intervention is performed over the guidewire. After the intervention, a retrieval catheter is advanced over the guidewire to collapse the filter and remove it along with retained contents. It is ease-of-use and antegrade blood flow during intervention is maintained to avoid ischemia allowing the ability to inject contrast media to facilitate accurate balloon inflation or stent placement. Distal filter systems may be preferred in high-risk patients who are at increased risk for hemodynamic instability such as patients with severe left ventricular dysfunction or last remaining conduit. These systems do need a high crossing profile (large diameter sheath approximately 3- to 4-F) and the maneuverability is poor. Moreover, the inability to completely entrap microparticles, possible occlusion of the filter due to large amounts of debris, and inability to use in very distal lesions because of the need for a landing zone to deploy the filter are some other disadvanteges. The FilterWire EX (Boston Scientific) and the FilterWire EX (Boston Scientific) both showed noninferiority to distal balloon occlusion devices. [195]

The Proxis embolic protection system (St. Jude Medical, Maple Groves, Minnesota), a proximal balloon occlusion device, employs a distal balloon to seals the SVG while a proximal balloon seals the inside of the guiding catheter. This secures the blood with debris from embolizing

downstream into the microvasculature. After the intervention, the blood with the debris can be aspirated with a suction catheter before deflating the balloon. The advantages are that protection from distal embolization of atheromatous debris can be established before crossing the lesion, side branches can be protected, and distal lesions that are not amenable to distal embolic protection because of lack of a landing zone can be treated. The device can not be used in ostial or very proximal lesions as approximately 15 mm of landing zone is required, and the device causes cessation of antegrade perfusion resulting in myocardial ischemia. The multicenter prospective randomized PROXIMAL trial determined outcomes of the Proxis embolic protection device compared to distal protection devices during stenting of degenerated SVG. [196] In a subset of 410 patients with lesions amenable to treatment with either proximal or distal protection devices the primary composite end point, death, MI, or target vessel revascularization at 30 days, occurred in 12.2% of distal protection patients and 7.4% of proximal protection patients.

The decision regarding whether or not to intervene in a diseased graft should be guided by the patient's symptoms, angiographic evidence of a significant stenosis, and noninvasive evidence of myocardial ischemia in the region subtended by the bypass graft. Fractional flow reserve (FFR) measurement to assess the significance of stenosis in a bypass graft can be performed in a similar fashion as in a native coronary vessel and guide decision making.

Moreover, risk-scoring models are considered to be valuable in predicting outcomes and guiding to appropriate treatment strategies for patients undergoing PCI. Although, the SYNTAX score, developed to characterize angiographic complexity, has been proposed to predict outcomes and select an optimal treatment strategy for patients with coronary artery disease, the score is complex and does not take into account patients with coronary bypass graft lesions. [197-199] The Duke myocardial jeopardy score was developed in the 1980s as a simple method to estimate the amount of myocardium at risk for ischemia on the basis of the location of a coronary lesion in non-surgically managed patients with coronary artery disease. [200] Recently, an adjustment was suggested to this score to include left main disease as well as the protective properties of patent bypass grafts, the modified Duke jeopardy score (Figure 1). [201] The same assumptions are used as in the original score, assigning greater prognostic significance to more proximal lesions than more distal lesions in the same vessel. Noteworthy, the modified Duke jeopardy score has not been validated yet.

Acute coronary syndrome - After CABG, progression of atherosclerosis occurs both in grafts and native coronary arteries, resulting in significant morbidity and mortality, especially in patients who present with acute ACS. Estimates from the Coronary Artery Surgery Study and Veteran's Affairs Cooperative Study of Coronary Bypass indicate a rate of MI of approximately 2% to 3% per year over the first 5 years after CABG, with recurrent infarction in as many as 36% of patients at 10 years and even higher rates of hospitalization for recurrent ischemia. [202-204] Although primary PCI is the preferred strategy for STEMI patients, current guidelines do not provide specific recommendations on the optimal reperfusion strategy in patients with prior CABG. [205] Compared to patient without prior CABG, patients with prior CABG presenting with ACS are older, have more cardiovascular risk factors, more frequent comorbidities, higher

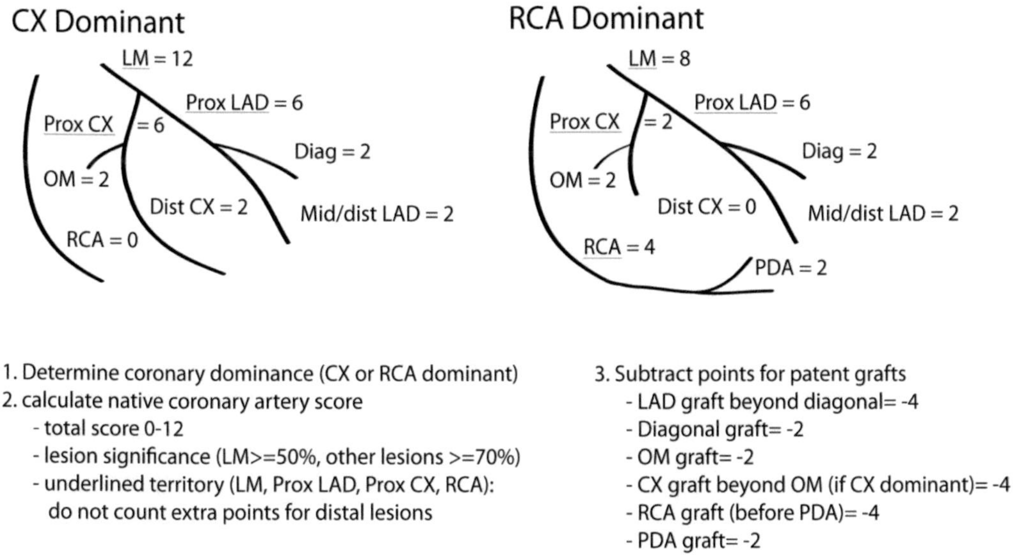

Figure 1. Modified Duke Jeopardy Score

TIMI risk score, lower left ventricular ejection fraction, had higher prevalence of previous treatment with evidence-based medications, were less likely to have ST-segment deviation or positive cardiac biomarker on presentation. [206-209] During hospitalization prior CABG patients experienced larger infarct size, were less likely to receive reperfusion therapy, early invasive therapy and were more likely to be managed medically when compared to non-CABG patients. [207,209] However, the efficacy of reperfusion therapy in patients with previous CABG is less well characterized. Given the large amount of atherosclerotic material and thrombus burden with limited runoff found in occluded SVG, it is suggested that reperfusion success rate is reduced. In the GUSTO-1 (Global Utilization of Streptokinase and TPA for Occluded Arteries I) trial a significantly increase in 30-day mortality was observed following reperfusion with tissue-type plasminogen activator in prior CABG patients compared to those without prior CABG (10.7% vs. 6.7%). [210] In addition, the prior CABG group also suffered more pulmonary edema, hypotension, or cardiogenic shock and a lower TIMI flow grade 3 rate was achieved (31% vs. 49.2%). In the PERSUIT (Platelet Glycoprotein IIb/IIIa in Unstable Angina: Receptor Suppression Using Integrilin Therapy) trial the efficacy of eptifibatide, a Glycoprotein IIb/IIIa antagonist, in patients with ACS was compared in patients with or without prior CABG. [88] After adjusting for differences in baseline characteristics and treatment, patients with prior CABG had a significantly higher mortality rates at 6 months. At 30 days, there was a similar effect on the primary end point of death or MI in the eptifibatide group versus the placebo group in prior CABG patients and in patients without a history of CABG. Finally, in the ACUITY (Acute Catheterization and Urgent Intervention Triage Strategy) Trial patients with prior CABG presenting with ACS were randomized to bivalirudin or heparin plus a glycoprotein IIb/IIIa inhibitor. [209] Bivalirudin monotherapy did not

improve short-term or long-term prognoses in ACS patients with prior CABG. Currently, the optimal antithrombotic therapy for patients with prior CABG presenting with ACS is not known, and existing data are conflicting.

As the non-invasive treatment did not significantly improve outcomes in patients with prior CABG presenting with ACS a percutaneous strategy was investigated. Invasive versus non-invasive treatment in ACS and prior CABG was evaluated in the GRACE (Global Registry of Acute Coronary Events), and 6-month mortality was lower in patients revascularized versus those treated medically by univariate but not by multivariable analysis. [211] Similarly, in a large Swedish registry of 10,837 patients with previous CABG, 1-year adjusted mortality was reduced with 50% with revascularization compared with medical management. [212]

Long-term clinical follow-up of ACS patients with prior CABG treated with PCI has been assessed in several studies. In a small study, 34 consecutive patients with ACS who underwent PCI with DES for occluded SVG, showed a procedural success rate of 81%. [213] At 3-year follow-up mortality was 42%, recurrent ACS was 41% and repeat intervention was 38%. In a recently published retrospective analysis, the outcomes after PCI with BMS or DES for ACS due to graft failure were evaluated. [214] Although the majority of the 92 patients included were treated with BMS (84%), the groups were comparable for baseline clinical and angiographic characteristics. Graft failure occurred mainly in the SVG (90%), but also arterial grafts (LIMA and RIMA) were treated (8.7%). The initial restoration of normal blood flow was approximately 80%. The primary endpoint of death, MI, target vessel revascularization at 5-year follow-up was 65.9% in the BMS group and 43.4% in the DES group, this difference did not reach statistical significance. Individual endpoints at 5 years were also comparable between BMS and DES groups (death 46% vs. 43%, MI 36% vs. 33%, target lesion revascularization 26% vs. 15%, respectively). Predictors for the composite endpoint were cardiac shock (HR= 6.13; 95%-CI:3.12-12.01), creatinin (HR=1.006; 95%-CI:1.001-1.011), and multi-vessel disease (HR= 4.64; 95%-CI:1.40-15.41). Cardiac shock and creatinin also predicted for death.

The beneficial effect of redo CABG over PCI was examined in the randomized AWESOME (Angina With Extremely Serious Operative Mortality Evaluation) trial in which 3-year survival and freedom from recurrent ACS was similar among patients with prior CABG and refractory myocardial ischemia, although patients favoured PCI. [215]

Patients with an acute MI / STEMI from a SVG culprit undergoing PCI are a high-risk subset of an already high-risk population. In the PAMI-2 (Second Primary Angioplasty in Myocardial Infarction) trial demonstrated lower angiographic success rates and higher mortality rates after BA in 58 patients with prior CABG compared with the 1068 patients without prior CABG. Primary PCI in patients with acute MI and prior CABG showed that patients treated with BA or BMS in SVG grafts compared to patients in whom a native vessel was treated had more no-reflow at initial treatment (8.9% vs. 1.6%) and significantly more MI at 1 year follow-up (26% vs. 11%). [130] In another study, outcomes of 192 patients with acute MI from a SVG culprit undergoing PCI were compared to patients with a native culprit. [216] After multivariable adjustment, SVG culprit remained significantly associated with lower levels of peak troponin. The likelihood of MACE was higher in SVG vs. native culprits in patients with small to modest

troponin elevations. Patients with a SVG culprit also suffered higher rates of mortality at 30 days (14.3% vs. 8.4%) and MACE at 1 year (36.8% vs. 24.5%). Finally, in the APEX-AMI trial, STEMI patients with prior CABG exhibited a smaller baseline territory at risk as measured by 12-lead ECG and had less myocardial necrosis. Moreover, in these patients receiving primary PCI, TIMI flow grade 3 was less frequently achieved and ST-segment resolution was less common but they have more frequent clinical comorbidities and increased 90-day clinical events including mortality. Risk factors for mortality were prior heart failure and age.

In conclusion, in patients with prior CABG presenting with ACS, PCI improves clinical outcomes compared to medical therapy alone. Redo CABG does not seem to further improve clinical outcomes.

11. Redo CABG for graft failure

Redo CABG is considered when revascularization of the LAD or a large area of the myocardium is required. Redo CABG is also preferred in patients with prior CABG with no patent grafts present but left main disease or 3-vessel disease, and in those with disabling angina, despite optimal non-surgical therapy, including lesions unsuitable for PCI. [217]

Surgeons are posed with a number of challenges in patients requiring redo CABG, including a higher likelihood of technical complications, incomplete revascularization, inadequate myocardial preservation, lack of suitable conduits, neurologic complications including major disabling stroke, renal failure, peri-operative bleeding and ischemia. [218,219] To help decrease the risks associated with redo CABG, a number of technical advances have been introduced in the surgical arena. The first challenge, safe sternal re-entry without damaging coronary bypass grafts and other retrosternal structures, has been described to be safely performed when using an oscillating or micro-oscillating saw. [220,221] Periodic deflating of the lungs will help prevent injury to the pulmonary parenchyme during re-entry. When a mammary artery was used in the first surgery, there are generally four types of mammary artery to sternal relationships that can be encountered. [219] The first: LIMA and RIMA are both used with the LIMA supplying the LAD and the RIMA reaching to the RCA or its branches. In this case, the risk of injury is relatively low, because the IMA grafts are parallel to the body of the sternum at a deeper plane and go through the pericardium (which is therefore open) directly away from the midline toward the target vessels. In a second situation, a pedicle LIMA graft crosses in front of the pleura, curves around and goes back laterally to reach the LAD, which is typically seen as a C-shaped curve on the angiogram. This type of LIMA grafting is particularly prone to injury during sternotomy because of its close proximity to the sternal body. In the third scenario, the RIMA graft is used and comes in front of the aorta across the midline and reaches the LAD. Although the graft crosses the midline the risk of injury is relatively low due to the close proximity to the aorta which lies deeper in the thorax and can be easily identified. Finally, the RIMA may go behind the aorta through the transverse sinus to reach the marginal branches of the Cx artery, which is very far away from the sternal re-entry area and poses therefore minimal risk for potential injury. The proximity of vein grafts to the sternum varies signifi-

cantly due to the large number of options for proximal as well as distal anastomosis sites. Careful review of the coronary angiogram or even cardiac/thoracic imaging to assess the relationship to the sternum and other anatomic structures is therefore warranted. Other structures at risk for injury during sternal re-entry include perforation of the right ventricle, and innominate vein. This is particularly true in patients where the pericardium was not closed. After sternal access, subsequent exposure of the heart can be completed by fibrosis which can be significant especially after pericarditis or radiation exposure. In patients requiring posterior vessel bypass, the entire heart should be cleared of fibrosis to allow surgical manipulation.

After sternal entry and inspection of the coronary vessels and branches, the second challenge is to assure adequate revascularization. Diffuse coronary artery disease poses a major problem in finding a suitable and satisfactory area for anastomosis. Thick plaque build-up and calcified coronary artery branches as well as calcification of the aortic arch make distal and proximal anastomosis of coronary bypass grafts hard and increase the chances of graft failure. [219] Additionally, the lack of satisfactory bypass conduits is common, because many patients undergoing redo CABG have very thin and dilated varicose veins, and small and calcified radial arteries. Risk factors for poor saphenous vein quality are age, obesity and diabetes, which are all more prominent in patients requiring redo CABG. In those patients the IMA may be small or even atherosclerotic.

Inadequate myocardial protection is an important cause of failure to wean patients off cardiopulmonary bypass. In the presence of degenerative old vein grafts, delivery of cardioplegia solution is considered safer through retrograde coronary sinus perfusion than anterograde delivery of cardioplegic solution because of the risk of atheromatous embolization from atherosclerotic vein grafts which can lead to acute occlusion of coronary artery branches. [222] Additional measures include a no touch approach regarding diseased vein grafts to minimalize the chance of distal embolization due to manipulation. [223] To assure a constant temperature in an attempt to minimize haematological abnormalities and tissue edema, some surgeons also occlude the IMA with a bulldog clamp to prevent the delivery of warm blood into the myocardium. In such a way, the entire myocardium is provided with continuous, cold cardioplegic solution through coronary sinus perfusion. [224,225] After placement of newly constructed coronary artery bypass grafts, anterograde cardioplegic solution can also be given.

Neurological complications and bleedings are common following redo CABG. Several techniques are used to decrease the risk of neurological complications. Most common are ischemic stroke or TIA due to cerebral embolization from a calcified ascending aorta, atheromatous plaques on the ascending aorta, and embolization from a jet phenomenon from aortic cannulation. Other causes for cerebal dysfunction are systemic inflammatory processes in response to cardiopulmonary bypass and gaseous microemboli. [226] Soft flow aortic cannulae, heparin-coated circuits, and administration of adenosine have proposed as techniques to lower neurological complications, but adequate studies and therefore evidence are lacking. [227-229] Bleeding is associated with an increased morbidity and mortality. Bleedings can be largely avoided by meticulous surgical dissection and careful catherization. Some studies using the application of fibrin glue suggest that this may help minimize peri-operative

bleeding. [230] Intraoperative blood loss is a major cause of post-operative bleeding from depleted coagulation factors and hemodilution. Consideration should be given to preoperative antiplatelet therapy including aspirin and clopidogrel. A low platelet count and other medical conditions that adversely affect the coagulation process should be carefully investigated.

Redo CABG for coronary bypass graft failure is not favoured by cardiologists and surgeons alike, due to the higher morbidity and mortality compared with primary CABG. Reported intraoperative mortality rates are 5.8-9.6%. [231] Other major complications include stroke (1.4-3.2%), non-fatal MI (3.0-9.6%), renal failure (2.4-11%) and post-operative bleeding (2.7-4.4%). [217,223] Following redo CABG, survival is 75–90% and 55–75% at 5- and 10-year follow-up, respectively. [231]

Redo CABG versus PCI - Available data comparing the outcomes of PCI to redo CABG in patients with prior CABG is limited. Initial studies evaluating BA versus CABG noted comparable long-term results except for a much higher rate of repeat revascularization in the BA group (BA 64% vs. redo CABG 8%). [232] Multivariate analysis identified age > 70 years, left ventricular ejection fraction < 40%, unstable angina, number of diseased vessels and diabetes mellitus as independent correlates of mortality for the entire group. Direct comparison between redo CABG and PCI was performed in the AWESOME trial. A total of 142 patients with refractory post-CABG ischemia and at least one of five high-risk features (i.e. prior open-heart surgery, age >70 years, left ventricular ejection fraction <35%, MI within seven days or intraaortic balloon pump required) amandable for either PCI or redo CABG were randomized. [17] Arterial grafts were used in 75% of redo CABG procedures and stents in 54% of PCI (approximately one-half with BMS). In-hospital mortality was higher after redo CABG (8% vs. 0%). At 3 years, there was no significant difference in overall patient survival (redo CABG 71% vs. PCI 77%), but there was a nonsignificant increase in survival free of unstable angina in the CABG group (65% vs. 48%). In the much larger retrospective observational study from the Cleveland Clinic of 2191 patients with prior CABG who underwent multivessel revascularization between 1995 and 2000 were evaluated. [233] A total of 1487 had redo CABG and 704 underwent PCI (77% with at least one stent). No difference was observed in 30-day mortality with redo CABG compared to PCI (2.8% vs. 1.7%) but as expected periprocedural Q wave MI occurred more often after redo CABG (1.4% vs. 0.3%). At 5-years follow-up, cumulative survival was similar with redo CABG and PCI (79.5% vs. 75.3%). After adjustment, PCI was associated with a nonsignificant increase in mortality risk (hazard ratio 1.47, 95% CI 0.94-2.28). The major predictors of mortality were higher age and lower LVEF, not the method of revascularization. Importantly, the choice of treatment strategy was largely determined by coronary anatomy wherein the most important factors to perform redo CABG were: 1) more diseased or occluded grafts, 2) absence of a prior MI, 3) lower left ventricular ejection fraction, 4) longer interval from first CABG (15 vs. 6 years), 5) more total occlusions in native coronary arteries, and 6) the absence of a patent mammary artery graft.

In diabetic patients with post-CABG angina, the outcomes after repeat revascularization were evaluated in an observational study in which 1123 such patients underwent PCI (75% BA, 25% stent palcement) and 598 underwent redo CABG. [234] Redo CABG was associated with increased in-hospital mortality (11.2% vs. 1.6%) and stroke (4.7% vs. 0.1%). At 10 years, there

http://dx.doi.org/10.5772/54928

was no significant difference in mortality between groups (redo CABG 74% vs. PCI 68%). Noteworthy, the available comparative studies were, however, conducted before the use of aggressive dual antiplatelet therapy with aspirin and clopidogrel after PCI with stenting and aggressive lipid-lowering with statins for secondary prevention.

In a recently published retrospective study, in which patients were prescribed aggressive dual antiplatelet therapy, 287 consecutive patients with graft failure were assigned by the heart-team to PCI or redo CABG. [235] A total of 243 patients underwent PCI (82% treated with BMS, 18% treated with DES) and 44 redo CABG. Patient selection was present as patients undergoing PCI more frequently presented with STEMI, multivessel disease, SVG failure, a history of MI, and shorter time-to-graft failure. At 5 year, the rate of composite all-cause death, MI or target vessel revascularization was comparable, 57.6% after PCI and 51% after redo CABG. Target lesion revascularization was 21.3% after PCI, and 3.2% following redo CABG. In the PCI group, BMS was associated with significantly higher rates of target lesion revascularization (24.8% vs. 7.6%), but the rate of death or MI compared with DES was similar. Independent predictors for the composite outcome were creatinine and peak creatine kinase MB. These results have to be confirmed in larger studies before definite conclusion can be drawn.

12. Conclusion

Patients with prior CABG remain at risk for future cardiac events, including graft failure. Stable patients with recurrence of angina following CABG can be treated medically for their symptoms and risk factor reduction. In all patients with coronary heart disease aggressive risk factor reduction is recommended which includes aspirin, treatment for hypertension and serum lipids, avoidance of smoking, and controlling serum glucose in diabetic patients. Evaluation for ischemia is as in other patients with stable angina without prior CABG. However, early diagnostic angiography is suggested as the different anatomic possibilities, i.e. graft stenosis or progression of native vessel disease in nonbypassed vessels can lead to recurrent ischemia. Revascularization of graft failure either by PCI or redo CABG is associated with worse acute and long-term outcomes compared to patients without prior CABG. The choice of treatment modality is influenced by clinical and angiographic characteristics. When multiple grafts are occluded or the graft or native coronary artery appears unsuitable for PCI, surgery should be favoured. The target for PCI is the body of the coronary artery of the arterial graft while freshly occluded SVG or the anastomosis itself should be targeted due to the risk of embolization or perforation. Whether specific stent platforms, polymers or drugs are more appropriate in SVG and arterial graft lesions has not been addressed at this time. Moreover, the role of various surgical techniques for graft revascularization, such as off-pump and minimal invasive CABG also remain unclear. Finally, factors including disease status of the native vessel, and patient characteristics such as left ventricular function, renal failure, diabetes and advanced age, as shown in our multivariate analysis are of influence on outcomes. Future prospective studies in the medical and invasive treatment of graft failure are therefore warranted. Those studies together with our growing understanding of the pathobiology of arterial and vein grafts will

ultimately result in practical patient-tailored therapeutic strategies to enhance graft function and control intimal hyperplasia and accelerated atherosclerosis.

Author details

M.A. Beijk[1] and R.E. Harskamp[1,2]

1 Academic Medical Center – University of Amsterdam, Amsterdam,, The Netherlands

2 Duke Clinical Research Institute – Duke University, Durham, North Carolina,, USA

References

[1] Beck CS. The development of a new blood supply to the heart by operation. Ann Surg 1935;102:801-13.

[2] Leighninger DS, Dalem J. Revascularization of the heart by anastomosis between aorta and coronary sinus; the Beck II operation, an experimental study. Ann Surg 1954;140:668-74.

[3] Effler DB, Groves LK, Sones FM, Jr., Shirey EK. Increased myocardial perfusion by internal mammary artery implant: Vineberg's operation. Ann Surg 1963;158:526-36.

[4] Mehta NJ, Khan IA. Cardiology's 10 greatest discoveries of the 20th century. Tex Heart Inst J 2002;29:164-71.

[5] Vineberg AM. Development of an anastomosis between the coronary vessels and a transplanted internal mammary artery. Can Med Assoc J 1946;55:117-9.

[6] Gibbon JH, Jr. The development of the heart-lung apparatus. Am J Surg 1978;135:608-19.

[7] Haller JD, Olearchyk AS. Cardiology's 10 greatest discoveries. Tex Heart Inst J 2002;29:342-4.

[8] Favaloro RG, Effler DB, Cheanvechai C, Quint RA, Sones FM, Jr. Acute coronary insufficiency (impending myocardial infarction and myocardial infarction): surgical treatment by the saphenous vein graft technique. Am J Cardiol 1971;28:598-607.

[9] Johnson WD, Flemma RJ, Lepley D, Jr., Ellison EH. Extended treatment of severe coronary artery disease: a total surgical approach. Ann Surg 1969;170:460-70.

[10] Bailey CP, Hirose T. Successful internal mammary-coronary arterial anastomosis using a "minivascular" suturing technic. Int Surg 1968;49:416-27.

[11] Kolessov VI. Mammary artery-coronary artery anastomosis as method of treatment for angina pectoris. J Thorac Cardiovasc Surg 1967;54:535-44.

[12] Curtis JJ, Stoney WS, Alford WC, Jr., Burrus GR, Thomas CS, Jr. Intimal hyperplasia. A cause of radial artery aortocoronary bypass graft failure. Ann Thorac Surg 1975;20:628-35.

[13] Acar C, Jebara VA, Portoghese M, et al. Revival of the radial artery for coronary artery bypass grafting. Ann Thorac Surg 1992;54:652-9.

[14] Epstein AJ, Polsky D, Yang F, Yang L, Groeneveld PW. Coronary revascularization trends in the United States, 2001-2008. JAMA 2011;305:1769-76.

[15] Fitzgibbon GM, Leach AJ, Keon WJ, Burton JR, Kafka HP. Coronary bypass graft fate. Angiographic study of 1,179 vein grafts early, one year, and five years after operation. J Thorac Cardiovasc Surg 1986;91:773-8.

[16] Hong MK, Mehran R, Dangas G, et al. Are we making progress with percutaneous saphenous vein graft treatment? A comparison of 1990 to 1994 and 1995 to 1998 results. J Am Coll Cardiol 2001;38:150-4.

[17] Morrison DA, Sethi G, Sacks J, et al. Percutaneous coronary intervention versus repeat bypass surgery for patients with medically refractory myocardial ischemia: AWESOME randomized trial and registry experience with post-CABG patients. J Am Coll Cardiol 2002;40:1951-4.

[18] Weintraub WS, Jones EL, Morris DC, King SB, III, Guyton RA, Craver JM. Outcome of reoperative coronary bypass surgery versus coronary angioplasty after previous bypass surgery. Circulation 1997;95:868-77.

[19] Motwani JG, Topol EJ. Aortocoronary saphenous vein graft disease: pathogenesis, predisposition, and prevention. Circulation 1998;97:916-31.

[20] Rogers WJ, Canto JG, Lambrew CT, et al. Temporal trends in the treatment of over 1.5 million patients with myocardial infarction in the US from 1990 through 1999: the National Registry of Myocardial Infarction 1, 2 and 3. J Am Coll Cardiol 2000;36:2056-63.

[21] Bryan AJ, Angelini GD. The biology of saphenous vein graft occlusion: etiology and strategies for prevention. Curr Opin Cardiol 1994;9:641-9.

[22] Davies MG, Hagen PO. Pathophysiology of vein graft failure: a review. Eur J Vasc Endovasc Surg 1995;9:7-18.

[23] Milroy CM, Scott DJ, Beard JD, Horrocks M, Bradfield JW. Histological appearances of the long saphenous vein. J Pathol 1989;159:311-6.

[24] Thiene G, Miazzi P, Valsecchi M, et al. Histological survey of the saphenous vein before its use as autologous aortocoronary bypass graft. Thorax 1980;35:519-22.

[25] Panetta TF, Marin ML, Veith FJ, et al. Unsuspected preexisting saphenous vein disease: an unrecognized cause of vein bypass failure. J Vasc Surg 1992;15:102-10.

[26] He GW. Vascular endothelial function related to cardiac surgery. Asian Cardiovasc Thorac Ann 2004;12:1-2.

[27] Angelini GD, Passani SL, Breckenridge IM, Newby AC. Nature and pressure dependence of damage induced by distension of human saphenous vein coronary artery bypass grafts. Cardiovasc Res 1987;21:902-7.

[28] Bush HL, Jr., Jakubowski JA, Curl GR, Deykin D, Nabseth DC. The natural history of endothelial structure and function in arterialized vein grafts. J Vasc Surg 1986;3:204-15.

[29] Mills NL, Everson CT. Vein graft failure. Curr Opin Cardiol 1995;10:562-8.

[30] Ohta O, Kusaba A. Development of vasa vasorum in the arterially implanted autovein bypass graft and its anastomosis in the dog. Int Angiol 1997;16:197-203.

[31] Shi Y, O'Brien JE, Jr., Mannion JD, et al. Remodeling of autologous saphenous vein grafts. The role of perivascular myofibroblasts. Circulation 1997;95:2684-93.

[32] Thatte HS, Khuri SF. The coronary artery bypass conduit: I. Intraoperative endothelial injury and its implication on graft patency. Ann Thorac Surg 2001;72:S2245-S2252.

[33] Rao GN, Berk BC. Active oxygen species stimulate vascular smooth muscle cell growth and proto-oncogene expression. Circ Res 1992;70:593-9.

[34] Zou Y, Dietrich H, Hu Y, Metzler B, Wick G, Xu Q. Mouse model of venous bypass graft arteriosclerosis. Am J Pathol 1998;153:1301-10.

[35] Barboriak JJ, Pintar K, Van Horn DL, Batayias GE, Korns ME. Pathologic findings in the aortocoronary vein grafts. A scanning electron microscope study. Atherosclerosis 1978;29:69-80.

[36] Vlodaver Z, Edwards JE. Pathologic changes in aortic-coronary arterial saphenous vein grafts. Circulation 1971;44:719-28.

[37] Waller BF, Roberts WC. Remnant saphenous veins after aortocoronary bypass grafting: analysis of 3,394 centimeters of unused vein from 402 patients. Am J Cardiol 1985;55:65-71.

[38] Bourassa MG, Campeau L, Lesperance J, Grondin CM. Changes in grafts and coronary arteries after saphenous vein aortocoronary bypass surgery: results at repeat angiography. Circulation 1982;65:90-7.

[39] Rosenfeldt FL, He GW, Buxton BF, Angus JA. Pharmacology of coronary artery bypass grafts. Ann Thorac Surg 1999;67:878-88.

[40] Tsui JC, Dashwood MR. Recent strategies to reduce vein graft occlusion: a need to limit the effect of vascular damage. Eur J Vasc Endovasc Surg 2002;23:202-8.

[41] Peykar S, Angiolillo DJ, Bass TA, Costa MA. Saphenous vein graft disease. Minerva Cardioangiol 2004;52:379-90.

[42] Nwasokwa ON. Coronary artery bypass graft disease. Ann Intern Med 1995;123:528-45.

[43] Schwartz SM, Deblois D, O'Brien ER. The intima. Soil for atherosclerosis and restenosis. Circ Res 1995;77:445-65.

[44] Zhang L, Peppel K, Brian L, Chien L, Freedman NJ. Vein graft neointimal hyperplasia is exacerbated by tumor necrosis factor receptor-1 signaling in graft-intrinsic cells. Arterioscler Thromb Vasc Biol 2004;24:2277-83.

[45] Leask RL, Butany J, Johnston KW, Ethier CR, Ojha M. Human saphenous vein coronary artery bypass graft morphology, geometry and hemodynamics. Ann Biomed Eng 2005;33:301-9.

[46] Butany JW, David TE, Ojha M. Histological and morphometric analyses of early and late aortocoronary vein grafts and distal anastomoses. Can J Cardiol 1998;14:671-7.

[47] Domanski MJ, Borkowf CB, Campeau L, et al. Prognostic factors for atherosclerosis progression in saphenous vein grafts: the postcoronary artery bypass graft (Post-CABG) trial. Post-CABG Trial Investigators. J Am Coll Cardiol 2000;36:1877-83.

[48] Mehta D, Izzat MB, Bryan AJ, Angelini GD. Towards the prevention of vein graft failure. Int J Cardiol 1997;62 Suppl 1:S55-S63.

[49] Shi Y, O'Brien JE, Fard A, Mannion JD, Wang D, Zalewski A. Adventitial myofibroblasts contribute to neointimal formation in injured porcine coronary arteries. Circulation 1996;94:1655-64.

[50] Ratliff NB, Myles JL. Rapidly progressive atherosclerosis in aortocoronary saphenous vein grafts. Possible immune-mediated disease. Arch Pathol Lab Med 1989;113:772-6.

[51] Hermiller JB, Tenaglia AN, Kisslo KB, et al. In vivo validation of compensatory enlargement of atherosclerotic coronary arteries. Am J Cardiol 1993;71:665-8.

[52] Atkinson JB, Forman MB, Vaughn WK, Robinowitz M, McAllister HA, Virmani R. Morphologic changes in long-term saphenous vein bypass grafts. Chest 1985;88:341-8.

[53] Lie JT, Lawrie GM, Morris GC, Jr. Aortocoronary bypass saphenous vein graft atherosclerosis. Anatomic study of 99 vein grafts from normal and hyperlipoproteinemic patients up to 75 months postoperatively. Am J Cardiol 1977;40:906-14.

[54] Amano J, Suzuki A, Sunamori M, Tsukada T, Numano F. Cytokinetic study of aorto-coronary bypass vein grafts in place for less than six months. Am J Cardiol 1991;67:1234-6.

[55] Dietrich H, Hu Y, Zou Y, et al. Rapid development of vein graft atheroma in ApoE-deficient mice. Am J Pathol 2000;157:659-69.

[56] Kockx MM, Cambier BA, Bortier HE, et al. Foam cell replication and smooth muscle cell apoptosis in human saphenous vein grafts. Histopathology 1994;25:365-71.

[57] Qiao JH, Walts AE, Fishbein MC. The severity of atherosclerosis at sites of plaque rupture with occlusive thrombosis in saphenous vein coronary artery bypass grafts. Am Heart J 1991;122:955-8.

[58] Walts AE, Fishbein MC, Matloff JM. Thrombosed, ruptured atheromatous plaques in saphenous vein coronary artery bypass grafts: ten years' experience. Am Heart J 1987;114:718-23.

[59] Goldman S, Zadina K, Krasnicka B, et al. Predictors of graft patency 3 years after coronary artery bypass graft surgery. Department of Veterans Affairs Cooperative Study Group No. 297. J Am Coll Cardiol 1997;29:1563-8.

[60] Mehta RH, Ferguson TB, Lopes RD, et al. Saphenous vein grafts with multiple versus single distal targets in patients undergoing coronary artery bypass surgery: one-year graft failure and five-year outcomes from the Project of Ex-Vivo Vein Graft Engineering via Transfection (PREVENT) IV trial. Circulation 2011;124:280-8.

[61] He GW, Yang CQ. Comparison among arterial grafts and coronary artery. An attempt at functional classification. J Thorac Cardiovasc Surg 1995;109:707-15.

[62] He GW, Acuff TE, Yang CQ, Ryan WH, Mack MJ. Middle and proximal sections of the human internal mammary artery are not "passive conduits". J Thorac Cardiovasc Surg 1994;108:741-6.

[63] He GW, Angus JA, Rosenfeldt FL. Reactivity of the canine isolated internal mammary artery, saphenous vein, and coronary artery to constrictor and dilator substances: relevance to coronary bypass graft surgery. J Cardiovasc Pharmacol 1988;12:12-22.

[64] Van Son JA, Smedts F, Vincent JG, van Lier HJ, Kubat K. Comparative anatomic studies of various arterial conduits for myocardial revascularization. J Thorac Cardiovasc Surg 1990;99:703-7.

[65] Luscher TF, Diederich D, Siebenmann R, et al. Difference between endothelium-dependent relaxation in arterial and in venous coronary bypass grafts. N Engl J Med 1988;319:462-7.

[66] Cameron AA, Green GE, Brogno DA, Thornton J. Internal thoracic artery grafts: 20-year clinical follow-up. J Am Coll Cardiol 1995;25:188-92.

[67] Loop FD, Lytle BW, Cosgrove DM, et al. Influence of the internal-mammary-artery graft on 10-year survival and other cardiac events. N Engl J Med 1986;314:1-6.

[68] Muneretto C, Negri A, Manfredi J, et al. Safety and usefulness of composite grafts for total arterial myocardial revascularization: a prospective randomized evaluation. J Thorac Cardiovasc Surg 2003;125:826-35.

[69] Merrilees MJ, Shepphard AJ, Robinson MC. Structural features of saphenous vein and internal thoracic artery endothelium: correlates with susceptibility and resistance to graft atherosclerosis. J Cardiovasc Surg (Torino) 1988;29:639-46.

[70] Berger PB, Alderman EL, Nadel A, Schaff HV. Frequency of early occlusion and stenosis in a left internal mammary artery to left anterior descending artery bypass graft after surgery through a median sternotomy on conventional bypass: benchmark for minimally invasive direct coronary artery bypass. Circulation 1999;100:2353-8.

[71] Tatoulis J, Buxton BF, Fuller JA. Patencies of 2127 arterial to coronary conduits over 15 years. Ann Thorac Surg 2004;77:93-101.

[72] Tatoulis J, Buxton BF, Fuller JA. The right internal thoracic artery: the forgotten conduit--5,766 patients and 991 angiograms. Ann Thorac Surg 2011;92:9-15.

[73] Achouh P, Boutekadjirt R, Toledano D, et al. Long-term (5- to 20-year) patency of the radial artery for coronary bypass grafting. J Thorac Cardiovasc Surg 2010;140:73-9, 79.

[74] Suma H, Tanabe H, Takahashi A, et al. Twenty years experience with the gastroepiploic artery graft for CABG. Circulation 2007;116:I188-I191.

[75] Khot UN, Friedman DT, Pettersson G, Smedira NG, Li J, Ellis SG. Radial artery bypass grafts have an increased occurrence of angiographically severe stenosis and occlusion compared with left internal mammary arteries and saphenous vein grafts. Circulation 2004;109:2086-91.

[76] Ruttmann E, Fischler N, Sakic A, et al. Second internal thoracic artery versus radial artery in coronary artery bypass grafting: a long-term, propensity score-matched follow-up study. Circulation 2011;124:1321-9.

[77] Suma H. Spasm of the gastroepiploic artery graft. Ann Thorac Surg 1990;49:168-9.

[78] He GW, Yang CQ, Starr A. Overview of the nature of vasoconstriction in arterial grafts for coronary operations. Ann Thorac Surg 1995;59:676-83.

[79] Fitzgibbon GM, Kafka HP, Leach AJ, Keon WJ, Hooper GD, Burton JR. Coronary bypass graft fate and patient outcome: angiographic follow-up of 5,065 grafts related to survival and reoperation in 1,388 patients during 25 years. J Am Coll Cardiol 1996;28:616-26.

[80] Grondin CM, Lesperance J, Bourassa MG, Campeau L. Coronary artery grafting with the saphenous vein or internal mammary artery. Comparison of late results in two consecutive series of patients. Ann Thorac Surg 1975;20:605-18.

[81] Desai ND, Cohen EA, Naylor CD, Fremes SE. A randomized comparison of radial-artery and saphenous-vein coronary bypass grafts. N Engl J Med 2004;351:2302-9.

[82] Barner HB, Barnett MG. Fifteen- to twenty-one-year angiographic assessment of internal thoracic artery as a bypass conduit. Ann Thorac Surg 1994;57:1526-8.

[83] Berger A, MacCarthy PA, Siebert U, et al. Long-term patency of internal mammary artery bypass grafts: relationship with preoperative severity of the native coronary artery stenosis. Circulation 2004;110:II36-II40.

[84] Shelton ME, Forman MB, Virmani R, Bajaj A, Stoney WS, Atkinson JB. A comparison of morphologic and angiographic findings in long-term internal mammary artery and saphenous vein bypass grafts. J Am Coll Cardiol 1988;11:297-307.

[85] Halabi AR, Alexander JH, Shaw LK, et al. Relation of early saphenous vein graft failure to outcomes following coronary artery bypass surgery. Am J Cardiol 2005;96:1254-9.

[86] Chen L, Theroux P, Lesperance J, Shabani F, Thibault B, De GP. Angiographic features of vein grafts versus ungrafted coronary arteries in patients with unstable angina and previous bypass surgery. J Am Coll Cardiol 1996;28:1493-9.

[87] Kleiman NS, Anderson HV, Rogers WJ, Theroux P, Thompson B, Stone PH. Comparison of outcome of patients with unstable angina and non-Q-wave acute myocardial infarction with and without prior coronary artery bypass grafting (Thrombolysis in Myocardial Ischemia III Registry). Am J Cardiol 1996;77:227-31.

[88] Labinaz M, Kilaru R, Pieper K, et al. Outcomes of patients with acute coronary syndromes and prior coronary artery bypass grafting: results from the platelet glycoprotein IIb/IIIa in unstable angina: receptor suppression using integrilin therapy (PURSUIT) trial. Circulation 2002;105:322-7.

[89] Alderman EL, Kip KE, Whitlow PL, et al. Native coronary disease progression exceeds failed revascularization as cause of angina after five years in the Bypass Angioplasty Revascularization Investigation (BARI). J Am Coll Cardiol 2004;44:766-74.

[90] Dunning J, Versteegh M, Fabbri A, et al. Guideline on antiplatelet and anticoagulation management in cardiac surgery. Eur J Cardiothorac Surg 2008;34:73-92.

[91] Gavaghan TP, Gebski V, Baron DW. Immediate postoperative aspirin improves vein graft patency early and late after coronary artery bypass graft surgery. A placebo-controlled, randomized study. Circulation 1991;83:1526-33.

[92] Goldman S, Copeland J, Moritz T, et al. Saphenous vein graft patency 1 year after coronary artery bypass surgery and effects of antiplatelet therapy. Results of a Veterans Administration Cooperative Study. Circulation 1989;80:1190-7.

[93] Hockings BE, Ireland MA, Gotch-Martin KF, Taylor RR. Placebo-controlled trial of enteric coated aspirin in coronary bypass graft patients. Effect on graft patency. Med J Aust 1993;159:376-8.

[94] Lorenz RL, Schacky CV, Weber M, et al. Improved aortocoronary bypass patency by low-dose aspirin (100 mg daily). Effects on platelet aggregation and thromboxane formation. Lancet 1984;1:1261-4.

[95] Sanz G, Pajaron A, Alegria E, et al. Prevention of early aortocoronary bypass occlusion by low-dose aspirin and dipyridamole. Grupo Espanol para el Seguimiento del Injerto Coronario (GESIC). Circulation 1990;82:765-73.

[96] Fremes SE, Levinton C, Naylor CD, Chen E, Christakis GT, Goldman BS. Optimal antithrombotic therapy following aortocoronary bypass: a meta-analysis. Eur J Cardiothorac Surg 1993;7:169-80.

[97] Sharma GV, Khuri SF, Josa M, Folland ED, Parisi AF. The effect of antiplatelet therapy on saphenous vein coronary artery bypass graft patency. Circulation 1983;68:II218-II221.

[98] Gurbuz AT, Zia AA, Vuran AC, Cui H, Aytac A. Postoperative clopidogrel improves mid-term outcome after off-pump coronary artery bypass graft surgery: a prospective study. Eur J Cardiothorac Surg 2006;29:190-5.

[99] Kulik A, Le May MR, Voisine P, et al. Aspirin plus clopidogrel versus aspirin alone after coronary artery bypass grafting: the clopidogrel after surgery for coronary artery disease (CASCADE) Trial. Circulation 2010;122:2680-7.

[100] Bhatt DL, Chew DP, Hirsch AT, Ringleb PA, Hacke W, Topol EJ. Superiority of clopidogrel versus aspirin in patients with prior cardiac surgery. Circulation 2001;103:363-8.

[101] Fox KA, Mehta SR, Peters R, et al. Benefits and risks of the combination of clopidogrel and aspirin in patients undergoing surgical revascularization for non-ST-elevation acute coronary syndrome: the Clopidogrel in Unstable angina to prevent Recurrent ischemic Events (CURE) Trial. Circulation 2004;110:1202-8.

[102] Harskamp RE, Beijk MA, Damman P, Tijssen JG, Lopés RD, de Winter RJ. Pre-hospitalization Antiplatelet Therapy and Outcomes following Saphenous Vein Graft Intervention. Accepted for publication 2012.

[103] Knatterud GL, Rosenberg Y, Campeau L, et al. Long-term effects on clinical outcomes of aggressive lowering of low-density lipoprotein cholesterol levels and low-dose anticoagulation in the post coronary artery bypass graft trial. Post CABG Investigators. Circulation 2000;102:157-65.

[104] Huynh T, Theroux P, Bogaty P, Nasmith J, Solymoss S. Aspirin, warfarin, or the combination for secondary prevention of coronary events in patients with acute coronary syndromes and prior coronary artery bypass surgery. Circulation 2001;103:3069-74.

[105] Becker RC, Meade TW, Berger PB, et al. The primary and secondary prevention of coronary artery disease: American College of Chest Physicians Evidence-Based Clinical Practice Guidelines (8th Edition). Chest 2008;133:776S-814S.

[106] The effect of aggressive lowering of low-density lipoprotein cholesterol levels and low-dose anticoagulation on obstructive changes in saphenous-vein coronary-artery bypass grafts. The Post Coronary Artery Bypass Graft Trial Investigators. N Engl J Med 1997;336:153-62.

[107] MRC/BHF Heart Protection Study of cholesterol lowering with simvastatin in 20,536 high-risk individuals: a randomised placebo-controlled trial. Lancet 2002;360:7-22.

[108] Campeau L, Hunninghake DB, Knatterud GL, et al. Aggressive cholesterol lowering delays saphenous vein graft atherosclerosis in women, the elderly, and patients with associated risk factors. NHLBI post coronary artery bypass graft clinical trial. Post CABG Trial Investigators. Circulation 1999;99:3241-7.

[109] Dotani MI, Elnicki DM, Jain AC, Gibson CM. Effect of preoperative statin therapy and cardiac outcomes after coronary artery bypass grafting. Am J Cardiol 2000;86:1128-30, A6.

[110] Shah SJ, Waters DD, Barter P, et al. Intensive lipid-lowering with atorvastatin for secondary prevention in patients after coronary artery bypass surgery. J Am Coll Cardiol 2008;51:1938-43.

[111] Zhou Q, Liao JK. Statins and cardiovascular diseases: from cholesterol lowering to pleiotropy. Curr Pharm Des 2009;15:467-78.

[112] Veillard NR, Braunersreuther V, Arnaud C, et al. Simvastatin modulates chemokine and chemokine receptor expression by geranylgeranyl isoprenoid pathway in human endothelial cells and macrophages. Atherosclerosis 2006;188:51-8.

[113] Steg PG, James SK, Atar D, et al. ESC Guidelines for the management of acute myocardial infarction in patients presenting with ST-segment elevation: The Task Force on the management of ST-segment elevation acute myocardial infarction of the European Society of Cardiology (ESC). Eur Heart J 2012;33:2569-619.

[114] McMurray JJ, Adamopoulos S, Anker SD, et al. ESC Guidelines for the diagnosis and treatment of acute and chronic heart failure 2012: The Task Force for the Diagnosis and Treatment of Acute and Chronic Heart Failure 2012 of the European Society of Cardiology. Developed in collaboration with the Heart Failure Association (HFA) of the ESC. Eur Heart J 2012;33:1787-847.

[115] Goyal A, Alexander JH, Hafley GE, et al. Outcomes associated with the use of secondary prevention medications after coronary artery bypass graft surgery. Ann Thorac Surg 2007;83:993-1001.

[116] Wijns W, Kolh P, Danchin N, et al. Guidelines on myocardial revascularization. Eur Heart J 2010;31:2501-55.

[117] Zhao DX, Leacche M, Balaguer JM, et al. Routine intraoperative completion angiography after coronary artery bypass grafting and 1-stop hybrid revascularization results from a fully integrated hybrid catheterization laboratory/operating room. J Am Coll Cardiol 2009;53:232-41.

[118] Brener SJ, Lytle BW, Casserly IP, Schneider JP, Topol EJ, Lauer MS. Propensity analysis of long-term survival after surgical or percutaneous revascularization in patients with multivessel coronary artery disease and high-risk features. Circulation 2004;109:2290-5.

[119] Patel MR, Dehmer GJ, Hirshfeld JW, et al. ACCF/SCAI/STS/AATS/AHA/ASNC/HFSA/SCCT 2012 appropriate use criteria for coronary revascularization focused update: a report of the American College of Cardiology Foundation Appropriate Use Criteria Task Force, Society for Cardiovascular Angiography and Interventions, Society of Thoracic Surgeons, American Association for Thoracic Surgery, American Heart Association, American Society of Nuclear Cardiology, and the Society of Cardiovascular Computed Tomography. J Thorac Cardiovasc Surg 2012;143:780-803.

[120] Sabik JF, III, Blackstone EH, Houghtaling PL, Walts PA, Lytle BW. Is reoperation still a risk factor in coronary artery bypass surgery? Ann Thorac Surg 2005;80:1719-27.

[121] Yau TM, Borger MA, Weisel RD, Ivanov J. The changing pattern of reoperative coronary surgery: trends in 1230 consecutive reoperations. J Thorac Cardiovasc Surg 2000;120:156-63.

[122] Morrison DA, Sethi G, Sacks J, et al. A multicenter, randomized trial of percutaneous coronary intervention versus bypass surgery in high-risk unstable angina patients. The AWESOME (Veterans Affairs Cooperative Study #385, angina with extremely serious operative mortality evaluation) investigators from the Cooperative Studies Program of the Department of Veterans Affairs. Control Clin Trials 1999;20:601-19.

[123] Dougenis D, Brown AH. Long-term results of reoperations for recurrent angina with internal mammary artery versus saphenous vein grafts. Heart 1998;80:9-13.

[124] Nguyen TT, O'Neill WW, Grines CL, et al. One-year survival in patients with acute myocardial infarction and a saphenous vein graft culprit treated with primary angioplasty. Am J Cardiol 2003;91:1250-4.

[125] Stone GW, Brodie BR, Griffin JJ, et al. Clinical and angiographic outcomes in patients with previous coronary artery bypass graft surgery treated with primary balloon an-

gioplasty for acute myocardial infarction. Second Primary Angioplasty in Myocardial Infarction Trial (PAMI-2) Investigators. J Am Coll Cardiol 2000;35:605-11.

[126] Brilakis ES, Wang TY, Rao SV, et al. Frequency and predictors of drug-eluting stent use in saphenous vein bypass graft percutaneous coronary interventions: a report from the American College of Cardiology National Cardiovascular Data CathPCI registry. JACC Cardiovasc Interv 2010;3:1068-73.

[127] Brodie BR, Wilson H, Stuckey T, et al. Outcomes with drug-eluting versus bare-metal stents in saphenous vein graft intervention results from the STENT (strategic transcatheter evaluation of new therapies) group. JACC Cardiovasc Interv 2009;2:1105-12.

[128] Foster ED, Fisher LD, Kaiser GC, Myers WO. Comparison of operative mortality and morbidity for initial and repeat coronary artery bypass grafting: The Coronary Artery Surgery Study (CASS) registry experience. Ann Thorac Surg 1984;38:563-70.

[129] Lytle BW, Loop FD, Cosgrove DM, et al. Fifteen hundred coronary reoperations. Results and determinants of early and late survival. J Thorac Cardiovasc Surg 1987;93:847-59.

[130] Al SJ, Velianou JL, Berger PB, et al. Primary percutaneous coronary interventions in patients with acute myocardial infarction and prior coronary artery bypass grafting. Am Heart J 2001;142:452-9.

[131] Brodie BR, Versteeg DS, Brodie MM, et al. Poor long-term patient and graft survival after primary percutaneous coronary intervention for acute myocardial infarction due to saphenous vein graft occlusion. Catheter Cardiovasc Interv 2005;65:504-9.

[132] O'Connor GT, Malenka DJ, Quinton H, et al. Multivariate prediction of in-hospital mortality after percutaneous coronary interventions in 1994-1996. Northern New England Cardiovascular Disease Study Group. J Am Coll Cardiol 1999;34:681-91.

[133] Thielmann M, Massoudy P, Jaeger BR, et al. Emergency re-revascularization with percutaneous coronary intervention, reoperation, or conservative treatment in patients with acute perioperative graft failure following coronary artery bypass surgery. Eur J Cardiothorac Surg 2006;30:117-25.

[134] Fellahi JL, Gue X, Richomme X, Monier E, Guillou L, Riou B. Short- and long-term prognostic value of postoperative cardiac troponin I concentration in patients undergoing coronary artery bypass grafting. Anesthesiology 2003;99:270-4.

[135] Force T, Hibberd P, Weeks G, et al. Perioperative myocardial infarction after coronary artery bypass surgery. Clinical significance and approach to risk stratification. Circulation 1990;82:903-12.

[136] Steuer J, Horte LG, Lindahl B, Stahle E. Impact of perioperative myocardial injury on early and long-term outcome after coronary artery bypass grafting. Eur Heart J 2002;23:1219-27.

[137] Jain U. Myocardial infarction during coronary artery bypass surgery. J Cardiothorac Vasc Anesth 1992;6:612-23.

[138] Rasmussen C, Thiis JJ, Clemmensen P, et al. Significance and management of early graft failure after coronary artery bypass grafting: feasibility and results of acute angiography and re-re-vascularization. Eur J Cardiothorac Surg 1997;12:847-52.

[139] Franke U, Wahlers T, Cohnert TU, et al. Retrograde versus antegrade crystalloid cardioplegia in coronary surgery: value of troponin-I measurement. Ann Thorac Surg 2001;71:249-53.

[140] Onorati F, De FM, Mastroroberto P, et al. Determinants and prognosis of myocardial damage after coronary artery bypass grafting. Ann Thorac Surg 2005;79:837-45.

[141] Thielmann M, Dorge H, Martin C, et al. Myocardial dysfunction with coronary microembolization: signal transduction through a sequence of nitric oxide, tumor necrosis factor-alpha, and sphingosine. Circ Res 2002;90:807-13.

[142] Fabricius AM, Gerber W, Hanke M, Garbade J, Autschbach R, Mohr FW. Early angiographic control of perioperative ischemia after coronary artery bypass grafting. Eur J Cardiothorac Surg 2001;19:853-8.

[143] Abdulmalik A, Arabi A, Alroaini A, Rosman H, Lalonde T. Feasibility of percutaneous coronary interventions in early postcoronary artery bypass graft occlusion or stenosis. J Interv Cardiol 2007;20:204-8.

[144] Virani SS, Alam M, Mendoza CE, Arora H, Ferreira AC, de ME. Clinical significance, angiographic characteristics, and short-term outcomes in 30 patients with early coronary artery graft failure. Neth Heart J 2009;17:13-7.

[145] Savage MP, Douglas JS, Jr., Fischman DL, et al. Stent placement compared with balloon angioplasty for obstructed coronary bypass grafts. Saphenous Vein De Novo Trial Investigators. N Engl J Med 1997;337:740-7.

[146] Stankovic G, Colombo A, Presbitero P, et al. Randomized evaluation of polytetrafluoroethylene-covered stent in saphenous vein grafts: the Randomized Evaluation of polytetrafluoroethylene COVERed stent in Saphenous vein grafts (RECOVERS) Trial. Circulation 2003;108:37-42.

[147] Stone GW, Goldberg S, O'Shaughnessy C, et al. 5-year follow-up of polytetrafluoroethylene-covered stents compared with bare-metal stents in aortocoronary saphenous vein grafts the randomized BARRICADE (barrier approach to restenosis: restrict intima to curtail adverse events) trial. JACC Cardiovasc Interv 2011;4:300-9.

[148] Turco MA, Buchbinder M, Popma JJ, et al. Pivotal, randomized U.S. study of the Symbiottrade mark covered stent system in patients with saphenous vein graft disease: eight-month angiographic and clinical results from the Symbiot III trial. Catheter Cardiovasc Interv 2006;68:379-88.

[149] Vermeersch P, Agostoni P, Verheye S, et al. Randomized double-blind comparison of sirolimus-eluting stent versus bare-metal stent implantation in diseased saphenous vein grafts: six-month angiographic, intravascular ultrasound, and clinical follow-up of the RRISC Trial. J Am Coll Cardiol 2006;48:2423-31.

[150] Vermeersch P, Agostoni P, Verheye S, et al. Increased late mortality after sirolimus-eluting stents versus bare-metal stents in diseased saphenous vein grafts: results from the randomized DELAYED RRISC Trial. J Am Coll Cardiol 2007;50:261-7.

[151] Brilakis ES, Lichtenwalter C, de Lemos JA, et al. A randomized controlled trial of a paclitaxel-eluting stent versus a similar bare-metal stent in saphenous vein graft lesions the SOS (Stenting of Saphenous Vein Grafts) trial. J Am Coll Cardiol 2009;53:919-28.

[152] Brilakis ES, Lichtenwalter C, bdel-karim AR, et al. Continued benefit from paclitaxel-eluting compared with bare-metal stent implantation in saphenous vein graft lesions during long-term follow-up of the SOS (Stenting of Saphenous Vein Grafts) trial. JACC Cardiovasc Interv 2011;4:176-82.

[153] Mehilli J, Pache J, bdel-Wahab M, et al. Drug-eluting versus bare-metal stents in saphenous vein graft lesions (ISAR-CABG): a randomised controlled superiority trial. Lancet 2011;378:1071-8.

[154] Hakeem A, Helmy T, Munsif S, et al. Safety and efficacy of drug eluting stents compared with bare metal stents for saphenous vein graft interventions: a comprehensive meta-analysis of randomized trials and observational studies comprising 7,994 patients. Catheter Cardiovasc Interv 2011;77:343-55.

[155] Lee MS, Yang T, Kandzari DE, Tobis JM, Liao H, Mahmud E. Comparison by meta-analysis of drug-eluting stents and bare metal stents for saphenous vein graft intervention. Am J Cardiol 2010;105:1076-82.

[156] Testa L, Agostoni P, Vermeersch P, et al. Drug eluting stents versus bare metal stents in the treatment of saphenous vein graft disease: a systematic review and meta-analysis. EuroIntervention 2010;6:527-36.

[157] Wiisanen ME, bdel-Latif A, Mukherjee D, Ziada KM. Drug-eluting stents versus bare-metal stents in saphenous vein graft interventions: a systematic review and meta-analysis. JACC Cardiovasc Interv 2010;3:1262-73.

[158] Papayannis AC, Michael TT, Yangirova D, et al. Optical coherence tomography analysis of the stenting of saphenous vein graft (SOS) Xience V Study: use of the everolimus-eluting stent in saphenous vein graft lesions. J Invasive Cardiol 2012;24:390-4.

[159] Lee MS, Hu PP, Aragon J, et al. Comparison of sirolimus-eluting stents with paclitaxel-eluting stents in saphenous vein graft intervention (from a multicenter Southern California Registry). Am J Cardiol 2010;106:337-41.

[160] Meier P, Brilakis ES, Corti R, Knapp G, Shishehbor MH, Gurm HS. Drug-eluting versus bare-metal stent for treatment of saphenous vein grafts: a meta-analysis. PLoS One 2010;5:e11040.

[161] Choussat R, Black AJ, Bossi I, Joseph T, Fajadet J, Marco J. Long-term clinical outcome after endoluminal reconstruction of diffusely degenerated saphenous vein grafts with less-shortening wallstents. J Am Coll Cardiol 2000;36:387-94.

[162] Leborgne L, Cheneau E, Pichard A, et al. Effect of direct stenting on clinical outcome in patients treated with percutaneous coronary intervention on saphenous vein graft. Am Heart J 2003;146:501-6.

[163] Gruberg L, Weissman NJ, Pichard AD, et al. Impact of renal function on morbidity and mortality after percutaneous aortocoronary saphenous vein graft intervention. Am Heart J 2003;145:529-34.

[164] Hong MK, Mehran R, Dangas G, et al. Creatine kinase-MB enzyme elevation following successful saphenous vein graft intervention is associated with late mortality. Circulation 1999;100:2400-5.

[165] Lee MS, Hu PP, Aragon J, et al. Impact of chronic renal insufficiency on clinical outcomes in patients undergoing saphenous vein graft intervention with drug-eluting stents: a multicenter Southern Californian Registry. Catheter Cardiovasc Interv 2010;76:272-8.

[166] Coolong A, Baim DS, Kuntz RE, et al. Saphenous vein graft stenting and major adverse cardiac events: a predictive model derived from a pooled analysis of 3958 patients. Circulation 2008;117:790-7.

[167] Kirtane AJ, Heyman ER, Metzger C, Breall JA, Carrozza JP, Jr. Correlates of adverse events during saphenous vein graft intervention with distal embolic protection: a PRIDE substudy. JACC Cardiovasc Interv 2008;1:186-91.

[168] Ahmed JM, Dangas G, Lansky AJ, et al. Influence of gender on early and one-year clinical outcomes after saphenous vein graft stenting. Am J Cardiol 2001;87:401-5.

[169] Gruberg L, Dangas G, Mehran R, et al. Percutaneous revascularization of the internal mammary artery graft: short- and long-term outcomes. J Am Coll Cardiol 2000;35:944-8.

[170] Crowley ST, Bies RD, Morrison DA. Percutaneous transluminal angioplasty of internal mammary arteries in patients with rest angina. Cathet Cardiovasc Diagn 1996;38:256-62.

[171] Dimas AP, Arora RR, Whitlow PL, et al. Percutaneous transluminal angioplasty involving internal mammary artery grafts. Am Heart J 1991;122:423-9.

[172] Hearne SE, Davidson CJ, Zidar JP, Phillips HR, Stack RS, Sketch MH, Jr. Internal mammary artery graft angioplasty: acute and long-term outcome. Cathet Cardiovasc Diagn 1998;44:153-6.

[173] Ishizaka N, Ishizaka Y, Ikari Y, et al. Initial and subsequent angiographic outcome of percutaneous transluminal angioplasty performed on internal mammary artery grafts. Br Heart J 1995;74:615-9.

[174] Popma JJ, Cooke RH, Leon MB, et al. Immediate procedural and long-term clinical results of internal mammary artery angioplasty. Am J Cardiol 1992;69:1237-9.

[175] Shimshak TM, Giorgi LV, Johnson WL, et al. Application of percutaneous transluminal coronary angioplasty to the internal mammary artery graft. J Am Coll Cardiol 1988;12:1205-14.

[176] Sharma AK, McGlynn S, Apple S, et al. Clinical outcomes following stent implantation in internal mammary artery grafts. Catheter Cardiovasc Interv 2003;59:436-41.

[177] Buch AN, Xue Z, Gevorkian N, et al. Comparison of outcomes between bare metal stents and drug-eluting stents for percutaneous revascularization of internal mammary grafts. Am J Cardiol 2006;98:722-4.

[178] Zavalloni D, Rossi ML, Scatturin M, et al. Drug-eluting stents for the percutaneous treatment of the anastomosis of the left internal mammary graft to left anterior descending artery. Coron Artery Dis 2007;18:495-500.

[179] Freixa X, Carpen M, Kotowycz MA, et al. Long-term outcomes after percutaneous intervention of the internal thoracic artery anastomosis: the use of drug-eluting stents is associated with a higher need of repeat revascularization. Can J Cardiol 2012;28:458-63.

[180] Akiyama T, Moussa I, Reimers B, et al. Angiographic and clinical outcome following coronary stenting of small vessels: a comparison with coronary stenting of large vessels. J Am Coll Cardiol 1998;32:1610-8.

[181] Elezi S, Kastrati A, Neumann FJ, Hadamitzky M, Dirschinger J, Schomig A. Vessel size and long-term outcome after coronary stent placement. Circulation 1998;98:1875-80.

[182] Savage MP, Fischman DL, Rake R, et al. Efficacy of coronary stenting versus balloon angioplasty in small coronary arteries. Stent Restenosis Study (STRESS) Investigators. J Am Coll Cardiol 1998;31:307-11.

[183] Virmani R, Farb A. Pathology of in-stent restenosis. Curr Opin Lipidol 1999;10:499-506.

[184] Goube P, Hammoudi N, Pagny JY, et al. Radial artery graft stenosis treated by percutaneous intervention. Eur J Cardiothorac Surg 2010;37:697-703.

[185] Ellis SG, Lincoff AM, Miller D, et al. Reduction in complications of angioplasty with abciximab occurs largely independently of baseline lesion morphology. EPIC and

EPILOG Investigators. Evaluation of 7E3 for the Prevention of Ischemic Complications. Evaluation of PTCA To Improve Long-term Outcome with abciximab GPIIb/IIIa Receptor Blockade. J Am Coll Cardiol 1998;32:1619-23.

[186] Mak KH, Challapalli R, Eisenberg MJ, Anderson KM, Califf RM, Topol EJ. Effect of platelet glycoprotein IIb/IIIa receptor inhibition on distal embolization during percutaneous revascularization of aortocoronary saphenous vein grafts. EPIC Investigators. Evaluation of IIb/IIIa platelet receptor antagonist 7E3 in Preventing Ischemic Complications. Am J Cardiol 1997;80:985-8.

[187] Roffi M, Mukherjee D, Chew DP, et al. Lack of benefit from intravenous platelet glycoprotein IIb/IIIa receptor inhibition as adjunctive treatment for percutaneous interventions of aortocoronary bypass grafts: a pooled analysis of five randomized clinical trials. Circulation 2002;106:3063-7.

[188] Jonas M, Stone GW, Mehran R, et al. Platelet glycoprotein IIb/IIIa receptor inhibition as adjunctive treatment during saphenous vein graft stenting: differential effects after randomization to occlusion or filter-based embolic protection. Eur Heart J 2006;27:920-8.

[189] Rha SW, Kuchulakanti PK, Pakala R, et al. Bivalirudin versus heparin as an antithrombotic agent in patients who undergo percutaneous saphenous vein graft intervention with a distal protection device. Am J Cardiol 2005;96:67-70.

[190] Kumar D, Dangas G, Mehran R, et al. Comparison of Bivalirudin versus Bivalirudin plus glycoprotein IIb/IIIa inhibitor versus heparin plus glycoprotein IIb/IIIa inhibitor in patients with acute coronary syndromes having percutaneous intervention for narrowed saphenous vein aorto-coronary grafts (the ACUITY trial investigators). Am J Cardiol 2010;106:941-5.

[191] Smith SC, Jr., Feldman TE, Hirshfeld JW, Jr., et al. ACC/AHA/SCAI 2005 guideline update for percutaneous coronary intervention: a report of the American College of Cardiology/American Heart Association Task Force on Practice Guidelines (ACC/AHA/SCAI Writing Committee to Update the 2001 Guidelines for Percutaneous Coronary Intervention). J Am Coll Cardiol 2006;47:e1-121.

[192] Lee MS, Park SJ, Kandzari DE, et al. Saphenous vein graft intervention. JACC Cardiovasc Interv 2011;4:831-43.

[193] Baim DS, Wahr D, George B, et al. Randomized trial of a distal embolic protection device during percutaneous intervention of saphenous vein aorto-coronary bypass grafts. Circulation 2002;105:1285-90.

[194] Carrozza JP, Jr., Mumma M, Breall JA, Fernandez A, Heyman E, Metzger C. Randomized evaluation of the TriActiv balloon-protection flush and extraction system for the treatment of saphenous vein graft disease. J Am Coll Cardiol 2005;46:1677-83.

[195] Halkin A, Masud AZ, Rogers C, et al. Six-month outcomes after percutaneous intervention for lesions in aortocoronary saphenous vein grafts using distal protection devices: results from the FIRE trial. Am Heart J 2006;151:915-7.

[196] Mauri L, Cox D, Hermiller J, et al. The PROXIMAL trial: proximal protection during saphenous vein graft intervention using the Proxis Embolic Protection System: a randomized, prospective, multicenter clinical trial. J Am Coll Cardiol 2007;50:1442-9.

[197] Kim YH, Park DW, Kim WJ, et al. Validation of SYNTAX (Synergy between PCI with Taxus and Cardiac Surgery) score for prediction of outcomes after unprotected left main coronary revascularization. JACC Cardiovasc Interv 2010;3:612-23.

[198] Ong AT, Serruys PW, Mohr FW, et al. The SYNergy between percutaneous coronary intervention with TAXus and cardiac surgery (SYNTAX) study: design, rationale, and run-in phase. Am Heart J 2006;151:1194-204.

[199] Sianos G, Morel MA, Kappetein AP, et al. The SYNTAX Score: an angiographic tool grading the complexity of coronary artery disease. EuroIntervention 2005;1:219-27.

[200] Califf RM, Phillips HR, III, Hindman MC, et al. Prognostic value of a coronary artery jeopardy score. J Am Coll Cardiol 1985;5:1055-63.

[201] Perera D, Stables R, Booth J, Thomas M, Redwood S. The balloon pump-assisted coronary intervention study (BCIS-1): rationale and design. Am Heart J 2009;158:910-6.

[202] Myocardial infarction and mortality in the coronary artery surgery study (CASS) randomized trial. N Engl J Med 1984;310:750-8.

[203] Murphy ML, Meadows WR, Thomsen J, et al. Veterans Administration Cooperative Study on medical versus surgical treatment for stable angina--progress report. Section 11. The effect of coronary artery bypass surgery on the incidence of myocardial infarction and hospitalization. Prog Cardiovasc Dis 1986;28:309-17.

[204] Peduzzi P, Detre K, Murphy ML, Thomsen J, Hultgren H, Takaro T. Ten-year incidence of myocardial infarction and prognosis after infarction. Department of Veterans Affairs Cooperative Study of Coronary Artery Bypass Surgery. Circulation 1991;83:747-55.

[205] Antman EM, Hand M, Armstrong PW, et al. 2007 Focused Update of the ACC/AHA 2004 Guidelines for the Management of Patients With ST-Elevation Myocardial Infarction: a report of the American College of Cardiology/American Heart Association Task Force on Practice Guidelines: developed in collaboration With the Canadian Cardiovascular Society endorsed by the American Academy of Family Physicians: 2007 Writing Group to Review New Evidence and Update the ACC/AHA 2004 Guidelines for the Management of Patients With ST-Elevation Myocardial Infarction, Writing on Behalf of the 2004 Writing Committee. Circulation 2008;117:296-329.

[206] Al-Aqeedi R, Sulaiman K, Al SJ, et al. Characteristics, management and outcomes of patients with acute coronary syndrome and prior coronary artery bypass surgery:

findings from the second Gulf Registry of Acute Coronary Events. Interact Cardiovasc Thorac Surg 2011;13:611-8.

[207] Al-Aqeedi R, Asaad N, Al-Qahtani A, et al. Acute coronary syndrome in patients with prior coronary artery bypass surgery: observations from a 20-year registry in a middle-eastern country. PLoS One 2012;7:e40571.

[208] Elbarasi E, Goodman SG, Yan RT, et al. Management patterns of non-ST segment elevation acute coronary syndromes in relation to prior coronary revascularization. Am Heart J 2010;159:40-6.

[209] Nikolsky E, McLaurin BT, Cox DA, et al. Outcomes of Patients With Prior Coronary Artery Bypass Grafting and Acute Coronary Syndromes: Analysis From the ACUITY (Acute Catheterization and Urgent Intervention Triage Strategy) Trial. JACC Cardiovasc Interv 2012;5:919-26.

[210] Labinaz M, Sketch MH, Jr., Ellis SG, et al. Outcome of acute ST-segment elevation myocardial infarction in patients with prior coronary artery bypass surgery receiving thrombolytic therapy. Am Heart J 2001;141:469-77.

[211] Gurfinkel EP, Perez de la HR, Brito VM, et al. Invasive vs non-invasive treatment in acute coronary syndromes and prior bypass surgery. Int J Cardiol 2007;119:65-72.

[212] Held C, Tornvall P, Stenestrand U. Effects of revascularization within 14 days of hospital admission due to acute coronary syndrome on 1-year mortality in patients with previous coronary artery bypass graft surgery. Eur Heart J 2007;28:316-25.

[213] bdel-karim AR, Banerjee S, Brilakis ES. Percutaneous intervention of acutely occluded saphenous vein grafts: contemporary techniques and outcomes. J Invasive Cardiol 2010;22:253-7.

[214] Harskamp RE, Kuijt WJ, Damman P, et al. Percutaneous coronary intervention for acute coronary syndrome due to graft failure; use of bare-metal and drug-eluting stents and subsequent long-term clinical outcome. Catheter Cardiovasc Interv 2012.

[215] Morrison DA, Sethi G, Sacks J, et al. Percutaneous coronary intervention versus coronary artery bypass graft surgery for patients with medically refractory myocardial ischemia and risk factors for adverse outcomes with bypass: a multicenter, randomized trial. Investigators of the Department of Veterans Affairs Cooperative Study #385, the Angina With Extremely Serious Operative Mortality Evaluation (AWESOME). J Am Coll Cardiol 2001;38:143-9.

[216] Gaglia MA, Jr., Torguson R, Xue Z, et al. Outcomes of patients with acute myocardial infarction from a saphenous vein graft culprit undergoing percutaneous coronary intervention. Catheter Cardiovasc Interv 2011;78:23-9.

[217] Christenson JT, Schmuziger M, Simonet F. Reoperative coronary artery bypass procedures: risk factors for early mortality and late survival. Eur J Cardiothorac Surg 1997;11:129-33.

[218] Jones JM, O'kane H, Gladstone DJ, et al. Repeat heart valve surgery: risk factors for operative mortality. J Thorac Cardiovasc Surg 2001;122:913-8.

[219] Machiraju VR. How to avoid problems in redo coronary artery bypass surgery. J Card Surg 2004;19:284-90.

[220] Elami A, Laks H, Merin G. Technique for reoperative median sternotomy in the presence of a patent left internal mammary artery graft. J Card Surg 1994;9:123-7.

[221] Grunwald RP. A technique for direct-vision sternal reentry. Ann Thorac Surg 1985;40:521-2.

[222] Mills NL, Everson CT, Hockmuth DR. Technical considerations for myocardial protection during the course of coronary artery bypass reoperation: the impact of functioning saphenous vein and internal mammary artery grafts. J Card Surg 1991;6:34-40.

[223] Mishra YK, Collison SP, Malhotra R, Kohli V, Mehta Y, Trehan N. Ten-year experience with single-vessel and multivessel reoperative off-pump coronary artery bypass grafting. J Thorac Cardiovasc Surg 2008;135:527-32.

[224] Menasche P, Tronc F, Nguyen A, et al. Retrograde warm blood cardioplegia preserves hypertrophied myocardium: a clinical study. Ann Thorac Surg 1994;57:1429-34.

[225] Salerno TA, Houck JP, Barrozo CA, et al. Retrograde continuous warm blood cardioplegia: a new concept in myocardial protection. Ann Thorac Surg 1991;51:245-7.

[226] Borger MA, Peniston CM, Weisel RD, Vasiliou M, Green RE, Feindel CM. Neuropsychologic impairment after coronary bypass surgery: effect of gaseous microemboli during perfusionist interventions. J Thorac Cardiovasc Surg 2001;121:743-9.

[227] Gu YJ, Van OW, Akkerman C, Boonstra PW, Huyzen RJ, Wildevuur CR. Heparin-coated circuits reduce the inflammatory response to cardiopulmonary bypass. Ann Thorac Surg 1993;55:917-22.

[228] Levy JH, Tanaka KA. Inflammatory response to cardiopulmonary bypass. Ann Thorac Surg 2003;75:S715-S720.

[229] Vinten-Johansen J, Thourani VH, Ronson RS, et al. Broad-spectrum cardioprotection with adenosine. Ann Thorac Surg 1999;68:1942-8.

[230] Spotnitz WD, Dalton MS, Baker JW, Nolan SP. Reduction of perioperative hemorrhage by anterior mediastinal spray application of fibrin glue during cardiac operations. Ann Thorac Surg 1987;44:529-31.

[231] Stamou SC, Pfister AJ, Dullum MK, et al. Late outcome of reoperative coronary revascularization on the beating heart. Heart Surg Forum 2001;4:69-73.

http://dx.doi.org/10.5772/54928

[232] Stephan WJ, O'Keefe JH, Jr., Piehler JM, et al. Coronary angioplasty versus repeat coronary artery bypass grafting for patients with previous bypass surgery. J Am Coll Cardiol 1996;28:1140-6.

[233] Brener SJ, Lytle BW, Casserly IP, Ellis SG, Topol EJ, Lauer MS. Predictors of revascularization method and long-term outcome of percutaneous coronary intervention or repeat coronary bypass surgery in patients with multivessel coronary disease and previous coronary bypass surgery. Eur Heart J 2006;27:413-8.

[234] Cole JH, Jones EL, Craver JM, et al. Outcomes of repeat revascularization in diabetic patients with prior coronary surgery. J Am Coll Cardiol 2002;40:1968-75.

[235] Harskamp RE, Beijk MA, Damman P, et al. Clinical outcome after surgical or percutaneous revascularization in coronary bypass graft failure. J Cardiovasc Med (Hagerstown) 2012.

Chapter 14

The Cardioprotection of Silymarin in Coronary Artery Bypass Grafting Surgery

D. Tagreed Altaei, D. Imad A. Jamal and
D. Diyar Dilshad

Additional information is available at the end of the chapter

http://dx.doi.org/10.5772/55125

1. Introduction

Coronary artery bypass grafting surgery (CABG) is one of the most effective therapies for coronary artery disease (CAD). CABG is conventionally performed with the use of cardiopulmonary bypass (CPB), which has been associated with an increased frequency of complications [1-3]. A variety of risk factors has been described to help delineate risk assessment of patients undergoing CABG, including preoperative left ventricular ejection fraction (LVEF) [4, 5] and postoperative increase in creatine kinase myocardial band (CK-MB) levels [6-11]. In patients undergoing coronary artery bypass grafting (CABG), the use of cardiopulmonary bypass (CPB) in combination with aortic clamping during coronary artery bypass grafting (CABG) elicits ischemic myocardial injury [12]. The vascular endothelium is a complex synthetic organ subject to injury from numerous potential insults, including oxidative stress [13, 14] modified lipoproteins [15], and hemodynamic forces [16]. Injured endothelial cells initiate a largely stereotyped, initially protective response. The concurrent uptake of low-density lipoproteins (LDLs) by monocyte-derived macrophages transforms them in to the lipid laden foam cells that constitute a key element of the fatty streak, the first recognizable progenitor of the advanced atherosclerotic lesion [17, 18].

Silymarin, a flavonolignan from 'milk thistle' (Silybum marianum) plant, is used from ancient times as a hepatoprotective, antioxidant, anti-lipid peroxidative, antifibrotic, anti-inflammatory, immunomodulatory and liver regenerating. Silymarin has cardioprotective activity against ischemia-reperfusion induced myocardial infarction in rats [19].

Protective efficacy of Silymarin treatment confirmed by anti-inflammatory and antioxidant actions against reperfusion injury and inflammation during CABG surgery [20].

This may represent a novel cardioprotective agent to be used pre CABG, to our knowledge; this is the first study of pretreatment Silymarin as cardioprotective agent in patients undergoing CABG.

2. Patients and methods

The local ethics committee approved the investigation, and informed written consent was obtained from all patients entering the study. 140 patients admitted to the hospital for the first time for elective coronary artery bypass surgery were invited to take part. They were randomized into three groups (G); G I: Administered Silymarin (Legalon® tablet), 140 mg×3; 1 day before surgery. G II: Administered Silymarin (Legalon® tablet), 140 mg×3; 3 days before surgery. G III: Control (no treatment). Patients receiving corticosteroids were deemed not eligible. Any drugs were withheld on the morning of surgery.

Surgical procedure: Specifications on the extracorporeal circulation circuit, cardiopulmonary bypass procedures and surgical procedures have been described previously [20].

At baseline, demographic data (age, sex, weight, BSA, BMI), and history of conventional vascular risk factors (hypertension, diabetes mellitus, hyperlipidemia, smoking habit, alcohol abuse) were obtained.

Routine laboratory investigations were performed the first day after admission to the hospital after overnight fasting and later before discharged. It included levels of WBCs; differential counts (Neutrophils, Monocytes, Lymphocytes), RBCs, ESR, total cholesterol, LDL, vLDL, HDL, triglycerides, SGOT, SGPT, B.urea, S.creatinin, alkaline phosphatase, serum bilirubin, blood sugar, HbA1c, & ESR. Blood samples for troponin I (T), & creatine kinase; (CK-MB) measurement were obtained within 24 hours before surgery, & 2 hr, 24 hr post CABG. All laboratory tests were performed according to companys' procedures. Laboratory staffs were blind to the tested drug and groups.

Statistical analysis

The present Data was analyzed using Student 't' test, one-way analysis of covariance. $P< 0.05$ was considered to be significant. All data were analyzed using the statistical package SPSS (version 10.0) Continuous data are presented as mean ± SD and categorical data as absolute numbers, or mean.

3. Results

One hundred and forty patients [105 (75%) males, and 35 (25%) females] with a mean age of 64.5 years were included in the study. All underwent on-pump CABG.

No significant differences were noted between the groups in age, body surface area, BMI, and operation data. The demographic data on the 140 patients completing the study are presented

in Table 1. Clinical & operative characteristics (Age, sex, body weight, smoking, left ventricular ejection fraction, usual administered drugs, other diseases, family history of coronary artery disease) were largely independent of silymarin treatment with no significance ($p>0.05$).

Variables	Silymarin (SM) Group (No. = 90)		Control Group (No. = 50)
	G I (n=40)	G II (n=50)	G III
Male/Female (No.)	68/22		37/13
Age (years) [a]	65		64
Body surface area (m^2) [b]	1.6 ± 0.2		1.7 ± 0.1
BMI (kg/m^2) [b]	42.3 ± 0.2		44.7 ± 0.2
Ejection fraction (%) [b]	58 ± 1		60 ± 1
Operative time (min) [b]	201 ± 16		200 ± 18
No. of grafts [a]	3		3.5
Hospitalization (days) [a]	4		7

Table 1. Clinical and Patients' data in Silymarin treated and control groups.

There was a significant decrease in post operative values of; WBCs counts, Neutrophil, monocytes, lymphocytes, RBCs, ESR (Figure1), total cholesterol, LDL, vLDL, & triglycerides (Figure 2), SGOT, SGPT, alkaline phosphatase (47%), showed in (Figure 3), B.urea, S.creatinine, serum bilirubin (48%) (Figure 4), blood sugar, HbA1c in diabetic patients (43%) as showed in figure 5, in SM treated group compared to baseline and control group; ($P=0.002$), while there was an elevation of postoperative HDL values in patients treated with SM compared to control, ($p=0.001$).

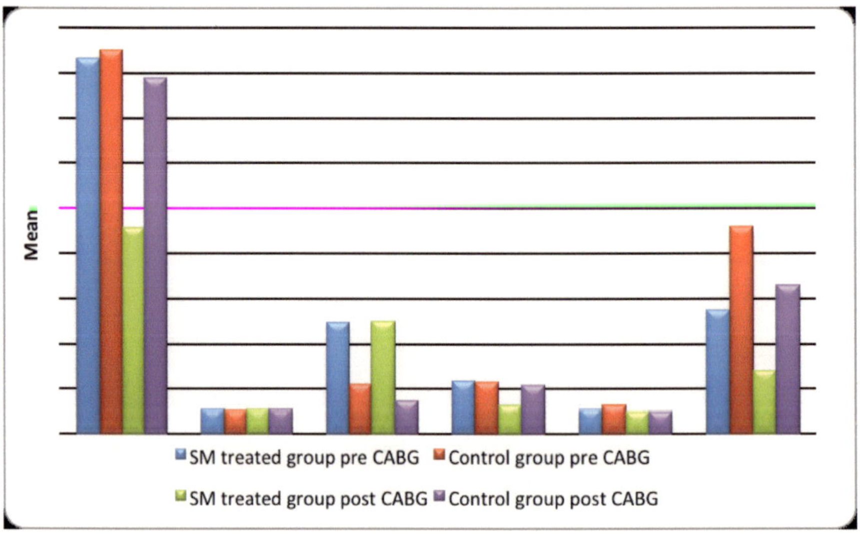

Figure 1. The mean values of Neutrophils, Monocytes, Lymphocytes, total WBCs, RBCs, and ESR for Silymarin treated and control groups pre and post CABG.

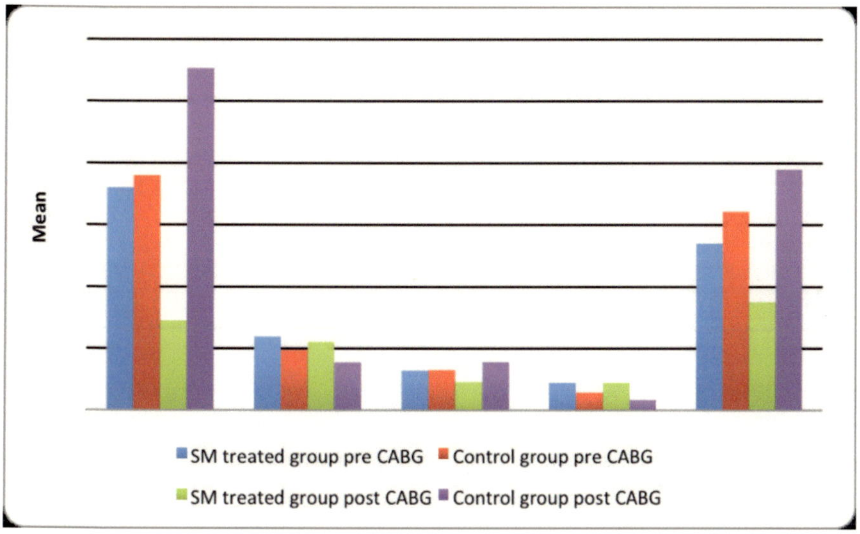

Figure 2. The mean values (mg/dL) of total cholesterol, LDL, vLDL, HDL, and triglycerides for Silymarin treated and control groups pre and post CABG.

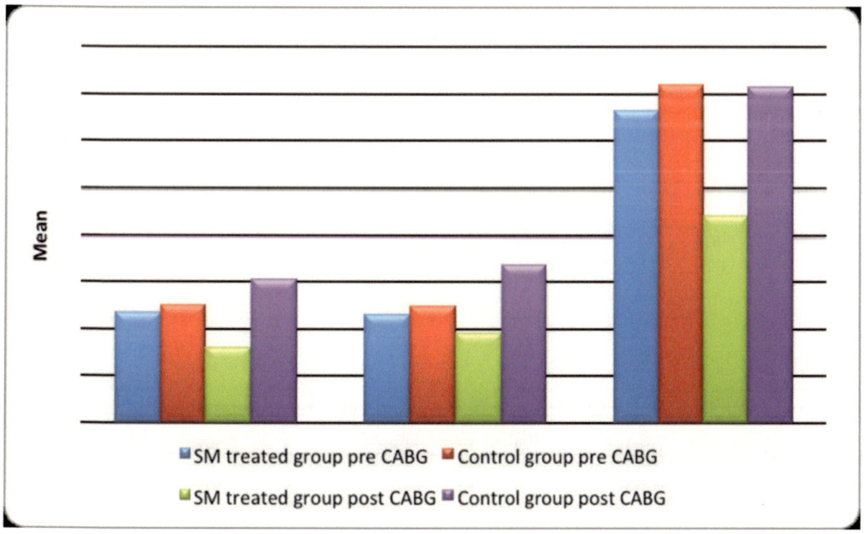

Figure 3. Mean values of SGOT, SGPT, & Alkaline phosphatase for both groups compared pre and post CABG.

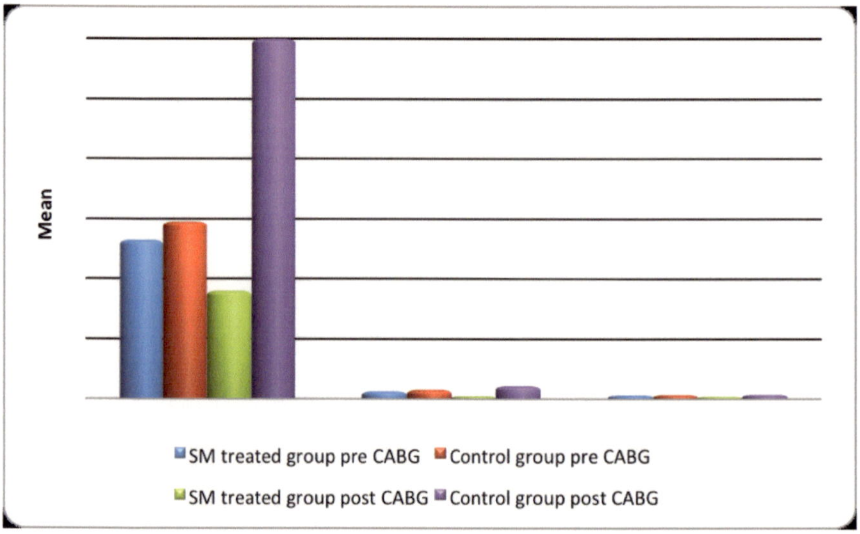

Figure 4. The mean values of blood urea & serum creatinin, & serum bilirubin in tested groups pre & post operation.

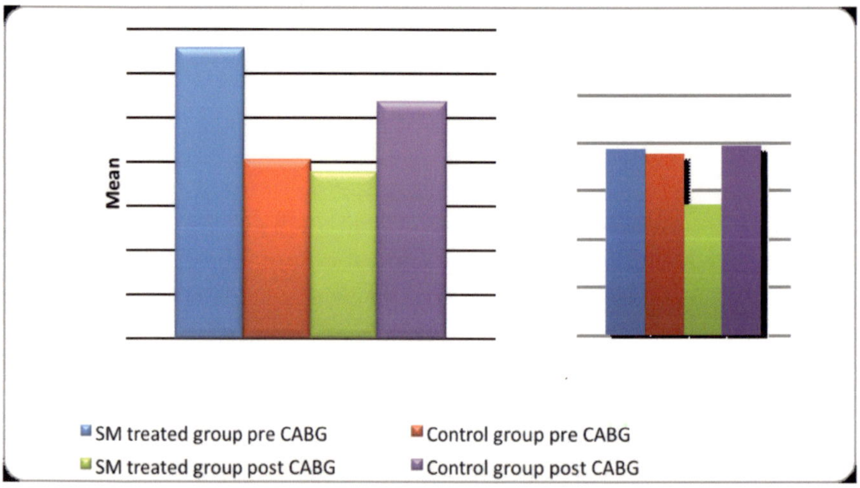

Figure 5. Mean values of fasting blood sugar, & glycosylated heamoglobin pre & post CABG for both groups.

Surgery was associated with a significant increase in troponin I (T1), CK-MB (CK1) in both groups, but after 24 hr post CABG there was a significant reduction of Troponin I (T2) values in SM treated group compared to baseline (T0), after 2 hour (T1), and control group, [p=0.001]. SM-treated patients released significantly less creatine kinase (CK)-MB than the control subjects postoperatively (CK1) after 2 hours, then back to normal levels after 24 hours (CK 2) [p = 0.004]; indicating less myocardial injury in patients receiving SM when compared to the control subjects (no significant change p > 0.05), as showed in figure 6.

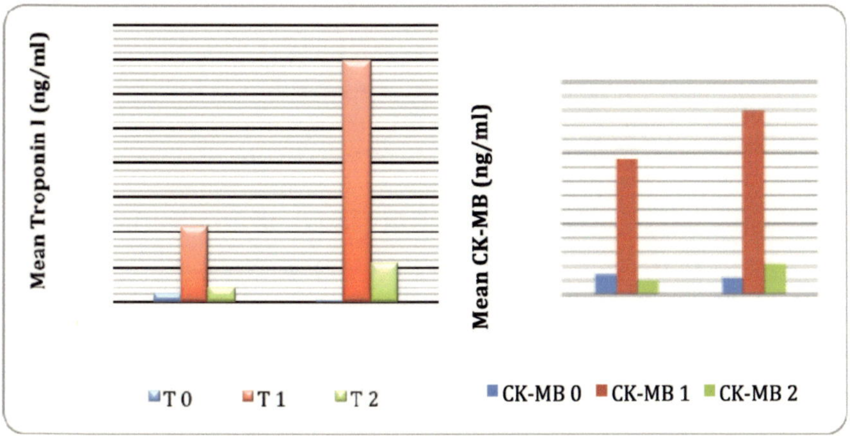

Figure 6. Mean Troponin I, & CK-MB values at different times in Silymarin (SM) treated patients and control groups. [T0=pre CABG, T1=2 hours after CABG, T2= 24 hours after CABG, CK-MB 0=pre CABG, CK-MB 1= 2 hours after CABG, CK-MB 2= 24 hours after CABG].

Patients treated with Silymarin before 3 days better than those treated before 1 day, but there was no statistical significant differences between them (G I & G II), $p>0.05$.

4. Discussion

Myocardial ischemia and reperfusion is a common occurrence in CABG patients. Reintroduction of oxygen to previously ischemic myocardium can result in irreversible tissue injury, and Ischemic myocardial damage is associated with inflammation [21, 22].

SM has been shown to have a potential positive effect on immune function by its ability to enhance neutrophil activity [23]. Silymarin & Silibinin by interacting with the lipid component of cell membranes can influence their chemical & physical properties. Studies in erythrocytes, mast cells, leucocytes, macrophages & hepatocytes have shown that SM renders cell membranes more resistant to lesions [24].

Studies have shown that silymarin exerts a number of effects, including inhibition of neutrophil migration [25, 24]. The inhibitory effects of silymarin on neutrophil function prevent post _ ischemic mucosal injury [26]. Activated neutrophils are thought to play a major role in ischemia-reperfusion injury [27]. This study agrees with that, SM treated groups showed a significant reduction of WBCs, neutrophils count post CABG, & ESR also. According to this, silymarin may prevent reperfusion injury so it may have a beneficial effect during CABG.

Milk thistle was able to inhibit the biosynthesis of cholesterol in the liver and reduce LDL cholesterol oxidation, one of the primary mechanisms of atherosclerosis [28,25]. This study agrees with it, SM treatment showed a significant reduction of total cholesterol, LDL, & vLDL, while HDL was elevated significantly.

http://dx.doi.org/10.5772/55125

SM interact directly with the cell membrane components to prevent any abnormalities in the content of lipid fraction responsible for maintaining normal fluidity [29].

Silymarin appears to act as an antioxidant not only because it acts as a scavenger of the free radicals that induce lipid peroxidation, but also because it influences enzyme systems associated with glutathione & superoxide dismutase [30]. Also, prevent damage to rat heart membrane primarily through a free radical scavenging mechanism [31]. This study agrees with previous mentioned studies, the antioxidant activity of Silymarin prevents vascular endothelium injury during CABG.

In the present study, all patients showed significantly higher plasma levels of markers of perioperative myocardial tissue injury early after the start of reperfusion. Silymarin treated group showed a significant reduction of all measured parameters compared to baseline and control.

Alkaline phosphatase, & serum bilirubin was elevated preoperatively in 47%, and 48% of enrolled patients, respectively, pretreatment with Silymarin showed a significant reduction post operatively because SM have the ability to prevent injury from different causes.

Blood sugar & HbA1c in diabetic patients (43%) were diminished significantly in those treated by SM.

SM counteracted the increase in the cardiac enzymes and cTnI concentration induced by cisplatin, toward near normal levels. Rao and Viswanath 2007 [19] reported that the administration of SM before ischemia–reperfusion-induced myocardial infarction maintained the levels of marker enzymes (LDH, CK and CK-MB) compared to isoproterenol-injected rats. A possible explanation is that silymarin, via its anti-lipid peroxidation activity, causes stabilization of cardiac membranes and prevents the leakage of cardiac enzymes [32]. Silibinin induced cardiac myocyte expression of Bcl-2 protein, which prevented permeability transition pore opening, and, therefore, cytochrome c release decreased. These events might be one of the mechanisms of silymarin-mediated stabilization of the mitochondrial membrane [33]. This study agrees with the above study in which Troponin I, and CK-MB diminished significantly in SM treated group compared to baseline and control.

The anti-inflammatory activity (significant reduction of cytokines post operatively), & antioxidant effects of SM during CABG [20], in addition to that, the highly significant reduction in serum levels of troponin I, & CK-MB, confirm the cardioprotection activity of SM during CABG. This mechanism of action may reduce ischemia-reperfusion injury, and protect the myocardium.

The results of this study indicate that SM pretreatment induces potent endogenous protection against subsequent ischemic stress in the human myocardium, and reduced the damage caused by reperfusion injury. SM has the ability to regulate membrane permeability and to increase membrane stability in the presence of xenobiotic damage, capacity to regulate nuclear expression by means of a steroid-like effect.

There was no statistically significant difference between the two treated groups, even the results of patients treated with SM before 3 days better than those treated before 1 day of CABG surgery. The data of this study needs further large-scale, randomized, double blind technique studies for other cardiovascular diseases to confirm the present study before clinical use of Silymarin.

5. Conclusion

The authors conclude that CABG surgery need using cardioprotective agent pre operation and suggest using other pharmaceutical preparation I.V. dosage form of SM and studying the pharmacokinetics during CABG surgery. The pre-operative administration of Silymarin may reduce perioperative morbidity and myocardial injury during CABG surgery. The authors suggest a large-scale, randomized, double blind study with cardiovascular events before Silymarin could be considered for clinical use.

Acknowledgements

The authors wish to thanks all patients who so kindly took part, and all staff.

Author details

D. Tagreed Altaei*, D. Imad A. Jamal and D. Diyar Dilshad

*Address all correspondence to: tagreedaltaei@yahoo.com

Dep. of Pharmacology and Toxicology, College of Pharmacy, Hawler Medical University, Erbil, Iraq

References

[1] Czerny, M, Baumer, H, Kilo, J, et al. Inflammatory response and myocardial injury following coronary artery bypass grafting with or without cardiopulmonary bypass. Eur J Cardiothorac Surg. (2000). , 17, 737-42.

[2] Wan, I. Y, Arifi, A. A, Wan, S, et al. Beating heart revascularization with or without cardiopulmonary bypass: evaluation of inflammatory response in a prospective randomized trial. J Thorac Cardiovasc Surg. (2004). , 127, 1624-31.

[3] Schulze, C, Conrad, N, Schutz, A, et al. Reduced expression of systemic proinflammatory cytokines after off-pump versus conventional coronary artery bypass grafting. Thorac Cardiovasc Surg. (2000). , 48, 364-9.

[4] Magovern, J. A, Sakert, T, Magovern, G. J, et al. A model that predicts morbidity and mortality after coronary artery bypass graft surgery. J Am Coll Cardiol. (1996). , 28, 1147-53.

[5] Provenchere, S, Berroeta, C, Reynaud, C, et al. Plasma brain natriuretic peptide and cardiac troponin I concentrations after adult cardiac surgery: association with post-operative cardiac dysfunction and 1-year mortality. Crit Care Med. (2006). , 34, 995-1000.

[6] Costa, M. A, Carere, R. G, Lichtenstein, S. V, et al. Incidence, predictors, and significance of abnormal cardiac enzyme rise in patients treated with bypass surgery in the arterial revascularization study (ARTS). Circulation. (2001)., 104, 2689-93.

[7] Klatte, K, Chaitman, B. R, Theroux, P, et al. Guardian Investigators (The GUARD during Ischemia Against Necrosis). Increased mortality after coronary artery bypass graft surgery is associated with increased levels of postoperative creatine kinase-myocardial band isoenzyme release: results from the guardian trial. J Am Coll Cardiol. (2001)., 38, 1070-7.

[8] Steuer, J, Horte, L. G, Lindahl, B, & Stahle, E. Impact of perioperative myocardial injury on early and long-term outcome after coronary artery bypass grafting. Eur Heart J. (2002)., 23, 1219-27.

[9] Brener, S. J, Lytle, B. W, Schneider, J. P, et al. Association between CKMB elevation after percutaneous or surgical revascularization and three-year mortality. J Am Coll Cardiol. (2002)., 40, 1961-7.

[10] Engoren, M. C, Habib, R. H, Zacharias, A, et al. The association of elevated creatine kinase-myocardial band on mortality after coronary artery bypass grafting surgery is time and magnitude limited. Eur J Cardiothorac Surg. (2005)., 28, 114-9.

[11] Ramsay, J, Shernan, S, Fitch, J, et al. Increased creatine kinase MK level predicts post-operative mortality after cardiac surgery independent of new Q waves. J Thorac Cardiovasc Surg. (2005)., 129, 300-6.

[12] Fransen, E. J, Maessen, J. G, & Hermens, W. T. Glatz JFC. Demonstration of ischemia-reperfusion injury separate from postoperative infarction in Coronary Artery Bypass Graft Patients. Ann Thorac Surg. (1998)., 65, 48-53.

[13] Gong, K. W, Zhu, G. Y, & Wang, L. H. Effect of active oxygen species on intimal proliferation in rat aorta after arterial injury. J Vasc Res. (1996)., 42-46.

[14] Liao, F, Andalibi, A, & Qiao, J. H. Genetic evidence for a common pathway mediating oxidative stress, inflammatory gene induction, and aortic fatty streak formation in mice. J Clin Invest. (1994)., 94, 877-84.

[15] Steinberg, D. Antioxidants and atherosclerosis: A current assessment. Circulation. (1991)., 84, 1420-25.

[16] Glagov, S, Zarins, C, & Giddens, D. P. Hemodynamics and atherosclerosis: Insights and perspectives gained from studies of human arteries. Arch Pathol lab Med. (1988)., 112, 1018-31.

[17] Aqel, N. M, Ball, R. Y, & Waldmann, H. Monocytic origin of foam cells in human atherosclerotic plaques. Atherosclerosis. (1984). , 53, 265-71.

[18] Stary, H. C. Evolution and progression of atherosclerotic lesions in coronary arteries of children and young adults, Arteriosclerosis. (1989). , 9, 119-32.

[19] Rao, P. R, & Viswanath, R. K. Cardioprotective activity of silymarin in ischemia-reperfusion-induced myocardial infarction in albino rats. Exp Clin Cardiol. (2007). , 12(4), 179-187.

[20] Altaei, Tagreed. Protective effect of Silymarin during coronary artery bypass grafting surgery. Exp Clin Cardiol. (2011). , 17(1), 34-38.

[21] Hawkins, H. K, Entman, M. L, Zhu, J. Y, et al. Acute inflammatory reaction after myocardial ischemic injury and reperfusion. Development and use of a neutrophil-specific antibody. Am J Pathol.(1996). , 148, 1957-1969.

[22] Entman, M. L, Michael, L, Rossen, R. D, et al. Inflammation in the course of early myocardial ischemia. FASEB J. (1991). , 5, 2529-2537.

[23] Kalmar, L. Silibinin (Legalon-70) enhances the motility of human neutrophils immobilizes by calcium ionophore, lymphokine, and normal human serum. Agents Actions. (1990).

[24] De La Puerta, R, Martinez, E, Bravo, L, et al. Effect of silymarin on different acute inflammation models and leukocyte migration. J Pharm Pharmacol. (1996).

[25] Skottova, N, & Krecman, V. Silymarin as a potential hypocholesterolaemic drug. Physiol Res. (1998). , 47, 1-7.

[26] Alarcon de la Lastra ACMartin MJ, Motilva V, Jimenez M, La Casa C, Lopez A. Gastroprotection induced by silymarin, the hepatoprotective principle of Silybum marianum in ischemia-reperfusion mucosal injury: role of neutrophils. Planta Med. (1995).

[27] Weiss, S. J. Tissue destruction by neutrophils. N Engl J Med. (1989). , 320, 365-376.

[28] Bialecka, M. The effect of bioflavonoids and lecithin on the course of experimental atherosclerosis. Acad Med Stetin. (1997).

[29] Muriel, P, & Mourelle, M. Prevention by silymarin of membrane alterations in acute CCl4 liver damage. J Appl Toxicol. (1990). , 10, 275-9.

[30] Letteron, P, Labbe, G, Degott, C, et al. Mechanism for the protective effects of silymarin against carbon tetrachloride-induced lipid peroxidation and hepatotoxicity in mice. Biochem Pharmacol. (1990).

[31] Psotova, J, Chlopcikova, S, Grambal, F, & Simanek, V. Ulrichova J; Influence of silymarin and its flavolignans on doxorubicin-iron induced lipid peroxidation in rat heart microsomes and mitochondria in comparison with quercetin: Phytother Res. (2002). Suppl 1: S63_7.

[32] Abu GhadeerA.R., Ali, S.E., Osman, S.A., Abu Bedair, F.A., Abbady, M.M., El-Kady, M.R. Antagonistic role of silymarin against cardiotoxicity and impaired antioxidation induced by adriamycin and/or radiation exposure in albino rats. Pakistan J.Biol. Sci. (2001). , 4, 604-607.

[33] Zhou, B, Wu, L, Tashiro, S, Onodera, S, Uchiumi, F, & Ikejima, T. Silibinin protect rat cardiac myocyte from isoproterenol-induced DNA damage independent on regulation of cell cycle. Biol. Pharm. Bull. (2006 a). , 29, 1900-1905.

Chapter 15

Pharmacology of Arterial Grafts for Coronary Artery Bypass Surgery

Oguzhan Yildiz, Melik Seyrek and Husamettin Gul

Additional information is available at the end of the chapter

http://dx.doi.org/10.5772/54723

1. Introduction

Interest has increased in the use of arterial conduits for CABG significantly in most major cardiac surgery centers around the world, because the number of patients receiving arterial grafts and our knowledge about the biologic characteristics of arterial grafts have increased. In addition, more advanced clinical protocols for the use of grafts have been developed and midterm results with alternative arterial grafts are encouraging.

The internal mammary artery (IMA) has been shown to have greater long-term patency for coronary artery bypass grafting when compared with the saphenous vein graft. Because of the superior long-term results of the IMA, other arterial grafts which have recently been advocated include the radial artery (RA), the gastroepiploic artery (GEA), the inferior epigastric artery (IEA), the splenic artery, the subscapular artery, the inferior mesenteric artery, the descending branch of lateral femoral circumflex artery, the intercostal artery and the ulnar artery. One of the various manifestations clinically observed among these arterial grafts is a different tendency to develop spasm during surgical dissection and during the perioperative period which could be the cause of perioperative morbidity and mortalitiy [1-8]. For example, there are reports of vasoactive drugs altering IMA graft flow [3,4]. Moreover, there is accumulating evidence that blood flow in arterial grafts is insufficient in some circumstances [6,7]. Many vasoconstrictors (spasmogens) may cause arterial grafts spasm. Accordingly, antispastic therapy is important in the development of arterial grafts and the nature of constrictor substances that cause arterial graft spasm needs to be determined. In recent years, the problem of graft spasm has become more frequent with the increasing use of new arterial grafts. Therefore, it is essential for surgeons to understand the causes of vascular graft spasm, to improve patency rates and to use the optimal vasodilator in the most appropriate way to counteract vasospasm.

Surgeons have studied graft pharmacology by measuring the effects of vasodilators on blood flow through arterial grafts before they were attached to the heart [9]. Pharmacologists have also joined the study of graft pharmacology by evaluating endothelial and smooth muscle function of bypass grafts using their standard in vitro method, the isolated vessel ring preparation in the organ bath. However, results from these in vitro studies need to be carefully extrapolated to the clinical situations, where the conditions of the arterial grafts are complicated. Even so, the organ bath method can provide very useful information about the effects of vasoactive substances in the arterial grafts.

Several vasodilators have been tested and various antispastic methods have been suggested to prevent graft spasm; including papaverine, phenoxybenzamine, calcium antagonists and nitrates etc. Choice of a pharmacological agent to overcome the vasospasm encountered in the arterial grafts must be on the basis of pharmacological studies. Accordingly, current state of knowledge based on experiments to study the pharmacological effect of a number of vasoconstrictor and vasodilator substances and the practical application of this knowledge can be outlined as following sections:

2. *In Vitro* pharmacology of blood vessels

Pharmacology of isolated blood vessel allows the researcher to investigate the mechanisms of effect of spasmogens or vasodilatory substances. Most studies use the isolated vessel ring preparation in the organ bath, studying removed segments from the grafts during surgery. This technique only requires basic pharmacological equipment, i.e. isolated organ baths, transducers, recorder system etc. An important advantage of this method is that the vessel segment is studied in the organ bath and concentration-response curves for each vasoactive substances to be obtained under controlled conditions without extrinsic neural factors, circulating hormones interacting, blood flow or shear stress. Therefore, dose and response relationships to drugs, either vasoconstrictor or vasodilator substances, can be assessed more readily and accurately than is possible than in vivo experiments. This methodology also enabled agents to be compared with each other, and combinations of vasoactive drugs to be tested [10,11-13]. In vitro measurement of response of vascular preparations may help to researcher to predict what can happen, not what does actually happen in integrative and complicated in vivo conditions. However, isolated organ bath methods cannot identify the actual cause of in vivo spasm. The next challenge is to determine in the body what combination of factors, i.e. extrinsic neural factors, circulating hormones interacting, blood flow or shear stress, influencing passive distension from arterial wall are present the vessel with spasm.

Isolated organ bath technique is a standard research approach which requires basic pharmacological equipment (Figure 1). Segments of human arteries obtained from patients undergoing CABG surgery are placed in oxygenated physiological solution, i.e. Krebs-Henseleit solution etc., at room temperature and transferred immediately to the laboratory. The arteries are dissected from adhering fat and connective tissue then cut into 3-4 mm length rings. The strips are mounted in an organ bath, containing physiological solution, on a L-shaped brace

http://dx.doi.org/10.5772/54723

for tension measurement along the former circumferential axis. The solution is gassed with % 95 O_2 and % 5 CO_2 at 37 ºC. Changes in arterial tensions are recorded isometrically by a force-displacement transducer by using a recording system, preferably a computer software. The segments are allowed to equilibrate under final resting force of 1-2 g for at least 1 to 1.5 h and they were washed every 10-20 minutes. After the equilibration period, arterial strips were challenged with a vasoconstrictor, i.e. phenylephrine, prostaglandin $F_{2\alpha}$ or potassium chloride (KCl) to test the viability of the vessel. After an additonal 30 min of equilibration period with repeated washing every 10 min, the tissues are challenged with increasing cumulative concentrations of the vasoconstrictor substance to be tested and responses are recorded.

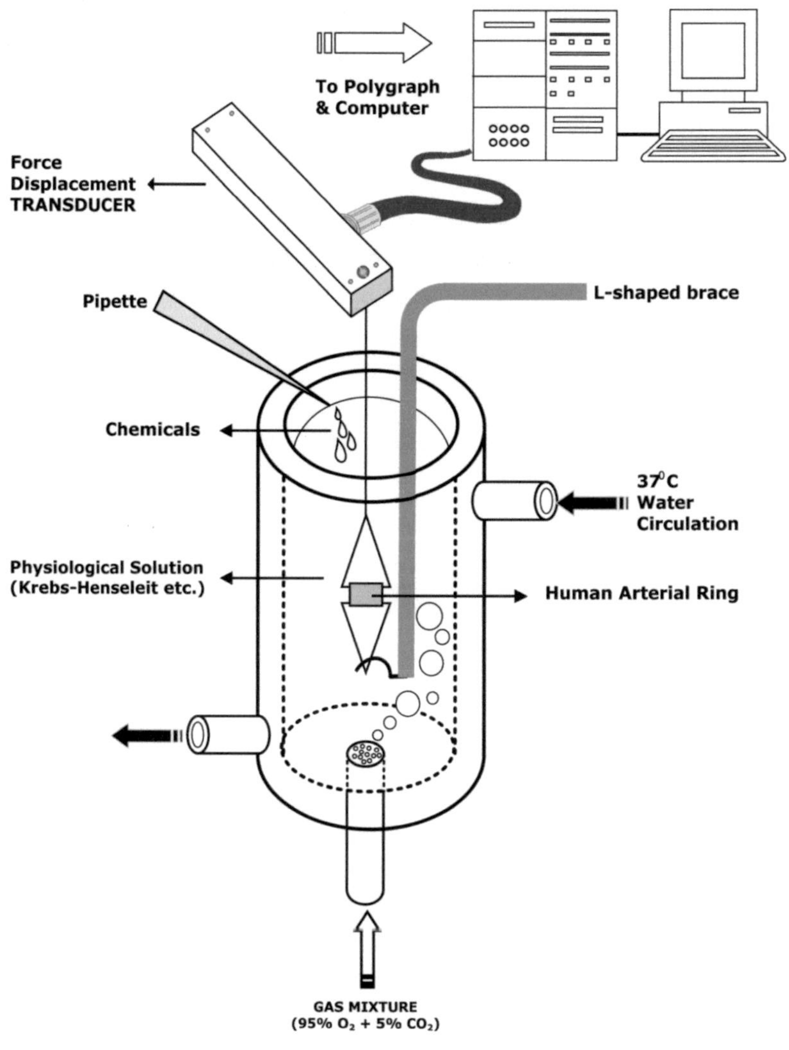

Figure 1. A schematic diagram of a human arterial ring preparation in an organ bath.

Each cumulative concentration is applied after the relaxation to previous concentration reached to a plateau. Vasoconstrictor substance -evoked responses are usually expressed as percentage of the maximum response in each corresponding tissue. Vasodilator agents are studied by establishing concentration-relaxation curves after precontracting the segments with a vasoconstrictor, i.e. phenylephrine, prostaglandin $F_{2\alpha}$ or potassium chloride (KCl). The relaxation is usually expressed as a percentage of the precontracting force. Potency, ie, sensitivity of the vessel to a drug is calculated as EC_{50} values (the concentrations of vasoconstrictor required to produce 50 % of the calculated maximum response). EC_{50} value is used to determine pEC_{50} value (negative $\log_{10}$ of the EC_{50} value). This value can differ considerably with the nature of the agent used for precontraction of the vessel and the amount of contraction that a particular concentration of vasoconstrictor substance will develop. The degree of relaxant effect of a dilator on a vessel precontracted by a particular vasoconstrictor agent, namely functional antagonism, is reflected by pEC_{50} value. Another important value is the maximal efficacy (E_{max}) which reflects the range of maximal response to the drug at high concentration.

A special method that measures the individual length-tension relationship curve for each vessel segment, cut to a precise length, has been developed [10]. This method, called as normalization technique, sets passive distension of the vessel segment to correspond with that caused transmural pressure experienced in vivo. The principal is to establish individual length-tension exponential curves for each vessel by relating the isometric tension, obtained from strain gauge transducers, with the corresponding diameter. This technique has been continously used by several researchers for studying CABG pharmacology [10,14-16].

2.1. Vasoconstrictor and vasodilator agents

Exogenous and endogenous vasoconstrictors are particularly important for vasoconstriction and its extreme form—vasospasm (Figure 2). Table 1 lists vasoconstrictor substances that are generally considered spasmogens for blood vessels and the receptors located on the cellular membrane of vascular smooth muscle, and of endothelium, which mediates vasodilatation. Most of these vasoconstrictor substances contract blood vessels through receptor-mediated mechanisms, i.e. internally secreted epinephrine and norepinephrine cause blood vessels to contract by stimulating α-adrenergic receptors on the vascular smooth muscle. Consequently, a selective α -receptor antagonist will be highly effective because the site of interaction is same. The contraction caused by epinephrine and norepinephrine is partly caused by depolarization of the tissue through voltage-operated calcium (Ca^{2+}) channels (VOCC) and partly caused by calcium release from intracellular sources. Thus, this mechanism would be more resistant to functional antagonist nifedipine. On the other hand, increased extracellular K^+ depolarizes smooth muscle membrane by closing of the hyperpolarizing K^+ channels. This effect allows VOCC to open and intracellular [Ca^{2+}] to rise, resulting in smooth muscle contraction. Therefore, a VOCC antagonist such as nifedipine would readily relax a tissue precontracted by potassium (K^+).

http://dx.doi.org/10.5772/54723

Vasoconstrictors	Vascular Smooth Muscle Contraction	Endothelium Relaxation
EDCFs		
Endothelin	ET_A, ET_B	ET_B
α-Adrenoceptor agonists		
Norepinephrine	α_1, α_2	α_2
Methoxamine	α_1	...
Phenylephrine	α_1	...
Dopamine	α_1***	...
Platelet-derived substances		
5-HT	$5\text{-}HT_2$	$5\text{-}HT_{1D}$
TxA_2 *	TP	TP (?)**
Prostanoids		
TxA_2 *	TP	TP (?)**
$PGF_{2\alpha}$	FP	FP (?)**
Substances released from mast cells and basophils		
Histamine	H (H_1, H_2)	H_1
Muscarinic receptor agonists		
Acetylcholine	$M_{3?}$	M_2
Renin-angiotensin system		
Angiotensin II	AII	AII
Vasopressin (ADH)	V_1****	...
Depolarizing agent		
Potassium		...

* TxA_2 is also considered as one of the endothelium-derived contracting factors; it is also derived from platelets.

** TP and FP receptors in endothelial cells to be clarified.

*** Dopamine also affects α_1 and α_2 receptors, exist in cardiac and bronchial cells respectively, it causes vasoconstriction at high dose.

**** Mainly effective in renal medulla, it also enhances sympathetic constriction,

EDCFs = Endothelium-derived contracting factors, ADH = antidiuretic hormone.

Table 1. Vasoconstrictors and their Receptors Involved in Vascular Smooth Muscle; Vasodilators in which Mediate Relaxation via Endothelium.

As stated above, vasodilator agents are usually studied by precontracting the vessel. The level of precontraction force should be chosen in the range of 60% to 80% of the maximum contraction of that agent. The precontractile tone should reach to a plateau and remain stable during the experimental period. The precontraction may dissipate in a time-dependent manner. This may lead researcher to ascribe decreased tone due to added drug instead of spontenaous relaxation. Therefore, a parallel time control is necessary to show that the precontraction is stable [11,17,18].

2.2. Influence of endothelial functions on contractility of arterial grafts

It has been well known that vascular endothelium plays an important role in maintaining vascular tone. Endothelium derives a number of vasoconstrictor as well as vasodilator substances. Vascular tone is maintained on the balance between vasoconstriction and vasodilatation caused by these substances. Endothelial cell produces endothelium- derived contracting factors (EDCFs) such as endothelin (ET) and thromboxane A_2 (TxA_2) that cause an increase in the intracellular calcium concentration and mediate contraction of the smooth muscle. Endothelium-dependent relaxation is known to be the effect of a variety of different endothelium-derived relaxing factors (EDRFs). These are endothelium-derived nitric oxide (NO) [19,20], prostacyclin (PGI_2) [21], and endothelium-derived hyperpolarizing factor (EDHF) [22-25]. These relaxing factors induce vasodilatation through different mechanisms by reducing the intracellular calcium concentration in the smooth muscle cell and cause relaxation. Spontaneous (basal) release of EDRF (NO) also depresses the contraction to some extent. As in other vessels, endothelium plays a modulatory role in contractility in CABGs [26]. Studies on endothelial function of CABGs have indicated that arterial endothelium has more ability to produce NO than venous endothelium (11-13, 26). EDHF also plays a role in arterial grafts [17].

Endothelin, prostanoids (TxA_2 and $PGF_{2\alpha}$) and α_1-adrenoceptor agonists are the most potent vasoconstrictors and they strongly contract arterial grafts even when endothelium is intact. On the other hand, some vasoconstrictors, i.e. serotonin (Serotonin (5-hydroxytryptamine, 5-HT)), have been demonstrated as being vasorelaxant agents through the mechanism of EDRF (NO). They induce contraction by their direct contractile effect on smooth muscle, and vasodilatation, induced by EDRF (NO) or EDRFs release due to its stimulation to endothelium. Therefore, these vasoconstrictors do not strongly contract the vessels in endothelium-intact blood vessels. However, when endothelium is damaged or denuded, they evoke a strong contraction.

3. Pharmacology of internal mammary artery

Vasoconstriction may be evoked by various stimuli such as vasoconstrictor substances, nerve stimulation and mechanical trauma. Clinically, although all arterial grafts may develop vasospasm, it develops less frequently in IMA and IEA than in GEA and RA [7,27]. Comparative functional studies have demonstrated that there are differences in arterial grafts with

regard to contractility and endothelial function. These differences, together with histological and anatomical diversity, may account for possible differences in the perioperative spasm.

The contractility of IMA to vasoconstrictors has been studied extensively [10,13]. TxA_2 is one of the several EDCFs, but it is also derived from platelets. Endothelin is also considered as one of the EDCFs. These two substances are two of the most potent vasoconstrictors known and they are very potent in IMA as well. Elevated plasma concentrations of ET [28] or TXA_2 [29] have been found during cardiopulmonary bypass. Therefore,.these vasoconstrictors are prime candidates as spasmogens for arterial grafts during CABG surgery.

Some receptors on the smooth muscle of IMA have been characterized. For example, IMA is an α_1-adrenoceptor-dominant artery with little α_2- or β -function [30,31]. Other receptors functionally demonstrated in IMA are ET_A, ET_B [32], 5-HT [33], angiotensin [34],TP (thromboxane-prostanoid) [35], vasopressin V_1 receptors [36,37], and vasoactive intestinal peptide [38] receptors. Dopaminergic receptors have also been demonstrated in the IMA [39]. The agonists for these receptors may also be spasmogenic agents for the IMA.

As stated above, some vasoconstrictors have been demonstrated as being vasorelaxant agents. 5-HT is an example of this type of vasoconstrictors and it directly contracts vascular smooth muscle through 5-HT_2 receptors [40] and relaxes blood vessels through endothelial NO release, mediated by 5-HT_{1D} receptors, [41] located in the endothelium. When endothelium is lost, perhaps also when it is damaged, platelets aggregate in the area where endothelium is denuded and release substances such as 5- HT (also TxA_2) that strongly contract smooth muscle. Accordingly, studies have shown 5-HT does not strongly contract IMA with intact endothelium [13,42]. However, its contracting effect is unmasked when endothelium is denuded [13,42].

The endothelium-dependent relaxation exists in IMA [43]. It has also been demonstrated that vascular endothelial growth factor may induce endothelium-dependent relaxation in the human IMA [44]; the relaxation has recently been demonstrated to be mediated by both NO and PGI_2 [45]. Further, physiological substances such as CRF induce both endothelium-dependent and -independent relaxation in the human IMA [46]. IMA releases both NO and EDHF [47]. Recent studies have demonstrated that the endothelium of the IMA releases more NO than the RA at both basal and stimulated levels [47]. Further, the IMA has a greater hyperpolarizing effect on bradykinin-stimulated release of EDHF than the RA does [47].

In addition, receptors, for common stimuli of EDRF such as acetylcholine, bradykinin, and substance P are present in the endothelium of arterial grafts [15,48,49]. The vascular endothelial growth factor (VEGF)-induced, endothelium- dependent relaxation, mediated by both NO and prostacyclin in the IMA, has been shown mainly through the KDR (kinase insert domain) receptors, rather than Flt-1 (fms-like thyrosine kinase-1) receptors [45]. Most recently, corticortropin-releasing factor (CRF) receptors CRF_1, $CRF_{2\alpha}$, and $CRF_{2\beta}$ have been shown to be present in the IMA [45]. The CRF urocortin- induced endothelium-dependent relaxation in the IMA is likely through CRF receptors allocated in the endothelium of the IMA [50].

3.1. Spasm of internal mammary artery

Compared to saphenous grafts, IMA is more resistant to ischaemic changes due to high content of elastin with a low metabolic rate. Occasionally, there is severe contraction (spasm), which may be visible or be inferred by minimal free flow. Spasm of IMA can cause inadequate blood flow, which may be detrimental during periods of increased nutritional demand such as weaning from cardiopulmonary bypass [51] or postoperative hypovolemia [52]. In addition, IMAs with poor perioperative flow rates are more likely to occlude [53]. Severe spasm may lead to graft malfunction and even mortality [11,54]. It is essential to to determine whether the IMA should be discarded or alternatively relegated to graft a minor vessel. Thus, a dilator drug, preferably a fast-acting one suitable for intraluminal injection, should be used for maximal pharmacologic dilation of the IMA, which allows the surgeon to evaluate the flow-carrying capacity of the IMA and provides a relaxed, dilated distal vessel that facilitates a precise anastomosis. Vasodilation of the IMA pedicle during CABG surgery may also unmask small bleeding points, improve hemostasis and facilitate placement of anastomotic sutures [9].

Vasoconstriction (or spasm) of IMA may be caused by multiple mechanisms. In addition, vasodilators relax vascular smooth muscle through a specific mechanism or mechanisms. Several vasodilators have been suggested to prevent graft spasm; including papaverine, phenoxybenzamine, calcium antagonists and nitrates. However, there is no "perfect" vasodilator which is effective for every situation.

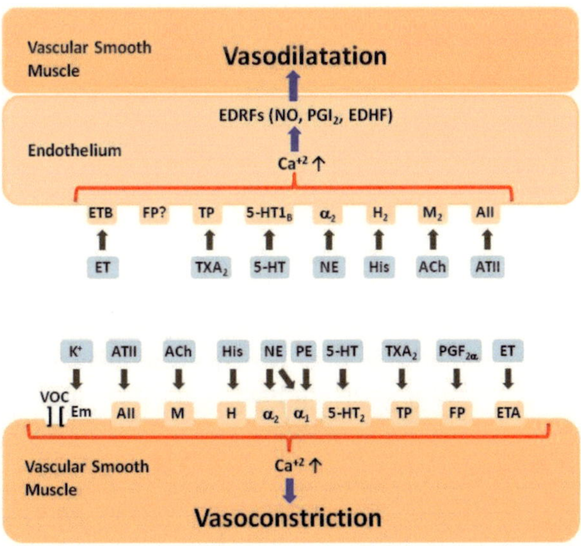

Figure 2. Endothelium-derived relaxing factor (EDRF) is produced and released by the endothelium to promote smooth muscle relaxation. NO, nitric oxide; AII, angiotensin II receptors; ACh, acetylcholine; EDHF, endothelium-derived hyperpolarizing factor; ET, endothelin; FP, $PGF_{2\alpha}$ receptors; H (H_2), histamine receptors; His, histamine; K, potassium; M (M_2), muscarinic receptors; NE, norepinephrine; PE, phenylephrine; PGI_2, prostacyclin; 5-HT, 5-hydroxytryptamine (serotonin); TP, thromboxane-prostanoid receptors; VOC, voltage operated channels; α, adrenergic receptors

3.2. Effect of vasodilator substances on IMA

To promote dilation of the IMA, some vasodilating substances have been applied to the outside of the pedicle [55-58] or injected intraluminally with or without hydrostatic dilation [9,55,56,58,59]. The vasodilator substances available are as follows:

Papaverine

The traditional topical vasodilator papaverine was first recommended by George Green, the pioneer IMA surgeon, in early days of IMA grafting to overcome spasm [60]. It is still widely used due to its satisfactory vasorelaxant effect in arterial grafts [61,62]. Papaverine is a non specific vasodilator substance which relaxes vessels via multiple mechanisms such as inhibition of phosphodiesterase [63], which increases cyclic guanosine monophosphate (cGMP) level in smooth muscle cells, decreasing calcium influx [64,65] or inhibition of release of intracellularly stored calcium [66]. Although hydrostatic dilation with papaverine dissolved in saline solution provides good dilation at high concentrations, it carries a potential risk of mechanical damage to the media and intima caused by cannulation and overstretching and by chemical damage as a result of the acidity of the solution [67-70]. The problem of acidity of papaverine solutions may be overcome by mixing the solutions with blood or albumin before its use [71]. However, the pharmacological action is uncertain in such a mixture. Additionally, papaverine has a slower onset of the vasodilating effect when compared to other vasodilators such as nitroglycerin (NTG) and verapamil [10,62,72]. However, once its effect reaches a plateau, it is sustained [10,62,72]. Papaverine hydrochloride is relatively unstable in non-acidic solutions and a white precipitate is sometimes formed when papaverine is added to the plasmalyte solution (pH approximately 7.4) [73]. In light of these points, papaverine is still an effective vasodilator for IMA. Its topical spray on the adventitia of the IMA may be effective but it is not recommended for systemic use.

Nitrovasodilators

Nitrovasodilators (organic nitrates), NTG, glyceryl trinitrate (GTN) and sodium nitroprusside (SNP), are a diverse group of pharmacological agents that produce vascular relaxation by releasing NO, which activates guanylate cyclase, resulting in an accumulation of cyclic GMP in the smooth muscle cell. This in turn reduces intracellular calcium concentrations and leads to vasodilatation. These drugs are effective against a range of constrictor stimuli and they are widely used in CABG patients. Nitrovasodilators have been shown to be potent vasodilators in the human IMA [55,61,74-79]. It has been demonstrated that NTG is compares favorably with diltiazem in the prevention of IMA spasm [80] and it is effective for either topical, intraluminal, or systemic use [78,81,82]. Although, nitrates are slightly more effective in blocking receptor operated channels, they are effective in treating established vascular spasm, regardless of the nature of contraction, i.e., either receptor mediated (TxA_2 receptors, α-adrenoceptors, or ET receptors) or depolarizing agent (K^+)- mediated contraction [10,54]. However, rapid tolerance (tachyphylaxis) of vessels develops to nitrovasodilators. Therefore, they are less potent in the prevention of vasospasm [54,74,75,83]. NTG is more potent in its

vasorelaxing effect when it is compared to SNP. However, SNP is more effective in inhibition ANGII and α-adrenoceptor-mediated contraction in the IMA [34].

Phosphodiesterase inhibitors

Phosphodiesterases (PDE) are a diverse family of enzymes that hydrolyse cyclic nucleotides and thus play a key role in regulating intracellular levels of the second messengers cyclic adenosine monophosphate (cAMP) and cGMP which modulate vascular smooth muscle tone. Concentrations of cAMP and cGMP are controlled through synthesis by cyclases and through hydrolysis by PDEs. Non-selective PDE inhibitors including papaverine have been injected routinely by surgeons, in and around the artery to prevent IMA spasm, but papaverine is not administered systemically. The discovery of eleven types of PDEs [84,85] provides an impetus for the development of isoenzyme selective inhibitors for the treatment of various diseases. Inamirinone (previously called amrirone) and milrinone are bipyridine compounds that inhibit phosphodiesterase (PDE) III, a form found in cardiac and smooth muscle. Therefore, they increase myocardial contractility and vasodilation, and they are called as 'inodilators'. These drugs are useful in postoperative management of patients who undergo open heart surgery, particularly in patients who present ventricular dysfunction and receive arterial grafts for coronary artery bypass surgery. Favorable effects of inamrinone on the IMA [76,86-88] have been reported. In addition, it has been demonstrated that inamrinone has a greater than additive vasodilatory effect when used in combination with NTG [76]. It was also demonstrated that systemically administered milrinone and nitroglycerin dilate the IMA after cardiopulmonary bypass [82]. Levosimendan is a new agent developed for the treatment of acute and decompensated heart failure. It exerts potent positive inotropic action and peripheral vasodilatory effects. The mechanism of vasodilation by levosimendan may involve reduction of Ca^{2+} sensitivity of contractile proteins in vascular smooth muscle, the lowering of intracellular free Ca^{2+}, the potential inhibition of PDE III, and an opening of K^+ channels [89,90]. We have recently shown that levosimendan effectively and directly decreases the tone of IMA [91]. Therefore, levosimendan may be a cardiovascular protective agent by its relaxing action on IMA.

Calcium antagonists

It has been known since the late 1800s that calcium influx was necessary for he contraction of smooth and cardiac muscle. The discovery of calcium channel in smooth and cardiac muscle was followed by the finding of several different types calcium channels including VOCC (L, T, N and P types) and receptor -operated calcium channels, (ROCC). The discovery of these channels made possible the development of clinically useful new generation calcium antagonists (calcium channel blockers). These drugs are consist of three chemically divergent groups: Dihydropyridine (nifedipine, etc.), phenylalkylamines (verapamil, etc.), and benzothiazepines (diltiazem, etc.). Important differences in vascular selectivity exist among the calcium antagonists. In general, nifedipin is the most potent. In addidion, verapamil is more potent than diltiazem. It has been demonstrated that nifedipine is more potent than diltiazem with regard to the vasorelaxant effect in the human IMA [54].

http://dx.doi.org/10.5772/54723

The degree of vasodilatory effect of calcium antagonists is dependent on the nature of contraction. Calcium antagonists are less effective in blocking receptor-operated than voltage-operated calcium channels. For example, increased extracellular K^+ depolarizes smooth muscle membrane by closing of the hyperpolarizing K^+ channels. This effect allows VOCC to open and intracellular [Ca^{2+}] to rise, resulting in smooth muscle contraction. Therefore, a VOCC antagonist such as nifedipine would readily relax a tissue precontracted by K^+. On the other hand, the contraction caused by receptor agonists is partly caused by calcium influx and partly caused by calcium release from intracellular sources. Consequently, calcium antagonists are weak in either preventing or treating TxA_2, α-adrenoceptor, or VP_1 receptor-mediated contraction, in comparison to K^+-mediated contraction [54,74,92,93].

Potassium (K^+) channel openers

Drugs that open potassium channels (potassium channel openers, KCOs) can exert antivasoconstrictor and vasorelaxant actions, that is, they reduce or prevent cellular response ro excitatory stimuli, repolarize or hyperpolarize the cell membrane, overcome a contraction once it has developed, and strengten the resting state of the vessel. KCOs are considered to comprise a heterogeneous group of organic compounds [94]. These are apricalim, bimakalim, celikalim, cromakalim, levokromakalim, diazoxide, L-27,152, P 1075, minoxidil sulphate, pinacidil, and nicorandil. KCOs act by stimulating ion flux through a distinct class of potassium channels which are inhibited by intracellular adenosine triphosphate (ATP) and activated by intracellular nucleoside diphosphates. They restrain the opening probability of voltage-dependent L- and T-type calcium-channels and decrease agonist-induced Ca^{2+} release from intracellular sources through inhibition of inositol trisphosphate (IP_3) formation, and lower the efficiency of calcium as an activator of contractile proteins [95]. Additionally, they may accelerate clearance of intracellular free calcium via the Na^+/Ca^{2+} exchange pathway [95]. The functional outcome of these effects is to reduce the membrane excitability and to drive vascular myocytes into a relaxed state. Particularly, vascular smooth muscle is sensitive to KCOs [96-99]. In view of these points, KCOs are of great value as therapeutic agents [98,99,] and aprikalim [100,102] have been studied in the human IMA and found to be potent vasodilators in a number of receptor-mediated contractions. Therefore, this group of drugs may become clinically useful antispastic agents by their relaxing action on IMA.

α-Adrenoceptor antagonists

IMA is an α_1-adrenoceptor-dominant artery with little α_2- or β -function [30,31,103]. Theoretically, a selective α -receptor antagonist may be a highly effective antispastic agent because the site of interaction is same. Herewith, the use of α-adrenoceptor antagonists such as phenoxybenzamine as an antispastic agent has a rationale. However, the nature of vasoconstriction is complex and may involve many other vasoconstrictors (Table 1). It has been demonstrated that, α- adrenoceptor antagonists are not effective in reversing the contraction evoked by other vasoconstrictors such as vasopressin, angiotensin II, endothelin-1, and KCl [104]. From pharmacological point of view, use of phenoxybenzamine is inappropriate as the sole antispastic agent in the arterial grafts. Moreover, a novel α_1-adrenergic receptor blocking substance with calcium antagonist with activity, AJ-2615, has been studied with regard to inhibition of

vasoconstriction in the IMA [44]. Further studies on this kind of substances may provide development of new antispastic protocols.

Vascular endothelial growth factor

Vascular endothelial growth factor (VEGF) has been studied in the human IMA and found to be a potent vasodilator through KDR receptors and NO -and PGI_2 -mediated mechanisms [44,45]. However, VEGF has potent hypotensive effect due to systemic vasodilaton [44,45]. Therefore, the use of VEGF as a vasorelaxant agent may not be the primary consideration for antispastic therapy in arterial grafts.

β-Adrenoceptor agonists: Dopamine and dobutamine

Albeit at least three distinct beta-adrenoceptors exist in IMA [105], β -receptor function is weak [31]. Consequently, it has been demonsted that use of β -adrenoceptor agonists is unlikely relax the IMA significantly [106]. Same study also indicated that beta-receptor agonist dobutamine exerts weak vasodilator effect in IMA. Dopamine-induced responses are complex and dose-dependent, inasmuch as the complexity of interaction between dopamine and dopamine receptors as well as α_1-adrenoceptors [107]. In IMA, dopamine induced a vasorelaxation on the norepinephrine contraction only at higher concentrations [107]. Similar to VEGF, the use of dopamine and dobutamine may not be the primary consideration for antispastic therapy. On the other hand, vasodilator effect of β-adrenoceptor agonists in IMA at high concentrations should be kept in mind when these agents are used primarily as inotropic agents.

TxA_2 antagonists

TxA_2 is one of the the most potent vasoconstrictors known and it is very potent in IMA as well [10,13]. Inasmuch as its importance in thrombosis together with its elevated plasma concentrations during cardiopulmonary bypass, specific TxA_2 antagonists may be useful in the antispastic therapy of IMA. Accordingly, specific TxA_2 antagonist GR30191 is a potent vasodilator for TxA_2-mediated contraction in IMA [86]. However, to date, no clinical data are available.

5-HT receptor antagonists

Studies on human IMA have shown that 5-HT directly contracts IMA through $5\text{-}HT_{1D}$ and $5\text{-}HT_2$ receptors [33,108-110]. In IMA, 5-HT receptor mediated contractions are unmasked when endothelium is denuded [13,42]. Additionally, studies have shown 5-HT may interact synergistically with other vasoconstrictor substances, such as TxA_2 released from platelets during thrombus formation, and 5-HT receptor mediated contractions may be unmasked or amplified [33,108-110]. $5\text{-}HT_{2A}$ receptor antagonist ketanserin has antihypertensive properties and it's recently used to reduce the severity and frequency of the vasospasm in Raynaud's phenomenon [111]. Therefore, it may have potential to overcome IMA spasm when it's applied topically.

Testosterone

Testosterone may exert vasorelaxant effects on several vascular tissues [112-119]. We have studied effects of testosterone in the human IMA and found that vasorelaxant re-

sponse to testosterone may occur in via large-conductance Ca^{2+}-activated K^+ channel-opening action [112]. Clinical studies of testosterone therapy in male patients with coronary artery disease raised promising results. Therefore, the use of testosterone, i.e. direct topical administration on adventitia, as a vasorelaxant agent may be considered for antispastic therapy in arterial grafts.

Iloprost and botilinum toxin

It has been demonstrated that botilinum toxin may prevent arterial spasm in vitro [120]. Iloprost, a PGI_2 analogue, may be considered as an alternative antispastic agent in arterial grafts [121].

4. Pharmacology of other arterial grafts

4.1. Radial artery

The use of the RA as a graft for coronary revascularization was already introduced in the 1970s, but shortly thereafter it was abandoned due to high incidence of vasospasm and comparatively poorer short-term and long-term patency rates than IMA [27,122-124]. This was partly due to the inability to recognize RA spasm, but it was also due to lack of proper pharmacological tools to prevent this. It was later noted that radial grafts were indeed patent in patients long after their surgery. Thereafter, the RA was reassessed and its role as an alternative arterial graft was re-established.

Because of the dual blood supply to the hand, RA occlusion is not associated with major clinical sequelae but prevention is important. RA spasm rarely leads to serious vascular complications but can cause patient discomfort and can result in prolonging or failure of the procedure. Several studies now suggest that the vasospastic tendency of RA grafts has been countered in the operating room (immediately after harvest) by treating the artery with papaverine or milrinone, or both, and placing it in a bath of heparinized saline containing NTG or a combination of NTG and a calcium channel blocker to prevent spasms. Similarly, protection from immediate postoperative and postdischarge vasospasm is sought through the use of intravenous or oral combinations of the aforementioned vasodilator drugs. However, clinical studies indicate that such vasodilatory precautions do not provide the expected protection from postoperative vasospasm of RA grafts. Although the patency rate of RA is debatable, mid-term and long-term patency rates may reach 90% and greater, that makes the RA a valuable addition in arterial grafting [125,126].

RA has less active endothelium compared to IMA and is stronger receptor-mediated contractions can be evoked in the RA than in the IMA [49,127], which presumably predisposes it to higher incidences of spasm. Additionally, it was previously reported that RA grafts are more sensitive to TxA_2 [13]. Furthermore, it has been reported that IMAs produce substantial amounts of both PGI_2 and TxA_2 [128]; nonetheless, the TxA_2 to PGI_2 ratio was significantly higher in the RA than in the IMA. Because PGI_2 antagonizes the actions of TxA_2, the higher TxA_2 to PGI_2 ratio implies that TxA_2 would exert greater effects in the RA. Contraction to KCl

in the RA is stronger than in the IMA or the GEA [16]. The RA is more reactive than the IMA to angiotensin II and ET-1, but the endothelial function of the RA is similar to the IMA [49].

Pharmacological and non-pharmacological strategies have been evaluated to prevent RA occlusion and RA spasm. A number of pharmacological 'cocktails' have been successfully tested but there is currently no agreement on the optimal combination of agents. RA studied in vitro was found to relax fully either to GV solution or to papaverine, but the relaxation to GV solution was more rapid in onset and of longer duration than for papaverine [62]. GV (GTN +Verapamil) solution has been found to be satisfactory when is used on the RA to dilate it during harvesting and preparation and it [11,129]. It can be argued that GV solution represents the optimum agent for RA spasm when used in the perioperative period [129]. It has been suggested that a 'cocktail' of agents may be given to counteract RA spasm before transradial coronary angiography or angioplasty [130]. A combination of heparin, NTG and verapamil seems to be associated with the best preventive outcome [130].

4.2. Gastroepiploic artery

Excellent long-term angiographic results have been reported with GEA [131], but its progressive loss of caliber with mobilization and its greater tendency for vasospasm compared with other arterial conduits both in in vitro testing [13] and in clinical practice [7] has limited its widespread use.

Spasm of the GEA is a well-described clinical phenomenon [7] Some studies have suggested that the GEA and the IMA have similar response to NE, phenylephrine, and 5-HT [132,133], and that the IMA is more reactive to the TXA_2 mimetic, U46619. On the other hand, Dignan and associates [15] have found that the GEA has a stronger contractility than the IMA and more reactive to K^+, NE, and 5-HT. He and Yang [13,134] compared the contractility of the GEA, the IMA, and the IEA and found that among arterial grafts the GEA has the highest contractility. Variation of techniques used in the studies may account for diverse results from different groups. Therefore, the above mentioned vasoconstrictors may be the spasmogenic agents for the GEA [15]. Additionally, relaxation of the GEA to SNP [15] or to endothelium-dependent vasodilators [134,135] appears to be similar to the IMA.

Several vasodiators have been studied to counteract GEA spasm [81,136]. It has been demonstrated that papaverine, when given externally on the perivascular fat of the GEA, prevents GEA spasm for up to 2 hr [136]. In contrast, intraluminally applied papaverine does not show graft protection against NE-induced spasm. In addition, nifedipine prevents NE-induced spasm only when given intraluminally. Same study has also shown that verapamil is the most potent and versatile vasodilator with effective graft protection of up to 2 hr whether applied externally or internally and is the preferred agent for protecting against GEA spasm [136]. During intraoperative preparation of the GEA graft, GTN and papaverine to a lesser extent, used as topical vasodilators, appear to be more efficient in external application to increase the free flow of the GEA [81]. GV solution has been suggested to be suitable to treat spasm of GEA [137] GTN has a more rapid onset and verapamil has a longer action than papaverine [11]. That should prevent spasm of conduit in the early postoperative hours [137].

4.3. Inferior epigastric artery

It has been demonstrated that there is no difference between the IEA and the IMA for some vasoconstrictors, such as ET, NE, K^+, and U46619 [48] However, a previous study showed that IEA contracted less in response to histamine, but relaxed more in response to endothelium-dependent vasodilators, compared with the IMA [138]. Different contractile responses to TXA_2 and NE between the IEA and the IMA have also been reported [139]. In general, it has been argued that the contractile response of the IEA is basically similar to that of the IMA [11].

It has been demonstrated that endothelium dependent relaxation is reduced in the IEA compared with the IMA [140]. Another report has shown that the non–receptor-mediated endothelium dependent relaxation (induced by calcium ionophore A23187) in the IEA is less than in the IMA, although the receptor-mediated endothelium-dependent relaxation induced by acetylcholine is similar [48]. This decreased endothelium-dependent relaxation may be an early sign of arteriosclerosis in the IEA [48], since non– receptor-mediated endothelium-dependent relaxation is impaired.

5. Conclusion

The problem of grafts spasm has become more obvious with the increasing use of new arterial grafts. Arterial spasm is a multifactor phenomenon modulated by different mechanism, such as drugs, temperature, endogenous catecholamine, and mechanical stimuli (surgical trauma), which is the most common cause. Surgical trauma can usually be minimized by harvesting the artery as a pedicle rather than skeletonizing it by careful surgical technique.

Antispastic management is an important part of technical considerations during CABG surgery. There is extensive evidence that the use of appropriate vasodilators during CABG surgery can facilitate the operative procedure as well as improve graft flow and reduce structural damage to the graft conduit. Spasm of arterial graft conduits is best managed by prevention rather than treatment after it has occurred. There are many dilators of arterial grafts that vary in potency, rapidity of onset, and duration of action as shown in organ bath studies. Using these findings to make a rational choice of type of dilator and optimal concentration for clinical use requires an understanding of the reactivity of that particular type of graft to vasoconstrictor and vasodilator agents. In addition, clinical choice of grafts must be based on consideration of many additional factors, including the systemic effects of the agent if it enters the circulation, the effect of the agent and its vehicle on the endothelium, convenience of preparation, and cost.

Acknowledgements

The authors thank Enis Macit, PhD, for his contribution in preparing this chapter.

Author details

Oguzhan Yildiz*, Melik Seyrek and Husamettin Gul

*Address all correspondence to: oyildiz@gata.edu.tr

Department of Medical Pharmacology, Gulhane School of Medicine, Ankara, Turkey

References

[1] Sarabu MR, McClung JA, Fass A, Reed GE. Early postoperative spasm in left internal mammary artery bypass grafts. Ann Thorac Surg. 1987;44(2):199-200.

[2] Houghton JL, Callaghan WE, Frank MJ. Disappearance of high-grade left anterior descending stenosis after revascularization. Cathet Cardiovasc Diagn. 1988;14(3): 169-171.

[3] McCormick JR, Kaneko M, Baue AE, Geha AS. Blood flow and vasoactive drug effects in internal mammary and venous bypass grafts. Circulation. 1975;52(2):72-80.

[4] Jett GK, Arcidi JM Jr, Dorsey LM, Hatcher CR Jr, Guyton RA. Vasoactive drug effects on blood flow in internal mammary artery and saphenous vein grafts. J Thorac Cardiovasc Surg. 1987;94(1):2-11.

[5] Kawasuji M, Tedoriya T, Takemura H, Sakakibara N, Taki J, Watanabe Y. Flow capacities of arterial grafts for coronary artery bypass grafting. Ann Thorac Surg. 1993;56(4):957-962.

[6] Loop FD, Thomas JD. Hypoperfusion after arterial bypass grafting. Ann Thorac Surg. 1993;56(4):812-813.

[7] Suma H. Spasm of the gastroepiploic artery graft. Ann Thorac Surg. 1990;49(1):168-169.

[8] Fisk RL, Brooks CH, Callaghan JC, Dvorkin J. Experience with the radial artery graft for coronary artery bypass. Ann Thorac Surg. 1976;21(6):513-518.

[9] Mills NL, Bringaze WL 3rd. Preparation of the internal mammary artery graft. Which is the best method? J Thorac Cardiovasc Surg. 1989;98(1):73-77.

[10] He GW, Angus JA, Rosenfeldt FL. Reactivity of the canine isolated internal mammary artery, saphenous vein, and coronary artery to constrictor and dilator substances: relevance to coronary bypass graft surgery. J Cardiovasc Pharmacol. 1988;12(1):12-22.

[11] Rosenfeldt FL, He GW, Buxton BF, Angus JA. Pharmacology of coronary artery bypass grafts. Ann Thorac Surg. 1999;67(3):878-888. Review.

[12] He GW, Yang CQ. Pharmacological studies and guidelines for the use of vasodilators for arterial grafts. In He GW (ed.) Arterial grafting for coronary artery bypass surgery. Springer; 2006. p38-47.

[13] He GW, Yang CQ, Starr A. Overview of the nature of vasoconstriction in arterial grafts for coronary operations. Ann Thorac Surg. 1995;59(3):676-683

[14] Angus JA, Cocks TM, Satoh K. Alpha 2-adrenoceptors and endothelium-dependent relaxation in canine large arteries. Br J Pharmacol. 1986;88(4):767-777.

[15] Dignan RJ, Yeh T Jr, Dyke CM, Lee KF, Lutz HA 3rd, Ding M, Wechsler AS. Reactivity of gastroepiploic and internal mammary arteries. Relevance to coronary artery bypass grafting. J Thorac Cardiovasc Surg. 1992;103(1):116-122.

[16] Chardigny C, Jebara VA, Acar C, Descombes JJ, Verbeuren TJ, Carpentier A, Fabiani JN. Vasoreactivity of the radial artery. Comparison with the internal mammary and gastroepiploic arteries with implications for coronary artery surgery. Circulation. 1993;88:115-127.

[17] He G-W, Yang C-Q, Acuff TE, Ryan WH, Mack MJ. Endothelium-derived hyperpolarizing factor (EDHF) plays a role in human coronary bypass grafts through Na^+-K^+ pump mechanism [Abstract]. Circulation 1994;90:242.

[18] Henry PJ, Drummer OH, Horowitz JD. S-nitrosothiols as vasodilators: implications regarding tolerance to nitric oxide-containing vasodilators. Br J Pharmacol. 1989;98(3): 757-766.

[19] Ignarro LJ, Buga GM, Wood KS, Byrns RE, Chaudhuri G. Endothelium-derived relaxing factor produced and released from artery and vein is nitric oxide. Proc Natl Acad Sci USA. 1987;84(24):9265-9269.

[20] Palmer RM, Ferrige AG, Moncada S. Nitric oxide release accounts for the biological activity of endothelium-derived relaxing factor. Nature. 1987;327(6122):524-526.

[21] Moncada S, Korbut R, Bunting S, Vane JR. Prostacyclin is a circulating hormone. Nature. 1978;273(5665):767-768.

[22] Feletou M, Vanhoutte PM. Endothelium-dependent hyperpolarization of canine coronary smooth muscle. Br J Pharmacol. 1988;93(3):515-524.

[23] Chen G, Suzuki H, Weston AH. Acetylcholine releases endothelium-derived hyperpolarizing factor and EDRF from rat blood vessels. Br J Pharmacol. 1988;95(4): 1165-1174.

[24] He GW, Yang CQ, Graier WF, Yang JA. Hyperkalemia alters EDHF-mediated hyperpolarization and relaxation in coronary arteries. Am J Physiol. 1996;271:H760-767.

[25] Ge ZD, Zhang XH, Fung PC, He GW. Endothelium-dependent hyperpolarization and relaxation resistance to N(G)-nitro-L-arginine and indomethacin in coronary circulation. Cardiovasc Res. 2000;46(3):547-556.

[26] Schoeffter P, Dion R, Godfraind T. Modulatory role of the vascular endothelium in the contractility of human isolated internal mammary artery. Br J Pharmacol 1988;95:531-543.

[27] Acar C, Jebara VA, Portoghese M, Beyssen B, Pagny JY, Grare P, Chachques JC, Fabiani JN, Deloche A, Guermonprez JL. Revival of the radial artery for coronary artery bypass grafting. Ann Thorac Surg. 1992;54(4):652-659.

[28] van Zwienen JCW, van der Linden CJ, Cimbrere JSF, Lacquet LK, Booij LHDJ, Hendriks T. Endothelin release during coronary artery bypass grafting [Abstract]. Chest 1993;103:176S

[29] Davies GC, Sobel M, Salzman EW. Elevated plasma fibrinopeptide A and thromboxane B_2 levels during cardiopulmonary bypass. Circulation. 1980;61(4):808-814.

[30] He GW, Shaw J, Hughes CF, Yang CQ, Thomson DS, McCaughan B, Hendle PN, Baird DK. Predominant alpha 1-adrenoceptor-mediated contraction in the human internal mammary artery. J Cardiovasc Pharmacol. 1993;21(2):256-263.

[31] He GW, Buxton B, Rosenfeldt FL, Wilson AC, Angus JA. Weak beta-adrenoceptor-mediated relaxation in the human internal mammary artery. J Thorac Cardiovasc Surg. 1989;97(2):259-266.

[32] Seo B, Oemar BS, Siebenmann R, von Segesser L, Lüscher TF. Both ET_A and ET_B receptors mediate contraction to endothelin-1 in human blood vessels. Circulation. 1994;89(3):1203 1208.

[33] Yildiz O, Ciçek S, Ay I, Tatar H, Tuncer M. 5-HT1-like receptor-mediated contraction in the human internal mammary artery. J Cardiovasc Pharmacol. 1996;28(1):6-10.

[34] He GW, Yang CQ. Comparison of nitroprusside and nitroglycerin in inhibition of angiotensin II and other vasoconstrictor-mediated contraction in human coronary bypass conduits. Br J Clin Pharmacol. 1997;44(4):361-367.

[35] He GW, Yang CQ. Effect of thromboxane A2 antagonist GR32191B on prostanoid and nonprostanoid receptors in the human internal mammary artery. J Cardiovasc Pharmacol. 1995;26(1):13-19.

[36] He GW, Yang Q, Yang CQ. Smooth muscle and endothelial function of arterial grafts for coronary artery bypass surgery. Clin Exp Pharmacol Physiol. 2002;29(8):717-720. Review.

[37] Liu JJ, Phillips PA, Burrell LM, Buxton BB, Johnston CI. Human internal mammary artery responses to non-peptide vasopressin antagonists. Clin Exp Pharmacol Physiol. 1994;21(2):121-124.

[38] Luu TN, Dashwood MR, Chester AH, Tadjkarimi S, Yacoub MH. Action of vasoactive intestinal peptide and distribution of its binding sites in vessels used for coronary artery bypass grafts. Am J Cardiol. 1993;71(15):1278-1282.

[39] Myers ML, Li GH, Yaghi A, McCormack D. Human internal thoracic artery reactivity to dopaminergic agents. Circulation. 1993;88[Part 2]:110-114.

[40] Cocks TM, Angus JA. Endothelium-dependent relaxation of coronary arteries by noradrenaline and serotonin. Nature. 1983;305(5935):627-630.

[41] Schoeffter P, Hoyer D. 5-Hydroxytryptamine (5-HT)-induced endothelium-dependent relaxation of pig coronary arteries is mediated by 5-HT receptors similar to the 5-$HT1_D$ receptor subtype. J Pharmacol Exp Ther. 1990;252(1):387-395.

[42] He GW, Yang CQ. "Vasoactivators"--a new concept for naturally secreted vasoconstrictor substances. Angiology. 1994;45(4):265-271.

[43] Luscher TF, Diederich D, Siebenmann R, Lehmann K, Stulz P, von Segesser L, Yang ZH, Turina M, Grädel E, Weber E. Difference between endothelium-dependent relaxation in arterial and in venous coronary bypass grafts. N Engl J Med. 1988;319(8): 462-467

[44] Liu MH, Jin H, Floten HS, Ren Z, Yim AP, He GW. Vascular endothelial growth factor-mediated, endothelium-dependent relaxation in human internal mammary artery. Ann Thorac Surg. 2002;73(3):819-824.

[45] Wei W, Jin H, Chen ZW, Zioncheck TF, Yim AP, He GW. Vascular endothelial growth factor-induced nitric oxide- and PGI_2-dependent relaxation in human internal mammary arteries: a comparative study with KDR and Flt-1 selective mutants. J Cardiovasc Pharmacol. 2004;44(5):615-621.

[46] Liu ZG, Ge ZD, He GW. Difference in endothelium-derived hyperpolarizing factor-mediated hyperpolarization and nitric oxide release between human internal mammary artery and saphenous vein. Circulation. 2000;102(19 Suppl 3):296-301.

[47] He GW, Liu ZG. Comparison of nitric oxide release and endothelium-derived hyperpolarizing factor-mediated hyperpolarization between human radial and internal mammary arteries. Circulation. 2001;104(12 Suppl 1):344-349.

[48] He GW, Acuff TE, Ryan WH, Yang CQ, Mack MJ. Functional comparison between the human inferior epigastric artery and internal mammary artery. Similarities and differences. J Thorac Cardiovasc Surg. 1995;109(1):13-20.

[49] He GW, Yang CQ. Radial artery has higher receptor-mediated contractility but similar endothelial function compared with mammary artery. Ann Thorac Surg. 1997;63(5): 1346-1352.

[50] Chen ZW, Huang Y, Yang Q, Li X, Wei W, He GW. Urocortin-induced relaxation in the human internal mammary artery. Cardiovasc Res. 2005;65(4):913-920.

[51] von Segesser L, Simonet F, Meier 8, Finci L, Faidutti B. Inadequate flow after internal mammaryxoronary artery anastomoses. Thorac Cardiovasc Surg 1987;35:352-354.

[52] von Segesser LK, Lehmann K, Turina M. Deleterious effects of shock in internal mammary artery anastomoses. Ann Thorac Surg. 1989;47(4):575-579.

[53] Huddleston CB, Stoney WS, Alford WC Jr, Burrus GR, Glassford DM Jr, Lea JW 4th, Petracek MR, Thomas CS Jr. Internal mammary artery grafts: technical factors influencing patency. Ann Thorac Surg. 1986;42(5):543-549.

[54] He GW, Rosenfeldt FL, Buxton BF, Angus JA. Reactivity of human isolated internal mammary artery to constrictor and dilator agents. Implications for treatment of internal mammary artery spasm. Circulation. 1989;80(3 Pt 1):I141-150.

[55] Cooper GJ, Wilkinson GA, Angelini GD. Overcoming perioperative spasm of the internal mammary artery: which is the best vasodilator? J Thorac Cardiovasc Surg. 1992;104(2):465-468.

[56] Dion RA, Verhelst R, Goenen M, Rousseau M, Baele P, Ponlot R, Schoevaerdts JC, Chalant CH. Sequential mammary artery grafts in one hundred and twenty consecutive patients: indications, operative technique, 6 months postoperative functional and angiographic controls. J Cardiovasc Surg (Torino). 1989;30(4):635-642.

[57] Dion R, Verhelst R, Rousseau M, Goenen M, Ponlot R, Kestens-Servaye Y, Chalant CH. Sequential mammary grafting. Clinical, functional, and angiographic assessment 6 months postoperatively in 231 consecutive patients. J Thorac Cardiovasc Surg. 1989;98(1):80-88.

[58] Galbut DL, Traad EA, Dorman MJ, DeWitt PL, Larsen PB, Kurlansky PA, Button JH, Ally JM, Gentsch TO. Seventeen-year experience with bilateral internal mammary artery grafts. Ann Thorac Surg. 1990;49(2):195-201.

[59] Eckel L, Skupin M, Schräder R, Gusic L, Beyersdorf F, Sarai K, Krause E. Adequate flow through the internal mammary artery graft achieved by a dilatation technique. Thorac Cardiovasc Surg. 1990;38(3):157-160.

[60] Green GE. Rate of blood flow from the internal mammary artery. Surgery. 1971;70(6): 809-813.

[61] He GW, Rosenfeldt FL, Angus JA. Pharmacological relaxation of the saphenous vein during harvesting for coronary artery bypass grafting. Ann Thorac Surg. 1993;55(5): 1210-1217.

[62] He GW, Yang CQ. Use of verapamil and nitroglycerin solution in preparation of radial artery for coronary grafting. Ann Thorac Surg. 1996;61(2):610-614.

[63] Martin W, Furchgott RF, Villani GM, Jothianandan D. Phosphodiesterase inhibitors induce endothelium-dependent relaxation of rat and rabbit aorta by potentiating the effects of spontaneously released endothelium-derived relaxing factor. J Pharmacol Exp Ther. 1986;237(2):539-547.

[64] Huddart H, Saad KH. Papaverine-induced inhibition of electrical and mechanical activity and calcium movements of rat ileal smooth muscle. J Exp Biol. 1980;86:99-114.

[65] Fujioka M. Lack of a causal relationship between the vasodilator effect of papaverine and cyclic AMP production in the dog basilar artery. Br J Pharmacol. 1984;83(1):113-124.

[66] Brading AF, Burdyga TV, Scripnyuk ZD. The effects of papaverine on the electrical and mechanical activity of the guinea-pig ureter. J Physiol. 1983;334:79-89.

[67] Boerboom LE, Olinger GN, Bonchek LI, Gunay II, Kissebah AH, Rodriguez ER, Ferrans VJ. The relative influence of arterial pressure versus intraoperative distention on lipid accumulation in primate vein bypass grafts. J Thorac Cardiovasc Surg. 1985;90(5): 756-764.

[68] Malone JM, Kischer CW, Moore WS. Changes in venous endothelial fibrinolytic activity and histology with in vitro venous distention and arterial implantation. Am J Surg. 1981;142(2):178-182.

[69] van Son JA, Tavilla G, Noyez L. Detrimental sequelae on the wall of the internal mammary artery caused by hydrostatic dilation with diluted papaverine solution. J Thorac Cardiovasc Surg. 1992;104(4):972-976.

[70] Constantinides P, Robinson M. Ultrastructural injury of arterial endothelium. 1. Effects of pH, osmolarity, anoxia, and temperature. Arch Pathol. 1969;88(2):99-105.

[71] Roberts AJ, Hay DA, Jawahar LM, et al. Biochemical and ultrastructural integrity of the saphenous vein conduit during CABG: preliminary results of the effect of papaverine. J Thorac Cardiovasc Surg 1984;88:39-48.

[72] He GW, Buxton BF, Rosenfeldt FL, Angus JA, Tatoulis J. Pharmacologic dilatation of the internal mammary artery during coronary bypass grafting. J Thorac Cardiovasc Surg. 1994;107(6):1440-1444.

[73] Cunningham JN Jr. Papaverine hydrochloride preservation of vein grafts. J Thorac Cardiovasc Surg. 1982;84(6):933.

[74] He GW, Yang CQ, Mack MJ, Acuff TE, Ryan WH, Starr A. Interaction between endothelin and vasodilators in the human internal mammary artery. Br J Clin Pharmacol. 1994;38(6):505-512.

[75] He GW, Shaw J, Yang CQ, Hughes C, Thomson D, McCaughan B, Hendle PN, Baird DK. Inhibitory effects of glyceryl trinitrate on alpha-adrenoceptor mediated contraction in the human internal mammary artery. Br J Clin Pharmacol. 1992;34(3):236-243.

[76] He GW, Yang CO, Gately H, Furnary A, Swanson J, Ahmad A, Floten S, Wood J, Starr A. Potential greater than additive vasorelaxant actions of milrinone and nitroglycerin on human conduit arteries. Br J Clin Pharmacol. 1996;41(2):101-107.

[77] He GW, Yang CQ. Comparison of the vasorelaxant effect of nitroprusside and nitroglycerin in the human radial artery in vitro. Br J Clin Pharmacol. 1999;48(1):99-104.

[78] Zabeeda D, Medalion B, Jackobshvilli S, Ezra S, Schachner A, Cohen AJ. Comparison of systemic vasodilators: effects on flow in internal mammary and radial arteries. Ann Thorac Surg. 2001;71(1):138-141.

[79] Shapira OM, Xu A, Vita JA, Aldea GS, Shah N, Shemin RJ, Keaney JF Jr. Nitroglycerin is superior to diltiazem as a coronary bypass conduit vasodilator. J Thorac Cardiovasc Surg. 1999;117(5):906-911.

[80] Shapira OM, Alkon JD, Macron DS, Keaney JF Jr, Vita JA, Aldea GS, Shemin RJ. Nitroglycerin is preferable to diltiazem for prevention of coronary bypass conduit spasm. Ann Thorac Surg. 2000;70(3):883-888.

[81] Chavanon O, Cracowski JL, Hacini R, Stanke F, Durand M, Noirclerc M, Blin D. Effect of topical vasodilators on gastroepiploic artery graft. Ann Thorac Surg. 1999;67(5): 1295-1298

[82] Lobato EB, Janelle GM, Urdaneta F, Martin TD. Comparison of milrinone versus nitroglycerin, alone and in combination, on grafted internal mammary artery flow after cardiopulmonary bypass: effects of alpha-adrenergic stimulation. J Cardiothorac Vasc Anesth. 2001;15(6):723-727.

[83] Cable DG, Caccitolo JA, Pearson PJ, O'Brien T, Mullany CJ, Daly RC, Orszulak TA, Schaff HV. New approaches to prevention and treatment of radial artery graft vasospasm. Circulation. 1998;98(19 Suppl):II15-21.

[84] Beavo JA, Reifsnyder DH. Primary sequence of cyclic nucleotide phosphodiesterase isozymes and the design of selective inhibitors. Trends Pharmacol Sci. 1990;11(4): 150-155. Review.

[85] Beavo JA. Multiple isozymes of cyclic nucleotide phosphodiesterase. Adv Second Messenger Phosphoprotein Res. 1988;22:1-38. Review.

[86] He GW, Yang CQ. Inhibition of vasoconstriction by phosphodiesterase III inhibitor milrinone in human conduit arteries used as coronary bypass grafts. J Cardiovasc Pharmacol. 1996;28(2):208-214.

[87] Liu JJ, Doolan LA, Xie B, Chen JR, Buxton BF. Direct vasodilator effect of milrinone, an inotropic drug, on arterial coronary bypass grafts. J Thorac Cardiovasc Surg. 1997;113(1):108-113.

[88] He GW. Effect of milrinone on coronary artery bypass grafts. J Thorac Cardiovasc Surg. 1997;114(2):302-304.

[89] Yildiz O, Nacitarhan C, Seyrek M. Potassium channels in the vasodilating action of levosimendan on the human umbilical artery. J Soc Gynecol Investig. 2006;13(4): 312-315.

[90] Yildiz O. Vasodilating mechanisms of levosimendan: involvement of K^+ channels. J Pharmacol Sci. 2007;104(1):1-5.

[91] Yildiz O, Seyrek M, Yildirim V, Demirkilic U, Nacitarhan C. Potassium channel-related relaxation by levosimendan in the human internal mammary artery. Ann Thorac Surg. 2006;81(5):1715-1719.

http://dx.doi.org/10.5772/54723

[92] He GW, Acuff TE, Ryan WH, Yang CQ, Douthit MB, Bowman RT, Mack MJ. Inhibitory effects of calcium antagonists on alpha-adrenoceptor-mediated contraction in the human internal mammary artery. Br J Clin Pharmacol. 1994;37(2):173-179.

[93] Wei W, Floten HS, He GW. Interaction between vasodilators and vasopressin in internal mammary artery and clinical significance. Ann Thorac Surg. 2002;73(2):516-522.

[94] Atwal KS. Pharmacology and structure-activity relationships for K_{ATP} modulators: tissue-selective K_{ATP} openers. J Cardiovasc Pharmacol. 1994;24 Suppl 4:S12-17. Review.

[95] Quast U, Guillon JM, Cavero I. Cellular pharmacology of potassium channel openers in vascular smooth muscle. Cardiovasc Res. 1994;28(6):805-810. Review.

[96] Lazdunski M, Allard B, Bernardi H, De Weille J, Fosset M, Heurteaux C, Honoré E. ATP-sensitive K+ channels. Ren Physiol Biochem. 1994;17(3-4):118-120.

[97] He GW, Yang CQ, Graier WF, Yang JA. Hyperkalemia alters EDHF-mediated hyperpolarization and relaxation in coronary arteries. Am J Physiol. 1996;271(2 Pt 2):760-767.

[98] He GW, Yang CQ. Superiority of hyperpolarizing to depolarizing cardioplegia in protection of coronary endothelial function. J Thorac Cardiovasc Surg. 1997;114(4): 643-650.

[99] He GW. Potassium-channel opener in cardioplegia may restore coronary endothelial function. Ann Thorac Surg. 1998;66(4):1318-1322.

[100] Liu MH, Floten HS, Furnary AP, Yim AP, He GW. Effects of potassium channel opener aprikalim on the receptor-mediated vasoconstriction in the human internal mammary artery. Ann Thorac Surg. 2001;71(2):636-641.

[101] Ren Z, Floten S, Furnary A, Liu M, Gately H, Swanson J, Ahmad A, Yim AP, He GW. Effects of potassium channel opener KRN4884 on human conduit arteries used as coronary bypass grafts. Br J Clin Pharmacol. 2000;50(2):154-160.

[102] He GW, Yang CQ. Inhibition of vasoconstriction by potassium channel opener aprikalim in human conduit arteries used as bypass grafts. Br J Clin Pharmacol. 1997;44(4):353-359.

[103] Yan M, Liu DL, Chua YL, Chen C, Lim YL. Tyrosine kinase inhibitors suppress alpha1-adrenoceptor mediated contraction in human radial, internal mammary arteries and saphenous vein. Neurosci Lett. 2002;333(3):171-174.

[104] Conant AR, Shackcloth MJ, Oo AY, Chester MR, Simpson AW, Dihmis WC. Phenoxybenzamine treatment is insufficient to prevent spasm in the radial artery: the effect of other vasodilators. J Thorac Cardiovasc Surg. 2003;126(2):448-454.

[105] Shafiei M, Omrani G, Mahmoudian M. Coexistence of at least three distinct beta-adrenoceptors in human internal mammary artery. Acta Physiol Hung. 2000;87(3): 275-286.

[106] Cracowski JL, Stanke-Labesque F, Chavanon O, Blin D, Mallion JM, Bessard G, Devillier P. Vasorelaxant actions of enoximone, dobutamine, and the combination on human arterial coronary bypass grafts. J Cardiovasc Pharmacol. 1999;34(5):741-748.

[107] Katai R, Tsuneyoshi I, Hamasaki J, Onomoto M, Suehiro S, Sakata R, Kanmura Y. The variable effects of dopamine among human isolated arteries commonly used for coronary bypass grafts. Anesth Analg. 2004;98(4):915-920, table of contents.

[108] Yildiz O, Ciçek S, Ay I, Demirkiliç U, Tuncer M. Hypertension increases the contractions to sumatriptan in the human internal mammary artery. Ann Thorac Surg. 1996;62(5):1392-1395.

[109] Yildiz O, Smith JR, Purdy RE. Serotonin and vasoconstrictor synergism. Life Sci. 1998;62(19):1723-1732. Review.

[110] Chen J, Yildiz O, Purdy RE. Phenylephrine precontraction increases the sensitivity of rabbit femoral artery to serotonin by enabling 5-HT1-like receptors. J Cardiovasc Pharmacol. 2000;35(6):863-870.

[111] Rego AC, Oliveira CR. Influence of lipid peroxidation on [3H]ketanserin binding to 5-HT_2 prefrontal cortex receptors. Neurochem Int. 1995;27(6):489-496.

[112] Yildiz O, Seyrek M, Gul H, Un I, Yildirim V, Ozal E, Uzun M, Bolu E. Testosterone relaxes human internal mammary artery in vitro. J Cardiovasc Pharmacol. 2005;45(6): 580-585.

[113] Yildiz O, Seyrek M, Un I, Gul H, Candemir G, Yildirim V. The relationship between risk factors and testosterone-induced relaxations in human internal mammary artery. J Cardiovasc Pharmacol. 2005;45(1):4-7.

[114] Seyrek M, Yildiz O, Ulusoy HB, Yildirim V. Testosterone relaxes isolated human radial artery by potassium channel opening action. J Pharmacol Sci. 2007;103(3):309-316.

[115] Yildiz O, Seyrek M. Vasodilating mechanisms of testosterone. Exp Clin Endocrinol Diabetes. 2007;115(1):1-6. Review.

[116] Irkilata HC, Yildiz O, Yildirim I, Seyrek M, Basal S, Dayanc M, Ulku C. The vasodilator effect of testosterone on the human internal spermatic vein and its relation to varicocele grade. J Urol. 2008;180(2):772-776.

[117] Seyrek M, Irkilata HC, Vural IM, Yildirim I, Basal S, Yildiz O, Dayanc M. Testosterone relaxes human internal spermatic vein through potassium channel opening action. Urology. 2011;78(1): 233.e1-5.

[118] Yildiz O, Seyrek M, Irkilata HC, Yildirim I, Tahmaz L, Dayanc M. Testosterone might cause relaxation of human corpus cavernosum by potassium channel opening action. Urology. 2009;74(1):229-232.

[119] Yildiz O, Seyrek M. Effects of testosterone on vascular tone. In Chichinadze K (ed.) Testosterone: Biochemistry, therapeutic uses and physiological effects. Nova Science Publishers; 2012. p159-183.

[120] Murakami E, Iwata H, Imaizumi M, Takemura H. Prevention of arterial graft spasm by botulinum toxin: an in-vitro experiment. Interact Cardiovasc Thorac Surg. 2009;9(3): 395-398.

[121] Ozdemir C, Ikizler M, Besogul Y, Karakaya A, Sirmagul B. An alternative agent for radial arterial graft spasm: application of topical iloprost. Scand Cardiovasc J. 2007;41(3):201-206.

[122] Mussa S, Choudhary BP, Taggart DP. Radial artery conduits for coronary artery bypass grafting: current perspective. J Thorac Cardiovasc Surg. 2005;129(2):250-253. Review.

[123] [123] Barner HB. The continuing evolution of arterial conduits. Ann Thorac Surg. 1999;68(3 Suppl):S1-8.

[124] Shah PJ, Bui K, Blackmore S, Gordon I, Hare DL, Fuller J, Seevanayagam S, Buxton BF. Has the in situ right internal thoracic artery been overlooked? An angiographic study of the radial artery, internal thoracic arteries and saphenous vein graft patencies in symptomatic patients. Eur J Cardiothorac Surg. 2005;27(5):870-875.

[125] Sahin MA, Guler A, Cingoz F, Yokusoglu M, Demirkol S, Ozal E, Demirkilic U, Arslan M. Mid-term results of radial artery grafts used in coronary bypass surgery. Gulhane Med J. 2012; 54(1): 7-13. Turkish.

[126] Possati G, Gaudino M, Prati F, Alessandrini F, Trani C, Glieca F, Mazzari MA, Luciani N, Schiavoni G. Long-term results of the radial artery used for myocardial revascularization. Circulation. 2003;108(11):1350-1354.

[127] Lockowandt U, Ritchie A, Grossebener M, Franco-Cereceda A. Endothelin and effects of endothelin-receptor activation in the mammary and radial artery. Scand Cardiovasc J. 2004;38(4):240-244.

[128] Gupte SA, Zias EA, Sarabu MR, Wolin MS. Role of prostaglandins in mediating differences in human internal mammary and radial artery relaxation elicited by hypoxia. J Pharmacol Exp Ther. 2004;311(2):510-518.

[129] Attaran S, John L, El-Gamel A. Clinical and potential use of pharmacological agents to reduce radial artery spasm in coronary artery surgery. Ann Thorac Surg. 2008;85(4): 1483-1489. Review.

[130] Vuurmans T, Hilton D. Brewing the right cocktail for radial intervention. Indian Heart J. 2010;62(3):221-225. Review.

[131] Suma H. Optimal use of the gastroepiploic artery. Semin Thorac Cardiovasc Surg. 1996;8(1):24-28.

[132] Koike R, Suma H, Kondo K, Oku T, Satoh H, Fukuda S, Takeuchi A. Pharmacological response of internal mammary artery and gastroepiploic artery. Ann Thorac Surg. 1990;50(3):384-386.

[133] Ochiai M, Ohno M, Taguchi J, Hara K, Suma H, Isshiki T, Yamaguchi T, Kurokawa K. Responses of human gastroepiploic arteries to vasoactive substances: comparison with

responses of internal mammary arteries and saphenous veins. J Thorac Cardiovasc Surg. 1992;104(2):453-438.

[134] He GW, Yang CQ. Comparison among arterial grafts and coronary artery. An attempt at functional classification. J Thorac Cardiovasc Surg. 1995;109(4):707-715.

[135] Yang Z, Siebenmann R, Studer M, Egloff L, Lüscher TF. Similar endothelium-dependent relaxation, but enhanced contractility, of the right gastroepiploic artery as compared with the internal mammary artery. J Thorac Cardiovasc Surg. 1992;104(2): 459-464.

[136] Ali AT, Montgomery WD, Santamore WP, Spence PA. Preventing gastroepiploic artery spasm: papaverine vs calcium channel blockade. J Surg Res. 199715;71(1):41-48.

[137] Formica F, Ferro O, Brustia M, Corti F, Colagrande L, Bosisio E, Paolini G. Effects of papaverine and glycerylnitrate-verapamil solution as topical and intraluminal vasodilators for internal thoracic artery. Ann Thorac Surg. 2006;81(1):120-124.

[138] Mügge A, Barton MR, Cremer J, Frombach R, Lichtlen PR. Different vascular reactivity of human internal mammary and inferior epigastric arteries in vitro. Ann Thorac Surg. 1993;56(5):1085-1089.

[139] Tadjkarimi S, O'Neil GS, Schyns CJ, Borland JA, Chester AH, Yacoub MH. Vasoconstrictor profile of the inferior epigastric artery. Ann Thorac Surg. 1993;56(5):1090-1095.

[140] Tadjkarimi S, Chester AH, Borland JA, Schyns CJ, O'Neil GS, Yacoub MH. Endothelial function and vasodilator profile of the inferior epigastric artery. Ann Thorac Surg. 1994;58(1):207-210.

Chapter 16

Surgical Treatment for Diffuse Coronary Artery Diseases

Cheng-Xiong Gu, Yang Yu and Chuan Wang

Additional information is available at the end of the chapter

http://dx.doi.org/10.5772/54416

1. Introduction

Currently coronary artery bypass grafting (CABG) is the most commonly used procedure for revascularization of coronary heart disease. However it may not be suitable for the patients with diffuse coronary artery lesions, for which endarterectomy is a way but it's not feasible to thin coronary artery without inner lumen or to the immature plaque. In this case, it may be a proper therapeutic option to achieve coronary revascularization by retrograde perfusion via cardiac venous system, namely retrograde coronary venous bypass grafting (CVBG). [1] Saphenous veins could be used to realize arterialization for great or middle cardiac vein by separate or sequential bypass grafting. But it would cause myocardial hemorrhage, edema and even heart failure due to excessive perfusion by high pressure [2]. However, internal mammary artery (IMA), as one kind of muscular artery materials, can enlarge or contract its lumen to adjust the blood flow with strong adaptability [3]. Off-pump coronary artery bypass surgery (OPCAB) has been widely applied as a less invasive method of myocardial revascularization in recent years. It could avoid the systemic inflammatory effects caused by cardiopulmonary bypass (CPB). OPCAB has more merits such as low mortality, low morbidity, and reduced costs, especially in high risk patients [4]. Therefore, sequential bypass of bilateral IMA combined with arterialization for middle cardiac vein were carried out during OPCAB for patients with diffuse lesions existing in right coronary artery.

2. Definition & anatomy

Diffuse CAD was defined as: length of significant stenoses ≥20 mm; multiple significant stenoses (≥70% narrowing) in the same artery separated by segments of apparently normal (but probably diseased) vessel; and significant narrowing involving the whole length of the coronary artery [5] (Figure 1). Provided a mature plaque is successfully endarterected through

the true arterial lumen (Figure 2)., patients with a long diffuse lesion can be treated very efficiently. But sometimes long, severe diffuse coronary artery stenosis isn't recommended for surgical treatment because of its low patency and more postoperative complications [6]. (Figure 3)

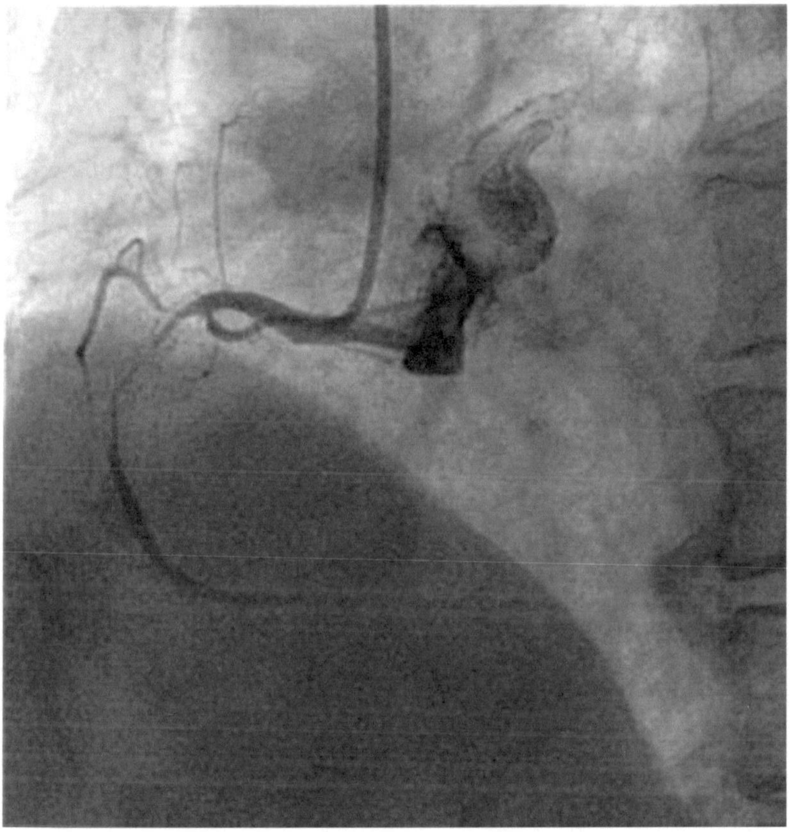

Figure 1. Diffuse CAD of the right coronary artery

3. History

The idea that the mammalian myocardium could be nourished by means of a flow of blood from the coronary venous system, acting as an alternative myocardial perfusion way because it would not be affected by atherosclerosis, was proposed by Pratt in 1898 [7]. However, few clinical trials and long-term outcome data have been presented and clinical use of venous arterialization has rarely been reported. Further experiments were made in 1943, in which the coronary sinus in a canine model was arterialized by using an autologous carotid artery as a conduit between the dogs descending aorta and the coronary sinus. In 1948, Beck and colleagues first carried out blobally retroperfusion by CVBG through coronary sinus[8]. These

http://dx.doi.org/10.5772/54416

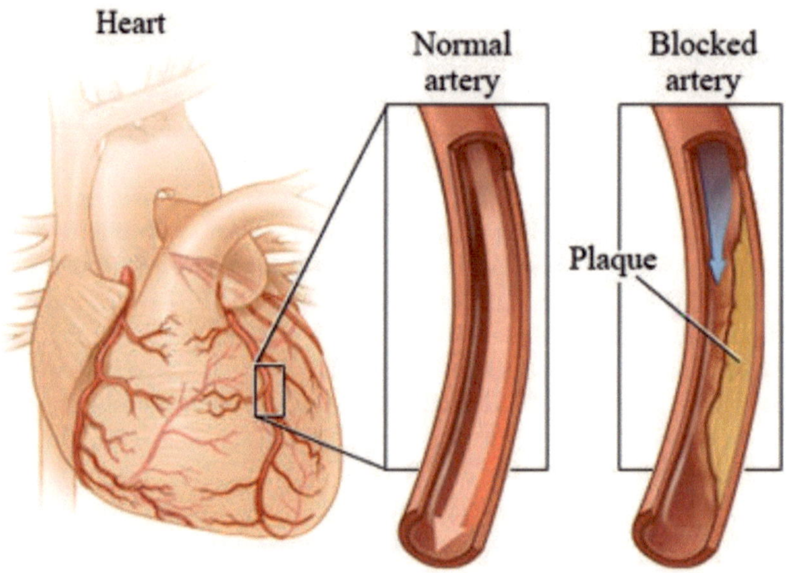

Figure 2. Mature plaque in the blocked coronary artery

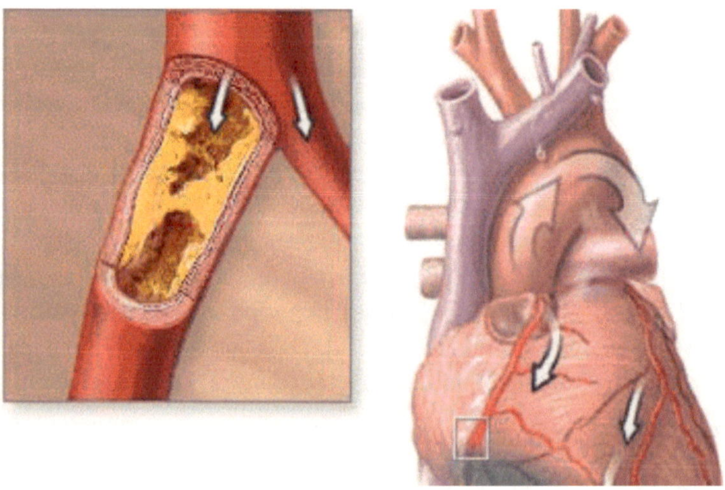

Figure 3. Diffuse coronary artery with immature plaque

findings led them to state that there are communications between the venous and arterial sides of the circulation which, in the dead specimen, allowed blood flow in a retrograde direction. The Beck II procedure afterwards consisted of a free vein graft from the aorta to the coronary sinus, with a second operation 2 to 3 weeks later to ligate the coronary sinus, which reported remarkable success in attempts to revascularize the heart. The effectiveness of reversing flow in the coronary venous system had been debated and this operation was gradually abandoned because of related mortality of 26.1% and development of CABG. However, CABG was soon discovered to have its own limitations, particularly in patients with diffuse atherosclerotic lesion and tiny coronary arteries. Arterialization of coronary veins therefore regained its appeal. Arealis and colleagues brought forth selective CVBG in 1973 which was made only for part of ischemic myocardium, while normal reflux was kept for the rest myocardial veins. Great cardiac vein parallel to LAD and middle cardiac vein parallel to PDA were selected as goal vessels. Eventually an ample report of CVBG animal trial was published by Dr. Hochberg in 1979which indicated CVBG's advantages, such as perfusion all layers of the myocardium, especially the subendocardium – the crucial layer of myocardial muscle[2]. However, this mechanism had been studied at the experimental level because its relatively high clinical mortality and was only theoretic until CVBG technique developed in the recent years.

4. Preclinical study and animal trials

Historically, most studies of revascularization have been based on and reported according to angiographic criteria. Some patients with significant arteriosclerosis of the heart are not amenable to revascularization of a coronary artery because they have a combination of microangiopathy and significant macroangiopathy. Therefore cardiac surgeons developed the technical approach of venous revascularization. Several systematic reviews have been conducted in an attempt to define the exact role of animal models as platforms for future human therapy [9-12].We investigated the benefit of arterialization of a cardiac vein under these circumstances in some animal models [13] which indicate retrograde venous revascularization is possible and improves cardiac function in a state of acute ischemia so we could find its way into practical use in coronary heart surgery. In experimental studies in a variety of animals and in human clinical studies, retroperfusion of the coronary sinus has been used to improve myocardial perfusion and postischemic systolic and diastolic function in many surgical procedures. In addition, animal trials, mostly involving sheep, dogs and pigs showed that arterialization of cardiac veins decreases infarct size as well[11,14]. These animal models are likely to be useful for pre-clinical evaluation of the functional effects of surgical therapy.

5. Surgical option – CVBG versus traditional CABG

There is no doubt that for patients with surgical triple-vessel coronary disease and a severely diseased left main artery, CABG appears to be preferable [15]. Despite constant advances in surgical and interventional therapy of coronary artery disease, there remains a group of

patients who are not amenable to these traditional treatment strategies. Many patients being referred for CABG nowadays have far advanced CAD, which is often diffuse and exhibits poor vessel runoff. The idea of myocardial revascularization by means of grafting the coronary venous system is more than a century old; in cases of diffuse coronary artery disease, this may represent a valid therapeutic option [16].

The lack of suitable targets vessels remains a challenge for aortocoronary bypass grafting in diffuse coronary heart disease. Although this figure approximates 20% to 50% frequency reported in many series [17], our study represents a highly selective group with diffuse coronary disease in which CABG was not feasible with or without an endarterectomy.

5.1. Data analysis

From March 2004 to August 2010, patients with diffuse right coronary lesions were studied retrospectively and divided into two groups (Table1). Informed consent and ethical review committee approval were obtained. Group 1 included seventeen patients who underwent selective CVBG during OPCAB while group 2 included twenty-one patients without right coronary artery surgical therapy. Group 1 included eleven male cases (64.7%), the mean age was (46.1±6.2) years, seven hypertension cases (41.2%) and ten diabetes mellitus (58.8%) cases were involved. The case number of cardiac function from II–IV grade was eight, eight, and one respectively. Left ventricular ejection fraction (LVEF) was 0.52±0.09 and left ventricular end diastolic diameter (LVEDD) was (52.7±5.1) mm. Group 2 included fourteen male cases (66.7%), the mean age was (45.9±5.7) years, nine hypertension cases (42.9%) and eleven diabetes mellitus (52.4%) cases were involved. The case number of cardiac function from II–IV level was twelve, seven, two respectively. LVEF was 0.52±0.11 and LVEDD was (51.9±5.2) mm. There was no significant difference between the two groups ($P > 0.05$). All the patients had angina pectoris symptom before operation. It was indicated by electrocardiogram that all the cases with old myocardial infarction had obvious ST-T changes. Coronary angiography showed that seven cases had double-vessel lesions and ten cases had triple-vessel lesions in group 1; nine cases had double-vessel lesions and twelve cases had triple-vessel lesions in group 2. Right coronary artery of all the patients took on diffuse lesions with vascular diameter <1 mm and length >20 mm. It was shown by vascular ultrasound examination that blood flow in bilateral mammary artery was smooth and vascular diameter >2 mm; and left subclavian artery was not narrow.

OPCAB was performed with an average of 3.6 grafts per patient, group 1 being (3.3±1.1) grafts and group 2 being (2.2±1.6) grafts respectively. These patients discharged eight to fourteen days after the operation. Determination of blood flow was made for eleven cases in group 1 and thirteen cases in group 2 which were (81.47±32.65) ml/min and (76.82±28.36) ml/min in trunk of IMA, (32.52±18.82) ml/min and (28.12±16.71) ml/min in trunk of left IMA, (39.63±19.02) ml/min and (35.92±18.34) ml/min in trunk of right IMA. The both groups had no death. Tracheal cannula was pulled out on the date of operation or one day after operation. Low-dose positive inotropic drugs were used as assistance for four cases postoperatively. All the patients had no brain complication and no infection of sternum and mediastinum.

	Group 1 N=17	Group 2 N=21
Gender (M/F)	11/6	14/7
Age (years)	46.1±6.2	45.9±5.7
Hypertension (yes/no)	7/10	9/12
Diabetes mellitus (yes/no)	10/7	11/10
LVEF	0.52±0.09	0.52±0.11
LVEDD (mm)	52.7±5.1	51.9±5.2
Coronary angiography		
Double-vessel lesions	7	9
Triple-vessel lesions	10	12

LVEF: Left ventricular ejection fraction; *LVEDD*, left ventricular end diastolic diameter.

Table 1. Characteristics of patients

5.2. Surgical procedure

5.2.1. General surgical procedure

In group 1, standard median sternotomy incision was applied for the exposure of the heart under general anesthesia. Bilateral IMAs were harvested as longer as possible and usually cut proximally at the starting position from subclavian artery and distally on the level of Xiphoid. Surrounding tissues of IMA were desected and removed so as to ensure enough length of IMA (generally 18–25 cm). The free right IMA was anastomosed with left IMA to form a bifurcation as "Y" type. The anastomotic position on the LIMA should be determined according to its length and the distance from the bypass grafting anastomosis between LIMA and LAD or diagonal. The position was usually selected at the location of 3–4 cm proximal to the first anastomotic site of left IMA, and 8-0 prolene suture was utilized in end-to-side anastomosis between two mammary arteries. Subsequently, CABG was carried out on beating heart. Left IMA was anastomosed to left anterior descending artery (LAD) and then right IMA was sequentially anastomosed with diagonal branch and circumflex artery (obtuse marginal and posterior branch of the left ventricle). Then the end of middle cardiac vein proximal to heart was blocked with 6-0 prolene suture so that blood can not reflow to coronary sinus in normal way. Finally, end-to-side anastomosis between middle cardiac vein parallel to right coronary post descending artery (PDA) and right IMA was performed with 8-0 prolene suture. When all the vessels were anastomosed and blood circulation was stable, blood flow of grafting vessels was determined by Transonic H1311 flowmeter (Transonic Systems, Inc., Ithaca, NY, USA). Incision was carefully washed before closing chest. In group 2, no branch of the right coronary artery was bypass grafted.

5.2.2. *Unique surgical procedure – Blood flow limitation*

Venous arterialization occurs when a vein segment is transposed as a bypass graft into the arterial circulation, and atherosclerosis is a common feature of autogenous vein bypass grafts resulting in their long-term failure [18-20]. Arterial pressure-induced distension is thought to play a major role in the wall thickening of vein grafts, which may in turn favor atherosclerotic complications [21,22]. Reduction of the wall distension by perfusion pressure reduction using blood flow limitation protected the vein grafts from atherosclerosis, possibly as a result of the decrease in wall thickening that occurred in response to arterialization [23,24].

Saphenous vein was commonly used to complete CVBG. After harvesting, meticulous care should be taken to avoid distention of the vein graft. An infusion pressure of no more than 100 mmHg is recommended for minimal endothelial damage [25]. In our previous study and emerged that ischemia and infarction of myocardium would happen if the blood flow in grafting vessel was less than 50 ml/min. The blood was delivered into the cardiac veins by the native arterial pressure, However when intravascular pressure reached 60 mm Hg (1 mmHg = 0.133 kPa) or higher, the risk of complications would increase such as myocardial edema and even intramural hemorrhage and so on [26]. In this case, we used to ligate the vein graft to 1.5 to 2 mm in diameter with two interrupted silk lines to control blood flow (Figure 4). It has been reported that infarct size can be reduced by which arterial blood is delivered retrogradely to the ischemic myocardium through the cardiac veins [27].

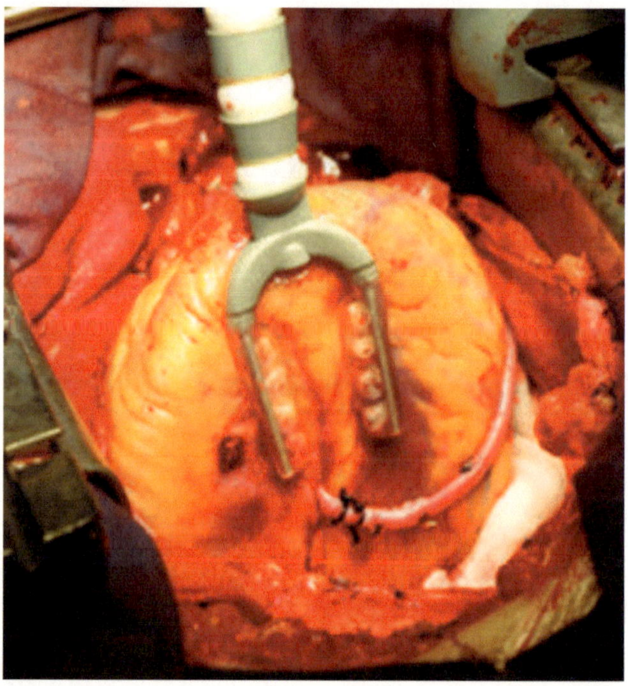

Figure 4. Flow-limited CVBG

5.3. Follow up

Three months after discharge, all the patients in group 1 had no preoperative symptom. Myocardial ischemia was not found by electrocardiogram in group 1. Postoperative angina was found in eight cases of group 2 and electrocardiogram showed inferior wall myocardial ischemia. There was significant difference between the two groups ($P < 0.05$). Cardiac function was improved to class I ($P < 0.001$), LVEF was increased to 0.60±0.08 ($P < 0.001$) in group 1 and 0.56±0.10 ($P < 0.001$) in group 2 which showed no preoperative differences and the postoperative LVEF of group 1 was superior to group 2 while there was no significant difference between these two groups. LVEDD decreased to (48.1±3.4) mm ($P < 0.001$) in group 1 and (47.2±3.5) mm ($P < 0.001$) in group 2. Patients underwent physical examination and echocardiography in our outpatient clinic periodically after discharge. These data were compared with the patients' preoperative variables. Several examination of myocardial nuclide imaging, coronary angiography (41 months postop.) and CT scanning (5 years postop.) were carried out (Figure 5).

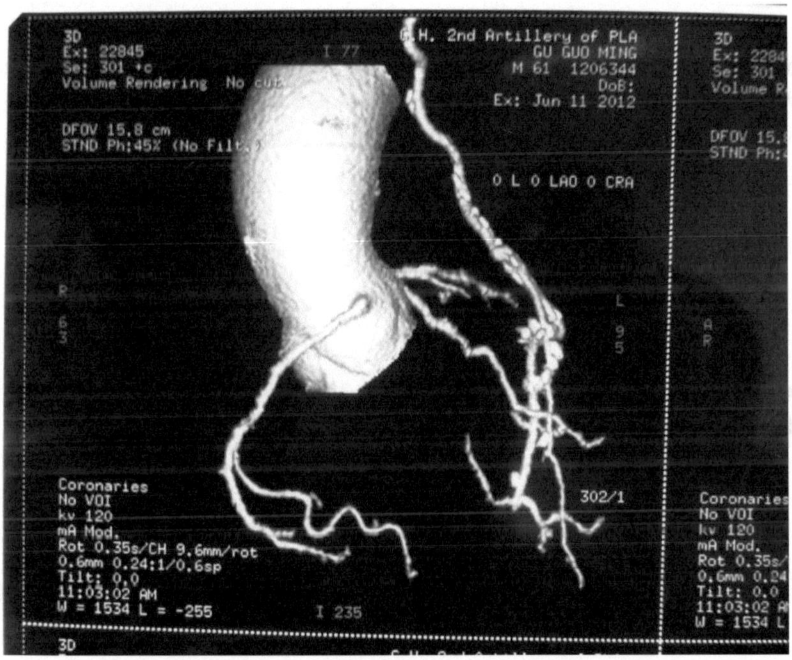

Figure 5. follow-up CT scanning data of CVBG.

6. Conclusion

In the past few decades, there was an increase in the number of patients with coronary heart disease who were not eligible for standard procedures including CABG and percutaneous coronary angioplasty, and diffuse coronary atherosclerosis occupies 12%–30% of patients

requiring further intervention [28]. Clinical trials investigating treatment with angiogenesis factors and gene therapy have been initiated, and new devices for creating cardiac arteriovenous fistulas percutaneously have also been introduced [29-32]. Whereas injection of growth factors require an adequate arterial inflow, which is not often existent in the hearts of these "no option patients". New catheter devices to create a fistula between a coronary artery and the accompanying vein or, as performed in animal experiments, a coronary vein and the left ventricle, are difficult to handle, and hold all the risks of catheterization of a severely altered vessel [33]. Before that, small numbers of reports of the clinical application had published, so no remarkable conclusions can be yet drawn [34-37]. As the efficiency of these new methods awaits the evaluation of long-term trials, we think that some patients might benefit from the revival of an "old" procedure that is retrograde venous revascularization. In both short and long-term experiments, effective selected area perfusion had been achieved.

Despite the successful and widespread application of these revascularization procedures, a large number of patients are not good candidates for either angioplasty or surgery. These "no-option" patients frequently have diffuse coronary disease without a discrete target for angioplasty, stenting, or surgical bypass [33].In clinical application, we draw some experiences as follows. Blood flow of IMA is important to ensure perfusion of myocardium after bypass grafting which can be determined by preoperative vascular ultrasound examination and intraoperative testing. It is also important to make sure the diameter of each anastomotic incision 1.5 times as that of IMA in order to keep adequate blood flow. For the patients with coronary vessel less than 1.5 mm in diameter, it is necessary to use 8-0 prolene suture in case of anastomotic stricture. Attention should be focused on not damaging the posterior wall of middle cardiac vein while opening it, because the vascular wall of coronary vein is obviously thinner than that of coronary artery. The graft should be fixed to myocardium on both sides because IMA and middle cardiac vein are prone to twist due to different thickness of vascular wall. It is valuable to observe the difference of color on both segments of middle cardiac vein in the ligation. If red and dark are distinctive, it is indicated the ligation is definite. Otherwise it is possible that there is some residue blood flow [38]. It is useful to measure blood flow of each graft with flowmeter after anastomosis in order to keep vessel grafting patent.

CVBG surgery is indicated for both the relief of symptoms and the improvement of life expectancy in patients suffering from diffuse coronary heart disease [39-41]. We believe the selective CVBG should be considered in cases of coronary artery disease not amenable to traditional revascularization strategies [42-45]. Indications of selective CVBG include the patients with tenuous right coronary artery or diffuse lesions. It is possibly fit for the patients who need reoperation of CABG as well [46-48]. A substantial improvement in the long-term prognosis may be expected with more precise anastomosis.

Author details

Cheng-Xiong Gu, Yang Yu and Chuan Wang

6 Department of Cardiac Surgery, Beijing An Zhen Hospital, Capital Medical University, Beijing, China

References

[1] YU Yang, YAN Xiao-lei, Gu cheng-xiong, et al. Off-pump sequential bilateral internal mammary artery grafting combined with selective arterialization of the coronary venous system. Chinese Medical Journal 2011;124(19):3017-3021

[2] Hochberg MS, Roberts WC, Morrow AG, Austen WG.. Selective arterialization of the coronary venous system. Encouraging long-term flow evaluation utilizing radioactive microspheres. J Thorac Cardiovasc Surg 1979; 77: 1-12.

[3] Rankin JS, Tuttle RH, Wechsler AS, Teichmann TL, Glower DD, Califf RM. Techniques and benefits of multiple internal mammary artery bypass at 20 years of follow-up. Ann Thorac Surg 2007; 83: 1008-1014.

[4] Guru V, Glasgow KW, Fremes SE, Austin PC, Teoh K, Tu JV. The real-world outcomes of off-pump coronary artery bypass surgery in a public health care system. Can J Cardiol 2007;23: 281-286.

[5] Di Sciascio G, Patti G, Nasso G, Manzoli A, D'Ambrosio A, Abbate A. Early and longterm results of stenting of diffuse coronary artery disease. Am J Cardiol 2000;86:1166–70.

[6] Jeffrey H. Shuhaiber, Alexander N. Evans, Malek G. Massad, Alexander S. Geha et al. Mechanisms and future directions for prevention of vein graft failure in coronary bypass surgery. European Journal of Cardio-thoracic Surgery 22 (2002) 387–396.

[7] Pratt FH. The circulation through the veins of Thebesius. J Boston Soc Med Sci 1897; 1: 29-34.

[8] Beck CS, Stanton E, Batiuchok W. Revascularization of the heart by graft or systemic artery into the coronary sinus. JAMA 1948; 137: 436-442.

[9] R.W. Eckstein, George Smith, Morton Eleff and James Demming. The Effect of Arterialization of the Coronary Sinus in Dogs on Mortality Following Acute Coronary Occlusion. Circulation 1952;6;16-20

[10] Mark S. Hochberg, and W. Gerald Austen, Selective Retrograde Coronary Venous Perfusion, Ann Thorac Surg 1980;29:578-588

[11] Peter Boekstegers, Wolfgang Peter, Georges Von Degenfeld, et al. Preservation of Regional Myocardial Function and Myocardial Oxygen Tension During Acute Ischemia in Pigs: Comparison of selective Synchronized Suction and Retroinfusion of Coronary Veins to Synchronized Coronary Venous Retroperfusion. J Awn Coll Cardiol 1994, 23 :45'9-69.

[12] Stephanie Kwei, George Stavrakis, Masaya Takahas, et al. Early Adaptive Responses of the Vascular Wall during Venous Arterialization in Mice. American Journal of Pathology, Vol. 164, No. 1, January 2004.

[13] Michaela Elisabeth Resetar, Cris Ullmann, Petra Broeske et al. Selective arterialization of a cardiac vein in a model of cardiac microangiopathy and macroangiopathy in sheep. The Journal of Thoracic and Cardiovascular Surgery. May 2007

[14] J. Kevin Drury, Shigeru Yamazaki, Michael C. Fishbein, et al. Synchronized Diastolic Coronary Venous Retroperfusion: Results of a Preclinical Safety and Efficacy Study, J Am Call Cardiol1985;6:328-35

[15] Donald E. Gregg and David C. Sabiston, JR. Current Research and Problems of the Coronary Circulation. Circulation 1956;13;916-927.

[16] J. Rafael Sadaba, FRCS, and Unnikrishnan R. Nair, FRCS. Selective Arterialization of the Coronary Venous System. Ann Thorac Surg 2004;78:1458–60

[17] Richard S. Hahn, Maurice Kim, Revascularization of the Heart Histologic Changes after Arterialization of the Coronary Sinus. Circulation 1952;5;810-815.

[18] Glen R. Rhodes, Donald C. Syracuse, and Charles L. McIntosh. Evaluation of Regional Myocardial Nutrient Perfusion Following Selective Retrograde Arterialization of the Coronary Vein. The Annals of Thoracic Surgery Vol 25 No 4 April 1978.

[19] Raymond C. Truex and Martin J. Schwartz, Venous System of the Myocardium with Special Reference to the Conduction System. Circulation 1951;4;881-889

[20] A Zalewski, S Goldberg, S Slysh and PR Maroko, Myocardial protection via coronary sinus interventions: superior effects of arterialization compared with intermittent occlusion. Circulation 1985;71;1215-1223.

[21] J. Rafael Sadaba, FRCS, and Unnikrishnan R. Nair, FRCS, Selective Arterialization of the Coronary Venous System, Ann Thorac Surg 2004;78:1458–60.

[22] Jean Batellier, Michel Wassef, Regine Merval, Micheline Duriez, and Alain Tedgui. Protection From Atherosclerosis in Vein Grafts by a Rigid External Support. Arteriosclerosis and Thrombosis Vol 13, No 3 March 1993.

[23] Stephanie Kwei, George Stavrakis, Masaya Takahas, George Taylor, et al. Early Adaptive Responses of the Vascular Wall during Venous Arterialization in Mice. AJP January 2004, Vol. 164, No. 1

[24] Adcock Jr OT, Adcock GL, Wheeler JR, et al. Optimal techniques for harvesting and preparation of reversed autogenous vein grafts for use as arterial substitutes: a review. Surgery 1984;96(5):886–894.

[25] Malte Meesmann, Hrayr S. Karagueuzian, Takeshi, et al. Selective Perfusion of Ischemic Myocardium During Coronary Venous Retroinjection: A Study of the Causative Role of Venoarterial and Venoventricular Pressure Gradients, J Am Coil Cardiol 1987;10:887-97.

[26] Andrew Zalewski, Sheldon Goldberg, Sonya Slysh, et al. Myocardial protection via coronary sinus interventions: superior effects of arterialization compared with intermittent occlusion. Circulation 71, No. 6, 1215-1223, 1985.

[27] Sherif E. Moustafa, Kenton Zehr, Martina Mookadam, et al. Anomalous interarterial left coronary artery: An evidence based systematic overview. International Journal of Cardiology 126 (2008) 13–20.

[28] Nabil Dib, Edward. Diethrich, Ann Campbell, Amir Gahremanpour, et al. A percutaneous swine model of myocardial infarction. Journal of Pharmacological and Toxicological Methods 53 (2006) 256– 263.

[29] Emerson. Perin, Guilherme. Silva, Yi Zheng, Human Hepatocyte Growth Factor (VM202) Gene Therapy via Transendocardial Injection in a Pig Model of Chronic Myocardial Ischemia. Journal of Cardiac Failure Vol. 17 No. 7 July 2011.

[30] Nabil Dib, Edward. Diethrich, Ann Campbell, Amir Gahremanpour, et al. A percutaneous swine model of myocardial infarction, / Journal of Pharmacological and Toxicological Methods 53 (2006) 256– 263.

[31] ML Marcus, WM Chilian, H Kanatsuka, KC Dellsperger, CL Eastham and KG Lamping, Understanding the coronary circulation through studies at the microvascular level, Circulation 1990;82;1-7.

[32] Stephen N. Oesterle, Nicolaus Reifart, Eugen Hauptmann,et al. Percutaneous In Situ Coronary Venous Arterialization Report of the First Human Catheter-Based Coronary Artery Bypass. Circulation 2001;103;2539-2543

[33] GM Hutchins, A Kessler-Hanna and GW Moore, Development of the coronary arteries in the embryonic human heart, Circulation 1988;77;1250-1257.

[34] Kurt Wallner, Chen Li, Michael C. Fishbein, Arterialization of Human Vein Grafts Is Associated With Tenascin-C Expression, Journal of the American College of Cardiology Vol. 34, No. 3, 1999.

[35] Alexander Kulik, Michael A. Borger and Hugh E. Scully, Aortovenous bypass graft to the posterior left ventricle in absence of an identifiable coronary artery, Ann Thorac Surg 2004;78:313-314

[36] Anke M. Smits1, Jos F.M. Smits, Ischemic heart disease: models of myocardial hypertrophy and infarction. Drug Discovery Today: Disease Models, Vol. 1. No. 3 2004.

[37] Harold L. Lazar, Coronary sinus retroperfusion: Can forward progress still be achieved by using a backward technique? The Journal of Thoracic and Cardiovascular Surgery. Volume 127, Number 6, June 2004.

[38] Karl Mischke, Christian Knackstedt, Georg Mühlenbruch, Thomas Schimpf, et al. Imaging of the coronary venous system: Retrograde coronary sinus angiography ver-

sus venous phase coronary angiograms. International Journal of Cardiology 119 (2007) 339–343.

[39] Tomoko Tani, Kazuaki Tanabe, Minako Tani, Fumie Ono, et al. Quantitative assessment of harmonic power doppler myocardial perfusion imaging with intravenous levovist in patients with myocardial infarction: comparison with myocardial viability evaluated by coronary flow reserve and coronary flow pattern of infarct-related artery. Cardiovascular Ultrasound 2005, 3:22.

[40] Michaela Elisabeth Resetar, Cris Ullmann, Petra Broeske, et al. Selective arterialization of a cardiac vein in a model of cardiac microangiopathy and macroangiopathy in sheep. The Journal of Thoracic and Cardiovascular Surgery, Volume 133, Number 5, May 2007.

[41] Egemen Tuzun, Eddie Oliveira, Cuneyt Narin, Hassan Khalil, et al. Correlation of Ischemic Area and Coronary Flow With Ameroid Size in a Porcine Model. Journal of Surgical Research Vol. 164, NO. 1, NOVEMBER 2010,164, 38–42 (2010)

[42] Aaron M. Abarbanell, Jeremy L. Herrmann, Brent R. Weil, et al. RESEARCH REVIEW Animal Models of Myocardial and Vascular Injury, Journal of surgical research: VOL. 162, NO. 2, aug 2010, 239–249.

[43] Masanori Fujita, Yuji Morimoto, Masayuki Ishihara, Masafumi Shimizu, et al. A New Rabbit Model of Myocardial Infarction without Endotracheal Intubation. Journal of Surgical Research: Vol. 116, No. 1, January 2004, 124–128116.

[44] Nabil Dib, Edward B. Diethrich, Ann Campbell, Amir Gahremanpour, et al. A percutaneous swine model of myocardial infarction, Journal of Pharmacological and Toxicological Methods 53 (2006) 256– 263.

[45] Alexander Kulik, Michael A. Borger, and Hugh E. Scully, Aortovenous Bypass Graft to the Posterior Left Ventricle in Absence of an Identifiable Coronary Artery. Ann Thorac Surg 2004;78:314–6

[46] E. Marc Jolicoeur, MSc, Christopher. Granger, Timothy. et al. Clinical and research issues regarding chronic advanced coronary artery disease: Part I: Contemporary and emerging therapies. American Heart Journal Volume 155, Number 3. March 2008.

[47] Armando Pérez de Prado, Carlos Cuellas-Ramón, Marta Regueiro-Purriños, J. Manuel Gonzalo-Orden, et al. Closed-chest experimental porcine model of acute myocardial infarction reperfusion. Journal of Pharmacological and Toxicological Methods. 60 (2009) 301–306.

[48] Yasuhiro Shudo, Shigeru Miyagawa, Satsuki Fukushima, Atsuhiro Saito, et al. Novel regenerative therapy using cell-sheet covered with omentum flap delivers a huge number of cells in a porcine myocardial infarction model. The Journal of Thoracic and Cardiovascular Surgery c Volume 142, Number 5 November 2011.

Chapter 17

The Antiagregant Treatment After Coronary Artery Surgery Depending on Cost – Benefit Report

Luminita Iliuta

Additional information is available at the end of the chapter

http://dx.doi.org/10.5772/54467

1. Introduction

Despite routine use of ASA before CABG, and lifelong following the revascularization, patients who undergo CABG remain at high risk of long-term events in any vascular bed (cerebrovascular, cardiovascular, peripheral). The handicap of management of antiplatelet agents in the perioperative period of cardiac surgery requires close collaboration between cardiologists, surgeons and anaesthesiologists. It is necessary to avoid thrombotic complications maintaining the antiagregation, but balancing bleeding complications. [1]

Combined antiplatelet therapy employing agents from different pharmacological classes is characterised by good safety and efficacy profiles.

Antiplatelet therapy and antithrombin therapy have been demonstrated to reduce the risk of cardiac events in patients presenting with acute coronary syndrome, yet all effective therapies also increase the risk of bleeding. Antiplatelet therapy and antithrombotic therapy have been demonstrated to favorably modify clinical outcome, and recent trials of revascularization in ACSs have demonstrated a reduction in the frequency of major cardiac events.[2-14]

Multiple clinical trials showed the favorable benefit/risk ratio of clopidogrel over aspirin justifying the indication for using clopidogrel in a wide range of at risk patients and in long-term prevention in various manifestations of atherosclerosis.[2-9]

Antiplatelet and antithrombin therapy can have synergistic actions that reduce the risk of spontaneous or revascularization, especially percutaneous coronary intervention (PCI)–related events. On the other hand, all effective antithrombotic agents also increase the risk of bleeding, especially bleeding that results from vascular access or associated with surgery, including coronary artery bypass grafting (CABG).

The Clopidogrel in Unstable angina to prevent Recurrent ischemic Events (CURE) trial demonstrated that the combination of clopidogrel and aspirin was superior to aspirin alone for patients hospitalized with non–ST-elevation ACSs.[5] The therapy was in addition to the current standard of care, including heparin or low-molecular-weight heparin, antianginal therapy, and revascularization.[5, 6, 15].

Actually the field of the indications of use of the Clopidogrel is being continuously updated. There are different type of patients who benefit from antiplatelet therapy [16, 17] Moreover the combination of two antiagregant drugs (mainly ASA and clopidogrel) in high risk patients is a practice more and more extended [18] and dual antiplatelet therapy is recommended and has to be maintained at least 12 months after drug eluting stent placement [19].

On the other hand, in patients undergoing coronary artery bypass grafting, immediate postoperative antiagregant regimens are only regulated for routinely use Aspirin.

Antiplatelet therapy is critical in the management of coronary artery disease. For patients undergoing coronary artery bypass graft surgery (CABG), controversy remains regarding the safety of preoperative antiplatelet therapy and the optimal postoperative antiplatelet regimen to maintain graft patency and reduce ischemic complications.

Despite > 30 years of experience with antiplatelet agents during CABG, questions remain regarding their perioperative safety and efficacy. The results of continuing randomized controlled trials should further clarify the role of perioperative aspirin and clopidogrel therapy and help redefine the modern antiplatelet management of coronary artery bypass patients.

Following surgery, extensive evidence supports the use of aspirin, in doses of 100 - 325 mg daily, to be administered in 48 h postoperatively and continued indefinitely. Less is known regarding the use of clopidogrel following CABG, although it is now recommended as postoperative antiplatelet therapy in patients with recent acute coronary syndromes.[20]

It is very important to identify the optimal timing and dose ofAaspirin following CABG, and to assess the role of postoperative Clopidogrel therapy.

The recommendations regarding the treatment with Clopidogrel in coronary artery sugery do not take into consideration the cost-benefit ratio which reflect the usefulness from economic point of view, probably because of a the complexity of factors of this equation.

2. Objectives

1. To compare the efficacy and safety of Clopidogrel with Aspirin and Aspirin plus Clopidogrel in patients undergoing surgical coronary revascularisation in the immediate postoperative period and 1 year after coronary artery bypass grafting depending on the type of the lesion, on the type of the surgical procedure and on the associated risk factors for gastrointestinal bleeding.

http://dx.doi.org/10.5772/54467

2. To evaluate the importance and utility of antiplatelet therapy with Clopidogrel early postoperatively in the intensive care unit (ICU) for the prevention of postoperative complications

3. To establish the prognostic implications of the type of the perioperative antiagregant regimen in patients with CABG and to determine which therapy can reduce hospital stay after cardiac surgery and improve the quality of life of these patients.

4. To determine the indications for using Clopidogrel or Aspirin or Aspirin plus Clopidogrel in coronary artery surgery depending on the cost-benefit ratio and its economic implications.

3. Methods and material

Randomized,, open label three years clinical trial with open study period, carried out on 1200 pts undergoing coronary artery bypass grafing divided in three parallel groups: Group A: Clopidogrel po 75 mg/day, Group B: Aspirin po 75 mg/day and Group C: Aspirin 75mg plus Clopidogrel 75mg once daily.

The main phases of the study protocol were: (Figure 1)

- Enrollment phase – there were enrolled one thousand and two hundred patients undergoing CABG, in the immediate postoperative period
- Active treatment phase – after randomisation all patients received antiagregant therapy:
  - Group A with Aspirin 75 mg daily
  - Goup B with Clopidogrel 75 mg daily
  - Group C with combination of Aspirin 75 mg with Clopidogrel 75 mg.

The treatment began the second day postoperatively and lasted no less than 1 year postoperatively.

- follow –up phase – all patients were evaluated clinically and paraclinically daily for the first ten days and at one, three, six months and one year postoperatively. Patients were followed for a minimum of 1 to a maximum of 3 years, regardless of discontinuation of the study drug. Follow-up assessments took place at 1, 3, 6, and 12 months for all patients and at 1, 2 and 3 years for patients randomized early in the study.

4. Eligibility criteria

The study included all patients undergoing coronary artery bypass grafting, who underwent surgery in an Emergency Institute for Cardiovascular Diseases between January 1st 2008 and May 1st 2011 who did not have the non – eligibility criterias.

Patients were over the age of 21, and able to provide informed consent and agreed to comply with all protocol-specified procedures.

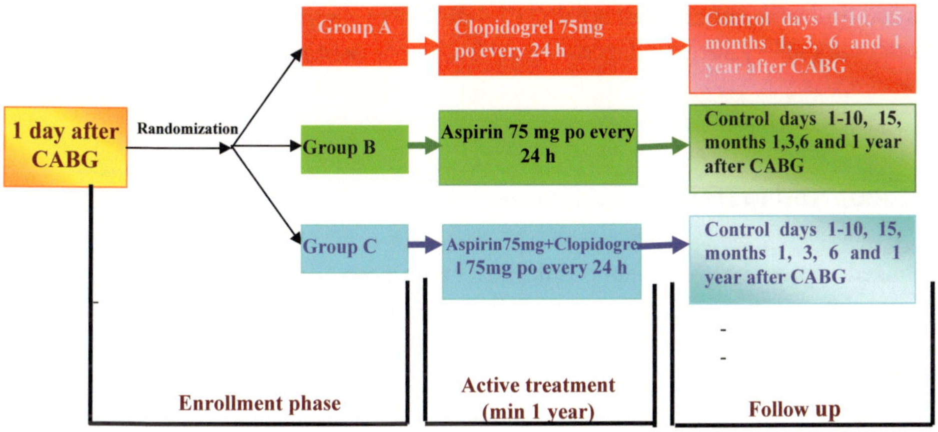

Figure 1. Treatment protocol phases

5. Non-eligibility criteria

Patients were excluded from enrolment in the study if any of the following criteria were met:

- Active internal bleeding or risk of hemorrhagic diathesis
- Q-wave myocardial infarction within 24 hours prior to randomization
- Cardiogenic shock.
- Serum Creatinine ≥ 3.0 mg/dl
- severe hepatic failure with ALT or AST > 3x ULN
- Previous use of a GPIIb/IIIa antagonist within 7 days
- Need for long-term anticoagulant or NSAID use
- Failed PCI within 2 weeks prior to randomization
- Active participation in another clinical trial
- Failure to comply with the hospital protocol

http://dx.doi.org/10.5772/54467

6. Study drop out criteria

The occurrence of adverse events (skin reactions, gastrointestinal symptoms, active internal bleeding)

Failure to comply with the hospital protocol/ absence to follow-up

The protocol was approved by the institute management, and every patient signed the informed consent form.

The essential inclusion criteria (gender,mean age, comorbidities, number of grafts per patient, the type of the grafts (arterial or venous) and the mean left ventricular ejection fraction, left ventricular diastolic performance and left atrial dimensions (diameters and area), the duration of treatment and assessment criteria were similar in the three treatment groups ($p<0.0001$). All patients received standard therapy including beta blockers, IEC, statins throughout the study period. The patients with exclusive arterial revascularisation also received calcium channel blockers agents but their number was similar in the three groups of study.

Clinical and laboratory parameters were initially assessed, at baseline and at each visit until the end of the study period.

The clinical measurements included: NYHA class for heart failure, presence of angina pectoris, ventricular rhytm, patient compliance and quality of life.

Laboratory parameters included: the usual blood tests (platelet count, hemoglobin, hematocrit, aminotransferases, LDH, biochemistry cholesterol and tryglycerides levels), electrocardiogram(with the evaluation of rhythm, frequence and ST-T elevation), 24 hours ECG Holter monitoring for silent ischemia, stress efort test at 1,3,6 months and 1 year postoperatively and when angina occurred (Bruce or Bruce modified protocol), echocardiography (with assessment of the LV dimensions, ventricular sistolic and diastolic performance, ventricular walls contractility - segmental kinetics, mitral regurgitation degree) and coronarography at 1 year when the other tests where positive for ischemia. Also, at each visit were recorded the occurrence of major and minor bleeding episodes, gastrointestinal symptoms, skin reactions, thrombocytopenia and lab tests abnormalities.

24 hours ECG Holter used a 12 channels monitoring with the evaluation of conduction or rhythm disturbances or occurrence of silent ischemia.

Treadmill stress test was done at 1, 3, 6 months and at 1 year postoperatively and used Bruce or Bruce modified protocol. If the stress test or Holter monitoring diagnosed ischemia at one follow up visit, this was the indication for performing coronarography.

Early development of graft occlusion was diagnosed based on clinical criteria and through electrocardiogram, Holter monitoring, thoracic and transesophageal echocardiography. The appearance of gastrointestinal bleeding was diagnosed using clinical evaluation, endoscopy and colonoscopy.

6.1. Primary and secondary endpoints

The looked at all-cause mortality and major cardiac events, namely cardiac mortality, myocardial infarction or need for target lesion revascularization. The most important endpoints used for the estimation of the medium term prognosis were:

The primary endpoint (efficacy endpoint) was a composite outcome cluster of 30-day mortality, myocardial infarction, in-hospital and at 1 year occurrence of graft occlusion (efficacy endpoints), total hospital stay and immobilization (measured in days), Intensive Care Unit length of stay and cost, quality of life. Quality of life was appreciated using a scale from one to ten calculated on the base of a questionnaire filled by the patients at each visit

The secondary endpoints at 30 days looked at in-hospital major peripheral or bleeding complications (including surgical bleeding complications, transfusion of at least two units of blood, intracranial bleeding, retroperitoneal bleeding, overt hemorrhage), neutropenia (<1.5 x 109 per litre), thrombocytopenia (<100 x 109 per litre), early discontinuation of the study drug due to a non-cardiac adverse event (including death of non-cardiac origin) (safety endpoint).

The data collected represented the fields of a database in the Visual Fox Pro computer program. Data were processed by means of computers, using the Excel, EpiInfo, Systat and SPSS programs for multivariate regression analysis and relative risk and correlation coefficient calculation

No confirmatory statistical hypothesis was pre-specified, but a detailed analysis plan was defined before the database was locked. This analysis plan was based on generating risk ratios and CIs (CI–confidence index) for the pairwise comparisons of primary interest. These comparisons were presented with the two - sided 95% CI of the relative risk and with normal p values. For the primary endpoints Kaplan-Meier curves were constructed and log-rank tests were done. For each endpoint, a two-sided 95% CI was also calculated and an overall Chi square test, comparing the three treatment groups was done [19, 21, 25].

The frequency of the primary efficacy plus safety endpoint for the Aspirin group as a reference group was 17,7%. On the basis of phase-II studies we assumed that the experimental groups with Clopidogrel and Aspirin plus Clopidogrel would result in better, or at least similar outcomes when compared with standard treatment. The sample size and power calculations were therefore based on non-inferiority of the experimental group versus the reference group. The study has 80% power to exclude, with 95% confidence (one-sided), a 1% higher rate of the primary endpoints compared with the reference group, provided the point estimate in the experimental treatment group was 1,7% lower for the efficacy endpoint and 2% lower for the efficacy and safety endpoint. [2-11, 13-18, 22]

7. Patients

The study included 1200 patients undergoing coronary artery bypass grafing with arteries (internal mammar, radial, gastroepiploic) or inverted saphenal veins. The patients were

http://dx.doi.org/10.5772/54467

randomised to receive Clopidogrel 75 mg daily or Aspirin 75 mg daily or Aspirin plus Clopidogrel 75mg daily one day after surgery and in the postoperative period for no less than 1 year.. The patients undergoing also venticular remodelling for aneurysms were not taken in our study.

The baseline characteristics were similar in the three arms of the study (Table 1). Overall, the study populations were similar to those of previous trials on antiagregants.

	Group A – 397 pts	**Group B- 401 pts**	**Group C- 402 pts**
Mean (SD) age (years)	62,3 (12)	62,5 (13)	62,4(12)
Age"/>70 years	13,85%	14,21%	14,43%
Women	25,94%	26,18%	26,62%
Family history of heart disease (%)	49,62%	50,12%	49,75%
Dislipidemia (%)	75,06%	75,81%	76,37%
Prior myocardial infarction (%)	33,50%	33,91%	34,58%
NYHA class "/>II	20,15%	20,70%	20,89%
Prior stroke (%)	6,29%	6,73%	6,96%
Peripheral arterial disease	9,82%	9,72%	10,45%
Atrial fibrillation	6,04%	6,48%	6,47%
Hypertension	65,49%	66,58%	64,92%
Diabetes mellitus	25,19%	25,43%	25,12%
Current smoker	26,45%	26,43%	25,87%
Re-intervention (previous coronary artery surgery)	8,82%	8,98%	8,95%

Table 1. Baseline characteristics

The medications used chronically by the patients at the time of randomization were similar in the Aspirin, Clopidogrel and Aspirin plus Clopidogrel treatment arms and are are listed in Table 2

	Group A – 397 pts	Group B- 401 pts	Group C- 402 pts
Digoxin	23,68%	23,94%	24,13%
ACE inhibitors	67,25%	68,58%	63,68%
Angiotensin II inhibitors	24,43%	23,69%	25,12%
Beta blockers	89,92%	89,28%	90,29%
Aspirin before surgery	61,46%	63,84%	65,17%
Calcium channel blockers	25,44%	25,93%	26,37%
Diuretics	19,90%	20,70%	20,39%
Aldactone	21,91%	21,94%	20,89%
Lipid lowering agents	89,92%	93,76%	94,28%

Table 2. Number of patients who received concomitant medications during stay in hospital

61,46% of patients received Aspirin before surgery in group A, respectively 63,84% in group B and 65,17% in group C.

The primary efficacy and efficacy plus safety endpoints and their individual components in the treatment groups are shown in Table 3.

The clinical diagnosis at the time of randomization was similar in the three treated arms of the study:

- Over half of the patients presented with unstable angina (49,62% in group A, 51,63% in group B and 53.48% respectively in group C).
- Approximately one in five-six patients had experienced a recent myocardial infarction (16.37% in group A, 21,94% in group B and 22.39% respectively in group C).
- About a third presented with stable angina or another diagnosis requiring antiagregant regimen (aproximatively 33,6% in each treatment arm - 33.75% in group A, 33,66% in group B, 33,58% in group C).

8. Statistics (Figure 2, 3)

The data base was done using Visual Fox Pro programme. The main variables used were:

http://dx.doi.org/10.5772/54467

- Prediction variables :
  - patient ID Data
  - preoperative diagnosis
  - surgical risk (calculated using a scale from 1 to 10 taking into account different preoperative parameters: age, co-morbidities, severity of cardiac lesions (NYHA class), type and duration of surgical intervention, associated risk factors)
  - type of surgical intervention
  - specific variables related to the surgical performance: duration of surgical intervention, intraoperative complications
  - ICU duration and complications occured
- • Outcomes variables:
  - presence and type of postoperative complications
  - death and its causes.

The statistical analysis was performed using the SYSTAT and SPSS programmes for:

- Measurement of the power of association between the prediction variables and outcomes using different tests depending on the type of variables:
  - for qualitative variables: CHI square test or Fischer exact test
  - for quantitative variables: T test (Student test), ANOVA test or U test depending on samples volumes and Kruskal Wallis nonparametric tests or other methods of statistical correlation as analysis of simple linear and multivariate regression
- Relative Risk calculation and the 95% confidence limits for treatment groups
- Cost-benefit ratio calculation for using different antiplatelets agents after coronary artery bypass grafting. It was determined using a special programme, which used the data from the database and different economic data from specialized departments from our Institute, in order to perform the assessment of the efficiency of different antiplatelet therapies following coronary artery surgery.

The calculation of the cost-benefit ratio for each type of treatment and for routinely use clopidogrel in CABG was done taking into account the following parameters:

- parameters related to the type of the treatment
  - cost of the treatment for each patient
  - number of supplementary echographic and endoscopic examinations per patient
  - number of bleeding episodes and cost per patient
  - global cost/ patient

- parameters related to surgical intervention
  - early postoperative mortality rates for surgical intervention (global and specific depending on individual risk and type of the antiagregant regimen)
  - in hospital and at 1 year graft occlusion/myocardial infarction/severe bleeding on subgroups of patients taking into account the individual risk
  - immediate and long term postoperative complications rates depending on the type of the antiagregant regimen
  - ICU length of stay and cost
  - quality of life at 1 month and 1 year postoperatively on risk subgroups and on type of surgical interventions depending on the type of the antiagregant regimen
- Parameters related to the patient
  - age
  - gender
  - co-morbidities
  - associated risk factors.

Using the above mentioned parameters, the special programme calculated a risk score per patient on types of treatment and the cost of routinely use clopidogrel in cabg patients, which was used then for estimation of the cost-benefit ratio associated with the type of the antiagregant regimen

Data were grouped on types of surgical interventions according to the exposure level to the risk factors. For each exposure level there were introduced the number of patients taking Clopidogrel (cases) and the number of patients who have not taken Clopidogrel (controls). The confounders were controlled by stratification.

Data interpretation was performed taking into account the following hypothesis:

- a cost-benefit report >1 was considered unfavourable from economic point of view; for these patients the routine use of Clopidogrel as antiplatelet therapy after coronary artery bypass surgery was considered as having uncertain indication;
- a cost-benefit report =1 was considered neutral and included the patients subgroups classified as relative indication for the routine use of clopidogrel as antiplatelet therapy after coronary artery bypass surgery, risks and benefits of using that therapy it being appreciated on case to case basis, depending on the risk and benefit for each patient;
- a cost-benefit report <1 was considered favourable from economic point of view; for these patients the routine use of Clopidogrel as antiplatelet therapy after coronary artery bypass surgery was considered as having a standard indication, being recommended in each case.

http://dx.doi.org/10.5772/54467

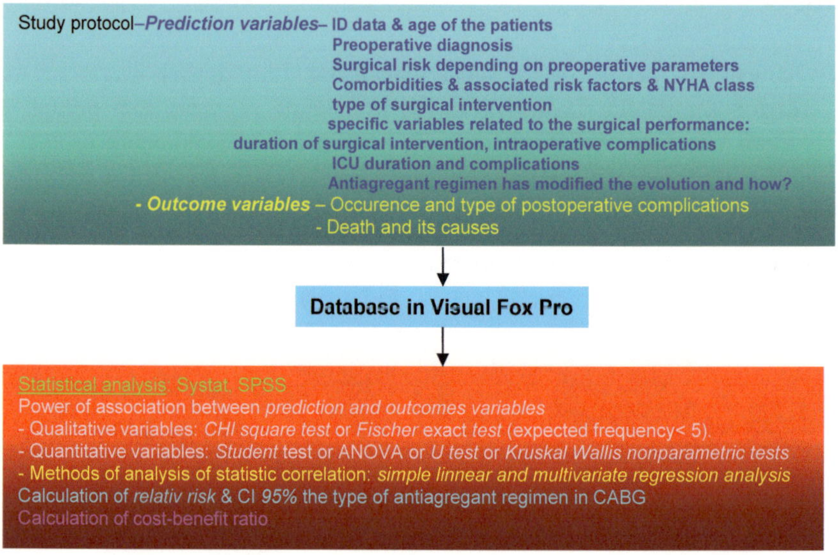

Figure 2. Statistic methodology

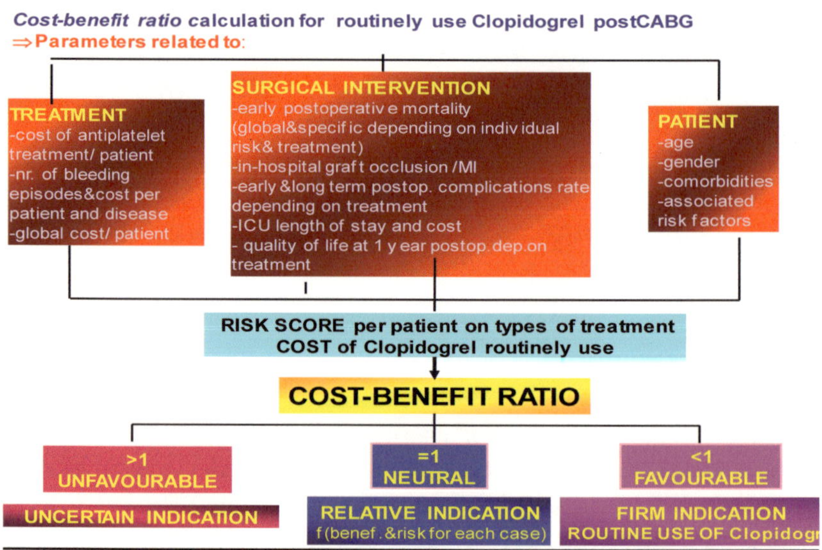

Figure 3. Statistical analysis and cost-benefit report calculation

9. Results

The main conclusion of our study was that using Clopidogrel single or associated with Aspirin for antiplatelet treatment in the immediate postoperative period in CABG patients is more effective than Aspirin alone, with a better cost-benefit report. The cost benefit report associated with using Aspirin plus Clopidogrel was almost two times higher than with Aspirin alone (Figure 4)

The incidence of myocardial infarction and death following graft thrombosis was 21% in Aspirin group,12% in Clopidogrel group and respectively 7% in aspirin plus Clopidogel group.

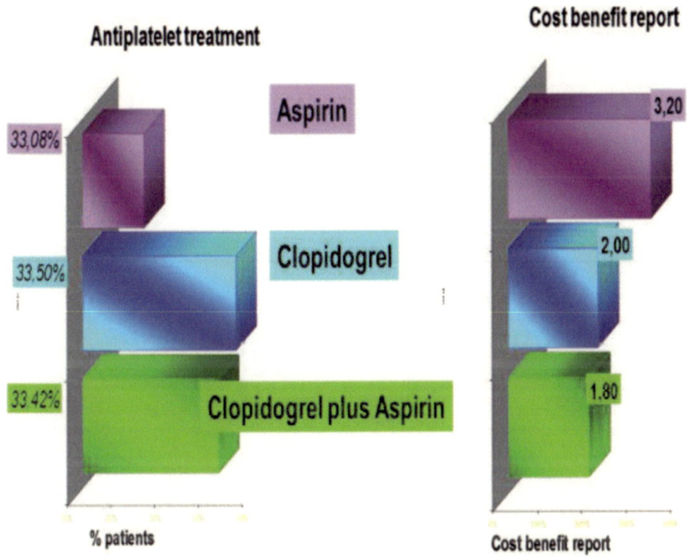

Figure 4. Cost-benefit report depending on the type of antiplatelet treatment in CABG patients

Relative risks and 95% confidence indexes for primary efficacy composite endpoints (30 days mortality, myocardial infarction, inhospital graft oclusion, hospital stay and immobilization (days), Intensive Care Unit length of stay and cost, quality of life) were different depending on the patients age, NYHA class, LVEF, the severity of associated MR, but, in all cases were lower among patients treated with Clopidogrel associated with Aspirin than among those treated with Aspirin alone

Also, there were different depending on the patients age, NYHA class, LVEF and associated severe mitral regurgitation.

Conventional statistical testing for Clopidogrel plus Aspirin versus Clopidogrel alone versus Aspirin alone resulted in p values of 0,0002 and 0,0003 respectively for the primary efficacy plus safety composite endpoints.

http://dx.doi.org/10.5772/54467

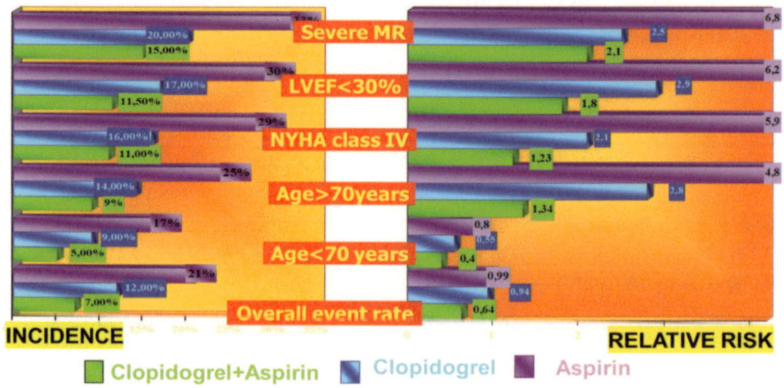

Figure 5. Relative risks and 95% Confidence Indexes for primary efficacy composite endpoints in the study groups

At hospital discharge and at 30 days, the combined efficacy and safety outcome endpoints were smaller in Clopidogrel plus Aspirin group.

For the primary efficacy plus safety endpoint (30 day mortality, inhospital graft oclusion or inhospital major bleeding), the rates were smaller for Clopidogrel plus Aspirin group, as the rates of in-hospital death

In-hospital graft oclusion and myocardial infarction occurred rarely in patients treated with Clopidogrel plus Aspirin compared with the patients treated with Aspirin alone. Major hemorrhagic events were similar in the study groups. Concerning the duration of the hospitalisation and imobilisation, there were a little bit smaller in Clopidogrel plus Aspirin group. (Figure 6)

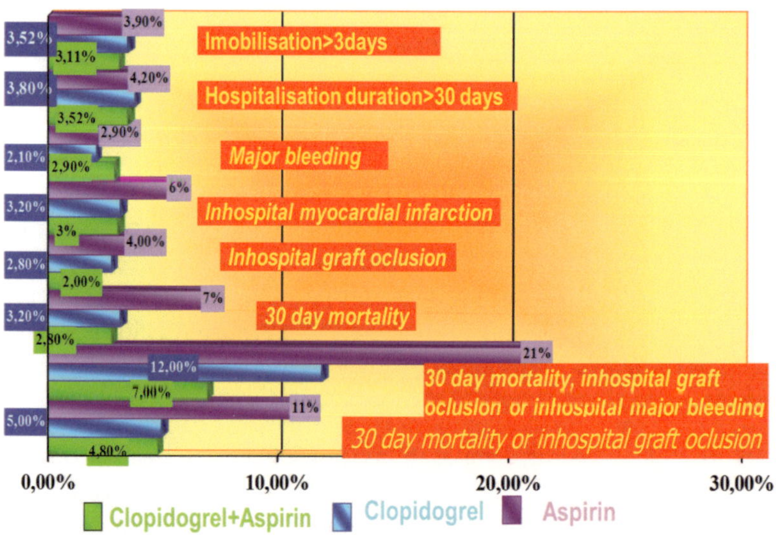

Figure 6. Frequency of composite and single endpoints at hospital discharge and at 30 days

On long term, the incidence of death, myocardial infarction, and revascularization occurring at one year following CABG was greater in Aspirin group compared with Clopidogrel and Clopidogrel plus Aspirin groups (15% versus 12% versus 10%)

The Kaplan Meier curves for primary efficacy and safety endpoints showed a smaller probability for death, myocardial infarction or graft oclusion in Clopidogrel plus Aspirin group (Figure 7).

Early after treatment, the curves for Clopidogel associated or not with Aspirin started to separate from the one of Aspirin alone. At 30 days, differences in the primary endpoints between the three groups were already present.

Until the end of the follow up, for the primary efficacy endpoint and for the primary efficacy plus safety endpoint, event rates were abut two times higher for Aspirin group compared with Clopidogrel plus Aspirin group with log rank tests highly significant and significant p values (p<0,0001).

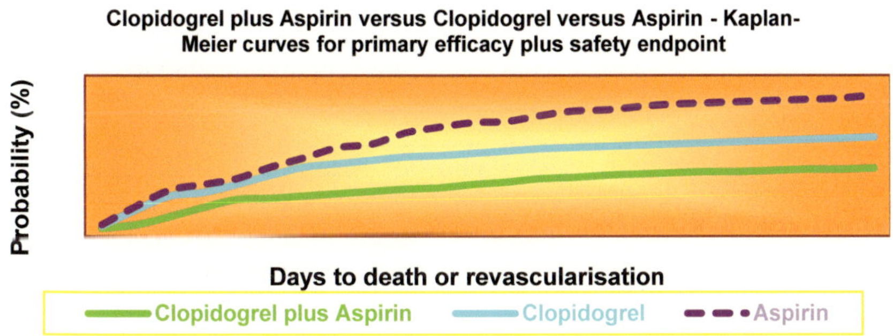

Figure 7. The Kaplan Meier curves for primary efficacy and safety endpoints

Concerning antiagregany therapy complications, the dates on in-hospital strokes are summarized in Figure 8.

There were no significant differences between the three groups regarding major hemorrhage and thrombocytopenia. Minor hemorrhage occurs more frequently in patients taking Aspirin. Total stroke and ischemic stroke rates were similar in the three groups. A few hemorrhagic conversions were seen in each of the tthree treatment groups. More minor or major bleeding complications and blood transfusions were also seen in the aspirin alone or associated with clopidogrel groups compared with clopidogrel alone group, although these differences were not significant.

Significantly more major bleeding complications (p=0,0001), more transfusions (p=0,002) and a higher rate of thrombocytopenia (p=0,001) were seen in patients with associated treatment with anticoagulants, in patients older than 75 years and in diabetics, the rate of major bleeding complications was three times higher in those with associated anticoagulant therapy (4%versus 14% and 2% versus 7% respectively

http://dx.doi.org/10.5772/54467

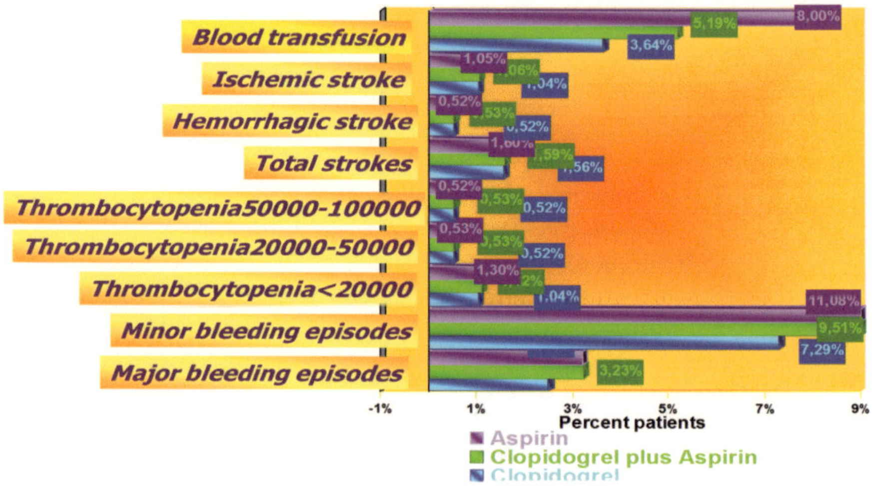

Figure 8. Hemorhagic and ischemic postoperative complications in the study groups.

The probability of early graft oclusion and perioperative myocardial infarction was smaller with Clopidogrel alone or associated with Aspirin versus Aspirin alone, the associated relative risks being negative because the studied drugs worked as protection factors for these perioperative complications. (Figure 9)

As we seen before, the relative risks for the most severe antiagregant therapy complications, hemoragic stroke were similar in the three study groups

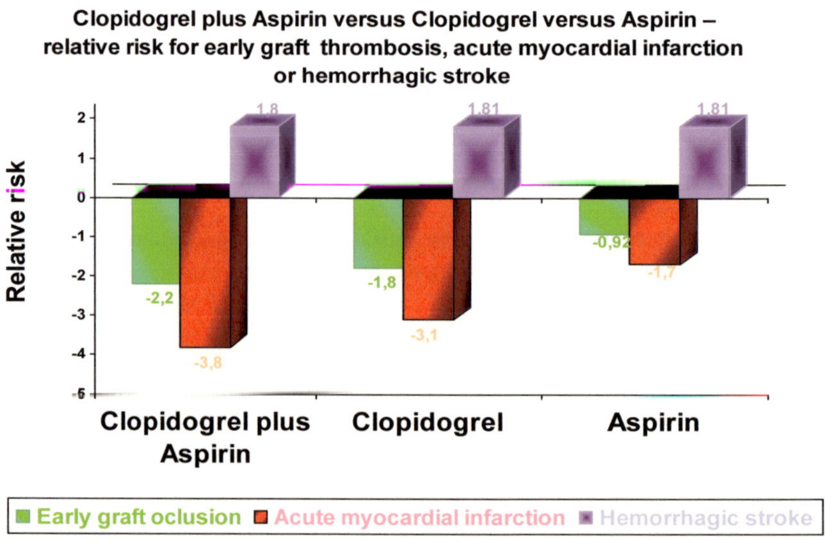

Figure 9. Relative risk for early graft thrombosis, acute myocardial infarction or hemorrhagic stroke

10. Discussions

Multiple clinical trials showed the favorable effects of Clopidogrel alone or combined with Aspirin extending the indication for using Clopidogrel in a wide range of at risk patients and in long-term prevention in various manifestations of atherosclerosis.

In recent years, enormous growth in the use of coronary stenting procedures has resulted in a significant decrease in restenosis rates, while acute and sub-acute stent thrombosis remain a significant potential complication. It has been shown, however, that the risk of acute and sub-acute stent thrombosis is greatly reduced by the administration of antiplatelet therapies following stenting. Much clinical experience with combination of aspirin and ticlopidine has been gained, however ticlopidine has been shown to be associated with rare risk of haematological adverse events.

The CLASSICS study demonstrated the safety and efficacy of clopidogrel (with or without loading dose) in combination with aspirin for use following coronary stenting.

A large randomized trial has demonstrated that the acute administration of clopidogrel—a long-acting antiplatelet therapy—to patients with non–ST-segment elevation acute coronary syndromes (NSTE ACS) can reduce subsequent risk for death, myocardial infarction, or stroke by 20% when continued for a mean duration of nine months [21]. However, single-center case series have demonstrated that, in patients requiring coronary artery bypass graft surgery, the use of Clopidogrel is associated with increased risk of perioperative bleeding and a need for transfusion [22- 26].

This risk appears to be time dependent. For example, post-hoc data analysis from the CURE (Clopidogrel in Unstable Angina to Prevent Recurrent Events) trial revealed that bleeding risks were increased when patients had CABG surgery within 5 days of clopidogrel treatment but not when surgery was delayed for >5 days after treatment with clopidogrel [21]

These findings are reflected in the American College of Cardiology/American Heart Association (ACC/AHA) guidelines for the acute management of patients with NSTE ACS, which endorse the acute use of clopidogrel but also recommend withholding clopidogrel for at least 5 days before CABG surgery (27).

Adherence in community practice to this guidelines recommendation is very unclear. has not been characterized previously. There are studies trying to characterize patterns of Clopidogrel use before CABG and to examine the time-dependent risks for postoperative transfusion among NSTE ACS patients treated at 264 hospitals participating in the CRUSADE (Can Rapid Risk Stratification of Unstable Angina Patients Suppress Adverse Outcomes With Early Implementation of the ACC/AHA Guidelines) National Quality Improvement Initiative [15, 28- 29].

Combined antiplatelet therapy was also studied in a lot of trials and most of them showed good safety and efficacy profiles. Antiplatelet therapy and antithrombin therapy have been demonstrated to reduce the risk of cardiac events in patients presenting with acute coronary syndrome, yet all effective therapies also increase the risk of bleeding. Antiplatelet therapy

http://dx.doi.org/10.5772/54467

and antithrombotic therapy have been demonstrated to favorably modify clinical outcome, and recent trials of revascularization in ACSs have demonstrated a reduction in the frequency of major cardiac events[2-14].

The benefits versus risks of early and long-term clopidogrel therapy (freedom from CV death, MI, stroke, or life-threatening bleeding) are similar in those undergoing revascularization (CABG or PCI) and in the study population as a whole. Overall, the benefits of starting clopidogrel on admission appear to outweigh the risks, even among those who proceed to CABG during the initial hospitalization.

Actually the field of the indications of use of the antiagregant therapy is being continuously updated.The role of the aspirin in the primary prevention has extended its prescription based on related factors of cardiovascular and/or neurological risk. Moreover the combination of two antiagregant drugs (mainly Aspirin and clopidogrel) in high risk patients is a practice more and more extended [18]. Dual antiplatelet therapy has to be maintained at least 12 months after drug eluting stent placement and, in this patient a specific protocol of antiaggregation in type, combination and duration need to be applied [30, 31].

For patients undergoing coronary artery bypass graft surgery, controversy remains regarding the safety of preoperative antiplatelet therapy and the optimal postoperative antiplatelet regimen to maintain graft patency and reduce ischemic complications. There are also of this systematic reviews trying to evaluate the risks and benefits of preoperative aspirin and clopidogrel therapy, to identify the optimal timing and dose of aspirin following CABG, and to assess the role of postoperative clopidogrel therapy.[20]Following surgery, extensive evidence supports the use of aspirin, in doses of 100 - 325 mg daily, to be administered in 48 h postoperatively and continued indefinitely. Less is known regarding the use of clopidogrel following CABG, although it is now recommended as postoperative antiplatelet therapy in patients with recent acute coronary syndromes.Despite > 30 years of experience with antiplatelet agents during CABG, questions remain regarding their perioperative safety and efficacy. The results of continuing randomized controlled trials should further clarify the role of perioperative aspirin and clopidogrel therapy and help redefine the modern antiplatelet management of coronary artery bypass patients.

Also, the optimal aspirin dose for the prevention of cardiovascular events remains controversial.[32]: Daily aspirin doses of 100 mg or greater were associated with no clear benefit in patients taking aspirin only and possibly with harm in patients taking clopidogrel. Daily doses of 75 to 81 mg may optimize efficacy and safety for patients requiring aspirin for long-term prevention, especially for those receiving dual antiplatelet therapy.

The response to aspirin and/or clopidogrel and its impact on graft patency after off-pump coronary artery bypass grafting is characterised by individual variability, but, overall combined clopidogrel and aspirin overcome single drug resistances, were are safe for bleeding and improve venous graft patency. [33]

At first sight, clopidogrel appears to be undesirable for cardiac surgeons: antiplatelet therapy can increase the risk of bleeding during coronary artery bypass graft surgery (CABG).1 Traditionally, many surgeons have felt that, with impeccable technique, their personally

constructed grafts would be nearly 'immune' to thrombosis, even without antiplatelet therapy. However, it could theoretically reduce the risk for early vein graft failure, which is predominantly thrombosis related.

There are three different principal mechanisms that play a role in vein graft failure during postoperative periods: early (<1 month): thrombosis; related to technical factors, Intermediate (1 to 12 months): intimal hyperplasia and Later postoperative (>12 months): accelerated atherosclerosis [34]

Concern about possible hemorrhagic complications arising from use of oral antiplatelet agents in immediate proximity to coronary artery bypass graft (CABG) surgery leads many clinicians to avoid or discontinue these agents preoperatively. Recent evidence suggests that.the modest hemorrhagic risk may be acceptable, given the clinical benefits of sustained antiplatelet therapy in preventing graft occlusion and ischemic complications pre- and post-CABG. [35]

Also, other analysis provide insight into patterns of clopidogrel use and outcomes in the setting of CABG performed on patients with NSTE ACS [36] and found that as many as 30% of patients currently receive clopidogrel before CABG surgery, and, of these, nearly 90% have surgery within 5 days of treatment, contrary to the ACC/AHA guidelines recommendations. These data demonstrating a modest increase in transfusion risk in part reflect a more stable estimate of risks based on a much larger case sample in the CRUSADE Initiative.

The benefits versus risks of early and long-term clopidogrel therapy (freedom from CV death, MI, stroke, or life-threatening bleeding) were similar in those undergoing revascularization (CABG or PCI) and in the study population as a whole. Overall, the benefits of starting clopidogrel on admission appear to outweigh the risks, even among those who proceed to CABG during the initial hospitalization.[26]

Data from the Antiplatelet Trialists' Collaboration support the use of antiplatelet therapy (mostly data for aspirin) after CABG and further data support the initiation of aspirin within 48 hours of CABG. The CURE trial provides the opportunity to explore the combined use of aspirin and clopidogrel for those undergoing CABG.[26]

Clopidogrel offers multiple advantages in acute and chronic use in coronary intervention. The favorable benefit/risk ratio of clopidogrel over aspirin established by CAPRIE, combined with its characteristics related to rapid onset of action, loading dose, pre-treatment efficacy and ease of use, justify the consideration of using clopidogrel in a wide range of at risk patients and in long-term prevention in various manifestations of atherosclerosis / atherothrombosis.

Combined antiplatelet therapy employing agents from different pharmacological classes after CABG was characterised by good safety and efficacy profiles. The absence of interaction, and the potential synergistic effect when used with other antithrombotic agents, will allow clinicians to optimise treatment in acute situations. Combination therapy, using clopidogrel and other drugs commonly administered for a range of cardiovascular and other disorders, appears safe after CABG.

Despite routine use of ASA before CABG, and lifelong following the revascularization, patients who undergo CABG remain at high risk of long-term events in any vascular

bed (cerebrovascular, cardiovascular, peripheral). The incidence of death, MI, and revascularization occurring at one and three-year following a CABG is greater than 15%. 3. Therefore, patients who undergo CABG could benefit from long-term therapy that provides improved protection against all types of atherothrombotic events such as myocardial infarction, ischemic strokes, and vascular death.

11. Study limitations

First, our comparisons of clinical outcomes by treatment strategy were observational. Although we adjusted all comparisons for baseline clinical factors, we cannot exclude any persistent unmeasured confounding. Nonetheless, because a randomized clinical trial evaluating the benefits and risks of different antiagregant regimen of patients undergoing CABG is unlikely to be undertaken, this study is the first to provide insight into the scope of this issue at a national level.we considered the diagnostic of ischemia using stress test, Holter monitoring and, in case of a positive result, invasive coronarography as sufficient. Second, we did not collect data on the incidence of re-exploration at 2 or three years after CABG, although we had some information about that and we did nor perform routinely coronarography at 1 year postoperatively to all patients.

12. Conclusions

1. Antiplatelet therapy with Clopidogrel plus Aspirin in the immediate postoperative period in patients with CABG was associated with an better cost-benefit report, proving to be more effective than Aspirin alone.

   Taking into account both efficacy and safety, the combined antiplatelet therapy with Clopidogrel and Aspirin emerged as the best treatment in this trial.

2. The favourable cost/benefit ratio of Clopidogrel over Aspirin established by this study, combined with its characteristics related to rapid onset of action, loading dose, pretreatment efficacy and ease of use, justify the consideration of routinely using Clopidogrel in CABg patients and in long-term prevention in various manifestations of atherosclerosis

3. Taking into account cost-benefit report when comparing antiplatelet strategies after CABG,treatment with Aspirin alone was associated with an cost benefit report almost 1 in terms of reducing mortality and graft oclusion, Clopidogrel alone with a little bit more than one and the asociated therapy had an cost benefit ratio about 3, emerged as the best treatment inthis trial. It should be regarded as an attractive alternative pharmacological antiplatelet strategy in the immediate postoperative period in CABG patients,deserving further studies

Acknowledgements

Special thanks to cardiac surgeons and anesthesiologists from the Emergency Institute for Cardiovascular Diseases „C.C.Iliescu", Bucharest, Romania

Author details

Luminita Iliuta

University of Medicine and Pharmacy "Carol Davila" – Bucharest, Romania

References

[1] Ferrandis, R, Llau, J. V, & Mugarra, A. Perioperative Management of Antiplatelet-Drugs in Cardiac Surgery; Curr Cardiol Rev. (2009). May; , 5(2), 125-132.

[2] Collaborative meta-analysis of randomized trials of anti-platelet therapy for prevention of deathmyocardial infarction, and stroke in high risk patients: Anti-Platelet Trialists' Collaboration. BMJ. (2002). Abstract/FREE Full Text, 324, 71-86.

[3] Kong, D. F, Califf, R. M, Miller, D. P, et al. Clinical outcomes of therapeutic agents that block the platelet glycoprotein IIb/IIIa integrin in ischemic heart disease. Circulation. (1998). Abstract/FREE Full Text, 98, 2829-2835.

[4] Boersma, E, Harrington, R. A, Moliterno, D. J, et al. Platelet glycoprotein IIb/IIIa inhibitors in acute coronary syndromes: a meta-analysis of all major randomised clinical trials. Lancet. (2002). CrossRefMedline, 359, 189-198.

[5] Clopidogrel in Unstable Angina to Prevent Recurrent Events Trial InvestigatorsEffects of clopidogrel in addition to aspirin in patients with acute coronary syndromes without ST-segment elevation. N Engl J Med. (2001). CrossRefMedline, 345, 494-502.

[6] Mehta, S, Yusuf, S, et al. Effects of pre-treatment with clopidogrel and aspirin followed by long-term therapy in patients undergoing percutaneous coronary intervention: the PCI-CURE study. Lancet. (2001). CrossRefMedline, 358, 527-533.

[7] PURSUIT Trial InvestigatorsInhibition of platelet glycoprotein IIb/IIIa with eptifibatide in patients with acute coronary syndromes. N Engl J Med. (1998). CrossRefMedline, 339, 436-443.

[8] PRISM Study InvestigatorsA comparison of aspirin plus tirofiban with aspirin plus heparin for unstable angina. N Engl J Med. (1998). CrossRefMedline, 338, 1498-1505.

[9] GUSTO-IV ACS InvestigatorsEffect of glycoprotein IIb/IIIa receptor blocker abciximab on outcome in patients with acute coronary syndromes without early coronary

revascularization: the GUSTO IV-ACS randomised trial. Lancet. (2001). CrossRefMedline, 357, 1915-1924.

[10] Invasive compared with non-invasive treatment in unstable coronary-artery disease: FRISC II prospective randomized multicentre study: Fragmin and Fast Revascularization During Instability in Coronary Artery Disease (FRISC II) InvestigatorsLancet. (1999). CrossRefMedline, 354, 708-715.

[11] Outcome at 1 year after an invasive compared with a non-invasive strategy in unstable coronary-artery disease: the FRISC II invasive randomised trial: FRISC II Investigators: Fast Revascularisation During Instability in Coronary Artery DiseaseLancet. (2000). CrossRefMedline, 356, 9-16.

[12] Cannon, C. P, Weintraub, W. S, Demopoulos, L. A, et al. Comparison of early invasive and conservative strategies in patients with unstable coronary syndromes treated with the glycoprotein IIb/IIIa inhibitor tirofiban. N Engl J Med. (2001). CrossRefMedline, 344, 1879-1887.

[13] Berkowitz, S. D, Granger, C. B, Pieper, K. S, et al. for the Global Utilization of Streptokinase and Tissue Plasminogen Activator for Occluded Coronary Arteries (GUSTO) I Investigators. Incidence and predictors of bleeding after contemporary thrombolytic therapy for myocardial infarction. Circulation. (1997). Abstract/FREE Full Text, 95, 2508-2516.

[14] Fox KAAPoole-Wilson PA, Henderson RA, et al, for the Randomized Intervention Trial of Unstable Angina (RITA) Investigators. Interventional versus conservative treatment for patients with unstable angina or non-ST-elevation myocardial infarction: the British Heart Foundation RITA 3 randomised trial. Lancet. (2002). CrossRefMedline, 360, 743-751.

[15] Fox, K. A. A, Mehta, S. R, Peters, R, Zhao, F, Lakkis, N, Gersh, B. J, & Yusuf, S. Benefits and Risks of the Combination of Clopidogrel and Aspirin in Patients Undergoing Surgical Revascularization for Non-ST-Elevation Acute Coronary Syndrome- The Clopidogrel in Unstable angina to prevent Recurrent ischemic Events (CURE) Trial; Circulation. (2004). , 110, 1202-1208.

[16] The Task Force on the use of antiplatelet agents in patients with atherosclerotic cardiovascular disease of the European Society of CardiologyEspert consensus document on the use of antiplatelet agents. Eur Heart J. (2004). PubMed], 25, 166-81.

[17] Guyatt, G, Schunëmann, H, Cook, D, et al. Grade of recommendation for antithrombotic agents. Chest. (2001). S-7S.[PubMed]

[18] Patrono, C, Coller, B, Fitzgerald, G. A, Hirsh, J, & Roth, G. Platelet active drugs: the relationships among dose, effectiveness and side effects. Chest. (2004). S-64S.[PubMed]

[19] Servin, F. Low-dose aspirin and clopidogrel: how to act in patients scheduled for day surgery. Curr Opin Anaesthesiol. (2007). PubMed], 20, 531-4.

[20] Kulik, A, Chan, V, & Ruel, M. Antiplatelet therapy and coronary artery bypass graft surgery: perioperative safety and efficacy; Expert Opinion on Drug Safety[(2009). DOI: 10.1517/14740330902797081

[21] Yusuf, S, Zhao, F, & Mehta, S. R. Clopidogrel in Unstable Angina to Prevent Recurrent Events Trial investigators et al. Effects of clopidogrel in addition to aspirin in patients with acute coronary syndromes without ST-segment elevation, N Engl J Med CrossRef, 345-2001.

[22] Hongo, R. H, Ley, J, Dick, S. E, & Yee, R. R. The effect of clopidogrel in combination with aspirin when given before coronary artery bypass grafting, J Am Coll Cardiol CrossRef, 40-2002.

[23] Yende, S, & Wunderink, R. G. Effect of clopidogrel on bleeding after coronary artery bypass surgery, Crit Care Med CrossRef, 29-2001.

[24] Chen, L, Bracey, A. W, Radovancevic, R, et al. Clopidogrel and bleeding in patients undergoing elective coronary artery bypass grafting, J Thorac Cardiovasc Surg CrossRef, 128-2004.

[25] Englberger, L, Faeh, B, Berdat, P. A, Eberli, F, Meier, B, & Carrel, T. Impact of clopidogrel in coronary artery bypass grafting, Eur J Cardiothorac Surg CrossRef, 26-2004.

[26] Fox, K. A. A, Mehta, S. R, Peters, R, et al. Benefits and risks of the combination of clopidogrel in patients undergoing surgical revascularization for non-ST elevation acute coronary syndromes. the Clopidogrel in Unstable Angina to Prevent Recurrent Ischemic Events (CURE) trial, Circulation CrossRef, 110-2004.

[27] Braunwald, E, Antman, E. M, Beasley, J. W, et al. ACC/AHA 2002 guideline update for the management of patients with unstable angina and non-ST-segment elevation myocardial infarction-summary article. a report of the American College of Cardiology/American Heart Association Task Force on Practice Guidelines (Committee on the Management of Patients With Unstable Angina), J Am Coll Cardiol CrossRef, 40-2002.

[28] Bhatt, D. L, Roe, M. T, Peterson, E. D, et al. Utilization of early invasive management strategies for high-risk patients with non-ST-segment elevation acute coronary syndromes. results from the CRUSADE Quality Improvement Initiative, JAMA CrossRef, 292-2004.

[29] Sonel, A. F, Good, C. B, Mulgund, J, et al. Racial variations in treatment and outcomes of black and white patients with high-risk non-ST-elevation acute coronary syndromes. insights from CRUSADE (Can Rapid Risk Stratification of Unstable Angina Patients Suppress Adverse Outcomes With Early Implementation of the ACC/AHA Guidelines?), Circulation , 111-2005.

[30] Albaladejo, P, Marret, E, Piriou, V, & Samama, C. M. Perioperative management of antiplatelet agents in patients with coornary stents: recommendations of a French Task Force. Br J Anaesth. (2006). PubMed], 97, 580-84.

[31] Dalal, A. R, Souza, D, & Shulman, S. RS. Brief review: Coronary drug-eluting stents and anesthesia. Can J Anesth. (2006). PubMed], 53, 1230-43.

[32] Steinhubl, S. R, Bhatt, D. L, Brennan, D. M, Montalescot, G, Hankey, G. J, Eikelboom, J. W, Berger, P. B, & Topol, E. J. CHARISMA Investigators. Aspirin to prevent cardiovascular disease: the association of aspirin dose and clopidogrel with thrombosis and bleeding; Annals of Internal Medicine[(2009).

[33] Mannacio, V. A. Di Tommaso L, Antignano A, De Amicis V, Vosa C; Aspirin plus clopidogrel for optimal platelet inhibition following off-pump coronary artery bypass surgery: results from the CRYSSA (prevention of Coronary arteRY bypaSS occlusion after off-pump procedures) randomised study Heart heartjnl-Published Online First: 2 September (2012). Heart doi:10.1136/heartjnl-2012-302449, 2012-302449.

[34] Elefteriades, J. A, & Meier, P. Clopidogrel and cardiac surgery: enemy or friend?. Heart 2012; heartjnl-2012-302822Published Online First: 9 October (2012). doi:10.1136/heartjnl-2012-302822, 98(20)

[35] Cannon, C. P, Mehta, S. R, & Aranki, S. F. Balancing the benefit and risk of oral antiplatelet agents in coronary artery bypass surgery; The Annals of Thoracic Surgery[(2005).

[36] Rajendra, H, Mehta, M. D, Facc, M. S, Matthew, T, & Roe, M. D. MHS, FACC; Jyotsna Mulgund, MS; E. Magnus Ohman, MD, FACC; Christopher P. Cannon, MD, FACC; W. Brian Gibler, MD; Charles V. Pollack, Jr, MD, MA; Sidney C. Smith, Jr, MD, FACC; T. Bruce Ferguson, MD; Eric D. Peterson, MD, MPH, FACC. Acute Clopidogrel Use and Outcomes in Patients With Non-ST-Segment Elevation Acute Coronary Syndromes Undergoing Coronary Artery Bypass Surgery J Am Coll Cardiol. (2006). doi:10.1016/j.jacc.2006.04.029, 48(2), 281-286.

Section 3

Percutaneous Coronary Intervention

Chapter 18

Multivessel Disease in the Modern Era of Percutaneous Coronary Intervention

Michael Tsang and JD Schwalm

Additional information is available at the end of the chapter

http://dx.doi.org/10.5772/55103

1. Introduction

The rapid evolution of medical therapy, percutaneous coronary interventional techniques and cardiac surgery along with the changing patient profile over the last few decades has required the clinician to make increasingly complex decisions. This has led to significant variations in practices that may be discordant with evidence based clinical practice guidelines. Such variations have an unclear clinical impact. There is hope that with growing efforts to apply multidisciplinary care to the management of complex coronary artery disease (CAD),that we will arrive at more consistent and balanced decisions.

In this chapter, we will explore (1) The history of angiography and angioplasty, (2) the current clinical dilemma (3) the evidence supporting the use of cardiac surgery to improve survival above medical therapy alone, (4) the role of percutaneous approach versus surgery in different populations, (5) the impact of changing technologies/techniques in revascularization, (6) the current discordance between guidelines and clinical practice, and (7) the potential role of a multidisciplinary Heart Team to create a more unified, balanced approach to the treatment of complex CAD.

2. The origins of the age of percutaneous revascularization

2.1. Cardiac catheterization

One of the earliest descriptions of cardiac catheterizations was done by Steven Hales, an English chemist, botanist and animal physiologist who cannulated the carotid artery and the jugular vein to access the left and right-sided chambers of the heart respectively in the 17th

century [1]. It was through some of this initial work, that he was able to make the first measurements of blood pressure, describe systole and diastole, characterize the volumes of the heart through wax cast work and correctly describe the function of the aortic and mitral valve [1]. Interestingly, the first human cardiac catheterization was by a Urologist by the name of Werner Forssmann [2]. He performed right heart catheterization on himself in 1929 by advancing a cannula through the left antecubital vein via cut-down access into the right atrium [2].

2.2. Selective coronary angiography and angioplasty

The credit of the first true selective coronary angiogram and much of the initial correlations between angina pectoris and coronary anatomy has to be granted to Mason Sones, a Pediatric Cardiologist, who at the time of discovery was working out of the Cleveland clinic [3-5]. In 1958, whilst performing non-selective aortogram on a patient, Sones inadvertently engaged the right coronary artery [2].

The original technique of angioplasty was born out earlier work by a Vascular Radiologist by the name of Charles Theodore Dotter [6]. Andreas Gruentzig, now known as the father of modern day coronary angioplasty, learned the Dotter technique from a German Radiologist Eberard Zeitler while doing a clinical fellowship in the Radiology Department of Aggertalclinic in Engelskirchen, Germany [6]. He had adopted the Dotter concept of using the balloon approach for angioplasty [6]. After experimenting with a number of materials performed the first procedure in 1977 in a man with stenosis of his left anterior descending artery (LAD) using a polyvinyl chloride balloon mounted onto the Dotter catheter [6].

3. The current dilemma

The treatment of coronary artery disease can be simplified into three major therapeutic approaches: medical therapy alone, percutaneous coronary intervention (PCI), and coronary artery bypass grafting (CABG). However, deciding on which approach is optimal for the individual patient is sometimes far from simple. This decision requires not only an in depth understanding of the evidence but also the applicability of this evidence to the individual patient considering the anatomic characteristics of the disease, the clinical context, the patient's preferences, social circumstances, and available resources [ie. local expertise and access to PCI and/or CABG]. Furthermore, because there has been evolution of all of these three approaches, interpretation of the evidence has become quite complex. Comparison of different modes of therapy (eg CABG versus medical therapy or CABG to balloon angioplasty) in the past may not be as relevant in the current clinical milieu.

3.1. Advances in medical therapy

Medical therapy has made remarkable advances from a time when patients may have been treated with nitrates alone to contemporary use of a combination of antiplatelets, lipid lowering therapy (statins), beta-blockers (BB) and Angiotensin Converting Enzyme- inhibitors

http://dx.doi.org/10.5772/55103

(ACEI)/Angiotensin Receptor Blocker (ARB). This combined therapy addresses not only patient symptoms but also modifies the disease process such that prognosis is vastly improved [7]. The growth in our understanding the impact of lifestyle modification has also played a central role in how we manage patients with CAD [8].

3.2. Changing clinical patient profile

Due to advances in medical therapy, patients that are now considered for revascularization are also older and have accrued more co-morbidities [9]. These co-morbidities render the interpretation of relevant symptoms more difficult. For example, in a diabetic patient with chronic obstructive lung disease (COPD), it may be difficult to distinguish between dyspnea as an anginal equivalent versus that caused by the underlying pulmonary pathology. The severity of the patients' COPD may also complicate the eligibility for CABG as a mode of revascularization [10, 11]. In fact, in a recent clinical trial comparing CABG versus PCI in complex CAD, significant burden of co-morbidities was the most common reason that patients were felt not to be suitable for CABG and hence entered into the PCI registry [9].

3.3. Advances in angioplasty

Angioplasty has significantly evolved over the last several decades with respect to four principle areas. First, operator training has advanced from informal training courses to 1-2 year formal clinical fellowships [12, 13]. Second, the equipment to perform PCI has significantly improved from plain old balloon angioplasty (POBA) to second-generation drug-eluting stents (DES) and supporting devices to improve PCI outcomes (filter wires, thrombectomy in ST elevation acute coronary syndrome (STEACS), and rotational arthrectomy) [14, 15]. Third, vascular access has evolved from brachial cut-downs with large caliber sheaths (7-8 FR) to increasingly common radial access with smaller caliber sheaths (5 and 6 FR) [5, 15-18]. Finally, concomitant medications have become more sophisticated, from Aspirin (ASA) alone to combination antiplatelets resulting in reduced stent thrombosis [19]. Restenosis has remained in the forefront of limitation to PCI[20]. However, the challenges with restenosis have been significantly reduced with advancement in DES technology [21-23]. Concerns with the thrombosis rates in the setting of discontinuation of dual antiplatelet therapy (DAPT) after DES have been addressed by second-generation DES, which have dramatically reduced this clinical problem [24]. These advances have been paralleled by an increasing use in complex coronary artery disease including left main (LM) disease[25].

3.4. Advances in surgical techniques

From the standpoint of CABG, we have over the years learned the benefits of arterial grafting with the internal mammary artery (IMA) in improving survival [26]. A high long-term patency rate of left internal mammary artery (LIMA) after revascularization of the LAD is well established and is estimated at 88 percent at 10 to 15 years [26]. More recently, to circumvent particular risks associated with sternotomy, there has been some investigation of revascularization of the LAD with the LIMA using a minimally invasive direct coronary artery bypass (MIDCAB) technique [26]. In the setting of multivessel disease (MVD), there has been some

discussion of a hybrid approach with MIDCAB for the LAD and PCI of the other vessels. However, the evidence supporting this approach is still limited; the most recent European Society of Cardiology (ESC) Guidelines give a *Class IIb recommendation* to this approach *(Level of Evidence B) for those "patients with conditions likely to prevent healing after sternotomy"* [26]. This approach does have significant promise and further research is required before it is adopted on a population level.

3.5. Evidence of survival benefit for revascularization in stable ischemic heart disease (SIHD)

The current framework for patient selection in treatment strategy for MVD is largely shaped by early studies comparing medical therapy and CABG. This body of evidence has been best synthesized by a meta-analysis performed by Yusuf et al in the Lancet in 1994 [27]. This meta-analysis was an individual patient data analysis of 2549 patients derived from three large randomized controlled trials, the Coronary Artery Surgery Study (CASS), Veterans Administration (VA) study and the European Coronary Surgery Study (ECSS) as well as four other smaller randomized studies [27]. The population studied consisted of patients with stable symptomatic coronary artery disease of a wide spectrum of severity [27]. However, only 10 percent were single vessel disease (1VD); the remainder consisted of MVD with 59.4% affecting the proximal LAD [27].

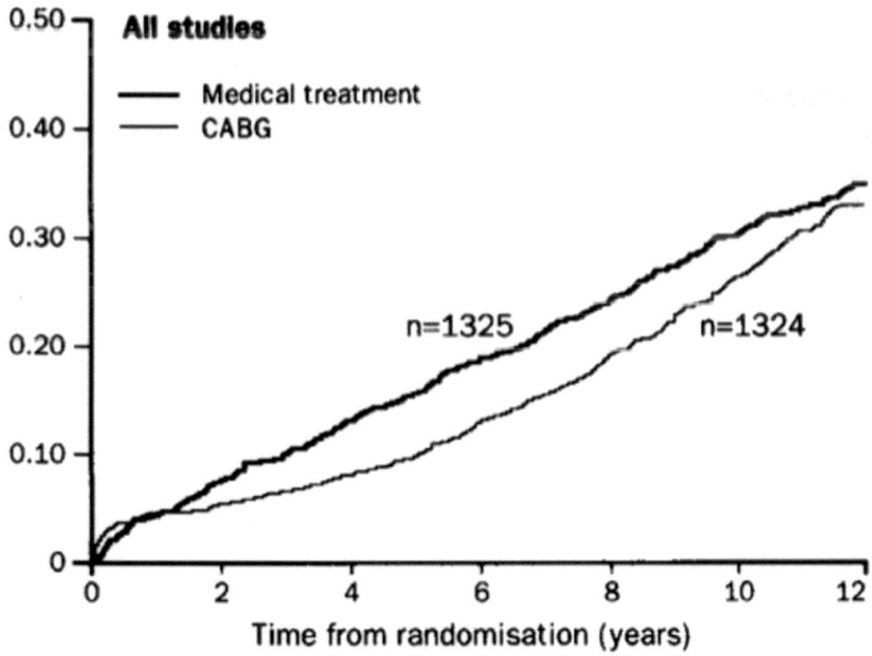

Figure 1. Survival curve for medical therapy versus coronary artery bypass grafting (CABG). Reproduced with permission from Yusuf S. et al. Lancet 1994. 344;8922:563-568

http://dx.doi.org/10.5772/55103

There was an overall statistically significant survival benefit with an **absolute risk reduction (ARR) 5.6% at 5 years, 5.9% at 7 years and 4.1% at 10 years** [Figure 1] [27]. This was likely an overall underestimate of the total treatment effect as there was a 36.4% cross over from the medical group to CABG over that time period whereas 93.7% of those assigned to the surgical group underwent CABG [27]. Subgroup analysis revealed that benefit was largely in those that had *three-vessel disease (3VD) and those with involvement of the proximal LAD* with each of those groups demonstrating a 42% relative risk reduction (RRR) in mortality [27]. In contrast, revascularization in two-vessel disease (2VD) in the absence of involvement of the proximal LAD did not result in a significant mortality benefit [27]. Randomized data is fairly consistent with that of registry data, demonstrating survival benefit for revascularization over medical therapy in those with 3VD; its support for benefit in those with 2VD even in those with proximal left anterior descending (LAD) involvement was non-significant [28]. The latter may be related to improvements in medical therapy.

4. Changing landscape in the treatment of CAD

Many of the earlier studies comparing surgical revascularization with medical therapy was during a period in cardiology where the BB and nitrates were the mainstay of medical therapy. Although antiplatelets were available, these were only taken by approximately 20% of the patients at the time [27]. It may hence be important to interpret these results in the context of current medical practice, which include contemporary treatments (standard secondary prevention with antiplatelets, statin therapy, BB and ACEi) that have all made further advancements in the survival and prognosis of patients with CAD [7].

ASA for secondary prevention has an estimated RRR of 18 percent in total serious vascular events (including stroke and major coronary event) with an **annual ARR of 1.5 percent**; the decrease in major coronary event (non-fatal myocardial infarction (MI) and cardiovascular death) is estimated at **annual ARR of 1.0 percent** [29]. As an adjunctive antiplatelet clopidogrel has further reduced death from cardiovascular causes, non-fatal MI and stroke in patients with Non ST elevation acute coronary syndromes (NSTEACS) with an **ARR of 2.1 percent** [30]. Most recently, newer agents such as prasugrel and ticagralor have both shown benefit compared to clopidogrel in patients with acute coronary syndromes (ACS). Prasugrel compared with clopidogrel in PCI treated ACS has demonstrated an **ARR of 2.2 percent** with regards to death from cardiovascular causes, nonfatal MI or non-fatal stroke over the 6-15 month follow up period [31]. Ticagralor has shown similar reduction in the same composite endpoint in patients with ACS over clopidogrel with an **ARR of 1.9 percent** [32]. In addition, ticagralor also showed an overall **reduction in all cause mortality with an ARR of 1.4 percent** [32].

BB's have a longstanding history in the management of CAD [7]. Although BB's can be used in patients post-MI with a normal ejection fraction (EF), the evidence for this is not as strong as that for those with significant Left Ventricular (LV) dysfunction [8]. It was previously shown that Carvedilol compared with placebo in patients with chronic heart failure (HF) and severe LV dysfunction (average EF 22-23 percent**) reduces all cause mortality with an ARR of 4.6 percent** [33].

The introduction of 3-hydroxyl-3-methyl-glutaryl-coenzyme A (HMG-CoA) reductase inhibitors otherwise known as the "statins," has significantly improved the care of patients with coronary artery disease [34, 35]. Simvastatin 40mg orally daily compared to placebo in patients with known vascular disease was shown in the Heart Protection Study (HPS) to *reduce all cause mortality with an ARR of 1.8 percent* over a five year period [34]. This was paralleled with a **reduction of coronary death with an ARR 1.2%** [34].

ACEi's have also been established to have a significant benefit towards long-term cardiovascular outcomes. It was shown in the Heart Outcomes Prevention Evaluation Study that in high-risk patients (vascular disease or diabetes plus one other risk factor) Ramipril compared with Placebo provides a *relative risk reduction* in myocardial infarction, stroke and death from cardiovascular causes of *21 percent* and *ARR of 3.8 percent* [36] over the mean follow up period of 5 years. There was also a *reduction in all cause death with an ARR of 1.8 percent* [36].

Concurrently, there was the advent and evolution of percutaneous approaches to revascularization. The first generation of angioplasty that truly adopted popular practice involved serial balloon inflations at the site of stenoses restore normal flow dynamics down the conducting epicardial vessels [6]. This approach, although promising was limited by a high rate of restenoses as a result of localized vascular recoil and epithelial hyperplasia [20, 37]. The bare metal stents (BMS) were created as a scaffolding technique that limited the degree of recoil but still faced significant re-stenosis rates due to mediated by injury to the medial layer, increased inflammation resulting from stent strut penetration into the lipid core and ultimately neointimal growth [38].

Pacitaxel and Sirolimus DES were developed in the next phase to overcome the challenge of restenosis requiring repeat intervention [20]. Although there was no difference in mortality or rates of myocardial infarction seen with DES compared with BMS, there were considerable reductions in restenosis rates with an estimated RRR of 0.44 [21, 22, 39-41].

Early enthusiasm for the use of drug eluting stents was curbed by a significantly higher rate of stent thrombosis, particularly in the face of an initially shorter duration (6 months) of dual antiplatelet therapy (DAPT) [22, 42, 43]. Currently the American College of Cardiology/American Heart Association (ACC/AHA) recommends at least *12 months of DAPT* in patients receiving DES for non-ACS indication and *12 months of DAPT* for ACS indication regardless of the stent type (BMS or DES) *(Class I recommendation, Level B evidence)* [14].

The most recent development in stent technology has been the introduction of second-generation (everolimus and zotarolimus) drug eluting stents. A large Swedish registry observational study containing 94, 384 patients demonstrated the advantage of the second-generation stents over its predecessors (first generation DES and BMS) both in terms of *restenosis* and *definite stent thrombosis* [44]. The second generation DES in this study was shown to have lower risk of restenosis compared with both BMS and the first generation DES with **Hazard Ratios (HR)** of **[0.29, 95% confidence interval (CI) 0.25-0.33]** and **[0.62, CI: 0.53 -0.72]** respectively [44]. The Cobalt Chromium Everolimus eluting stents (CoCr EES) have shown the most promise in reducing stent thrombosis. In a recent network meta-analysis of 50844 patients, the CoCr EES was shown to have a lower rate of 1 year definite stent thrombosis compared to both paclitaxel DES and sirolimus DES with odds ratio (OR) of **[0.41 95% CI 0.24-0.70]** and **[0.28 95% CI 0.16-0.48]** respectively [24]. The CoCr EES also had a lower rate of definite stent thrombosis compared with BMS at 1 year and 2 years with an odds ratio [OR] of

[0.23 95% CI 0.13-0.41) and [0.35, 95% CI 0.17-0.69] respectively [24]. Finally, compared to even the zotarolimus second generation DES, the CoCr EES still demonstrated a robust reduction in stent thrombosis with an OR **[0.21, 95% CI 0.17-0.69]** at one year [24].

5. PCI versus CABG in SIHD

There have been numerous randomized studies comparing PCI with surgical revascularization in MVD. A recent systematic review including 10 major trials over and the individual data from over 7800 patients found similar mortality in patients treated with CABG (15%) compared to patients treated with angioplasty (16%) over median survival of 5.9 years (p=0.12) [45]. There was, however a significantly lower rate of death or repeat revascularization in those treated with CABG (9.9%) compared with those treated with PCI (24.5%) [45]. This suggests that in fact the major benefit seen in CABG over PCI in this comparison is a lower need for repeat revascularization and is paralleled by a lower incidence of angina in the CABG group (14%) compared to the PCI group (26%) at one year (p<0.0001) [45]. The major caveat to this data is that stenting (which is known to reduce restenosis rates) only represented 37 percent of the total angioplasty group [45].

Subgroup analysis revealed that patients with diabetes have overall *better survival* when treated with surgical revascularization than when treated with angioplasty **with an ARR of 7.7% over 5 years** [45]. More definitive data supporting the use of CABG in patients with diabetes will be presented in *Section 6.2.* Interestingly, there was also a graded age interaction that was significant (p=0.002) [45]. For patients younger than 55 years of age, mortality was lower with PCI (8%) than CABG (10%). In patients between ages 55-64, PCI and CABG had similar mortality rates at 15 and 14 percent respectively [45]. And for patients older than 65 years of age, CABG had a lower overall mortality (20%) compared with PCI (24%) [45]. Prior to this study, this interaction had not been previously reported and we can only speculate whether the effect is a true function of age.

Other subgroups did not prove to contribute any significant interaction to the overall treatment effect [45]. Six of the trials included had POBA as the main mode of PCI whereas four trials used BMS; neither of these groups had significantly different survival rates when compared with surgery [45]. There was no overall interaction contributed by the presence/absence of proximal LAD disease, 3VD, abnormal LV function, previous MI or unstable symptoms [45].

6. Factors favoring surgery as the mode of revascularization

6.1. LV dysfunction

LV function has never been shown to have a significant interaction with mode of revascularization (PCI versus CABG) with regard to survival. In fact, the majority of studies comparing PCI with CABG enrolled a low percentage of patients with abnormal LV function *(20 percent or less)* [45]. However, it has been considered an important variable that favors revascularization with surgery due to historical data showing that patients with significant LV dysfunction

have improved survival with CABG compared to medical therapy. An initial signal for preferential benefit of revascularization in patients with mild to moderate LV dysfunction (*LV EF of 35-49%*) was seen in subgroup analyses of the CASS randomized study and the VA study [46, 47]. This was further supported by a meta-analysis demonstrating a significantly longer survival time in 10-year follow up with surgical revascularization over medical therapy in patients with LV dysfunction [10.6 months] compared with those with normal LV function [2.3 months] [27]. These studies however did not address whether a similar effect would be seen in severe LV dysfunction.

The Surgical Treatment for Ischemic Heart Failure (STITCH) trial published recently in 2011, designed to address this question in a randomized comparison of medical therapy versus surgical revascularization in patients with an *EF of 35 percent or less [48]*. There was a non-statistically significant trend (p=0.12) towards decreased all-cause mortality in the surgical group with an relative reduction of 24% and an ARR of 5 percent over the six year follow up period [48]. The lack of statistical significance, in the context of intention to treat analysis, may be related to the disproportionate crossover rate with 17 percent of the patients assigned to medical therapy ultimately receiving coronary bypass surgery [48]. Nevertheless, there was still a significant relative reduction of death from cardiovascular causes of 19 percent (p=0.05) and a significant relative reduction in death from any cause and hospitalization from cardio-vascular causes of 26 percent (p<0.001)[48].

It is unclear why surgical revascularization confers clear benefit in mild to moderate LV dysfunction, and only modest benefit severe LV dysfunction, but there are possible explana-tions. Medical therapy has advanced tremendously since the initial comparisons between medical therapy and surgery, which may decrease the relative mortality benefit between the two treatments during this more contemporary comparison. One could also hypothesize that the beneficial effect of revascularization plateaus at the extremes of LV dysfunction due to irreversible remodelling and/or the progressive increase in associated procedural risk.

There is currently limited data in how revascularization with PCI would affect prognosis in the setting of LV dysfunction[14]. As a result, the most recent ACC/AHA guidelines still recommend CABG for patients with LV EF 35-50 percent with a *IIa recommendation (Grade B evidence)* and a *IIb recommendation (Grade B evidence)* for those with a LV EF of less than 35 percent [49]. And currently, the ACC/AHA guidelines state that there is *insufficient data* to make a recommendation for revascularization with PCI in patients with LV dysfunction [49]. In practice however, if a patient does require revascularization but is not a surgical candidate, that natural decision is that if percutaneous intervention is feasible, that option should be entertained.

6.2. Diabetes favoring surgical revascularization

The Bypass Angioplasty Revascularization Investigation (BARI) was one of the first major landmark studies comparing angioplasty versus coronary bypass in patients with both stable anginal symptoms and unstable angina with MVD. Although there was no significant difference between the two treatments in the overall survival, patients with diabetes tended to have a significantly lower mortality rate with CABG (19.4%) compared with angioplasty (34.5%) with an **ARR of 15.1%** [50]. This finding was further confirmed with a meta-analysis comparing angioplasty with CABG in MVD, albeit with a smaller ARR of 7.7% [45]. In contrast,

in non-diabetics there was no overall benefit of surgery over angioplasty[45]. This relationship was corroborated by significant interaction found for the diabetic subgroup (p=0.014) [45]. The interaction was robust and was present even after excluding the data contributed by BARI and when adjusted for various clinical parameters (age, sex, smoking, hypertension, history of MI, heart failure and 3VD) [45].

One hypothesis that may explain why diabetics may have a better outcome with surgery than angioplasty is that restenosis may be more aggressive in this group of patients [20]. It has been well established that one major drawback of percutaneous coronary intervention is the need for repeat revascularization due to restenosis [20]. While restenosis itself may not incur an increased risk of mortality, the repeat exposure to the inherent risk of intervention may be additive. The need for repeat revascularization was certainly more striking in the earlier trials where POBA was used (54 percent within 5 years for the BARI trial) [50]. There has been considerable improvement to both the techniques and technology of PCI first with the development of BMS and now DES which are intended to reduced restenosis rates have been integrated into common practice. However, even in more contemporary trials such as *Synergy between PCI with Taxus and Cardiac Surgery* (SYNTAX), DES conferred a 13.5% need for revascularization compared with 5.9% in patients treated with CABG over a one-year period [51].

BARI 2D is a contemporary trial evaluating revascularization (both PCI and CABG) with intensive medical therapy for SIHD in diabetic patients. No significant difference emerged overall between the two groups in terms of overall mortality, cardiac death or myocardial infarction over the 5-year follow up period [52]. The mode of revascularization was at the discretion of the treating physician and the burden of disease tended to be higher in the CABG group than the PCI group with a mean number of lesions being 5.6 versus 4.3 respectively [52]. Although not specifically designed to compare PCI and CABG as a mode of revascularization, it is still noteworthy that there was a significant difference in death and MI for those revascularized with CABG compared to medical therapy (21.1% versus 29.2% p=0.010); the same comparison in the PCI stratum revealed no difference [52].

To date, the trial most relevant in determining whether the difference between PCI and CABG for revascularizing SIHD in diabetic patients in a randomized fashion is the *FREEDOM* trial [53]. There are 1900 diabetic patients with multivessel disease (defined by >70% stenosis in 2 or more epicardial vessels supplying different vascular territories) that were randomized to CABG versus PCI with DES (Paclitaxel or Sirolimus eluting stent at the discretion of treating physician) with a background of guideline supported optimal medical therapy. The primary endpoint is a composite of all-cause mortality, non-fatal MI or stroke over the mean follow up period of 4.37 years [53]. This consists of a high-risk population with 83% having 3-vessel disease and a significant proportion (32%) requiring insulin therapy [53]. The study results showed that there was a reduction in *primary endpoint all cause death, non-fatal MI and stroke in the CABG group*, with an **ARR of 7.9%** (26.6% in the PCI group and 18.7% in the CABG group, **p=0.005) and a Number Needed to Treat (NNT) of 12.5 [Figure 2] [53]**. There was also a reduction in *all-cause mortality* which was 16.3% in the PCI arm and 10.9% in the CABG arm with an **ARR = 5.4% and NNT of 19 [Figure 2] [53]**. This was at the cost of an increase in stroke, as might be expected in the CABG arm of **2.8% Number Needed to Harm (NNH) of 36 [53]**.

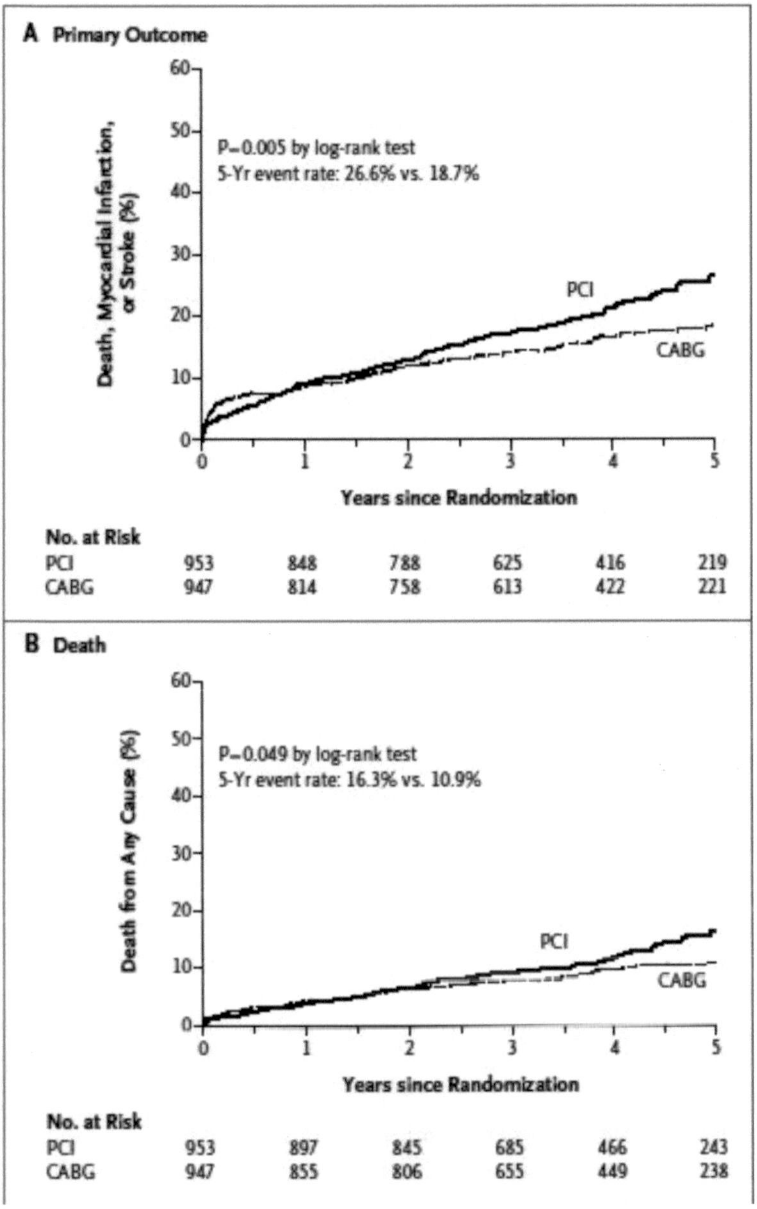

Figure 2. Kaplan-Meier Curves for composite primary outcome (all cause death, non-fatal myocardial infarction or stroke) and all cause death in a comparison between PCI with DES compared with CABG for multivessel disease in diabetic patients. Reproduced with permission from Farkough ME et al. NEJM 2012. DOI 10.1056/NEJMoa1211585.

http://dx.doi.org/10.5772/55103

6.3. Degree of ischemia and revascularization: Is the effect independent of symptoms?

Although there is paucity of randomized data addressing the question of how the degree of functional ischemia relates to the benefit of revascularization, there is observational data that suggests a strong relationship [54, 55]. Adjusted risk models have suggested that patients with *less than a 10-12.5% threshold* of ischemia as demonstrated by stress myocardial perfusion imaging, the survival profile of those treated with medical therapy were similar or even perhaps slightly better than those who are treated with revascularization [54]. However *above the threshold of 10-12.5% of ischemia,* there was a graded incremental survival benefit of revascularization over medical therapy, with a risk adjusted relative risk reduction of 50% [Figure 3] [54].

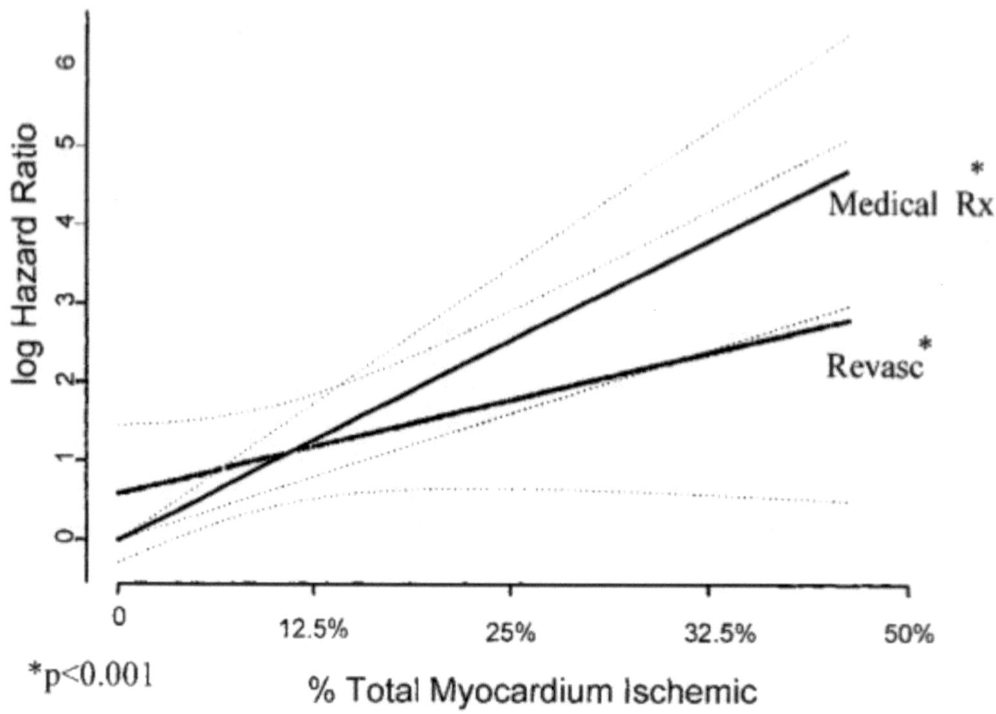

Figure 3. Log hazard ratio for revascularization (Revasc) versus medical therapy (Medical Rx) as a function of % myocardium ischemia based on final cox proportional hazards model. Model, P< 0.0001; interaction, P=0.0305 (Reproduced with permission from Hachamovitch et al. Circulation 2003. 107: 2900-2906).

This data was further corroborated by another observational study demonstrating a similar effect in a group of asymptomatic diabetic patients [55]. This study found a *14% survival benefit* in patients with a high-risk myocardial perfusion scan treated with CABG over medical therapy [55]. Patients treated with PCI in the high-risk scan group did not achieve a survival benefit over medical therapy [55]. This may be due to the fact that, this treatment group consisted of only 10.7% three vessel disease and no patients with left main disease whereas in the CABG group, this was 52.1% and 20.8% respectively [55]. The other caveat to this data is

the low overall use of optimal medical therapy, which may overestimate the effect size of revascularization in some anatomic subgroups. The use of ASA, ACEi's and BB's were all 40% or less with no mention of statin therapy [55].

In summary, patients with moderate to high-risk scans by myocardial perfusion have significant survival advantage if treated with revascularization over medical therapy alone *even in the absence of symptoms* [54, 55]. This benefit has more convincingly been demonstrated in patients undergoing CABG [54, 55]. Although the current standard and use of optimal medical therapy has improved over time, this effect is likely still significant. This survival benefit in the high-risk scans has not been clearly demonstrated in patients treated with PCI in stable coronary disease. Recently, the COURAGE trial involving over 2000 patients, which compared optimal medical therapy plus PCI with optimal medical therapy alone in stable CAD included a high prevalence of MVD (over two thirds) associated with the same proportion of multiple reversible defects by myocardial perfusion imaging [56]. This study showed, after exclusion of patients with high-risk anatomy (LM) and markedly positive exercise stress testing (substantial ST depression or hypotensive response in stage I Bruce protocol), no significant difference in all cause death and non-fatal myocardial infarction between the medical therapy and PCI groups [56].

6.4. Impact of complexity of disease

6.4.1. The synergy between PCI with taxus and cardiac surgery (SYNTAX) score

The SYNTAX score was designed as a comprehensive tool to classify the anatomic complexity and functional severity of a patients' coronary anatomy [57]. It is in fact an amalgamation of five different scoring/classification systems which can be distilled into three basic guiding principles: the first which describes the segments of the coronary artery tree; the second which describes the relative importance of the lesion based on the location and vascular territory to which the lesion impedes flow; the third which describes the complexity of the lesion [Table 1].

6.4.2. The SYNTAX trial

As techniques and technology for percutaneous coronary intervention have evolved, there has been an increasing number of patients with multivessel disease treated with percutaneous intervention [58]. The SYNTAX trial has evaluated the PCI versus CABG in patients with highly complex disease in the contemporary context of paclitaxel drug eluting stenting [51]. At 12 months there was a significantly lower incidence of the primary outcome of major cardiac and cerebrovascular events (MACCE) (ie. all cause death, stroke myocardial infarction or repeat revascularization) CABG group compared than the PCI group with an **ARR of 5.4% or NNT 19** [51]. This was largely driven by an increase need for repeat revascularization as the rates of *all cause death, MI or stroke was similar between the two groups* [51]. In the initial subgroup analysis at 12 months, while there was a trend towards lower MACCE in the CABG group compared to the PCI group as the SYNTAX scores increased, a significantly lower rate of the primary outcome could only be demonstrated at the highest SYNTAX scores (>33) [Figure 4] [51].

http://dx.doi.org/10.5772/55103

Principle	Description
Definition and segmentation of the coronary artery tree	1. The coronary tree can be divided into 16 major segments
Functional significance	2. Functional importance of the particular epicardial vessel is weighted according to the percentage of the left ventricle to which it supplies. For example the left main supplies 5 times the vascular territory compared to that of a dominant RCA; hence the LM will be given a score of 5 whereas the RCA will be given a score of 1.
Lesion Complexity	3. The complexity of the lesion itself can be described in terms of a. Degree of involvement of side branches, anatomic configuration of lesions b. Presence or absence of a total occlusions and presence of collaterals c. Lesion length d. Tortuousity of vessel e. Presence or absence of heavy calcification f. Presence or absence of Thrombus g. Presence or absence of diffuse disease

Table 1. Principles underlying the development of the SYNTAX score

The 3-year follow-up for this study more definitively demonstrated that PCI and CABG tended to have similar cardiovascular outcomes in patients with lower complexity while at higher levels of anatomical complexity, patients that underwent CABG faired better [Figure 5] [59]. At three-year follow-up, patients with 3VD in the CABG group versus the PCI group with intermediate complexity (SYNTAX Score 23-32) had overall **decrease in MI with an ARR of 5.8%** and those with the highest complexity (SYNTAX Score >33) had a decrease in **all cause mortality (ARR of 6.6%) and a decrease in MI (ARR of 5.3%)** [51, 59]. This was also reflected in an *overall lower all-cause death* in the 3VD patients treated with CABG versus PCI with an *ARR of 3.8% (p=0.02)* and a *lower rate of cardiac death* in those treated with CABG versus PCI *ARR 3.3% (p=0.01) [59].* Interestingly, there was no significant difference for all-cause death or cardiac death between the CABG group versus the PCI group among patients with LM disease [59]. In contrast to those with 3VD, there were only significantly lower MACCE rates among patients with LM disease treated with CABG compared with PCI at the highest SYNTAX scores (>33) [59]. Although it is difficult to make precise conclusions regarding the subgroup analyses, the overall trends are certainly compelling.

The recent SYNTAX trial has heralded a new era in revascularization. The recent European Guidelines have responded to the findings by giving a **IIa recommendation (level B evidence)** to PCI for revascularization in 3VD with low angiographic complexity (SYNTAX score ≤22) while giving a **class III recommendation (level A evidence)** for revascularization of such patients moderate to high angiographic complexity (SYNTAX score >22) [26]. The most recent ACC/AHA PCI guidelines state that in patients with 3VD with or without proximal LAD, revascularization with PCI for the purposes of prognosis is of **uncertain benefit (IIb recommendation, level B evidence)** [14]. In these populations, CABG is still given **Class I recommendation (level B evidence)** [Table 2 and 3] [14, 26].

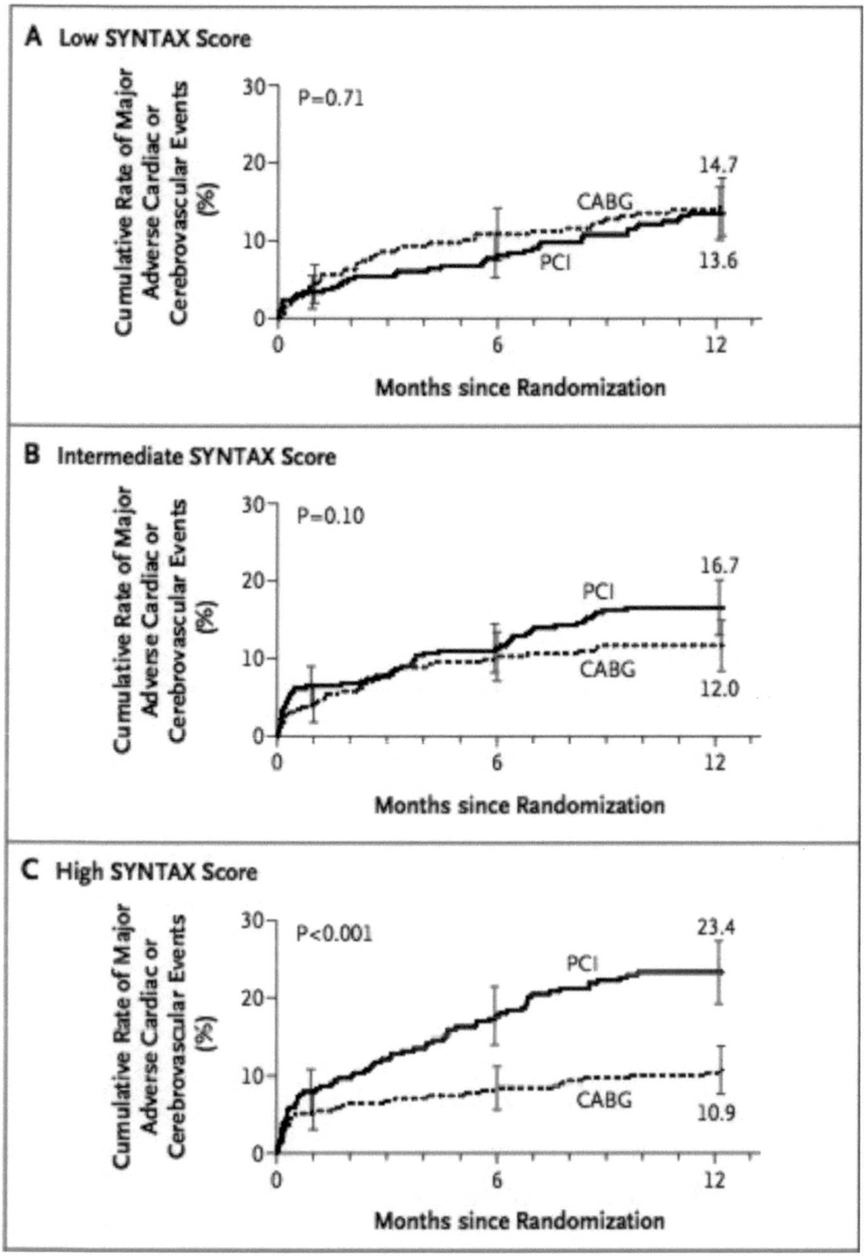

Figure 4. 12-month Subgroup analysis of the rates of (all cause death, stroke, myocardial infarction and repeat revascularization) between those treated by CABG versus PCI stratified by SYNTAX score. A significant difference in the overall rates was not significantly different at low (<22) and intermediate (23-32) SYNTAX scores. At the highest SYNTAX score (>33), there was a significantly lower rate of major cardiac and cerebrovascular events. Reproduced with permission from Serruys PW et al. NEJM 2009. 360;10: 961-972.

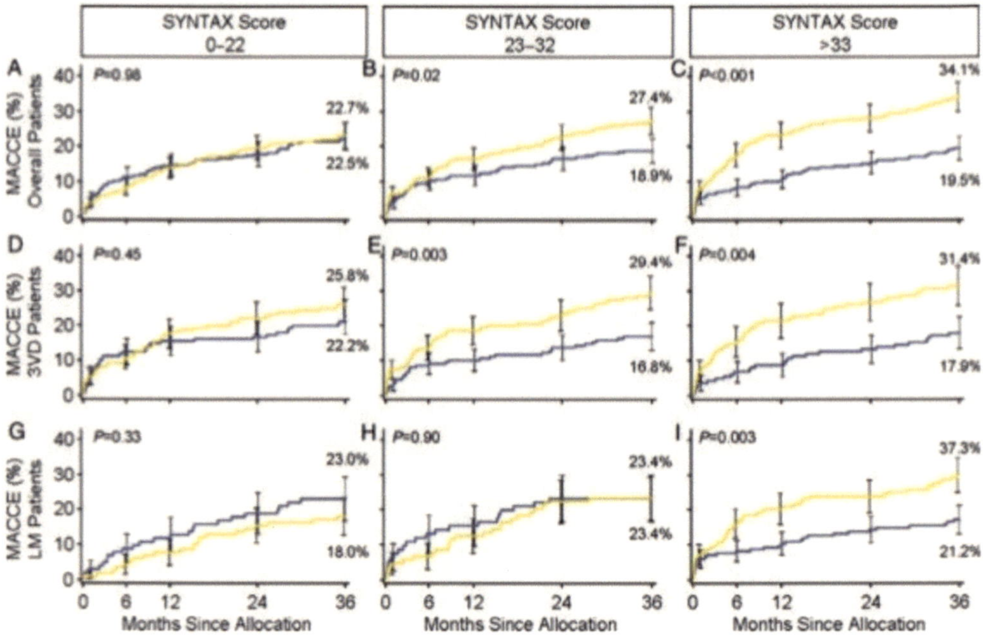

Figure 5. 3-year subgroup analysis of the rates of MACCE (all cause death, stroke, myocardial infarction and repeat revascularization) between those treated by CABG (blue line) versus PCI (yellow line) stratified by SYNTAX score: Low SYNTAX Score (0-22), Intermediate SYNTAX Score (23-32), High SYNTAX Score (>33). Results are provided for overall group (A-C), 3VD patients (D-F) and LM patients (G–I). Reproduced with permission from Kappetein et al. European Heart Journal 2011. 32: 2125-2134.

Subset of CAD by anatomy	Favours CABG	Favours PCI
1VD or 2VD - non-proximal LAD	IIb C	I C
1VD or 2VD - proximal LAD	I A	IIa B
3VD simple lesions, full functional revascularization achievable with PCI, SYNTAX score ≤22	I A	IIa B
3VD complex lesions, incomplete revascularization achievable with PCI, SYNTAX score >22	I A	III A
Left main (isolated or 1VD, ostium/shaft)	I A	IIa B
Left main (isolated or 1VD, distal bifurcation)	I A	IIb B
Left main + 2VD or 3VD, SYNTAX score ≤32	I A	IIb B
Left main + 2VD or 3VD, SYNTAX score ≥33	I A	III B

Table 2. ESC Guidelines on revascularization for complex coronary disease. Indications for CABG and PCI are tabulated for stable patients with low predicted surgical mortality and lesions suitable for either modes of revascularization. CABG= coronary artery bypass grafting; CAD= coronary artery disease; LAD = left anterior descending; PCI= percutaneous coronary intervention; VD= vessel disease. Reproduced with permission from Wijns W et al. European Heart Journal 2010. 31: 2501-2555.

http://dx.doi.org/10.5772/55103

Anatomical Setting	Class of Recommendation	Level of Evidence
UPLM or complex CAD		
CABG and PCI	I—Heart Team approach recommended	C
CABG and PCI	IIa—Calculation of STS and SYNTAX scores	B
UPLM*		
CABG	I	B
PCI	IIa—For SIHD when *both* of the following are present • Anatomic conditions associated with a low risk of PCI procedural complications and a high likelihood of good long-term outcome (eg, a low SYNTAX score of ≤22, ostial or trunk left main CAD) • Clinical characteristics that predict a significantly increased risk of adverse surgical outcomes (eg, STS-predicted risk of operative mortality ≥5%)	B
	IIa—For UA/NSTEMI if not a CABG candidate	B
	IIa—For STEMI when distal coronary flow is TIMI flow grade <3 and PCI can be performed more rapidly and safely than CABG	C
	IIb—For SIHD when *both* of the following are present • Anatomic conditions associated with a low to intermediate risk of PCI procedural complications and an intermediate to high likelihood of good long-term outcome (eg, low-intermediate SYNTAX score of <33, bifurcation left main CAD) • Clinical characteristics that predict an increased risk of adverse surgical outcomes (eg, moderate-severe COPD, disability from prior stroke, or prior cardiac surgery; STS-predicted risk of operative mortality >2%)	B
	III: Harm—For SIHD in patients (versus performing CABG) with unfavorable anatomy for PCI and who are good candidates for CABG	B
3-vessel disease with or without proximal LAD artery disease*		
CABG	I	B
	IIa—It is reasonable to choose CABG over PCI in patients with complex 3-vessel CAD (eg, SYNTAX score >22) who are good candidates for CABG	B
PCI	IIb—Of uncertain benefit	B
2-vessel disease with proximal LAD artery disease*		
CABG	I	B
PCI	IIb—Of uncertain benefit	B
2-vessel disease without proximal LAD artery disease*		
CABG	IIa—With extensive ischemia	B
	IIb—Of uncertain benefit without extensive ischemia	C
PCI	IIb—Of uncertain benefit	B
1-vessel proximal LAD artery disease		
CABG	IIa—With LIMA for long-term benefit	B
PCI	IIb—Of uncertain benefit	B
1-vessel disease without proximal LAD artery involvement		
CABG	III: Harm	B
PCI	III: Harm	B
LV dysfunction		
CABG	IIa—EF 35% to 50%	B
CABG	IIb—EF <35% without significant left main CAD	B
PCI	Insufficient data	
Survivors of sudden cardiac death with presumed ischemia-mediated VT		
CABG	I	B
PCI	I	C
No anatomic or physiologic criteria for revascularization		
CABG	III: Harm	B
PCI	III: Harm	B

Table 3. ACC Guidelines on revascularization for complex coronary disease to improve survival. Indications for CABG and PCI are tabulated. CABG = coronary artery bypass grafting; COPD= chronic obstructive pulmonary disease; EF= ejection fraction; LAD=left anterior descending artery; LIMA= left internal mammary artery; LV =left ventricular; N/A= not applicable; PCI = percutaneous coronary intervention; SIHD = stable ischemic heart disease; STEMI= ST-elevation myocardial infarction; STS= Society of Thoracic Surgeons; SYNTAX = Synergy between percutaneous coronary intervention with TAXUS and Cardiac Surgery; TIMI= Thrombolysis in myocardial infarction; UA/NSTEMI =unstable angina/ non-ST elevation myocardial infarction; UPLM= unprotected left main disease; VT=ventricular tachycardia. Reproduced with permission from Levine GN et al. Circulation 2011. 124: e574-e651.

For those with unprotected left main disease (UPLM), both the ACC and ESC guidelines still give a **Class I** ***recommendation for CABG in all cases*** **(Classified as Grade A evidence for ESC and Grade B evidence for ACC)** [14, 26]. They have both also given a **IIa recommendation for PCI in Stable Ischemic Heart Disease (SIHD) in UPLM when the SYNTAX is 22 or less (eg isolated ostial or main trunk LM)** and **IIb recommendation for PCI for low or intermediate SYNTAX score (<33) (Level B evidence)** [14, 26]

It is recognized however, that some populations are not expected to derive prognostic benefit from revascularization. In such groups for the purposes of alleviating symptoms refractory to optimal medical therapy, CABG and PCI have equivalent **Class I recommendation (level A evidence)** unless **SYNTAX is >22 in which case CABG is still favored (Class IIa recommendation, level B evidence)** [14].

7. PCI versus CABG in acute coronary syndromes versus stable ischemic coronary artery disease

7.1. Non-ST-elevation acute coronary syndromes (NSTEACS)

Although there are limited studies designed to address this specific question, it is generally accepted that the same considerations that are used to decide between PCI and CABG in stable ischemic coronary artery disease would be applied when faced with an NSTEACS **(Class I recommendation, Level B evidence)** [14]. Comparisons between PCI and CABG have typically included a mixture of patients with stable and unstable symptoms [45]. The ERACI II study contained the highest proportion of patients with unstable symptoms constituting 92% of the randomized patients whereas MASS II included the least with 0% having unstable symptoms [60, 61]. However in a large meta-analysis including individual patient data from 10 large randomized studies (n=7812) did not reveal any significant interaction between the presence or absence of unstable symptoms and mode of revascularization (PCI vs CABG) with respect to mortality outcomes over a 5 year period [45].

The optimal approach to PCI in the setting of a NSTEACS and MVD is still somewhat uncertain. There are currently no randomized trials in the literature comparing the multivessel PCI to culprit only PCI in NSTEACS [62].

7.2. ST -elevation acute coronary syndromes (STEACS)

Primary PCI remains the main modality of revascularization in STEACS *(Class I recommendation, Level A evidence)*. It is common to encounter MVD during the index angiogram for STEACS having an estimated incidence of up to 40-50 percent [62]. Current evidence supports primary PCI of the culprit vessel only, in the absence of hemodynamic instability, as the optimal approach [14, 62, 63]. *Multivessel PCI in this setting has been associated with a higher mortality and is not recommended (Class III recommendation, Level B evidence) [14, 62, 63].* The approach to residual coronary disease has been a subject of controversy and the decisions are likely made clinically on an individual basis.

7.3 Cardiogenic shock

The optimal mode of revascularization in patients with multivessel disease and cardiogenic shock is still under debate due to lack of supporting evidence for or against either PCI or CABG. It has been previously shown in the **Should We Emergently Revascularize Occluded Arteries for Cardiogenic Shock (SHOCK) Trial** that urgent revascularization with PCI or CABG for cardiogenic shock in the setting of STEACS has *mortality benefit* with an **ARR of 13 percent** or **NNT of 8** at 6 months compared with medical management [64]. This difference continued out to one year and remained stable at long-term follow up [Figure 6] [65, 66]. In the revascularization group, 64 percent were treated with angioplasty whereas 36 percent were treated with CABG [64]. Interestingly, because the mode of revascularization was at the discretion of the treating physicians, patients treated with CABG compared with those that received PCI tended to more often have LM disease and 3VD [64]. Nevertheless, there was no significant difference between patients treated with PCI versus CABG at either 30 days or at 1 year [64]. Certainly the advantage of PCI for revascularization over CABG would be a reduced time required to achieve revascularization; the time of randomization to first revascularization attempt was 0.9 hour for PCI and 2.7 hours for CABG [64].

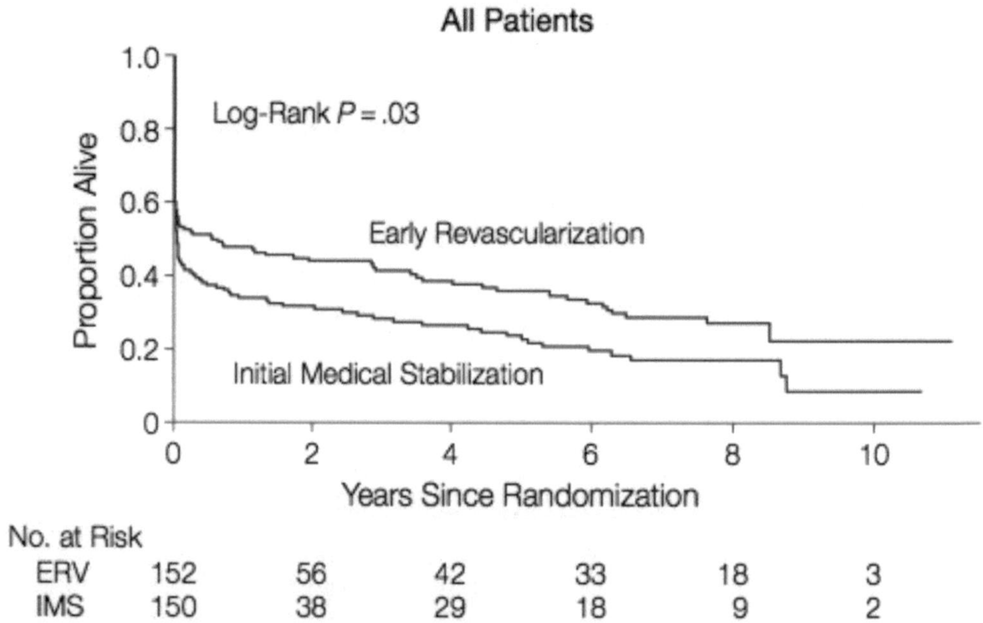

Figure 6. Kaplan-Meier Survival Curves For Early Revascularization Versus Initial Medical Stabilization in Long Term Follow-Up. ERV= Early Revascularization; IMS =Initial Medical Stabilization. Reproduced with permission from Hochman JS. et al. JAMA 2006. 295;21: 2511-2515.

There is a lack of randomized data regarding the optimal mode of revascularization in cardiogenic shock for acute coronary syndromes [67]. Currently, both the ACC and ESC

guidelines recommend that PCI (or emergency CABG) should be performed on patients who candidates for revascularization in the setting of STEMI and severe heart failure or cardiogenic shock *(Class I recommendation, Level B evidence)* [14, 26]. Although the data upon which this recommendation is based does not show a preferential benefit to either mode of revascularization, both guidelines favor PCI as the primary mode of revascularization in cardiogenic shock [14, 26]. The ACC guidelines do recognize however, that "select patients with severe 3VD or LM disease can benefit from emergency CABG" [14].

8. Treatment of hemodynamically significant disease

Currently, the ACC/ AHA defines a significant stenosis as "Greater than or equal to 70% luminal diameter narrowing, by visual assessment, of an epicardial stenosis measured in the "worst view" angiographic projection [68]." The exception is the left main artery in which a significant stenosis is defined as " greater or equal to 50% luminal diameter narrowing [68]." A challenge in the interpretation of the data surrounding comparisons of PCI versus CABG the variability in definitions of "significant disease." Interestingly, many of the landmark trials comparing PCI versus CABG actually defined a significant stenosis as greater or equal to 50% [27, 45, 51].

Even in the presence of a significant stenosis, myocardial blood flow can be maintained by compensatory mechanisms at rest [69]. Consequently, hemodynamically significant disease has been defined by those lesions, which produce a reduction in coronary flow reserve under conditions of maximal hyperemia [69, 70]. Reduction of coronary flow reserve is generally observed in lesions with as little as 50 percent stenosis but progressively worsens with the degree of narrowing [70]. There are two implications of this clinically. First, there is a significant interobserver and intraobserver variability in the degree of angiographic stenosis [69]. Second, the hemodynamic significance of a given lesion is dependent on the severity of the stenosis, the length of the lesion as well as the presence of collateral blood flow [71].

Aims to quantify the functional significance of coronary stenosis lead to the development of the concept Fractional Flow Reserve (FFR) [72]. FFR is a hemodynamic construct defined as the maximal blood flow distal to a stenosis compared with the maximal blood flow in the same vessel, hypothetically in the absence of any stenosis, conditions of maximal hyperemia [72]. Flow can be characterized by the following equation: Pressure (P) = Flow (Q) * Resistance (R) [72]. For a given lesion, the FFR is the maximal flow for the stenotic vessel (Qs)/ maximal flow if the vessel were normal (Qn). Since, under maximal hyperemia, the resistance becomes a constant, Q is only dependent on the pressure and fractional flow reserve can be defined by a ratio of aortic pressure (Pa)/ pressure distal to the lesion (Pd) [Figure 7] [72]. FFR allows for the functional assessment of ischemia at the time of coronary angiogram [72].

http://dx.doi.org/10.5772/55103

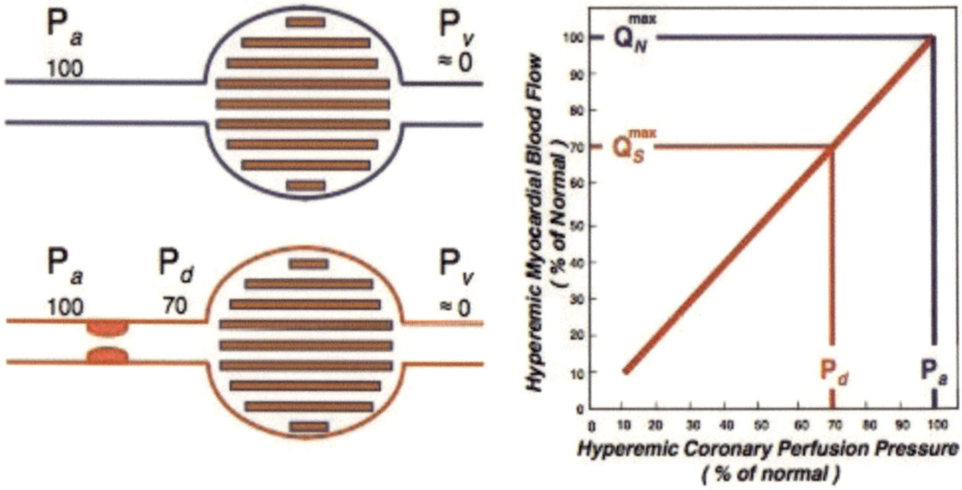

Figure 7. A schematic depiction of the concept of fractional flow reserve. On the right is the graphical correlation between Flow Q and perfusion pressure P under conditions of maximal hyperemia. The maximal blood flow in the stenotic vessel Q_S (Red Lines) is directly proportional to the perfusion pressure distal to the lesion. The maximal blood flow in the same vessel hypothetically without the stenosis Q_N (Blue Lines) is proportional to the perfusion pressure proximal to the stenosis Pa which is the same as aortic pressure. Q_S/Q_N is therefore equal to Pd/Pa. Reproduced with permission from Pijls NHJ et al. JACC 2012. 59: 1045-57.

The use of FFR will be come increasingly more relevant in the assessment of patients with multivessel disease. The **Fractional Flow Reserve Versus Angiography for Multivessel Evaluation (FAME)** was a study randomizing 1005 patients to either angiographically guided PCI or PCI guided by fractional flow reserve in patients with multivessel disease of at least moderate severity (greater or equal to 50%) [73]. Patients in the angiographic group were revascularized if PCI was indicated based on visual assessment of angiographic data and clinical data; patients in the FFR group only had PCI if the FFR was < 0.80 [73]. The combined outcome of death, myocardial infarction and repeat revascularization was significantly less in those treated with FFR guided PCI (18.3%) than the angiographically guided PCI (13.2%) [Figure 8] [73]. Death and myocardial infarction, although not a pre-specified outcome, was also significantly less in the FFR group (11.1%) versus the angiographic group (7.3%) [73]. This difference persisted to the two-year follow-up [74].

Although FFR is early in its development, certainly it has the potential to play a role in classifying the severity of disease for decision-making in MVD. Consider a patient with 3VD with a 50 percent lesion at the proximal LAD. If the proximal LAD lesion is FFR is greater than 0.80, this patient may in fact be classified as two vessel disease with no hemodynamic involvement of the proximal LAD and hence should receive PCI. While there is limited research exploring the use of FFR in determining the mode of revascularization, this is certainly an area worthy of further study. Currently the ACC advocates the use of FFR guiding revascularization decisions in stable ischemic heart disease with moderate lesions with 50-70% stenosis (**IIa recommendation, level A evidence**) [14].

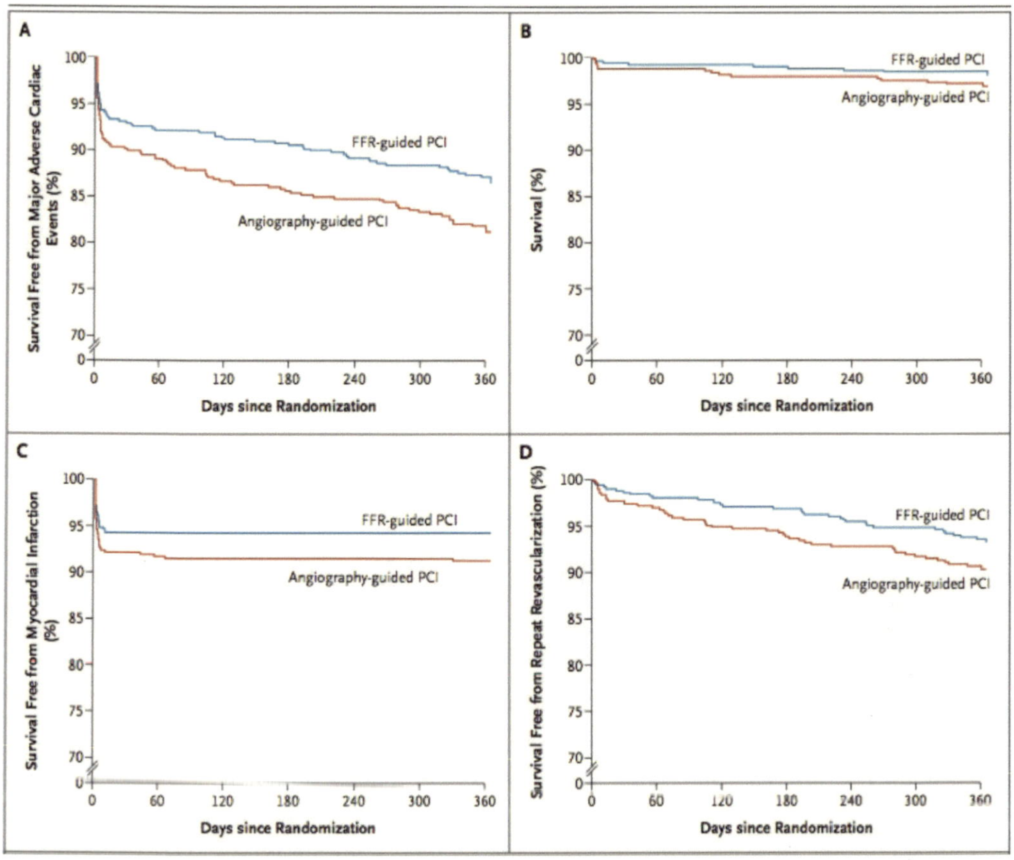

Figure 8. Kaplan-Meier Survival Curves according to study group PCI guided by angiography alone versus PCI guided by FFR in addition to angiography. FFR=fractional flow reserve, PCI=percutaneous coronary intervention. Reproduced with permission from Tonino PAL et al. Fractional flow reserve versus angiography or guiding percutanous coronary intervention. NEJM 2009. 360(3):213-224.

9. Current trends in PCI versus CABG in North America

The practice patterns regarding PCI and CABG have changed dramatically within the last 10-15 years. In the earlier part of this last decade, rates of PCI have been observed to be on the rise both in the United States and in Canada despite relatively more static rates of CABG over that same period [75, 76]. Furthermore, although there is some signal that the trend in PCI rates have begun to plateau or reverse in the latter part of this decade both in the United states and in Canada, there is still a consistent increase in the overall PCI: CABG ratio [77, 78].

These recent trends have been an area of increasing research interest, as it seems paradoxical in the context of relatively consistent practice guidelines from the ACC and the ESC supporting the use of CABG as the first line mode of revascularization in prognostically important stable

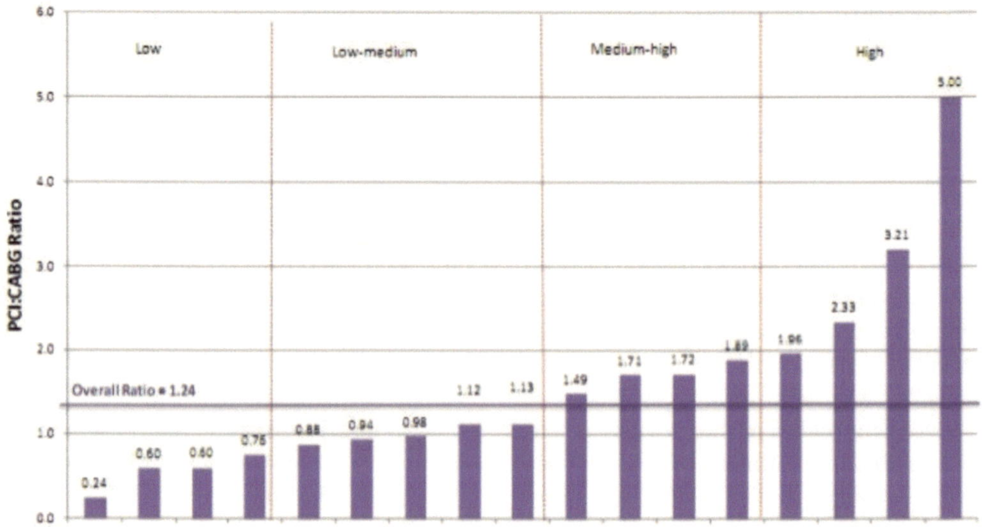

Figure 9. Variation in Revascularization for Multivessel Disease Across 17 Cardiac Centers in Ontario. Reproduced with permission from Schwalm JD et al. SYNTAX Score and Real World Revascularization Patterns. Canadian Cardiovascular Congress 2011 Vancouver, BC. Abstract Presentation.

ischemic coronary artery disease [Figure 9] [14, 26]. In fact, recent data has demonstrated a rise in PCI with DES in patients with Class I recommendation for surgery [25].

Significant variability in PCI: CABG ratio between provinces/states, between hospitals and even between individual interventionalists suggests that the trends in revascularization practices are not entirely explained by changes in population or advancements in revascularization techniques [76-80]. In Ontario, Canada, PCI to CABG ratios vary considerably between hospitals from 1.3 to 6.1 [81]. In multivessel disease, this ratio ranges from 0.24 to 5.0 [figure 9] [82]. The physician performing the diagnostic catheterization (interventional cardiologist versus non-interventional cardiologist), the coronary anatomy (LM, 3VD, 2VD), and the treating hospital were the three strongest determinants of the ultimate therapeutic strategy [58].

Two possible hypotheses for the presence of such dramatic variability in the management of multi-vessel disease include misinterpretation of the evidence and misclassification of disease complexity at the time of diagnostic angiogram. There are complex interacting variables upon which the final therapeutic decision is based, including: (1) complexity of coronary anatomy, (2) presence or absence of prognostically important factors favoring surgery, (3) degree of active functional ischemia, (4) complex co-morbid state of patient, (5) patient preferences and social factors, (6) local resources and expertise. All of these factors may affect the patient's suitability for CABG and likelihood to benefit prognostically from surgical revascularization. Application of the large body of evidence in this variable clinical milieu is a complex process. The management algorithm is further complicated when considering the patient's role in the decision-making process and the steps required to ensure truly "informed" patient consent.

10. Angioplasty versus bypass surgery: An evolving complex decision analysis

10.1. Establishing a general approach

Decisions regarding revascularization are complex and have been founded on decades of evidence. This body of evidence has evolved in parallel with advances in treatment but also a patient population with increasing medical complexity. Therefore, a contemporary approach to MVD and revascularization must be founded on an understanding of the wide spectrum of disease severity, advances in medical/surgical therapy, diversity in patient populations, patient preference and social circumstances. Optimal treatment strategies must apply the most current evidence in an appropriate clinical context. Furthermore, guiding principles of management with a multidisciplinary 'Heart Team' approach should be the cornerstone of state of the art treatment of multivessel coronary artery disease as supported by recent revascularization guidelines [14]. The basic approach should address a number of basic clinical questions which address the (1) therapeutic goals of the case, (2) the presence or absence of clinical evidence to support revascularization, (3) the presence/absence of prognostic factors that may make surgical revascularization more favorable, (4) whether the anatomy favor PCI or CABG, (5) is the patient a good surgical candidate should prognostic disease be present, (6) does the patient have any particular preferences and (7) are there ambiguities that would benefit from further discussion by a Heart Team [Table 4].

Fundamental Question	
Therapeutic Goals:	● Can we improve survival? ● Can we improve symptoms? ● Can we improve both?
Clinical Evidence to support revascularization	● Severity of disease ● Severity of Symptoms ● Degree of Ischemia ● Degree of Medical Optimization
Prognostic Factors that may make surgical revascularization more favorable?	LM, 3VD, or 2VD with proximal LAD with ● DM ● LV dysfunction ● High burden of ischemia ("/≥12.5 percent)
Does anatomy favor one mode of revascularization versus the other?	● Surgical targets ● Diffuseness of disease ● Complexity
Is the patient a good surgical candidate?	Consider: ● Age ● Co-morbidities ● Anatomy
Patient Preference and Social Factors	Discussed off the catheterization table
Ambiguities in Case?	Would this benefit from discussion with the Heart Team?

Table 4. Key clinical questions forming the basis of the therapeutic decision for management of multivessel coronary artery disease.

http://dx.doi.org/10.5772/55103

The fundamental basis of our decisions rest on what therapeutic goals can be achieved: *improvement of survival, improvement of symptoms or both.* It is important to make this distinction because although the goal would naturally to improve on both; consider the following two clinical scenarios:

- In a 50 year-old asymptomatic patient with 70% distal LM, CABG is the treatment of choice regardless of his symptom profile because of known survival benefit with surgical revascularization **(Class I, Level A evidence)**[14]
- In a 90 year-old, medically optimized, CCS class III patient who has 3VD and normal ejection fraction, his age may undermine any treatment for the purposes of prognosis, hence PCI may be favored if technically feasible as the overriding goal is for relief of symptoms. **(Class I, Level A evidence)**[14]

If the intent is to improve survival, there is good evidence that supports revascularization in certain patient populations: significant left main (>50%) or 3VD, 2VD with proximal LAD with diabetes LV dysfunction and/or high burden of functional ischemia).

If the intent is primarily to *improve symptoms (eg. The clinical profile undermines the prognostic benefit of surgical revascularization)*, there is good evidence that revascularization with PCI is of benefit in those who are symptomatic despite optimal medical therapy if technically feasible. But with advances in medical therapy, it is reasonable to maximize medical treatment before considering revascularization [56].

10.2. The decision algorithm

Based on existing evidence and guidelines, we have developed an algorithm that may help guide decision-making in the management of MVD [Figure10]. There are a number of factors that support surgical revascularization in SIHD for improving survival over medical therapy or PCI, namely: 1) LM disease, 3VD and likely some subsets of 2VD with proximal LAD; 2) MVD in the presence of mild to moderate LV dysfunction (35-49%) 3) MVD in the presence of diabetes 4) coronary anatomy of intermediate to high level of complexity (SYNTAX >22) and 5) high burden of ischemia (>12.5%). If these are present, then surgery should be considered first unless patient preference dictates otherwise **(Class I recommendation, Level B Evidence).**

If the patient does have prognostic disease, then considering the overall coronary anatomy, patients clinical profile and co-morbidities must be considered to ultimately guide the appropriate therapeutic decision. These factors may alter the likelihood of benefit from revascularization and also affect the patients' potential eligibility CABG and PCI.

If the patient does not appear to have prognostic disease and is not likely to prognostically benefit from revascularization, then the primary goal of treatment would be symptoms. The first goal of alleviating symptoms is medical optimization. If the patient has unacceptable symptoms despite optimal medical therapy, then revascularization (PCI or CABG) would be indicated **(Class I recommendation, Level A Evidence).**

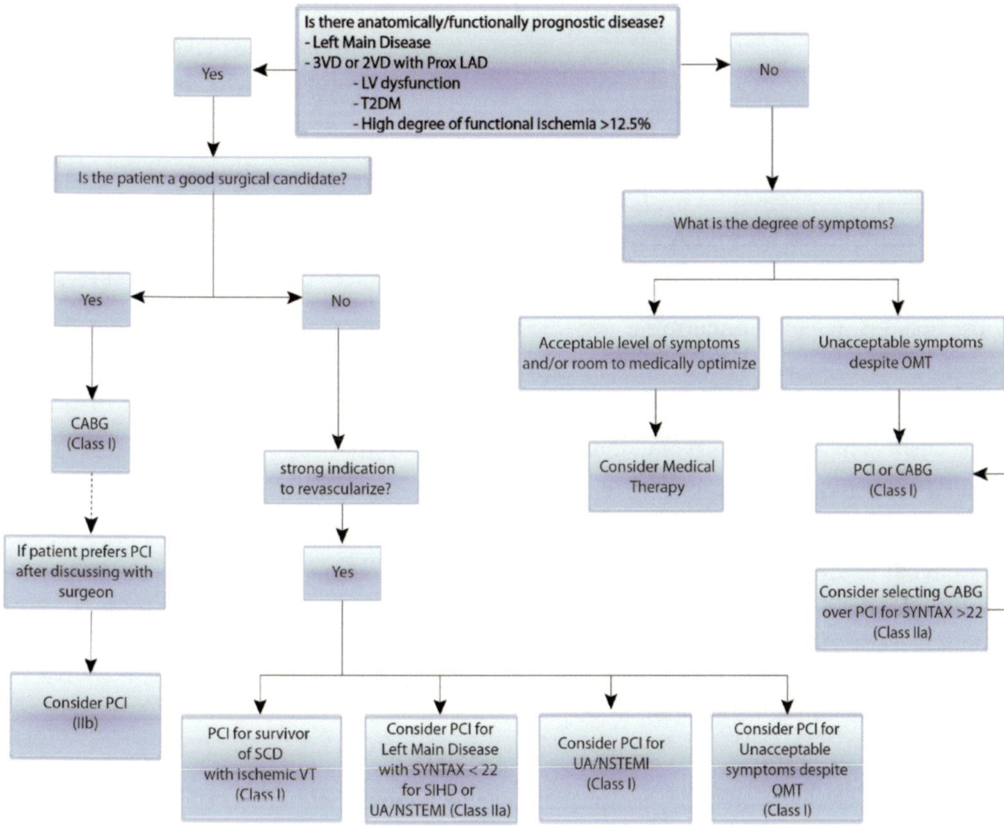

Figure 10. Suggested approach for decision making in multivessel coronary artery disease. CAD= coronary artery disease; CABG= coronary artery bypass grafting; LAD= left anterior descending artery; LM = left main disease; LV= Left Ventricular; OMT= optimal medical therapy; PCI= percutaneous coronary intervention; SCD= sudden cardiac death; SYNTAX = The Synergy between PCI with Taxus and Cardiac Surgery; T2DM= Type 2 Diabetes Mellitis; UA/NSTEMi = unstable angina/Non ST elevation myocardial infarction; VT= ventricular tachycardia; 3VD = Three vessel disease; 2VD = two vessel disease.

11. The Role of the heart team in the future of multivessel disease

The management of CAD with the advances in revascularization techniques and medical therapy, changing patient population and constantly expanding body of knowledge is becoming increasingly more complex. Such complexity would intuitively benefit from a broad spectrum of expertise. There is currently increasing interest in the area of multidisciplinary decision-making and both ACC and ESC have recommended that a Heart Team approach be implemented in the management of UPLM disease or complex CAD *(Class I recommendation, Level C Evidence)* [14, 26]. It is envisioned that with the joint involvement of the interventional cardiologist, the cardiac surgeon and a non-invasive cardiologist, there will be a more balanced, consistent management of these complex cases. From the patient's perspective, this approach would conceivably allow them to be more informed and involved in the ultimate

http://dx.doi.org/10.5772/55103

treatment decision. There is currently limited data on the true impact of the Heart Team and this is certainly an area of worthy future research.

12. The future of research in complex coronary artery disease

The approach to the management of complex CAD will continue to change with exponential growth of knowledge in this area. The majority of clinical trials involving CABG and PCI were largely based on complete revascularization of lesions greater than 50 percent [45]. Use of FFR has shown that PCI with DES of moderately severe lesions (50-70 percent) guided by angiography alone compared with PCI of lesions guided by both angiography and hemodynamic significance (FFR< 0.80) may actually confer a higher rate of death and MI [73]. Given our knowledge of this finding, the SYNTAX trial (where the threshold for revascularization was also a stenosis of 50 percent or greater) may conceivably have different results if FFR was used to guide therapy. Furthermore, investigations with the new second-generation DES, a now better understanding of how to utilize FFR and definition of the impact of coronary complexity may serve as a guide to better define the populations that may benefit from PCI versus CABG.

The other area requiring more research is in the arena of collaboration for decision-making in multivessel disease. The Heart Team, although a promising concept would benefit from formal validation. We also need to better define what type of institutions and what type of cases would most benefit from formal evaluation with a Heart Team approach. Furthermore as these decisions become more complex, we will also need to find better methods/mechanisms of informed balanced patient involvement in the final management decision.

Complex CAD remains a challenging area both from the scientific and the clinical point of view. The goal should be to build on the research foundations in the management of MVD CAD thus far and continue to improve our understanding of how to better manage and care for patients with complex CAD.

Abbreviations

ACC	American College of Cardiology
ACEi	Angiotensin Converting Enzyme inhibitor
ARB	Angiotensin Receptor Blocker
AHA	American Heart Association
ARR	Absolute risk reduction
ASA	Aspirin
BB	Beta Blocker
BMS	Bare metal stent

CABG	Coronary artery bypass grafting
CAD	Coronary artery disease
CI	95% Confidence interval
COPD	Chronic obstructive pulmonary disease
DAPT	Dual antiplatelet therapy
DES	Drug eluting stent
ESC	European Society of Cardiology
HMG-CoA	3-hydroxyl-3-methyl-glutaryl-coenzyme A
LAD	Left anterior descending artery
LIMA	Left internal mammary artery
LM	Left main
MID CAB	minimally invasive direct coronary artery bypass
NNH	Number Needed to Harm
NNT	Number Needed to Treat
NSTEACS	Non ST elevation acute coronary syndrome
NSTEMI	Non ST elevation myocardial infarction
PCI	Percutaneous coronary intervention
POBA	Plain old balloon angioplasty
RRR	Relative Risk Reduction
SCD	Sudden cardiac death
SIHD	Stable ischemic heart disease
STEACS	ST elevation acute coronary syndrome
STEMI	ST elevation myocardial infarction
SYNTAX	Synergy between PCI with Taxus and Cardiac Surgery
UA	Unstable angina
UPLM	Unprotected left main disease
VT	Ventricular tachycardia
3VD	Three vessel disease
2VD	Two vessel disease

Author details

Michael Tsang and JD Schwalm

Department of Medicine, Division of Cardiology, McMaster University, Hamilton Health Sciences, Population Health Research Institute, Hamilton, Ontario, Canada

http://dx.doi.org/10.5772/55103

References

[1] Macklem, P.T., *Stephen Hales, an unrecognized giant of medicine.* Osler Libr Newsl, 2010(114): p. 1-4.

[2] Bourassa, M.G., *The history of cardiac catheterization.* Can J Cardiol, 2005. 21(12): p. 1011-4.

[3] Proudfit, W.L., E.K. Shirey, and F.M. Sones, Jr., *Selective cine coronary arteriography. Correlation with clinical findings in 1,000 patients.* Circulation, 1966. 33(6): p. 901-10.

[4] Sones, F.M.J. and E.K. Shirey, *Cine coronary arteriography.* Mod Con Cardiov Dis, 1962. 31: p. 735.

[5] Mueller, R.L. and T.A. Sanborn, *The history of interventional cardiology: cardiac catheterization, angioplasty, and related interventions.* Am Heart J, 1995. 129(1): p. 146-72.

[6] Berry, D., *The unlocking of the coronary arteries: origins of angioplasty. A short historical review of arterial dilatation from Dotter to the creative Gruentzig.* Eur Heart J, 2009. 30(12): p. 1421-2.

[7] Nabel, E.G. and E. Braunwald, *A tale of coronary artery disease and myocardial infarction.* N Engl J Med, 2012. 366(1): p. 54-63.

[8] Smith, S.C., Jr., et al., *AHA/ACCF Secondary Prevention and Risk Reduction Therapy for Patients with Coronary and other Atherosclerotic Vascular Disease: 2011 update: a guideline from the American Heart Association and American College of Cardiology Foundation.* Circulation, 2011. 124(22): p. 2458-73.

[9] Head, S.J., et al., *Risk profile and 3-year outcomes from the SYNTAX percutaneous coronary intervention and coronary artery bypass grafting nested registries.* JACC Cardiovasc Interv, 2012. 5(6): p. 618-25.

[10] Fuster, R.G., et al., *Prognostic value of chronic obstructive pulmonary disease in coronary artery bypass grafting.* Eur J Cardiothorac Surg, 2006. 29(2): p. 202-9.

[11] Ried, M., et al., *Mild-to-moderate COPD as a risk factor for increased 30-day mortality in cardiac surgery.* Thorac Cardiovasc Surg, 2010. 58(7): p. 387-91.

[12] Hirshfeld, J.W., Jr., et al., *American College of Cardiology training statement on recommendations for the structure of an optimal adult interventional cardiology training program: a report of the American College of Cardiology task force on clinical expert consensus documents.* J Am Coll Cardiol, 1999. 34(7): p. 2141-7.

[13] Ryan, T.J., K. F.J., and R. W.A., *Clinical competence in percutaneous transluminal coronary angioplasty. A statement for physicians from the ACP/ACC/AHA Task Force on Clinical Privileges in Cardiology.* Circulation, 1990. 81(6): p. 2041-6.

[14] Levine, G.N., et al., *2011 ACCF/AHA/SCAI Guideline for Percutaneous Coronary Intervention: a report of the American College of Cardiology Foundation/American Heart Associa-*

tion Task Force on Practice Guidelines and the Society for Cardiovascular Angiography and Interventions. Circulation, 2011. 124(23): p. e574-651.

[15] Holmes, D.R., Jr., *Creativity, ingenuity, serendipity.* Can J Cardiol, 2005. 21(12): p. 1061-5.

[16] Campeau, L., *Entry sites for coronary angiography and therapeutic interventions: from the proximal to the distal radial artery.* Can J Cardiol, 2001. 17(3): p. 319-25.

[17] Gruntzig, A.R., A. Senning, and W.E. Siegenthaler, *Nonoperative dilatation of coronary-artery stenosis: percutaneous transluminal coronary angioplasty.* N Engl J Med, 1979. 301(2): p. 61-8.

[18] Molajo, A.O., et al., *Comparison of the performance of superflow (5F) and conventional 8F catheter for cardiac catheterization by the femoral route.* Cathet Cardiovasc Diagn, 1987. 13(4): p. 275-6.

[19] Chhatriwalla, A.K. and D.L. Bhatt, *Should dual antiplatelet therapy after drug-eluting stents be continued for more than 1 year?: Dual antiplatelet therapy after drug-eluting stents should be continued for more than one year and preferably indefinitely.* Circ Cardiovasc Interv, 2008. 1(3): p. 217-25.

[20] Farooq, V., B.D. Gogas, and P.W. Serruys, *Restenosis: delineating the numerous causes of drug-eluting stent restenosis.* Circ Cardiovasc Interv, 2011. 4(2): p. 195-205.

[21] Trikalinos, T.A., et al., *Percutaneous coronary interventions for non-acute coronary artery disease: a quantitative 20-year synopsis and a network meta-analysis.* Lancet, 2009. 373(9667): p. 911-8.

[22] Kastrati, A., et al., *Analysis of 14 trials comparing sirolimus-eluting stents with bare-metal stents.* N Engl J Med, 2007. 356(10): p. 1030-9.

[23] Stone, G.W., et al., *Comparison of a polymer-based paclitaxel-eluting stent with a bare metal stent in patients with complex coronary artery disease: a randomized controlled trial.* JAMA, 2005. 294(10): p. 1215-23.

[24] Palmerini, T., et al., *Stent thrombosis with drug-eluting and bare-metal stents: evidence from a comprehensive network meta-analysis.* Lancet, 2012. 379(9824): p. 1393-402.

[25] Frutkin, A.D., et al., *Drug-eluting stents and the use of percutaneous coronary intervention among patients with class I indications for coronary artery bypass surgery undergoing index revascularization: analysis from the NCDR (National Cardiovascular Data Registry).* JACC Cardiovasc Interv, 2009. 2(7): p. 614-21.

[26] Wijns, W., et al., *Guidelines on myocardial revascularization.* Eur Heart J, 2010. 31(20): p. 2501-55.

[27] Yusuf, S., et al., *Effect of coronary artery bypass graft surgery on survival: overview of 10-year results from randomised trials by the Coronary Artery Bypass Graft Surgery Trialists Collaboration.* Lancet, 1994. 344(8922): p. 563-70.

[28] Dzavik, V., et al., *Long-term survival in 11,661 patients with multivessel coronary artery disease in the era of stenting: a report from the Alberta Provincial Project for Outcome Assessment in Coronary Heart Disease (APPROACH) Investigators.* Am Heart J, 2001. 142(1): p. 119-26.

[29] Baigent, C., et al., *Aspirin in the primary and secondary prevention of vascular disease: collaborative meta-analysis of individual participant data from randomised trials.* Lancet, 2009. 373(9678): p. 1849-60.

[30] Yusuf, S., et al., *Effects of clopidogrel in addition to aspirin in patients with acute coronary syndromes without ST-segment elevation.* N Engl J Med, 2001. 345(7): p. 494-502.

[31] Wiviott, S.D., et al., *Prasugrel versus clopidogrel in patients with acute coronary syndromes.* N Engl J Med, 2007. 357(20): p. 2001-15.

[32] Wallentin, L., et al., *Ticagrelor versus clopidogrel in patients with acute coronary syndromes.* N Engl J Med, 2009. 361(11): p. 1045-57.

[33] Packer, M., et al., *The effect of carvedilol on morbidity and mortality in patients with chronic heart failure. U.S. Carvedilol Heart Failure Study Group.* N Engl J Med, 1996. 334(21): p. 1349-55.

[34] *MRC/BHF Heart Protection Study of cholesterol lowering with simvastatin in 20,536 high-risk individuals: a randomised placebo-controlled trial.* Lancet, 2002. 360(9326): p. 7-22.

[35] LaRosa, J.C., et al., *Intensive lipid lowering with atorvastatin in patients with stable coronary disease.* N Engl J Med, 2005. 352(14): p. 1425-35.

[36] Yusuf, S., et al., *Effects of an angiotensin-converting-enzyme inhibitor, ramipril, on cardiovascular events in high-risk patients. The Heart Outcomes Prevention Evaluation Study Investigators.* N Engl J Med, 2000. 342(3): p. 145-53.

[37] Liu, M.W., G.S. Roubin, and S.B. King, 3rd, *Restenosis after coronary angioplasty. Potential biologic determinants and role of intimal hyperplasia.* Circulation, 1989. 79(6): p. 1374-87.

[38] Farb, A., et al., *Pathology of acute and chronic coronary stenting in humans.* Circulation, 1999. 99(1): p. 44-52.

[39] Colombo, A., et al., *Randomized study to assess the effectiveness of slow- and moderate-release polymer-based paclitaxel-eluting stents for coronary artery lesions.* Circulation, 2003. 108(7): p. 788-94.

[40] Morice, M.C., et al., *A randomized comparison of a sirolimus-eluting stent with a standard stent for coronary revascularization.* N Engl J Med, 2002. 346(23): p. 1773-80.

[41] Moses, J.W., et al., *Sirolimus-eluting stents versus standard stents in patients with stenosis in a native coronary artery.* N Engl J Med, 2003. 349(14): p. 1315-23.

[42] Stone, G.W., et al., *Safety and efficacy of sirolimus- and paclitaxel-eluting coronary stents.* N Engl J Med, 2007. 356(10): p. 998-1008.

[43] Pfisterer, M., et al., *Late clinical events after clopidogrel discontinuation may limit the benefit of drug-eluting stents: an observational study of drug-eluting versus bare-metal stents.* J Am Coll Cardiol, 2006. 48(12): p. 2584-91.

[44] Sarno, G., et al., *Lower risk of stent thrombosis and restenosis with unrestricted use of 'new-generation' drug-eluting stents: a report from the nationwide Swedish Coronary Angiography and Angioplasty Registry (SCAAR).* Eur Heart J, 2012. 33(5): p. 606-13.

[45] Hlatky, M.A., et al., *Coronary artery bypass surgery compared with percutaneous coronary interventions for multivessel disease: a collaborative analysis of individual patient data from ten randomised trials.* Lancet, 2009. 373(9670): p. 1190-7.

[46] Passamani, E., et al., *A randomized trial of coronary artery bypass surgery. Survival of patients with a low ejection fraction.* N Engl J Med, 1985. 312(26): p. 1665-71.

[47] Scott, S.M., et al., *VA Study of Unstable Angina. 10-year results show duration of surgical advantage for patients with impaired ejection fraction.* Circulation, 1994. 90(5 Pt 2): p. II120-3.

[48] Velazquez, E.J., et al., *Coronary-artery bypass surgery in patients with left ventricular dysfunction.* N Engl J Med, 2011. 364(17): p. 1607-16.

[49] Gersh, B.J., et al., *2011 ACCF/AHA Guideline for the Diagnosis and Treatment of Hypertrophic Cardiomyopathy: a report of the American College of Cardiology Foundation/American Heart Association Task Force on Practice Guidelines. Developed in collaboration with the American Association for Thoracic Surgery, American Society of Echocardiography, American Society of Nuclear Cardiology, Heart Failure Society of America, Heart Rhythm Society, Society for Cardiovascular Angiography and Interventions, and Society of Thoracic Surgeons.* J Am Coll Cardiol, 2011. 58(25): p. e212-60.

[50] *Comparison of coronary bypass surgery with angioplasty in patients with multivessel disease. The Bypass Angioplasty Revascularization Investigation (BARI) Investigators.* N Engl J Med, 1996. 335(4): p. 217-25.

[51] Serruys, P.W., et al., *Percutaneous coronary intervention versus coronary-artery bypass grafting for severe coronary artery disease.* N Engl J Med, 2009. 360(10): p. 961-72.

[52] Chaitman, B.R., et al., *The Bypass Angioplasty Revascularization Investigation 2 Diabetes randomized trial of different treatment strategies in type 2 diabetes mellitus with stable ischemic heart disease: impact of treatment strategy on cardiac mortality and myocardial infarction.* Circulation, 2009. 120(25): p. 2529-40.

[53] Farkouh, M.E., et al., *Strategies for Multivessel Revascularization in Patients with Diabetes.* N Engl J Med, 2012.

[54] Hachamovitch, R., et al., *Comparison of the short-term survival benefit associated with revascularization compared with medical therapy in patients with no prior coronary artery dis-*

ease undergoing stress myocardial perfusion single photon emission computed tomography. Circulation, 2003. 107(23): p. 2900-7.

[55] Sorajja, P., et al., *Improved survival in asymptomatic diabetic patients with high-risk SPECT imaging treated with coronary artery bypass grafting.* Circulation, 2005. 112(9 Suppl): p. I311-6.

[56] Boden, W.E., et al., *Optimal medical therapy with or without PCI for stable coronary disease.* N Engl J Med, 2007. 356(15): p. 1503-16.

[57] Sianos, G., et al., *The SYNTAX Score: an angiographic tool grading the complexity of coronary artery disease.* EuroIntervention, 2005. 1(2): p. 219-27.

[58] Tu, J.V., et al., *Determinants of variations in coronary revascularization practices.* CMAJ, 2011.

[59] Kappetein, A.P., et al., *Comparison of coronary bypass surgery with drug-eluting stenting for the treatment of left main and/or three-vessel disease: 3-year follow-up of the SYNTAX trial.* Eur Heart J, 2011. 32(17): p. 2125-34.

[60] Rodriguez, A.E., et al., *Five-year follow-up of the Argentine randomized trial of coronary angioplasty with stenting versus coronary bypass surgery in patients with multiple vessel disease (ERACI II).* J Am Coll Cardiol, 2005. 46(4): p. 582-8.

[61] Hueb, W., et al., *Ten-year follow-up survival of the Medicine, Angioplasty, or Surgery Study (MASS II): a randomized controlled clinical trial of 3 therapeutic strategies for multivessel coronary artery disease.* Circulation, 2010. 122(10): p. 949-57.

[62] Hsieh, V. and S.R. Mehta, *How Should We Treat Multi-Vessel Disease in STEMI Patients?* Curr Treat Options Cardiovasc Med, 2012.

[63] Vlaar, P.J., et al., *Culprit vessel only versus multivessel and staged percutaneous coronary intervention for multivessel disease in patients presenting with ST-segment elevation myocardial infarction: a pairwise and network meta-analysis.* J Am Coll Cardiol, 2011. 58(7): p. 692-703.

[64] Hochman, J.S., et al., *Early revascularization in acute myocardial infarction complicated by cardiogenic shock. SHOCK Investigators. Should We Emergently Revascularize Occluded Coronaries for Cardiogenic Shock.* N Engl J Med, 1999. 341(9): p. 625-34.

[65] Hochman, J.S., et al., *One-year survival following early revascularization for cardiogenic shock.* JAMA, 2001. 285(2): p. 190-2.

[66] Hochman, J.S., et al., *Early revascularization and long-term survival in cardiogenic shock complicating acute myocardial infarction.* JAMA, 2006. 295(21): p. 2511-5.

[67] Mehta, R.H., et al., *Percutaneous coronary intervention or coronary artery bypass surgery for cardiogenic shock and multivessel coronary artery disease?* Am Heart J, 2010. 159(1): p. 141-7.

[68] Patel, M.R., et al., *ACCF/SCAI/STS/AATS/AHA/ASNC/HFSA/SCCT 2012 Appropriate use criteria for coronary revascularization focused update: a report of the American College of Cardiology Foundation Appropriate Use Criteria Task Force, Society for Cardiovascular Angiography and Interventions, Society of Thoracic Surgeons, American Association for Thoracic Surgery, American Heart Association, American Society of Nuclear Cardiology, and the Society of Cardiovascular Computed Tomography.* J Am Coll Cardiol, 2012. 59(9): p. 857-81.

[69] Baim, D.S., *Anatomy, Angiograpic Views and Quantitation of Stenosis.* Cardiac Catheterization, Angiography and Intervention, ed. D.S. Baim. Vol. Seventh Edition. 2006: Lippincott Williams and Wilkins.

[70] Uren, N.G., et al., *Relation between myocardial blood flow and the severity of coronary-artery stenosis.* N Engl J Med, 1994. 330(25): p. 1782-8.

[71] Pijls, N.H., et al., *Experimental basis of determining maximum coronary, myocardial, and collateral blood flow by pressure measurements for assessing functional stenosis severity before and after percutaneous transluminal coronary angioplasty.* Circulation, 1993. 87(4): p. 1354-67.

[72] Pijls, N.H. and J.W. Sels, *Functional measurement of coronary stenosis.* J Am Coll Cardiol, 2012. 59(12): p. 1045-57.

[73] Tonino, P.A., et al., *Fractional flow reserve versus angiography for guiding percutaneous coronary intervention.* N Engl J Med, 2009. 360(3): p. 213-24.

[74] Pijls, N.H., et al., *Fractional flow reserve versus angiography for guiding percutaneous coronary intervention in patients with multivessel coronary artery disease: 2-year follow-up of the FAME (Fractional Flow Reserve Versus Angiography for Multivessel Evaluation) study.* J Am Coll Cardiol, 2010. 56(3): p. 177-84.

[75] Ko, D.T., et al., *Temporal trends in the use of percutaneous coronary intervention and coronary artery bypass surgery in New York State and Ontario.* Circulation, 2010. 121(24): p. 2635-44.

[76] Hassan, A., et al., *Increasing rates of angioplasty versus bypass surgery in Canada, 1994-2005.* Am Heart J, 2010. 160(5): p. 958-65.

[77] McMurtry, M.S., et al., *Recent Temporal Trends and Geographic Distribution of Cardiac Procedures in Alberta.* Can J Cardiol, 2012.

[78] Riley, R.F., et al., *Trends in coronary revascularization in the United States from 2001 to 2009: recent declines in percutaneous coronary intervention volumes.* Circ Cardiovasc Qual Outcomes, 2011. 4(2): p. 193-7.

[79] Mercuri, M., et al., *An even smaller area variation: Differing practice patterns among interventional cardiologists within a single high volume tertiary cardiac centre.* Health Policy, 2012. 104(2): p. 179-85.

[80] Brown, R., et al., *Variation in Interventional Cardiac Care in Michigan.* Center for Healthcare research and Transformation, Ann Arbor, MI., 2012.

[81] Tu, J.V., et al., *Determinants of variations in coronary revascularization practices.* CMAJ, 2012. 184(2): p. 179-86.

[82] Schwalm, J., Lai, TF, Al-Haarbi, A, Karl D, Guo H, Kingsbury K, Tu JV, Natarajan MK, *Comparison of abstracted chart review and core-lab angiogram review on coronary angiography interpretation - an analysis from the variation in revascularization practice in ontario angiographic sub-study.* Canadian Cardiovascular Congress, 2010. Abstract presentation.

Chapter 19

Artery Bypass Versus PCI Using New Generation DES

Mohammed Balghith

Additional information is available at the end of the chapter

http://dx.doi.org/10.5772/54029

1. Introduction

Stents have substantially improved the safety and efficacy of percutaneous revascularization of atherosclerotic coronary arteries. The attendant risk of emergency referral for Coronary artery bypass graft surgery (CABG) and the need for subsequent revascularization procedures have been reduced by more than 50% since the use of new generation stents i.e drug eluted stents (DES) starting 2002. Comparisons of Percatouneous coronary intervention (PCI) and CABG have been made in 7 randomized trials designed to identify the most effective alternative for selected patients with multivessel CAD of whom both methods were deemed feasible. [1,2]. The individual results of these trials and a meta-analysis of their combined results have consistently shown equivalent survival rates with use of the 2 strategies over approximately 5 years of follow-up.

2. Coronary artery bypass graft surgery

A coronary artery bypass surgery is a surgical procedure performed to relieve angina and reduce the risk of death from coronary artery disease. Arteries or veins from elsewhere in the patient's body are grafted to the coronary arteries to bypass atherosclerotic narrowings and improve the blood supply to the coronary circulation supplying the myocardium (heart muscle). Example, Left internal mammary artery (LIMA) graft to LAD and SVG to OM and RCA (figure 1). The operation is usually performed with the heart stopped, requiring the usage of cardiopulmonary bypass; other methods are available to achieve CABG on a beating heart, so-called "off-pump" surgery. [3].

3. Advantages of CABG

Over the last 4 decades, surgical coronary artery revascularization techniques and technology have advanced significantly. As a result, despite an increasingly older and sicker patient population, CABG outcomes continue to improve. For example, the predicted mortality of CABG patients has increased steadily over the past decade, yet observed operative mortality rates have decreased, [4]. This is partly because advances in preoperative evaluation, including more precise coronary artery and myocardial imaging and diagnostic techniques, have allowed more appropriate patient selection and surgical planning. In addition, preoperative, intraoperative, and postoperative monitoring and therapeutic interventions have made CABG safer, even for critically ill and high-risk patients. Improvements in cardiopulmonary perfusion and careful myocardial protection, as well as the use of off-pump and on-pump beating-heart techniques in selected patients, have also decreased perioperative morbidity and mortality rates. [5,6].

Use of the bilateral IMAs offers the possibility of constructing various configurations, making total arterial myocardial revascularisation possible with a minimum number of arterial conduits. Use of the skeletonised RIMA through the transverse sinus and eventually retrocavally can reach most branches of the circumflex system and is associated with an excellent patency rate. Patients who received bilateral IMA grafts for left coronary system revascularisation had improved early and late outcomes and decreased risk of death, reoperation, and angioplasty. [7].

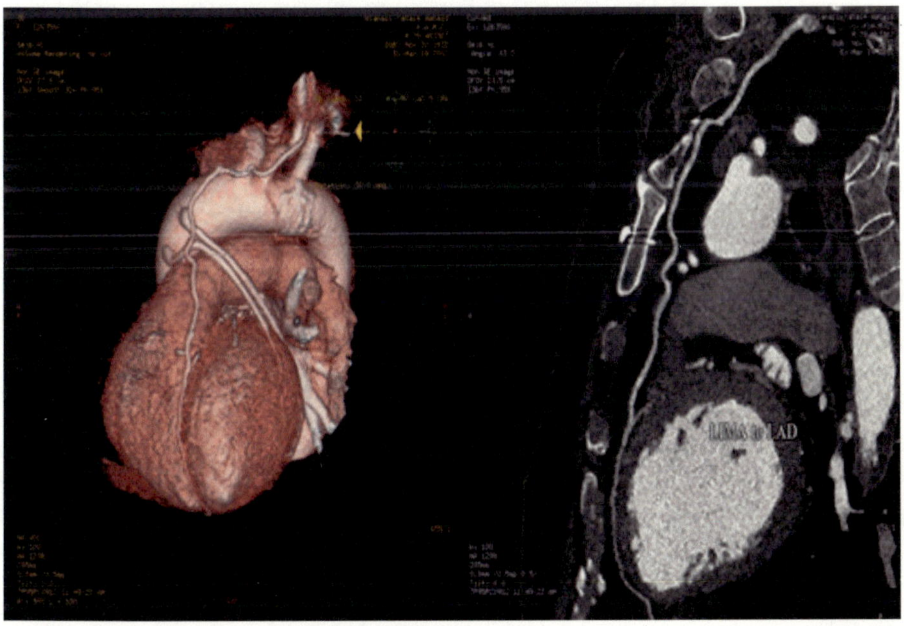

Figure 1. CT coronary angiogram, showing a CABG done 5 years ago with LIMA to LAD artery and SVG to OM and RCA.

http://dx.doi.org/10.5772/54029

4. Percutaneous coronary intervention using drug eluted stents

Percutaneous coronary intervention (PCI) involves dilatation of an obstructed or narrowed coronary artery, using a balloon catheter to dilate the artery from within. After balloon dilatation, a stainless steel stent is usually placed in the coronary artery. Antiplatelet agents like aspirin or clopidogrel are mandatory to be used after stenting. Stents may be either bare metal (BMS) or drug-eluting stents (DES). Indications for PCI might be elective or emergency according to the clinical presentations of the patients. Primary PCI in the setting of ST segment elevation myocardial infarction (STEMI): When the catheterization lab including the team and facility is available, angioplasty with stenting is the optimal method of reperfusion for STEMI. The target "door to balloon time" is 90 minutes, [8]. Rescue PCI is considered as a treatment in patients with thrombolysis - if there is failure to reperfuse, further ischaemia with persistant chest pain, or continuous ST elevation. PCI is considered also as an early invasive strategy in Acute coronary syndrome, Non-ST elevation myocardial infarction (NSTEMI) and unstable angina: [9]., or conservative strategy for patients who are at medium-to-high risk of subsequent cardiac events. Elective PCI for patient with Stable angina or positive stress test: with single or double vessel disease, where optimal medical therapy fails to control symptoms. Patients with triple vessel disease, who are unsuitable for CABG, [10].

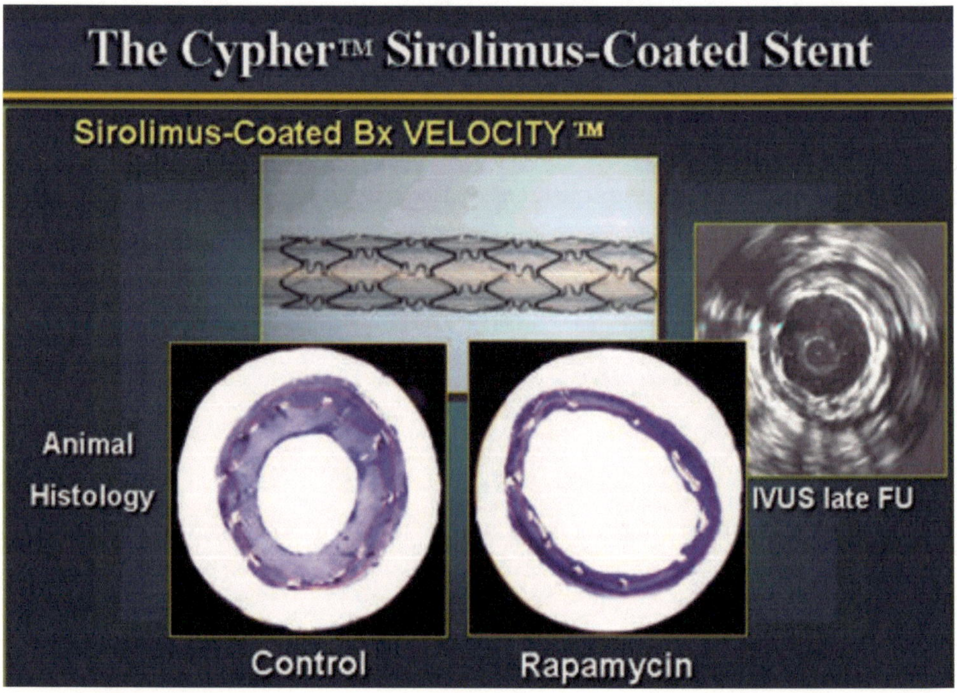

Figure 2. Cypher Stent- Siroliums eluted stent

A drug-eluting stent presents or releases single or multiple bioactive agents into the blood stream. The drug can deposit in and/or affect blood vessels, cells, plaque, or tissues either adjacent to the stent or at a distance. The drug can be embedded and released from within ("matrix-type") or surrounded by and released through ("reservoir-type") polymer materials that coat ("strut-adherent") or span ("strut-spanning") the struts of the stents. These agents prevent in-stent restenosis by reducing the intimal hyperplasia, [11].

The advantages and a lower cost compared to CABG makes DES an attractive option to treat coronary artery disease. Currently, five DESs are available in the USA: the CYPHER sirolimus-eluting stent from Cordis (approved by FDA on 24 April 2003), Figure 2, 3. The TAXUS Express and Liberté paclitaxel-eluting stents from Boston Scientific (approved by FDA on 4 March 2004 and 10 October 2008, respectively) (TAXUS Express is referred to as TAXUS) Figure 4, the ENDEAVOR zotarolimus-eluting stent from Medtronic (approved by FDA on 1 February 2008), and the XIENCE V Figure 5, everolimus-eluting stent from Abbott Vascular (approved by FDA on 2 July 2008). [12].

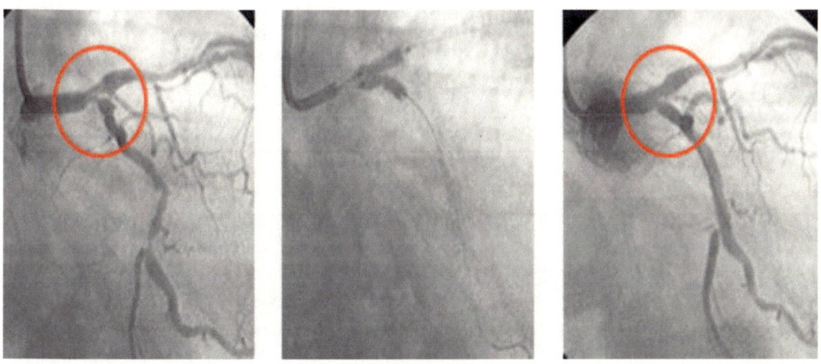

Figure 3. Complex case with LM disease treated by 2 Cypher stents

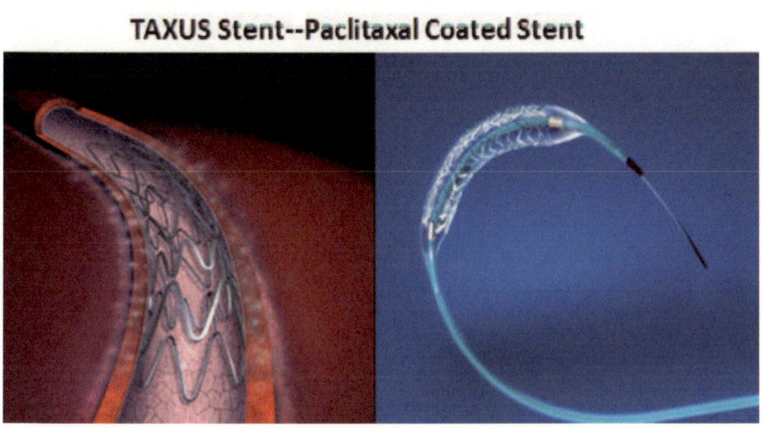

Figure 4. Taxus stent-Paclitaxal eluted stent

http://dx.doi.org/10.5772/54029

RCA 99% stenosis treated by Xience stent

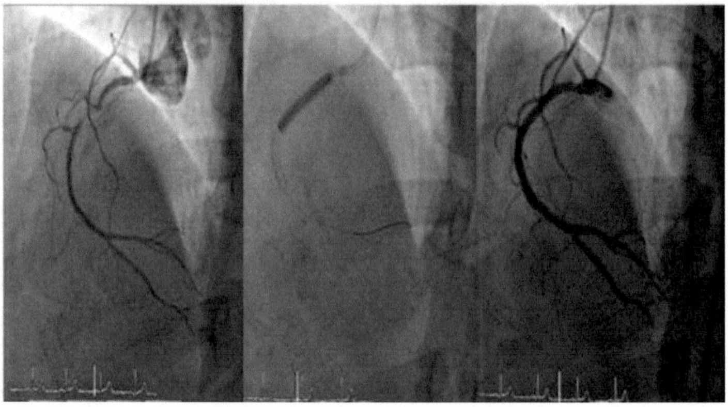

Figure 5. Significan disease of proximal RCA treated by Xience stent

5. Outcomes of coronary-artery bypass grafting versus bare metal stent implantation

The New York's cardiac registries were one of the largest studies which identify 37,212 patients with multivessel disease who underwent CABG and 22,102 patients with multivessel disease who underwent PCI using BMS from January 1, 1997, to December 31, 2000. They determined the rates of death and subsequent revascularization within three years after the procedure in various groups of patients according to the number of diseased vessels and presence or absence of involvement of the left anterior descending coronary artery LAD.

Risk-adjusted survival rates were significantly higher among patients who underwent CABG than among those who received a stent in all of the anatomical subgroups studied. For example, the adjusted hazard ratio for the long-term risk of death after CABG relative to stent implantation was 0.64 (95 percent confidence interval, 0.56 to 0.74) for patients with three-vessel disease with involvement of the proximal LAD and 0.76 (95 percent confidence interval, 0.60 to 0.96) for patients with two-vessel disease with involvement of the non-proximal LAD. Also, the three-year rates of revascularization were considerably higher in the stenting group than in the CABG group (7.8 percent vs. 0.3 percent for subsequent CABG and 27.3 percent vs. 4.6 percent for subsequent PCI), [13].

Texas Heart Institute Cardiovascular Research Database retrospectively identified patients who had undergone their 1st revascularization procedure with coronary artery bypass surgery (CABG; n=2,826) or coronary stenting (n=2,793) between January 1995 and December 1999. They have found that in-hospital mortality was significantly greater in patients undergoing CABG than in those undergoing stenting (3.6% vs 0.75%; adjusted OR 8.4; P <0.0001). At a mean 2.5-year follow-up, risk-adjusted survival was equivalent (CABG 91%, stenting 95%;

adjusted OR 1.26; $P = 0.06$). When subgroups matched for severity of disease were compared, no differences in risk-adjusted survival were seen, [14].

6. Drug-eluting stents vs coronary artery bypass surgery for the treatment of multivessel coronary disease

A Chinese study identified 3720 consecutive patients with multivessel disease who underwent isolated CABG surgery or received drug-eluting stents between April 1, 2004, and December 31, 2005, which compared safety (total mortality, myocardial infarction, and stroke) and efficacy (target-vessel revascularization) during a 3-year follow-up. These outcomes were compared after adjustment for the differences in baseline risk factors. Patients who underwent CABG (n=1886) were older and had more comorbidities than patients who received drug-eluting stents (n=1834). Patients receiving drug-eluting stents had considerably higher 3-year rates of target-vessel revascularization. Drug-eluting stents were also associated with higher rates of death (adjusted hazard ratio, 1.62; 95% confidence interval, 1.07 to 2.47) and myocardial infarction (adjusted hazard ratio, 1.65; 95% confidence interval, 1.15 to 2.44). The risk adjusted rate of stroke was similar in the 2 groups (hazard ratio, 0.92; 95% confidence interval, 0.69 to 1.51). [15]

In a Korean study, a 5-year clinical follow-up of 395 patients with unprotected LMCA disease who underwent PCI with drug-eluting stents (DES) (n = 176) or CABG (n = 219) was preformed from January 2003 to May 2004. In the 5-year follow-up, cohort of DES and concurrent CABG, there had not been a significant difference in the adjusted risk of death (HR: 0.83; 95% CI: 0.34 to 2.07; $p = 0.70$) or the risk of the composite outcome (HR: 0.91; 95% CI: 0.45 to 1.83; $p = 0.79$). The rates of TVR were also higher in the DES group than the CABG group (HR: 6.22; 95% CI: 2.26 to 17.14; $p < 0.001$), [16].

In an Italian study, 249 patients: 107 of whom were treated with PCI along with DES implantation and 142 treated with CABG. At 5-year clinical follow-up, no difference was found between PCI and CABG in the occurrence of cardiac death (adjusted odds ratio [OR]: 0.502; 95% confidence interval [CI]: 0.162 to 1.461; $p = 0.24$). The PCI group showed a trend toward a lower occurrence of the composite end point of cardiac death and MI (adjusted OR: 0.408; 95% CI: 0.146 to 1.061; $p = 0.06$). Percutaneous coronary intervention was associated with a lower rate of the composite end point of death, MI, and/or stroke (OR: 0.399; 95% CI: 0.151 to 0.989; $p = 0.04$). Indeed, CABG was correlated with lower target vessel revascularization (adjusted OR: 4.411; 95% CI: 1.825 to 11.371; $p = 0.0004$). No difference was detected in the occurrence of major adverse cardiac and cerebrovascular events (adjusted OR: 1.578; 95% CI: 0.825 to 3.054; $p = 0.18$) [17].

In a Meta-analysis of clinical studies comparing CABG with DES in patients with unprotected left main coronary artery narrowing, the analysis included 2,905 patients from 8 clinical studies (2 randomized trials and 6 nonrandomized studies). At 1-year follow-up, there was no significant difference between the CABG and DES groups in the risk for death (odds ratio [OR] 1.12, 95% confidence interval [CI] 0.80 to 1.56) or the composite

end point of death, myocardial infarction, or stroke (OR 1.25, 95% CI 0.86 to 1.82). The risk for target vessel revascularization was significantly lower in the CABG group compared to the PCI group (OR 0.44, 95% CI 0.32 to 0.59). In conclusion, PCI with DES is safe and could represent a good alternative to CABG for selected cases in patients with ULMCA disease, [18].

In the SYNTAX trial, 1,800 patients with three-vessel and/or LM disease were randomized to either CABG or PCI; of these, 271 LM patients were prospectively assigned to receive a 15-month angiogram. The primary endpoint for the CABG arm was the ratio of ≥50% to <100% obstructed/occluded grafts bypassing LM lesions to the number placed. The primary endpoint for the PCI arm was the proportion of patients with ≤50% diameter stenosis ('patent' stents) of treated LM lesions. Per protocol, no formal comparison between CABG and PCI arms was intended based on the differing primary endpoints. Available 15-month angiograms were analyzed for 114 CABG and 149 PCI patients. At 15 months, 9.9% (26/263) of CABG grafts were 100% occluded and an additional 5.7% (15/263) were ≥50% to <100% occluded. Overall, 27.2% (31/114) of patients had ≥1 obstructed/occluded graft. The 15-month CABG MACCE rate was 8.8% (10/114) and MACCE at 15 months was not significantly associated with graft obstruction/occlusion (p=0.85). In the PCI arm, 92.4% (134/145) of patients had ≤50% diameter LM stenosis at 15 months (89.7% [87/97] distal LM lesions and 97.9% [47/48] non-distal LM lesions). The 15-month PCI MACCE rate was 12.8% (20/156) and this was significantly associated with lack of stent patency at 15 months (p<0.001), mainly due to repeated revascularization. [19].

The results of the SYNTAX trial confirm that at 3 years CABG remains the treatment of choice for most patients with three-vessel and LMS disease and especially in those with the most severe disease. SYNTAX will have a profound effect on practice recommendations for the foreseeable future and has already had a major effect on the new European Society for Cardiology/European Association for Cardiothoracic Surgery guidelines for myocardial revascularization, [20].

At four years follow-up of SYNTAX trial which presented at TCT in 2011, there was no difference in MACCE between CABG and PCI in those with a SYNTAX score of 0 to 22, (26.1% vs 28.6%; p=0.57). This is good, and would legitimize the use of PCI in this kind of patient". But for those with an intermediate SYNTAX score of 23 to 32, "You see immediately a highly significant difference" in MACCE rate (21.5% for CABG vs 32% for PCI; p=0.006). For those with a high SYNTAX score (≥33), "mortality is double in the PCI group compared with CABG (16.1% vs 8.4%; p=0.04) in addition to MI is two to three times higher with PCI than with CABG (9.3% vs 3.9%; p=0.01).

In this highest-risk group, even the end point of death/stroke/MI becomes significantly higher with PCI, (22.7% vs 14.6%; p=0.01), and MACCE were much higher (40.1% vs 23.6%; p<0.001), driven in large part by a 17% higher rate of revascularization in this high-risk group at four years. Figures 6& 7

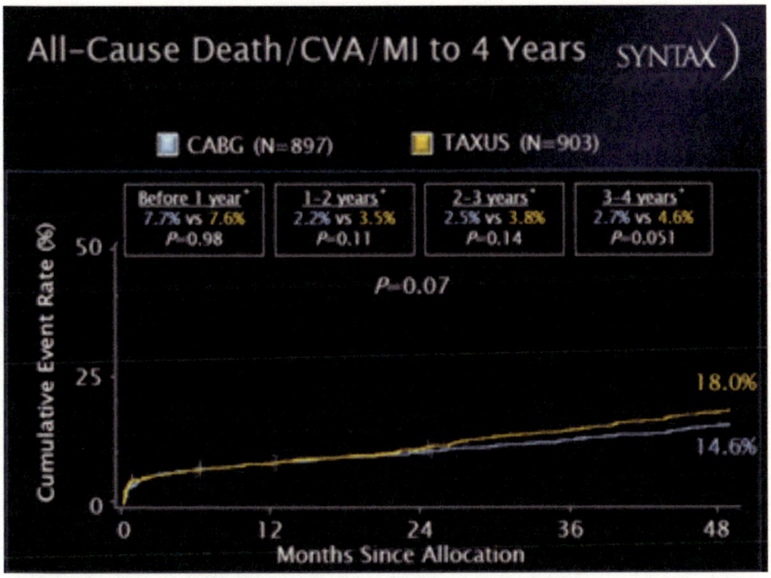

Figure 6. years follow up in Syntax study, demonstrate all cause death/CVA/MI up to 4 years

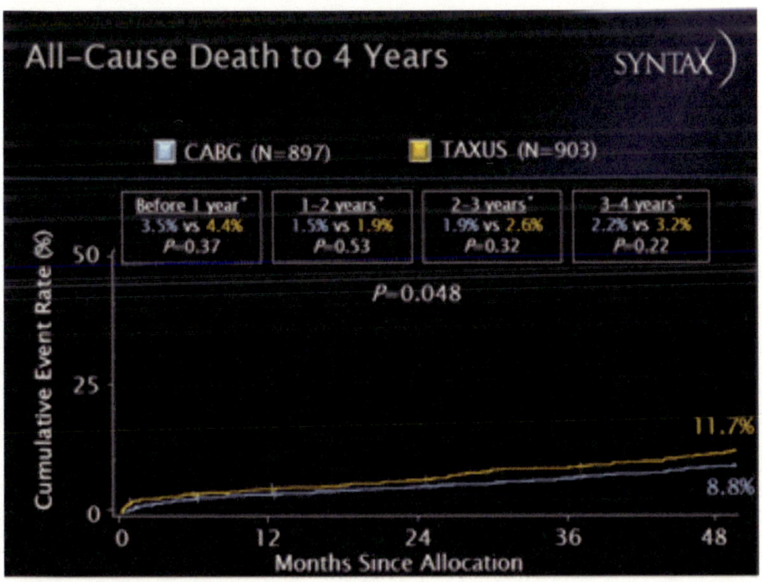

Figure 7. years follow up in Syntax study, demonstrate all cause death up to 4 years

http://dx.doi.org/10.5772/54029

7. Revascularization for patients with diabetes mellitus and multivessel CAD

In the BARI 2D trial, the selected revascularization strategy, CABG or PCI, was based on physician discretion, declared independent of randomization to either immediate or deferred revascularization if clinically warranted. They analyzed factors favoring selection of CABG versus PCI in 1,593 diabetic patients with multivessel CAD enrolled between 2001 and 2005. The majority of diabetic patients with multivessel disease were selected for PCI rather than CABG. Preference for CABG over PCI was largely based on angiographic features related to the extent, location, and nature of CAD, as well as geographic, demographic, and clinical factors. [21]

However, with each intervention the benefit is less and the risks and complications are greater than in patients without diabetes. Revascularization for treatment of ST elevation myocardial infarction increases survival. Both interventions relieve symptoms, but neither improves survival except in patients at high risk. In patients with clinically stable chronic coronary disease, survival after CABG or PCI is comparable with that in patients treated with optimal medical therapy alone. Accordingly, evaluation for revascularization can be deferred until signs and symptoms worsen except in patients at high risk. In patients at high risk survival after promptly implemented CABG is greater than that with optimal medical therapy, especially when the diabetes is being treated with insulin sensitizing agents. [22]

8. Quality of life after PCI with DES or CABG

Among patients with three-vessel or left main coronary artery disease who were suitable candidates for either PCI using DES or CABG, both strategies resulted in significant relief from angina and improvements in overall health status over the first year of follow-up. At both 6 and 12 months, there was a small but significant reduction in angina frequency with CABG as compared with PCI in the overall population. These symptomatic benefits of CABG were counterbalanced by the more rapid recovery and improved short-term health status achieved with PCI. [23]

9. Future study with the second generation des and other bioabsorbable stents

EXCEL is a 2600-patient study comparing patients with left main disease randomized to bypass surgery or PCI with the Xience stent and followed for at least three years. The primary end point is death, stroke, and MI; repeat revascularization is a secondary end point. EXCEL results awaited. Figure (8)

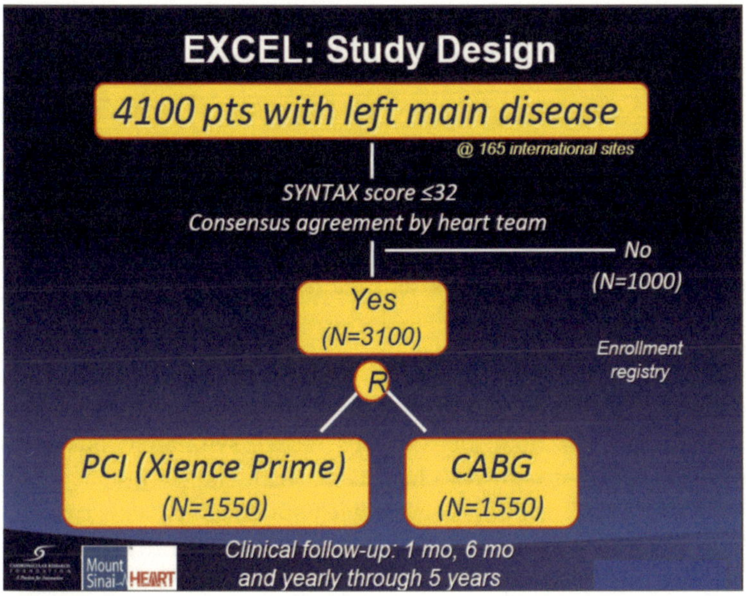

Figure 8. EXCEL study protocol comparing Xience stent with CABG

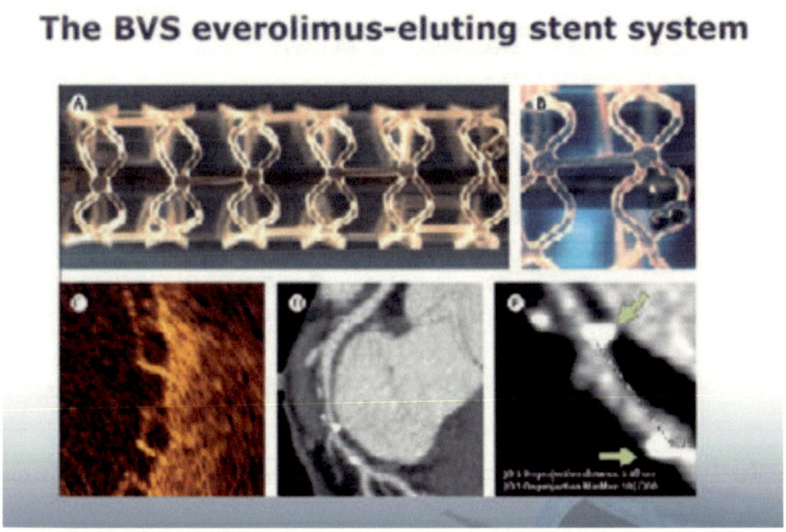

Figure 9. Absorb Stent- Bioabsorbale everolimus eluted stent

Stents composed of bioabsorbable/biodegradable materials represent an attractive alternative revascularization modality; the justification stems from the short-term need for vessel scaffolding and avoidance of the potential long-term complications of metallic stents. Compared with

metallic stents, there are several potential advantages, including complete absorption of stent material, [24], Abbott Vascular ABSORB Everolimus Eluting Bioresorbable Vascular Scaffold System"These outcomes suggest that a temporary scaffold like ABSORB provides durable results over the long term and a permanent implant may not be necessary to effectively treat patients with coronary artery disease". ABSORB II trial is ongoing. Figure (9)

10. Combining the best of both worlds hybrid coronary revascularization

As PCI technology improves and techniques of LIMA-to-LAD grafting become less invasive, hybrid coronary revascularization is becoming a distinct possibility. For example, a minimally invasive, off-pump, direct LIMA-to-LAD anastomosis can be combined with DES placement in a focal mid-right-coronary-artery lesion in a patient with complex proximal LAD lesions. Hybrid coronary revascularization procedures are currently being performed, with promising early results. A few centers, now have hybrid operating rooms with cardiac surgical and coronary angiographic capabilities that make it possible to perform simultaneous hybrid coronary revascularizations. Staged hybrid revascularizations are performed in standard catheterization laboratories and operating rooms. [25,26].

11. Conclusion

Each strategy can have great outcomes in appropriately selected patients. Hard clinical outcomes (death/MI/CVA) are generally similar, need to weigh the risk of potential repetition of procedures with PCI using DES vs. the greater morbidity of CABG. The 3VD and LMCA Disease are high-risk coronary lesions and the least stable subtypes of "stable CAD" PCI and CABG have very similar rates of hard clinical endpoints. Greater rates of recurrent revascularization with PCI, especially in complex disease, Patient selection and patient preference will generally dictate the best and most appropriate care. The so-called SYNTAX score, evolved for the trial, offers a grading system, based on patient anatomy, to help surgeons and interventionalists make this decision. As PCI and CABG are refined further, surgeons and cardiologists will no doubt learn to use these improved interventional techniques and surgical procedures in a way that will optimize the treatment of each individual patient.

Author details

Mohammed Balghith

King Saud Bin Abdulaziz University for Heath Sceinces, KACC, National Guard , Riyadh, Saudi Arabia

References

[1] Rodriguez A, Boullon F, Perez-Balino N, Paviotti C, Liprandi MI, Palacios IF. Argentine randomized trial of percutaneous transluminal coronary angioplasty versus coronary artery bypass surgery in multivessel disease (ERACI): in-hospital results and 1-year follow-up. ERACI Group. J Am Coll Cardiol 1993;22:1060–7.

[2] Hamm CW, Reimers J, Ischinger T, Rupprecht HJ, Berger J, Bleifeld W. A randomized study of coronary angioplasty compared with bypass surgery in patients with symptomatic multivessel coronary disease. German Angioplasty Bypass Surgery Investigation (GABI). N Engl J Med 1994;331: 1037–43

[3] Kolessov et al, "Mammary artery-coronary artery anastomosis as method of treatment for angina pectoris". J Thorac Cardiovasc Surg VI (October 1967). 54 (4): 535–44

[4] Ferguson TB Jr, Hammill BG, Peterson ED, DeLong ER, Grover FL, STS National Database Committee. A decade of change: risk profiles and outcomes for isolated coronary artery bypass grafting procedures, 1990–1999: a report from the STS National Database Committee and the Duke Clinical Research Institute. Society of Thoracic Surgeons. Ann Thorac Surg 2002;73:480–9.

[5] Al-Ruzzeh S, Ambler G, Asimakopoulos G, Omar RZ, Hasan R, Fabri B, et al. Off-pump coronary artery bypass (OPCAB) surgery reduces risk-stratified morbidity and mortality: a United Kingdom multi-center comparative analysis of early clinical outcome. Circulation 2003;108 Suppl 1:II1–8.

[6] Puskas JD, Williams WH, Mahoney EM, Huber PR, Block PC, Duke PG, et al. Off-pump vs conventional coronary artery bypass grafting: early and 1-year graft patency, cost, and quality-of-life outcomes: a randomized trial. JAMA 2004;291:1841–9.

[7] M Bonacchi, Battaglia F, Prifti E, Leacche M, Nathan N S, Sani G, and Popoff G,Early and late outcome of skeletonised bilateral internal mammary arteries anastomosed to the left coronary system Heart. 2005 February; 91(2): 195–202. Ratcliffe A T, C Pepper. Thrombolysis or primary angioplasty? Reperfusion therapy for myocardial infarction in the UK, Postgrad Med J2008;84:73-77

[8] Ratcliffe A T , C Pepper . Thrombolysis or primary angioplasty? Reperfusion therapy for myocardial infarction in the UK, Postgrad Med J2008;84:73-77

[9] McCullough PA, Gibson CM, Dibattiste PM, et al. Timing of angiography and revascularization in acute coronary syndromes: an analysis of the TACTICS-TIMI-18 trial. J Interv Cardiol 2004;17:81-6

[10] Levine GN, Bates ER, Blankenship JC, et al. 2011 ACCF/AHA/SCAI guideline for percutaneous coronary intervention: A report of the American College of Cardiology Foundation/American Heart Association Task Force on Practice Guidelines and the

Society for Cardiovascular Angiography and Interventions. J Am Coll Cardiol 2011;08.007

[11] Robert S. Schwartz, MD; Elazer R. Edelman, MD, PhD; Andrew Carter, DO; Nicolas Chronos, MD; Campbell Rogers, MD; Keith A. Robinson, PhD; Ron Waksman, MD; Judah Weinberger, MD; Robert L. Wilensky, MD; Donald N. Jensen, DVM; Bram D. Zuckerman, MD; Renu VirmaniDrug-Eluting Stents in Preclinical Studies, Recommended Evaluation From a Consensus Group, Circulation. 2002; 106: 1867-1873

[12] Doostzadeh J, Clark LN, Bezenek S, Pierson W, Sood PR, Sudhir K. Recent progress in percutaneous coronary intervention: evolution of the drug-eluting stents, focus on the XIENCE V drug-eluting stent. Coron Artery Dis. 2010 Jan;21(1):46-56.

[13] Hannan EL, Racz MJ, Walford G, Jones RH, Ryan TJ, Bennett E, Culliford AT, Isom OW, Gold JP, Rose EA, N Engl J Med. Long-term outcomes of coronary-artery bypass grafting versus stent implantation. 2005 May 26;352(21):2174-83.

[14] Rollo P. Villareal, MD, Vei-Vei Lee, MS, MacArthur A. Elayda, MD, PhD, and James M. Wilson, MD Coronary Artery Bypass Surgery versus Coronary Stenting, Risk-Adjusted Survival Rates in 5,619 Patients. Tex Heart Inst J. 2002; 29(1): 3–9

[15] Li Y, Zheng Z, Xu B, Zhang S, Li W, Gao R, Hu S.Comparison of drug-eluting stents and coronary artery bypass surgery for the treatment of multivessel coronary disease: three-year follow-up results from a single institution. Circulation. 2009 Apr 21;119(15):2040-50

[16] Park DW, Kim YH, Yun SC, Lee JY, Kim WJ, Kang SJ, Lee SW, Lee CW, Kim JJ, Choo SJ, Chung CH, Lee JW, Park SW, Park SJ. Long-term outcomes after stenting versus coronary artery bypass grafting for unprotected left main coronary artery disease: 10-year results of bare-metal stents and 5-year results of drug-eluting stents from the ASAN-MAIN (ASAN Medical Center-Left MAIN Revascularization) Registry. J Am Coll Cardiol. 2010 Oct 19;56(17):1366-75.

[17] Chieffo A, Magni V, Latib A, Maisano F, Ielasi A, Montorfano M, Carlino M, Godino C, Ferraro M, Calori G, Alfieri O, Colombo A. 5-year outcomes following percutaneous coronary intervention with drug-eluting stent implantation versus coronary artery bypass graft for unprotected left main coronary artery lesions the Milan experience. JACC Cardiovasc Interv. 2010 Jun;3(6):595-601.

[18] Lee MS, Yang T, Dhoot J, Liao H. Meta-analysis of clinical studies comparing coronary artery bypass grafting with percutaneous coronary intervention and drug-eluting stents in patients with unprotected left main coronary artery narrowings. Am J Cardiol. 2010 Apr 15;105(8).

[19] Morice MC, Feldman TE, Mack MJ, Ståhle E, Holmes DR, Colombo A, Morel MA, van den Brand M, Serruys PW, Mohr F, Carrié D, Fournial G, James S, Leadley K, Dawkins KD, Kappetein AP. Angiographic outcomes following stenting or coronary artery bypass surgery of the left main coronary artery: fifteen-month outcomes from

the synergy between PCI with TAXUS express and cardiac surgery left main angiographic substudy (SYNTAX-LE MANS). EuroIntervention. 2011 Oct 30;7(6):670-9.

[20] Taggart DP. Lessons learned from the SYNTAX trial for multivessel and left main stem coronary artery disease. Curr Opin Cardiol. 2011 Nov;26(6):502-7.

[21] Kim LJ, King SB 3rd, Kent K, Brooks MM et al; BARI 2D (Bypass Angioplasty Revascularization Investigation Type 2 Diabetes) Study Group.Factors related to the selection of surgical versus percutaneous revascularization in diabetic patients with multivessel coronary artery disease in the BARI 2D (Bypass Angioplasty Revascularization Investigation in Type 2 Diabetes) trial. JACC Cardiovasc Interv. 2009 May; 2(5):384-92.

[22] Sobel BE.Coronary revascularization in patients with type 2 diabetes and results of the BARI 2D trial. Coron Artery Dis. 2010 May;21(3):189-98.

[23] David J. Cohen, M.D., Ben Van Hout, Ph.D., Patrick W. Serruys, M.D., Ph.D., for the Synergy between PCI with Taxus and Cardiac Surgery (SYNTAX) Investigators, Quality of Life after PCI with Drug-Eluting Stents or Coronary-Artery Bypass Surgery. N Engl J Med 2011; 364:1016-1026March 17, 2011

[24] Waksman R, Erbel R, Di Mario C, et al; PROGRESS-AMS (Clinical Performance Angiographic Results of Coronary Stenting with Absorbable Metal Stents) Investigators. Early- and long-term intravascular ultrasound and angiographic findings after bioabsorbable magnesium stent implantation in human coronary arteries. JACC Cardiovasc Intervent. 2009;2:312-320

[25] de Canniere D, Jansens JL, Goldschmidt-Clermont P, Barvais L, Decroly P, Stoupel E. Combination of minimally invasive coronary bypass and percutaneous transluminal coronary angioplasty in the treatment of double-vessel coronary disease: two-year follow-up of a new hybrid procedure compared with "on-pump" double bypass grafting. Am Heart J 2001;142:563–70.

[26] Lee MS, Wilentz JR, Makkar RR, Singh V, Nero T, Swistel D, et al. Hybrid revascularization using percutaneous coronary intervention and robotically assisted minimally invasive direct coronary artery bypass surgery. J Invasive Cardiol 2004;16:419–25.

Chapter 20

Generating Graphical Reports on Cardiac Catheterization

Yuki Igarashi, Takeo Igarashi, Ryo Haraguchi and Kazuo Nakazawa

Additional information is available at the end of the chapter

http://dx.doi.org/10.5772/54235

1. Introduction

Electronic medical recording systems [1-4] have become widespread due to the improvement in hardware performance and user interfaces. Some recent systems are designed to support doctor–patient communication using a tablet PC [5-6]. However, usability is still an issue and medical professionals need more such user-friendly interfaces. To make these systems accessible to inexperienced users and to reduce the overhead of data entry, we have been developing various pen-based electronic medical recording systems [7-8]. Pen-based computing is an active research area for both user interfaces and computer graphics. Our work is based on recent advances in this area, especially the freeform user interfaces proposed by Igarashi [9]. Using this approach, the user draws freehand lines on the screen assisted by the system, and the result is directly stored as a vector image. Our systems feature special purpose functions for pen input including three-dimensional (3D) sketching, user-identification, and handwritten character recognition and search [8]. They are designed to help medical professionals to think more freely when working on difficult problems without being constrained by cumbersome interfaces.

One problem with these freeform pen-based systems, however, is that their output does not easily fit into a structure that lends itself to further machine processing or interface with other more traditional recording systems. Our goal in the project was to bridge this gap between freeform diagramming and more structured recording.

One strength of pen-based systems is that they make it easy to draw and add diagrams to medical records. This is particularly useful in ophthalmology, otolaryngology, and dentistry in which diagrams play an important role in medical records. Indeed, the frequent use of

diagrams makes it difficult to use traditional GUI-based medical recording systems in these areas [10]. Cardiac catheterization is one of these areas in which the diagram is an indispensable tool for medical recording. Existing electronic medical recording systems rely on structured templates, but it is difficult to create an appropriate report of findings or treatment plan using these predefined templates. Most existing diagram editors are implemented as bitmap paint tools, not vector graphics. This makes it difficult to edit the geometry afterward and requires that a large amount of data be transmitted and stored

We therefore developed a pen-based interface for graphical reporting of findings in cardiac catheterization (Figure 1) [11]. Figure 2 shows an illustration of the human heart. The target of our system is the coronary arteries. Figure 3 shows a screenshot of our system. The user can freely "sketch" coronary arteries and stenoses on the screen using a pen on a template of coronary features. The location and degree of each stenosis, and various treatments such as bypass and stents, are visually represented. We developed an algorithm that can extract semantic information from the graphical representation and store it in XML format. The system can also generate a table in the format specified in the AHA (American Heart Association) committee report [12]. This system is useful not only as a tool for efficiently generating reports of findings but also as an effective explanation tool for patients.

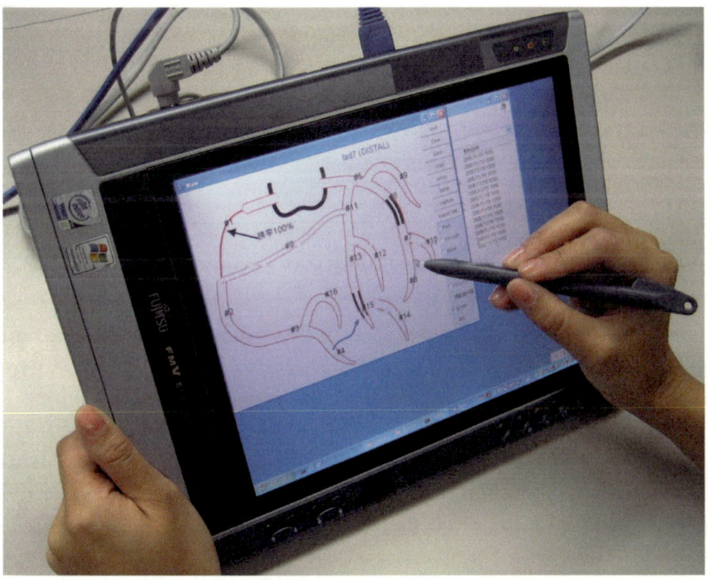

Figure 1. A screenshot of our system in use.

http://dx.doi.org/10.5772/54235

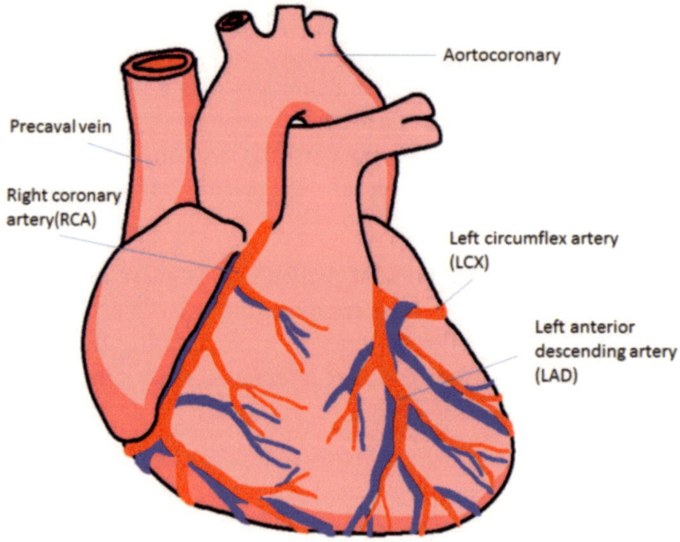

Figure 2. An illustration of the human heart. The target of our system is the coronary arteries (the red vessels shown in this figure).

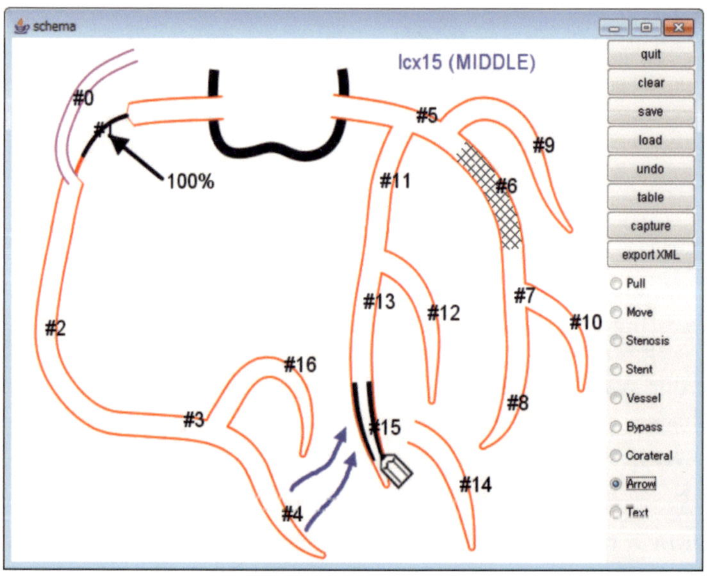

Figure 3. Recording an example of cardiac catheterization.

2. User Interface

The user can draw on the diagram template using a pen as if drawing on real paper. Our system shows the name of each coronary artery and segment (e.g., proximal, middle, or distal) at the upper right of the screen when the cursor is over any vessel. We use the naming scheme defined in the AHA committee report. The system can show border lines of coronary artery segments if required.

Our system is a Windows application that provides a familiar interface to permit new users to work with it without extensive training. For example, the system displays a pop-up menu when the user clicks on a window while pressing the barrel button on the pen (Figure 4). This section describes the user interaction steps one by one. The next section describes our algorithm.

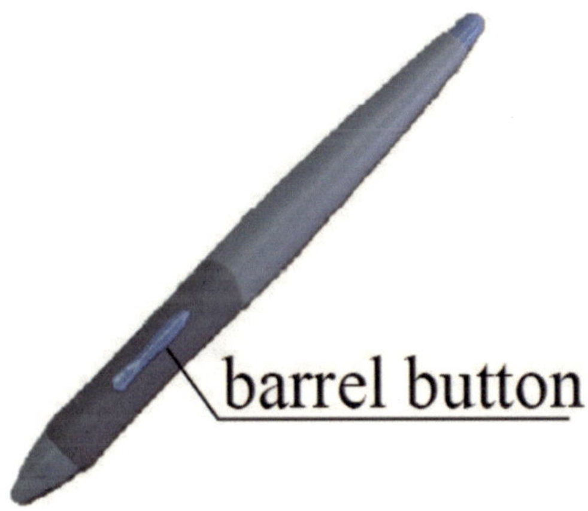

Figure 4. Barrel button on pen.

2.1. Insertion / editing of a vessel

Upon start-up, our system displays a default cardiac catheterization coronary schema. The user can then draw a finding report or a treatment plan on the schema. The system provides several functions for editing the geometry on screen, including adding, deleting, and deforming arteries.

The user can draw a new coronary artery with the pen after choosing the "draw coronary artery" mode from the tool palette on the right (Figure 5 (a)). The system automatically creates an appropriate junction where the new artery is connected to another, and tapers the free end. The user can delete a vessel by clicking on it while holding the barrel button down and choosing "delete" from a pop-up menu. The system automatically updates the display on the screen. The user can move an artery by dragging it with the pen after choosing the

http://dx.doi.org/10.5772/54235

"move coronary artery" mode from the tool palette (Figure 5 (b)). The user can deform an artery by dragging it with the pen (Figure 5 (c)) after choosing the "pull coronary artery" mode from the tool palette. We use a pulling interface for a curve that was introduced in [13]. It deforms a curve while preserving the local geometry. The user can also set the line width to small, normal, or large, using a pop-up panel (Figure 6). This system also supports the `absent' display, as shown in Figure 7.

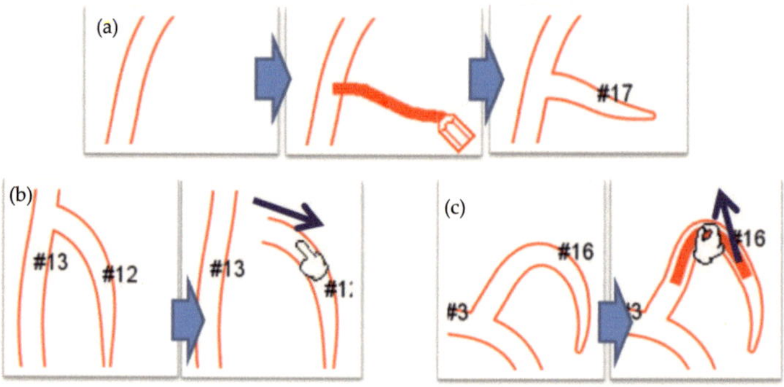

Figure 5. Editing operations on a coronary artery. (a) Draw a new coronary artery; (b) Move a coronary artery; (c) Pull a coronary artery

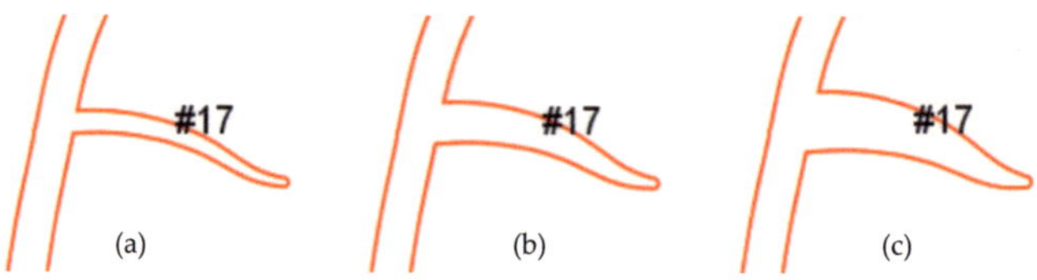

Figure 6. The user can set the line width to small, normal, or large, using a pop-up panel. (a) Small; (b) Normal; (c) Large

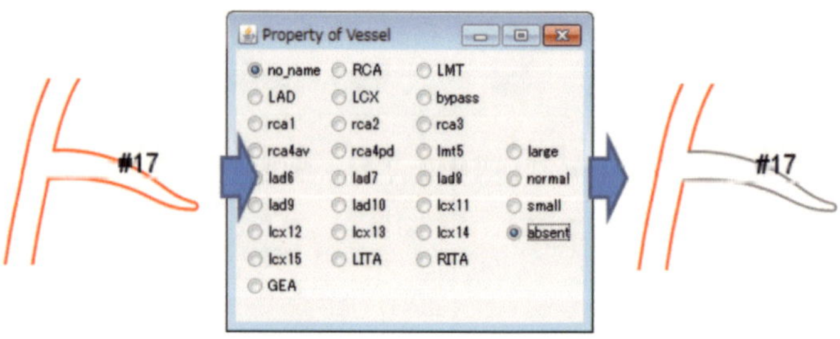

Figure 7. The system also supports the `absent' display

2.2. Recording of stenoses

Once the user has sketched the geometry of the coronary arteries, he or she can record stenoses. To do this, the user chooses the "draw stenosis" mode from the tool palette and draws the stenosis on the target artery with the pen (Figure 8 (a)). When the user completes drawing and lifts the pen from the screen, the system displays a dialog box to specify the type and severity of the stenosis (Figure 8 (b)). If the user wants to change the properties of an existing stenosis, he or she can open the properties window by clicking on the affected artery while holding the barrel button down. The display of each stenosis on the screen includes the severity specified by the user (Figure 8 (c)).

The user can also move an existing stenosis by dragging it along the coronary artery (Figure 9). The stenosis snaps to the border of the appropriate section of the artery as it moves.

If the severity of a stenosis is set to 100%, the portion of the artery beyond the stenosis is shown as a thin line (Figure 10 (a)) representing a complete blockage where no blood flows. The system automatically analyzes the tree structure of arteries and closes any downstream vessels as well.

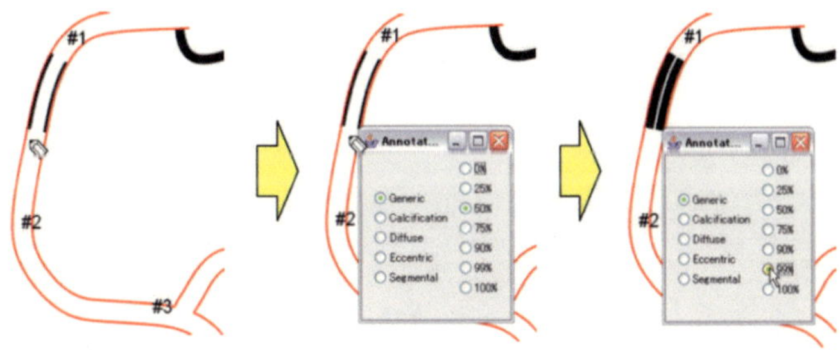

(a) (b) (c)

Figure 8. Recording a stenosis. When the user draws a stenosis (a), the system displays a dialog box to specify the type and severity of the stenosis (b, c).

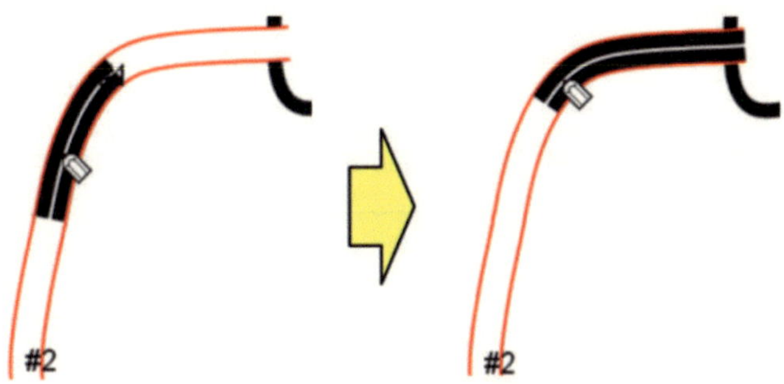

Figure 9. The user can move an existing stenosis by dragging it along the coronary artery.

http://dx.doi.org/10.5772/54235

2.3. Bypasses and collateral

The user can add a bypass to the schema by drawing a line connecting coronary arteries. If the bypass connects an open artery to a closed one, the system automatically opens the blockage to indicate that blood flow has been restored (Figure 10 (b)). The user can place a stenosis on a bypass just like on a coronary artery and can also delete, move, and pull a bypass.

The user can draw a collateral (new blood vessels that reroute blood flow around a stenosis) by drawing a line between coronary arteries. This appears as an arrow in the schema (Figure 11). Our current implementation does not modify the blood flow automatically in response to a new collateral.

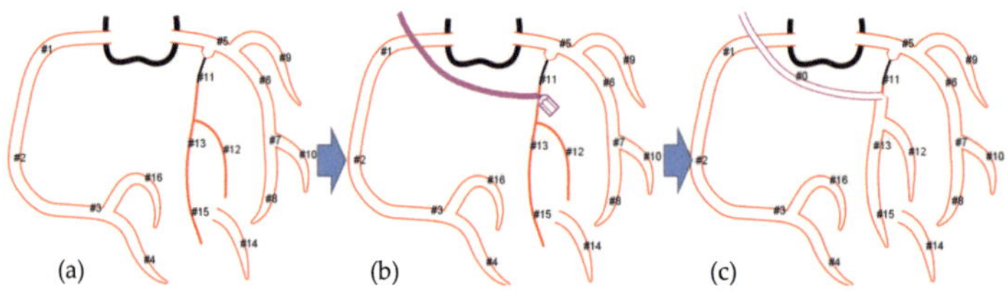

Figure 10. Drawing a bypass. If the bypass connects an open coronary artery to a closed one (a), the system automatically opens the closed coronary artery to indicate that blood flow has resumed (b, c).

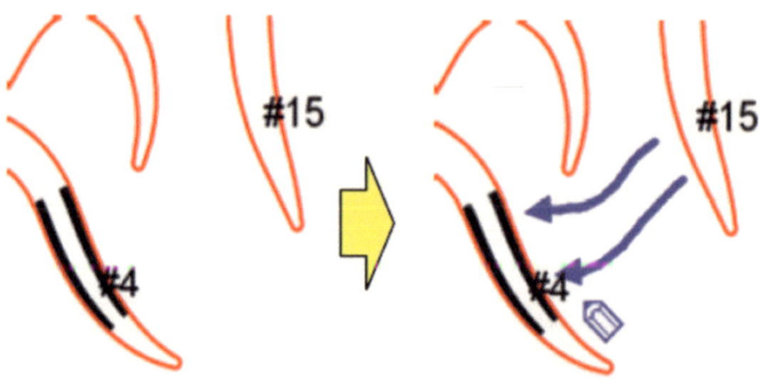

Figure 11. Example of recording a collateral.

2.4. Stent

The user can place a stent in a coronary artery (Figure 12). Recording of stents is very important for documenting the treatment of the stenosis. The procedure for editing a stent is identical to that for editing a stenosis. The user creates and moves a stent by dragging it along a coronary artery and deletes it using a pop-up menu. The stent also snaps to the borders of the artery segments.

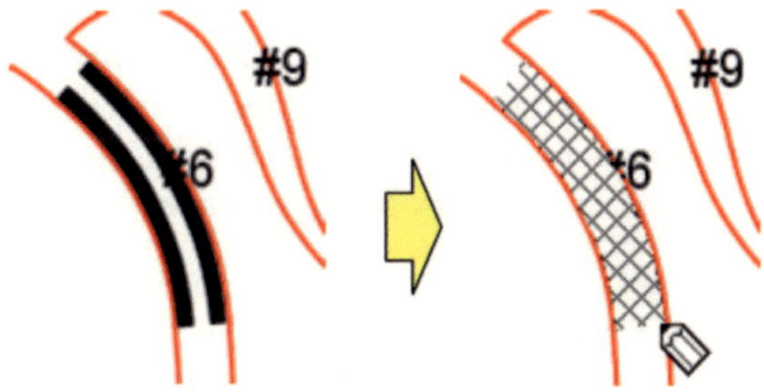

Figure 12. Example of placing a stent.

2.5. Other Functions

The user can annotate the schema as a record of miscellaneous medical diagnosis and treatment. Our current implementation supports text and arrow marks in annotations (Figure 13). Unconstrained annotation encourages the user to think freely, similar to handwriting notes on traditional paper medical records. It is also helpful to remind the user of miscellaneous details associated with specific treatments.

The system can save an edited coronary schema, and then load it again for review or further editing. The schema is stored as vector graphics to reduce file size and facilitate editing. The system can export a schema in PNG image format for import into another system.

The user can create a new schema starting from a default coronary schema template and can also specify any schema to be the default template.

When the user places the mouse cursor on a vessel, the system displays the name of the vessel at the top right corner of the screen, as shown in Figure 14. The system displays not only the name of the vessel, but also its position ('PROXIMAL', 'MIDDLE' or 'DISTAL') in each blood vessel. Moreover, segment border lines are displayed when the user enables this feature in the pop-up menu shown in Figure 15.

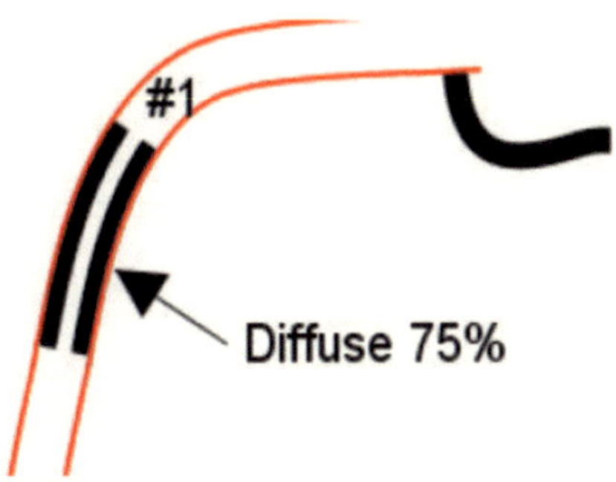

Figure 13. Example of recording text and arrow marks as an annotation.

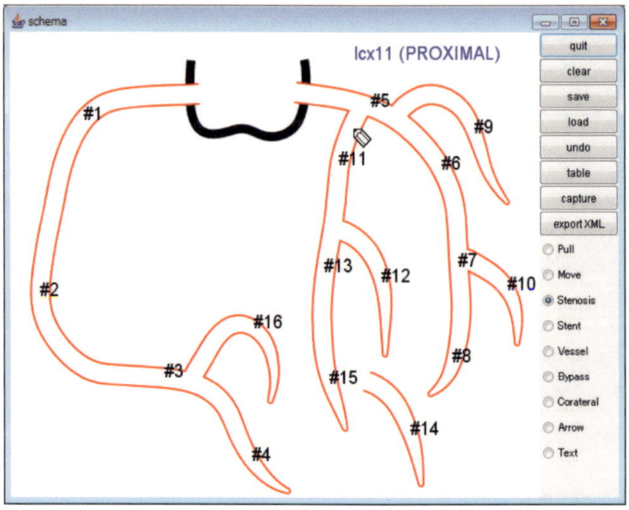

Figure 14. The system displays the name of the vessel at the top right of the screen when the user places the mouse cursor over it.

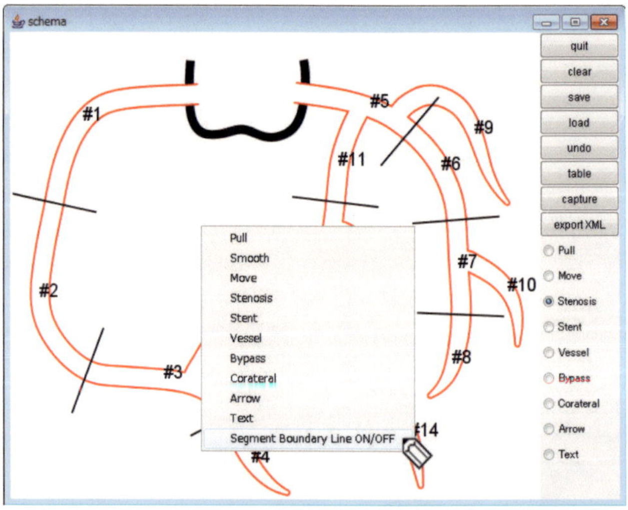

Figure 15. The system displays segment border lines when the user enables this feature in the pop-up menu.

3. Dataset structure and cooperation with other systems

Many doctors use coronary angiography (CAG) to represent coronary stenosis pathology. CAG compactly shows the location and severity of stenoses. Our system supports the conversion of the graphical record to a CAG-compliant table dataset. The table is represented in

the format specified in the AHA committee report and stored as an XML file. Figure 16 shows the relationship between our system and CAG. The top screen in Figure 16 (a) presents an example of recording stenoses using our system; the middle screen of Figure 16 (a) shows the CAG dataset it produces. Any other system that supports this format can use the data file as shown in the bottom screen of Figure 16 (a).

The user can also edit the exported CAG table. When this happens, our system automatically updates the corresponding stenosis on the coronary diagram including the information on the severity and character of the stenosis (Figure 16 (b)).

When a stenosis is straddling two or more segments, it is considered to belong to two or more segments. The stenosis drawn on LAD7 and LAD8 amid the strangulation shown in Figure 17 is an example.

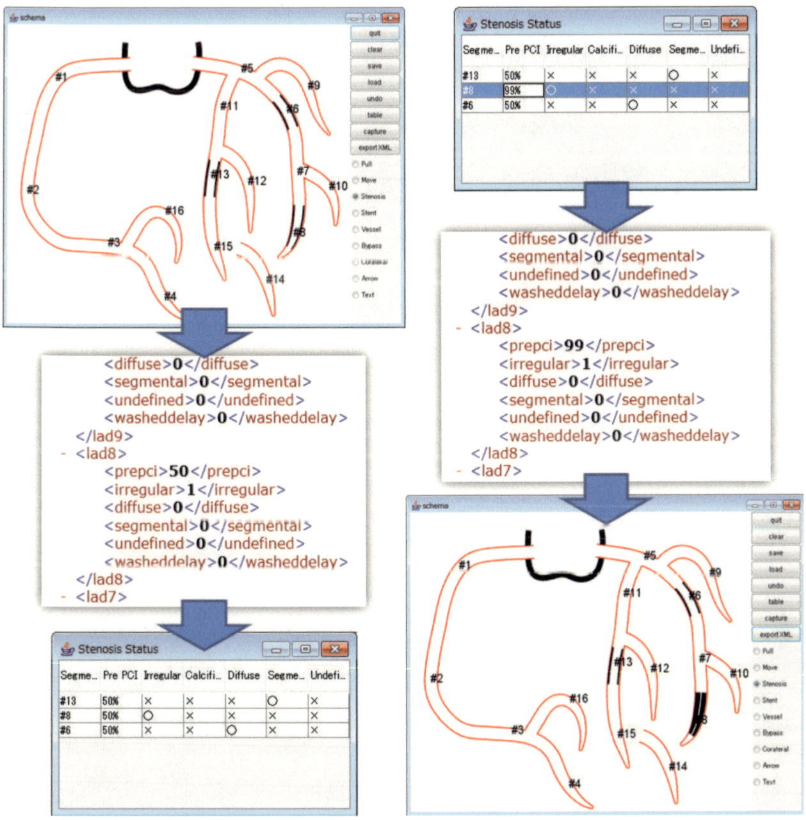

(a) (b)

Figure 16. Example of the automatic relationship between the coronary diagram and the CAG table. (a) The system automatically generates a CAG table from a graphical coronary schema by checking the existence of a stenosis in each segment of the coronary arteries, and stores the results in XML format. (b) The system can automatically update the stenoses on the coronary schema from the corresponding CAG table.

http://dx.doi.org/10.5772/54235

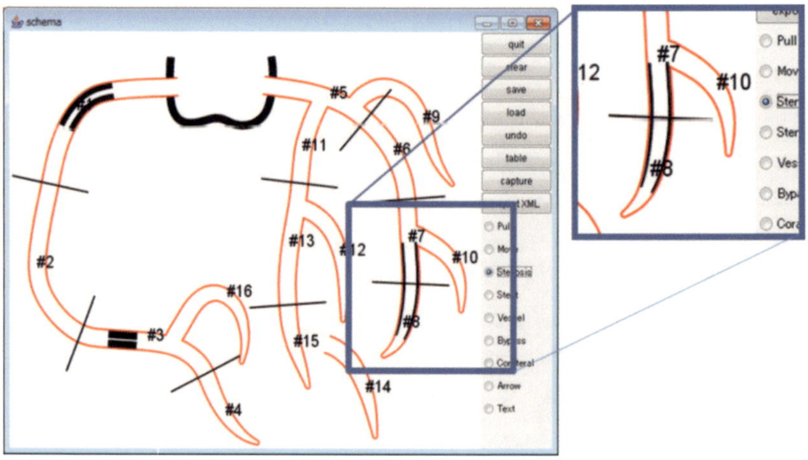

Figure 17. Example of a stenosis over two divisions.

4. Implementation

We designed our system as a platform-independent Java™ program using the Java2D™ graphics application programming interface. This section describes the implementation details of the current prototype.

4.1. On-screen displays

The system displays coronary arteries as two parallel lines and handles the branches appropriately (Figure 18 (a)). A vessel is a polyline composed of small line segments. The system first draws a wide red line and then a narrow white line inside (Figure 18 (b1), (b2)). The width of these lines decreases toward the non-connected end of a vessel to represent the taper (Figure 18 (c1), (c2)).

A stenosis is displayed in a similar manner. The system first draws a wide black line inside the vessel and then a narrow white line inside that. A stent is rendered by drawing a hatching pattern after setting a stencil inside the stent area.

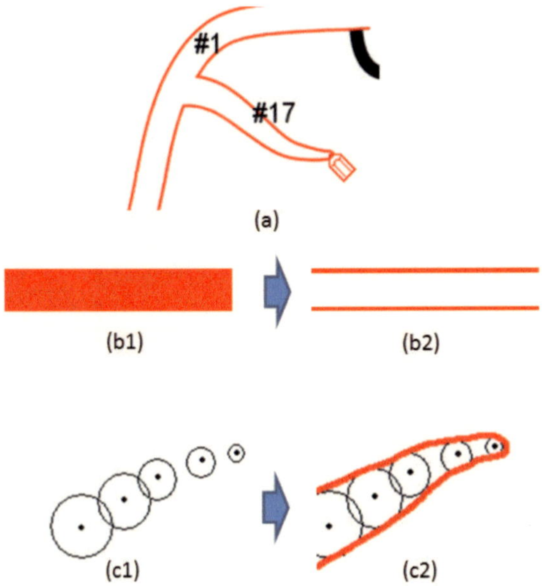

Figure 18. Vessel representation. The system displays coronary arteries as two parallel lines and handles the branches appropriately (a). The system first draws a wide red line (b1), and then a narrow white line inside (b2). The width of these lines decreases toward the non-connected end of a vessel to represent the taper (c1, c2).

4.2. Geometry editing

The pulling interface deforms the curve while maintaining its local details (Figure 5 (c)) [13]. The system first generates triangles by connecting sets of three neighboring points on a polyline. As the user pulls a point along the curve, the system determines the location of free vertices so as to minimize the distortion of the triangles. We also used the peeling interface introduced in [13] to adjust the size of the region to be deformed, so that a larger area is deformed as the user pulls more. As the user pulls the curve further away, the influence region grows (Figure 19, left to right).

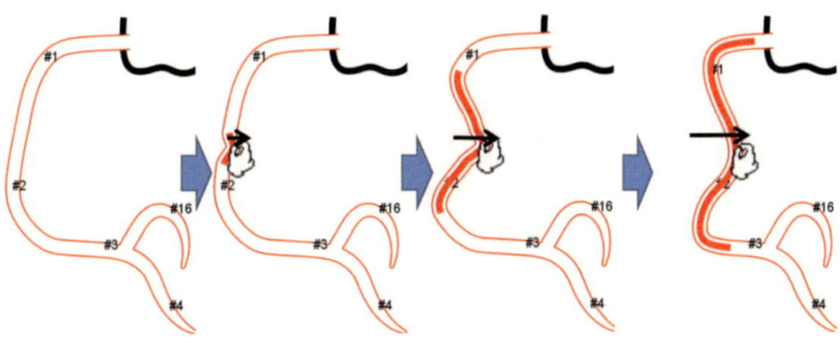

Figure 19. We use the pulling and peeling interface introduced in [13]. As the user pulls the curve further away, the influence region grows (left to right).

http://dx.doi.org/10.5772/54235

4.3. Generation of the CAG table

The CAG table stores the following information for each segment of a coronary artery: the presence or absence of a stenosis, the severity of the stenosis, and the type of stenosis (Figure 16 (a), bottom). The system automatically generates a CAG table from a graphical coronary schema by checking for the existence of a stenosis in each segment. It stores the result in XML format (Figure 16 (a), middle and bottom).

When the user edits the CAG table, the system first finds the corresponding stenosis in the XML file (Figure 16 (b), top and middle). It then obtains the information for that stenosis and changes it on the coronary schema. In this way, the system automatically updates the stenoses on the coronary schema from the corresponding CAG table (Figure 16 (b), bottom).

5. Case report using our system

We illustrate the effectiveness of our system, utilizing two cases of coronary artery bypass surgery as examples. These examples were only described (not illustrated) in the original papers.

The first example is Case 1 of [14]. The paper describes it as follows:

`A man, 45 years of age, had suffered attacks of angina pectoris during many years. He had had infarction of the myocardium. During the operation it was noted that the left coronary artery and the initial portions of its main branches were calcified. We also noted density of the right coronary artery. Anastomosis was applied between the inner thoracic artery and the circumflex branch of the left coronary artery.'

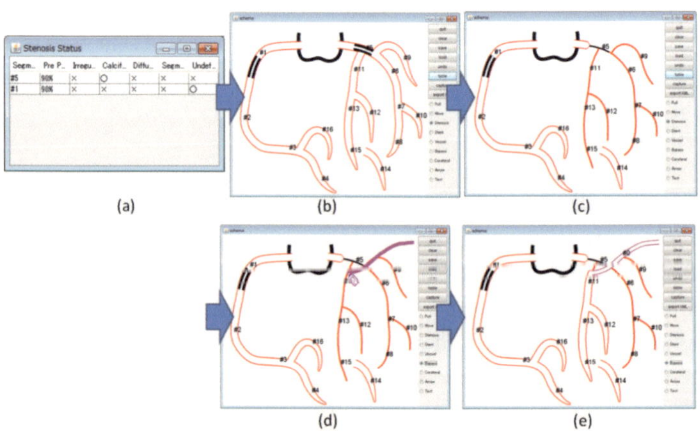

Figure 20. Case 1 of the report [14] using our system.

Figure 20 shows how to illustrate this process using our system. First, the user inputs a CAG table, as shown in Figure 20 (a). With our system, the user can set the type of the corresponding stenosis, as shown in the CAG table. The system then automatically generates a graphical coronary schema, as shown in Figure 20 (b). Figure 20 (c) shows the result of setting the severity of a stenosis of the left coronary artery to 100%.

The bypass connects an open vessel to the closed coronary artery, and the system automatically opens the closed coronary artery to indicate that blood flow is recovered, as shown in Figure 20 (d, e).

The second example is Case 3 of the report [14]. The paper describes it as follows:

'A male patient (40 years of age), had suffered from generalized atherosclerosis. (...) During the operation calcification and complete occlusion of the initial portion of both branches of the left coronary artery were found. An end-to-end anastomosis between the inner thoracic and interventricular arteries was made.'

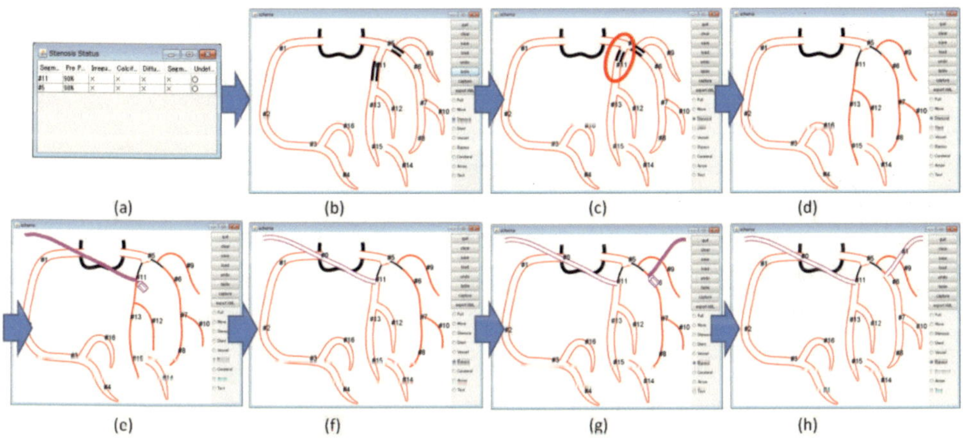

Figure 21. Case 3 of the report [14] using our system.

Figure 21 shows how to illustrate this process using our system. First, the user inputs a CAG table, as shown in Figure 21 (a). The system then automatically generates a graphical coronary schema, as shown in Figure 21 (b). By default, the system automatically generates the stenosis in the middle portion of the corresponding vessel, as shown in Figure 21 (b). The user can move the stenosis to the initial portion, as shown in Figure 21 (c). Figure 21 (d) shows the result of setting the severity of the stenosis to 100%.

The bypass connects an open vessel to the closed coronary artery, and the system automatically opens the closed coronary artery to indicate that blood flow is recovered, as shown in Figure 21 (e, f) and (g, h).

http://dx.doi.org/10.5772/54235

6. Discussion

Our current implementation is a research prototype and is not yet being used in clinical practice. However, we have already demonstrated it to medical professionals and confirmed the following benefits:

1. The user can easily modify the geometry of coronary arteries for individual patients.
2. The system can store the data compactly using vectors instead of bitmaps, which significantly improves the network response when storing information on a remote server.
3. The system can export the CAG table based on the AHA committee report in XML format. Therefore, the system can easily exchange data with other existing systems.
4. The user can edit a coronary schema while viewing a reference image on the same display.
5. The user can draw diagrams and text freely in our system, which allows the recording of new anomalies that have never been previously observed.

In addition, we received the following comment from another heart surgeon: `This is a user-friendly system. It is particularly effective for inexperienced doctors. Diagnosis is performed by a heart physician. But, I think that it is useful also for a young surgeon's training. '

The correspondence between a diagnosis and a dissection, as well as comparison between the diagnosis and a CT scan image, are important to a surgeonpreparing for an operation. However, even though there is an AHA standard that defines how to verbalize diagnosis results, there is significant variation in the way surgeons describe diagnosis results, even among experts. Accordingly, one specialist commented that it is useful to have a link between CT scan images of the circumflex branches to the corresponding locations in the schema. The specialist also commented that two-dimensional (2D) representation is sufficient if the purpose of the target system is diagnosis, but 3D representation is desirable for training purposes.

An issue with the current implementation is that it is limited by the AHA standards. The manner of recording schemas for cardiac catheterization varies widely among users and facilities. As the AHA committee report was designed more than 30 years ago, it cannot handle many cases well. Therefore, a more powerful and flexible representation is needed.

7. Conclusion and future work

We developed an effective interface for reporting graphical findings in cardiac catheterization using hand-drawn diagrams. The user can easily record the position and degree of a stenosis on a coronary schema template, and can also record treatments such as bypasses and stents. Once a bypass is added, the system automatically displays the resumption of blood flow. This type of automatic adaptation is not possible with paper-based medical re-

cords. Our system can store the data as a CAG table in an XML file in the AHA format for exchanging data with other existing systems. Our system makes it easier to handle graphical schemas in medical recording systems, encouraging the spread of medical recording systems in general.

Our system operates independently and does not require any other special infrastructure. Therefore, it can be easily introduced at low cost. We hope to put our system into actual clinical practice to make improvements based on feedback from actual users. We also plan to experiment with 3D schemas because 3D images are becoming increasingly widespread. We are also currently working with methods pertaining to 3D images. For example, Nakao et al. proposed a 3D cardiovascular modeling system based on neonatal echocardiographic images [15]. Using this system, medical doctors can interactively construct patient-specific cardiovascular models, and share the complex topology and shape information. Bo et al. introduced a lightweight sketching system that enables interactive illustration of complex fluid systems [16]. Users can sketch on a 2.5D canvas to design the shapes and connections of a fluid circuit. Ijiri et al. developed an efficient and robust framework for simulating the cardiac beating motion [17]. The global cardiac motion is generated by the accumulation of local myocardial fiber contractions. They compute such local-to-global deformations using a kinematic approach, dividing a heart mesh model into overlapping local regions, contracting them independently according to fiber orientation, and computing a global shape that fits the contracted shapes of all local regions as well as possible.

The interactive graphical schemas introduced in this paper should be useful in not only cardiac catheterization but also other areas that use schemas, for example, ophthalmology, otolaryngology, and dentistry. Such interactive schemas are useful not only for efficiently generating finding reports but also as an effective explanation tool for patients.

Author details

Yuki Igarashi[1], Takeo Igarashi[2], Ryo Haraguchi[3] and Kazuo Nakazawa[3]

1 University of Tsukuba, Japan

2 The University of Tokyo, Japan

3 National Cerebral and Cardiovascular Center Reserch Institute, Japan

References

[1] Takashi Matsumura. Electronic Medical Record and Hospital Information System . Comprehensive Management of Patient Information--. Japan Journal of Medical Informatics, 21(3), 2001, 211-222 (in Japanese).

[2] Yasushi Matsumura. Current Status of Electronic Medical Record and its Tasks. The Medical Frontline, 2003; 58(8): 46-51 (in Japanese).

[3] Dean F. Sitting, Gilad J. Kuperman, Julie Fiskio. Evaluating Physician Satisfaction Regarding User Interactions with an Electronic Medical Record System. Proceedings of AMIA Annual Symposium 99, 1999, 400-404.

[4] Mark Ginsburg. Pediatric Electronic Health Record Interface Design: The PedOne System. Proceedings of the 40th Hawaii International Conference on System Sciences, 2007, 139.

[5] Erik K. Fromme, Tawni Kenworthy-Heinige and Michelle Hribar. Developing an easy-to-use tablet computer application for assessing patient-reported outcomes in patients with cancer. Supportive Care in Cancer, Volume 19, Number 6 (2011), 815-822.

[6] Ole Andreas Alsos, Anita Das, Dag Svanæs. Mobile health IT: The effect of user interface and form factor on doctor–patient communication. International Journal of Medical Informatics, 81(1), 12-28, 2012.

[7] Kazuo Nakazawa, Takeo Igarashi. A Comprehensive Computer Interface for the Spreading of Electronic Medical Recording Systems Supporting Hand-writing Inputs by Pen Device. New Medicine in Japan, 2003; 345: 74-77 (in Japanese).

[8] Kazuo Nakazawa, Ryo Haraguchi, Takenori Yao, Satoru Nagata, Yoshihisa Sugimoto, Takashi Ashihara, Masahiro Takada, Hirokazu Namikawa, Yasushi Okada, Kohei Yoshimoto, Naomi Furuya, Shuji Senda, Yoshiyuki Uematsu, Takeo Igarashi. Pen-based Interface for Electronic Medical Record System with Advanced Recognition and Search Engine for the Hand-written Characters. Japan Journal of Medical Informatics, 2005; 25(2), 81-86 (in Japanese).

[9] Takeo Igarashi, "Freeform User Interfaces for Graphical Computing", Proceedings of 3rd International Symposium on Smart Graphics, Lecture Notes in Computer Science, Springer, 39-48, 2003.

[10] Sakabe Nagamasa, Arai Kazuo, Abe Kazuya, Inoue Hideo, Sakai Shunichi, Watanabe Yukio. A Survey of demerits of Electronic Medical Record in the Ear-Nose and Throat Department. Japan Journal of Medical Informatics, 2001; 21(1): 131-136 (in Japanese).

[11] Yuki Mori, Takeo Igarashi, Ryo Haraguchi, and Kazuo Nakazawa. A Pen-based Interface for Generating Graphical Reports of Findings in Cardiac Catheterization. Methods of Information in Medicine, 2007;46(6) pp.694-699.

[12] Austen G. W, Eswards J, Frye R. L., et al. "A Reporting System on Patients Evaluated for Coronary Artery Disease", Circulation, 1975; 51(4 Suppl.): 5-40.

[13] Igarashi T, Moscovich T, Hughes J F. As-Rigid-As-Possible Shape Manipulation. ACM Transactions on Computer Graphics 2005; 24(3): 1134-1141

[14] Kolessov, V. I. Mammary artery-coronary artery anastomosis as method of treatment for angina pectoris. The Journal of Thoracic and Cardiovascular Surgery. 1967; 54(4): 535-544.

[15] Megumi Nakao, Kazuma Maeda, Ryo Haraguchi, Ken-ichi Kurosaki, Koji Kagisaki, Isao Shiraishi, Kazuo Nakazawa, Kotaro Minato. "Cardiovascular Modeling of Congenital Heart Disease Based on Neonatal Echocardiographic Images", IEEE Transactions on Information Technology in BioMedicine, 16(1), 70-79, 2012.

[16] Bo Zhu, Michiaki Iwata, Ryo Haraguchi, Takashi Ashihara, Nobuyuki Umetani, Takeo Igarashi, Kazuo Nakazawa. Sketch-based Dynamic Illustration of Fluid Systems. ACM Transactions on Graphics (Proceedings of SIGGRAPH Asia 2011), 30(6), Article No. 134, 2011.

[17] Ijiri T, Ashihara T, Umetani N, Igarashi T, Haraguchi R, et al. (2012) A Kinematic Approach for Efficient and Robust Simulation of the Cardiac Beating Motion. PLoS ONE 7(5): e36706.

Section 4

Peripheral and Cerebral Vascular Disease Intervention

Chapter 21

Management of Carotid Artery Disease in the Setting of Coronary Artery Disease in Need of Coronary Artery Bypass Surgery

Aditya M. Sharma and Herbert D. Aronow

Additional information is available at the end of the chapter

http://dx.doi.org/10.5772/55669

1. Introduction

Coronary artery bypass graft surgery (CABG) is one of the most commonly performed major surgeries in the United States with over 397,000 CABG's performed in 2010.(Go, Mozaffarian et al. 2012) One of the most dreadful adverse sequelae of CABG is stroke which is also the 2nd most common major post-operative complication seen with CABG, occurring in 1 to 5% of patients.(Furlan, Sila et al. 1992; Brown, Kugelmass et al. 2008) Patients suffering from postoperative stroke have a very high incidence of in-hospital mortality.(Hogue, Murphy et al. 1999) Studies have shown that presence of extracranial carotid artery stenosis (ECAS) is a strong risk factor for post-operative morbidity and mortality due post-CABG strokes.(Brown, Kugelmass et al. 2008) In this book chapter, we will review the epidemiology of concomitant coronary and carotid artery disease, the association with post-operative stroke, recommendations for pre-operative ECAS screening and management options for patients in whom ECAS is identified.

Co-prevalence of carotid and coronary artery disease and its implications on perioperative and postoperative morbidity and mortality: Atherosclerosis is a systemic disease which is usually present in multiple vascular beds simultaneously.(Beique, Ali et al. 2006) In a recent study from the Cleveland Clinic involving 45,432 patient's, presence of carotid artery disease was confirmed as a significant risk factor for perioperative stroke after CABG. (Tarakji, Sabik et al. 2011) In the REACH Registry which was comprised of 67,888 patients, 10% of patients had concomitant coronary artery disease (CAD) and cerebrovascular disease (CVD). Anastasiasdis et al evaluated carotid arteries in 307 patients undergoing CABG and reported that while 3 out of 4 patients undergoing CABG had carotid atherosclerosis, the majority of these (63%) had <

50% ECAS. (Anastasiadis, Karamitsos et al. 2009). Various studies have reported the incidence of ECAS with varies degree of stenosis among the patient populations undergoing CABG which are summarized in table 1.

Study	Number of patients undergoing CABG being evaluated for ECAS	Prevalence of ECAS %
Wanamaker et al	559	ECAS >50% : 36%
Shirani et al	1045	ECAS > 60% : 6.9%
Anastasiadis et al	307	ECAS > 70% : 13%
Cornily et al	205	ECAS >70% : 5.8%
Salasidis et al	387	ECAS > 80% : 8.5%
Schwartz et al	582	ECAS > 50% : 22% ECAS > 80% : 12%

Abbreviations: CABG, coronary artery bypass grating'; ECAS, extracranial carotid artery stenosis.

Table 1. Prevalence of extracranial carotid artery stenosis among patients undergoing coronary artery bypass grafting.

Salasidis et al identified increasing age, history of previous carotid revascularization and presence of PAD in addition to severe ECAS as risk factors for neurological events after cardiac surgery, highlighting that ECAS is only 1 of a number of factors that drives peri-operative stroke risk.(Salasidis, Latter et al. 1995)

Interestingly, the likelihood of having ECAS increases with the underlying severity of CAD (Table 2).

Severity of CAD	Prevalence of Significant Carotid Atherosclerosis (%)
1- vessel CAD	5.3%
2- vessel CAD	13.5%
3- vessel CAD	24.5%
Left main disease	40%
3-vessel CAD or left main disease	24%

Table 2. Prevalence of significant carotid artery stenosis (extracranial carotid artery stenosis ≥ 50%) among patients with different severity of coronary artery disease based on number of vessels involved or left main disease.

It was postulated that increasing degree of stenosis was associated with increased risk of perioperative stroke by Naylor et al who reported that among 5,453 patients undergoing CABG, the risk of perioperative stroke was <2%, 3%, 5% and 7-11% among patients who had < 50% ECAS, 50-99% unilateral ECAS, 50-99% bilateral ECAS and occluded carotid artery respectively.(Naylor, Mehta et al. 2002)

http://dx.doi.org/10.5772/55669

2. Screening for carotid artery disease

Screening for carotid artery disease is usually performed with carotid duplex ultrasound. Screening recommendations for carotid artery disease are somewhat controversial and vary across medical societies.(Goldstein, Adams et al. 2006; Bates, Babb et al. 2007; Qureshi, Alexandrov et al. 2007; 2008; Brott, Halperin et al. 2011) The most widely accepted multisocietal vascular practice guidelines involving 14 different vascular societies including the American College of Cardiology Foundation, American Heart Association Task Force on Practice Guidelines, the American Stroke Association, American Association of Neuroscience Nurses, American Association of Neurological Surgeons, American College of Radiology, American Society of Neuroradiology, Congress of Neurological Surgeons, Society of Atherosclerosis Imaging and Prevention,Society for Cardiovascular Angiography and Interventions, Society of Interventional Radiology, Society of NeuroInterventional Surgery, Society for Vascular Medicine, and Society for Vascular Surgery recommend screening for patients with carotid bruit or patients with CAD or symptomatic PAD or atherosclerotic aortic aneurysm as well those who may not have evidence of atherosclerosis but have 2 or more cardiovascular risk factors such as hypertension, dyslipidemia, tobacco smoking, family history of premature atherosclerosis or family history of ischemic stroke.(Brott, Halperin et al. 2011). The US Preventive Service Task Force recommended against screening as it was not cost-effective in asymptomatic patients.(Bates, Babb et al. 2007) The American Society of Neuroimaging recommended against the screening of unselected populations but advised the screening of adults older than 65 years of age who have 3 or more cardiovascular risk factors (Qureshi, Alexandrov et al. 2007)

For patients undergoing elective CABG, the multi-societal guidelines recommend screening for carotid artery disease in patients older than 65 years of age and in those with left main stenosis, PAD, history of cigarette smoking, history of stroke or TIA or carotid bruit. The American Heart Association and American College of Cardiology CABG guidelines offer recommendations consistent with the multi-societal vascular guidelines, however they also recommend that patients who have history of hypertension or diabetes mellitus also undergo preoperative carotid duplex scanning.(Hillis, Smith et al. 2011)

3. Utility of advanced imaging carotid artery beyond carotid duplex ultrasound

Duplex ultrasound is an excellent tool to diagnose ECAS.(Eagle, Guyton et al. 1999) However there are certain inherent errors that can occur with duplex. The presence of calcification at the site of stenosis may cause underestimation of degree of stenosis; similarly contralateral occlusion may lead to falsely elevated velocities in the ipsilateral carotid artery leading to overestimation of the degree of stenosis. (Mitchell E 2004) In such situations additional imaging with computed tomography angiography (CTA) or magnetic resonance angiography (MRA) may further characterize the degree of stenosis as well as provide insight on plaque charac-

teristics, aortic pathology and intracranial ICA abnormalities. Given the excellent images rendered by CTA or MRA, conventional angiography is rarely required for determining degree of stenosis among those with normal or minimally impaired renal function. For those with moderate to severe chronic kidney disease, MRI may be relatively contraindicated due to the risk of nephrogenic systemic sclerosis and invasive angiography favored over CTA given its lower relative contrast volume and risk of contrast-induced acute kidney injury.

Other factors that may lead to increased stroke risk beyond degree of stenosis, including cerebrovascular reserve (CVR). Severe ECAS reduces cerebral perfusion pressure. Autoregulation of the cerebral vasculature dilates the cerebral arterioles maximally, and with further reduction in cerebral perfusion, blood flow will eventually decrease, causing impairment in cerebral perfusion leading to stroke. CVR can be assessed by two approaches. the first, CVR can be determined through direct measurements of brain tissue with flow-sensitive imaging through positron emission tomography, CT perfusion or MR perfusion before and after vasodilator stimulation. A second, indirect approach utilizes transcranial Doppler to assess flow velocities distal to the lesion, typically in the middle cerebral artery before and after vasodilatory stimulation, with increase in flow velocities used to indirectly measure CVR. (Gupta, Chazen et al. 2012) In a meta-analysis of patients with severe ECAS, there was an association between impaired CVR and increased stroke risk.(Gupta, Chazen et al. 2012) An incomplete circle of Willis has also been associated with increased ipsilateral cerebral ischemia during carotid cross clamping with CEA.(Manninen, Makinen et al. 2009) and as a risk factor for ischemic stroke (Hoksbergen AW et al. Cerebrovasc Dz 2003;16:191-8) Current guidelines do not comment on use of cerebral perfusion imaging when assessing stroke risk due to insufficient evidence available so far.(Brott, Halperin et al. 2011; Hillis, Smith et al. 2011)

4. Treatment

Treatment options for ECAS consist of medical therapy and in some cases, revascularization.

Medical therapy for carotid artery disease: Medical therapy is the cornerstone of treatment for atherosclerotic disease. Medical therapy for ECAS comprises of treatment of risk factors such as hypertension, dyslipidemia, diabetes mellitus, and tobacco use and use of antiplatelet therapy. Consensus societal class I recommendations for treatment of atherosclerotic carotid artery disease appear in Table 1 (Brott, Halperin et al. 2011).

Treatment of hypertension: Hypertension increases risk of stroke significantly. For each 10 mm Hg rise in blood pressure, the stroke risk increases by 30 to 45%. This risk significantly is significantly reduced with antihypertensive therapy. A systemic review of 7 randomized controlled trials (RCT) showed that treatment with antihypertensive agents reduced the risk of recurrent stroke by 24%. A meta-analysis of 40 studies with > 188,000 patients reported a 33% decreased risk of stroke with a 10 mm Hg reduction in BP.(Lawes, Bennett et al. 2004; Brott, Halperin et al. 2011) Hypertension should be treated to maintain a goal blood pressure (BP) < 140/90 mm Hg for all patients with ECAS except those with diabetes mellitus (DM) and chronic

http://dx.doi.org/10.5772/55669

Recommendation	Class of Indication	Level of Evidence
Antihypertensive treatment is recommended for patients with hypertension and asymptomatic extracranial carotid or vertebral atherosclerosis to maintain blood pressure below 140/90 mm Hg	I	A
Treatment with a statin medication is recommended for all patients with extracranial carotid or vertebral atherosclerosis to reduce low-density lipoprotein (LDL) cholesterol below 100 mg/dl	I	B
Patients with extracranial carotid or vertebral atherosclerosis who smoke cigarettes should be advised to quit smoking and offered smoking cessation interventions to reduce the risks of atherosclerosis progression and stroke	I	B
Antiplatelet therapy with aspirin, 75 to 325 mg daily, is recommended for patients with obstructive or nonobstructive atherosclerosis that involves the extracranial carotid and/or vertebral arteries for prevention of MI and other ischemic cardiovascular events, although the benefit has not been established for prevention of stroke in asymptomatic patients	I	A
In patients with obstructive or nonobstructive extracranial carotid or vertebral atherosclerosis who have sustained ischemic stroke or TIA, antiplatelet therapy with aspirin alone (75 to 325 mg daily), clopidogrel alone (75 mg daily), or the combination of aspirin plus extended-release dipyridamole (25 and 200 mg twice daily, respectively) is recommended (*Level of Evidence: B*) and preferred over the combination of aspirin with clopidogrel	I	B
Aspirin (81 to 325 mg daily) is recommended before CEA and may be continued indefinitely postoperatively	I	A
Beyond the first month after CEA, aspirin (75 to 325 mg daily), clopidogrel (75 mg daily), or the combination of low-dose aspirin plus extended-release dipyridamole (25 and 200 mg twice daily, respectively) should be administered for long-term prophylaxis against ischemic cardiovascular events	I	B
Administration of antihypertensive medication is recommended as needed to control blood pressure before and after CEA.	I	C
The findings on clinical neurological examination should be documented within 24 hours before and after CEA.	I	C
Before and for a minimum of 30 days after CAS, dual-antiplatelet therapy with aspirin (81 to 325 mg daily) plus clopidogrel (75 mg daily) is recommended. For patients intolerant of clopidogrel, ticlopidine (250 mg twice daily) may be substituted.	I	C
Administration of antihypertensive medication is recommended to control blood pressure before and after CAS.	I	C

Table 3. Recommendations from multisocietal guidelines for extracranial carotid artery stenosis.

kidney disease (CKD) in whom goal BP is < 130/80 mm Hg.(Chobanian, Bakris et al. 2003). These guidelines are applicable to all patients except those in the hyperacute period after stroke. The type of agent utilized should be based on presence of other co-morbid conditions (e.g., diabetes, CKD, CAD, etc.) and not on presence of carotid disease.(Chobanian, Bakris et al. 2003).

Management of Diabetes Mellitus: Presence of diabetes mellitus is associated with increased stroke risk. In the Rotterdam study, diabetes was the only risk factor independently associated with severe progression of carotid stenosis.(van der Meer, Iglesias del Sol et al. 2003). Although glycemic control is necessary, intensive control may not be of incremental benefit. In the UKPDS study, intensive glucose control compared to conventional glucose control did not reduce stroke risk. Similarly, in the ACCORD and ADVANCE trials, intensive glucose control to lower hemoglobin A1c <6 or <6.5, respectively, did not reduce stroke risk when compared to conventional treatment.(Gerstein, Miller et al. 2008; Patel, MacMahon et al. 2008) Intensive control of other risk factors in patients with diabetes is also beneficial, such as administering statins in patients with diabetes even with 'normal' serum cholesterol. Doing so may lower the risk of stroke by as much as 48%.(Colhoun, Betteridge et al. 2004). All diabetic patients with atherosclerotic ECAS should be treated with diet, exercise and glucose lowering drugs as needed to maintain hemoglobin A1c <7. All patients should be treated with statins regardless of cholesterol levels and LDL cholesterol goal should be < 100mg/dl.(Brott, Halperin et al. 2011)

Treatment of dyslipidemia: Dyslipidemia isn't as strongly associated with ischemic stroke as hypertension or diabetes mellitus. In the MR-FIT trial which involved over 350,000 men, the relative risk of death was 2.5 times higher in men with highest vs. the lowest cholesterol levels. (Iso, Jacobs et al. 1989) In the ARIC study, dyslipidemia weakly correlated with ischemic stroke. (Shahar, Chambless et al. 2003); however in the Women's Health Study which evaluated over 27,000 women, total and LDL cholesterol were associated with increased risk of stroke.(Kurth, Everett et al. 2007). The lipid lowering agents of choice are the statins which in addition to lowering cholesterol, work through so-called provide pleotropic effects such as plaque stabilization and reduction in inflammation which may help reduce overall cardiovascular events. A metanalysis comprising of 26 trials with > 90,000 patients found that statins reduce stroke risk by 21%; With every 10% reduction of serum LDL cholesterol, there was a 15.6% reduction in stroke.(Amarenco, Labreuche et al. 2004). The SPARCL trial randomized patients with recent stroke or TIA to atorvastatin 80 mg daily or placebo and found that atorvastatin reduced the incidence of ischemic stroke by 22%.(Amarenco, Bogousslavsky et al. 2006) All patients with atherosclerotic carotid artery disease should be treated with statin to maintain an LDL cholesterol < 100 mg/dl and it is reasonable to maintain LDL cholesterol < 70 mg/dl, especially in high risk patients such as those with ECAS and one or more cardiac risk factors such as current smoker or diabetes mellitus. If the goal LDL cholesterol is not achieved with statin therapy, other lipid lowering agents such as bile acid sequestrants, niacin or ezetimibe can be added to statin therapy.(Brott, Halperin et al. 2011)

Smoking Cessation: Smoking is strongly associated with increased stroke risk. Cigarette smoking is associated with 50% increase in relative risk of ischemic stroke.(Howard, Wagenknecht et al. 1998) Even patients who are past cigarette smokers have a 25% higher risk of stroke compared to lifelong non-smokers.(Howard, Wagenknecht et al. 1998) The Framingham

http://dx.doi.org/10.5772/55669

Heart Study and Cardiovascular Health Study both have reported an association between quantity and period of time an individual smoked and increased risk of stroke.(Tell, Rutan et al. 1994; Wilson, Hoeg et al. 1997). All smokers should be asked about smoking status on every visit and if currently smoking should be counseled on every visit. Every vascular specialist should assist these patients in developing a plan to quit smoking which would include behavioral and pharmacological interventions.(Rooke, Hirsch et al. 2012)

Antiplatelet therapy: Patients undergoing CABG should be on antiplatelet therapy regardless of the presence or absence of ECAS. The benefits of antiplatelet therapy are well-defined in patients with symptomatic ECAS. (2002), and it appears that clopidogrel is superior to aspirin in preventing death, MI or stroke among those with a history of PAD (CAPRIE PAD subgroup analysis/paper). The benefit of dual antiplatelet therapy over monotherapy in this sub-group of patients is not as well-defined and was not proven in the MATCH or in the overall CHARISMA trial.(Diener, Bogousslavsky et al. 2004; Bhatt, Fox et al. 2006) However, in the CHARISMA trial, dual antiplatelet therapy with aspirin and clopidogrel did reduce the incidence of death, MI or stroke among those with established atherosclerotic vascular disease at baseline.(Bhatt, Fox et al. 2006). The ESPS-2 trial demonstrated that extended-release dipyridamale 200 mg twice daily along with aspirin 25 mg once daily (aggrenox) was superior to aspirin alone in secondary prevention of ischemic strokes.(Diener, Cunha et al. 1996) The PROFESS trial compared aggrenox to clopidogrel for secondary prevention of ischemic stroke and found no difference in recurrent stroke reduction in both groups.(Sacco, Diener et al. 2008). Anticoagulant therapy was evaluated in the WARSS study where aspirin was compared to warfarin for stroke prevention in patients with recent stroke, No added benefit was observed with warfarin compared to aspirin in patients with large-vessel atherosclerosis.(Mohr, Thompson et al. 2001). Patients undergoing CABG who have atherosclerotic ECAS will benefit from antiplatelet monotherapy with at aspirin at a minimum; whether dual antiplatelet therapy is incrementally beneficial is less well established.

In summary, it is recommended that all patients with ECAS, regardless of whether they are to undergo CABG receive aggressive risk factor modification in addition to statins, beta-blockers, angiotensin converting enzyme inhibitors or angiotensin receptor blockers and antiplatelet therapy unless contraindicated.

Revascularization: The overall goal of carotid artery revascularization is to reduce the incidence of stroke beyond that afforded by medical therapy alone. In the perioperative setting, the decision about whether to perform carotid artery revascularization, which revascularization modality to pursue and when to revascularize (e.g., CEA or CAS preceded by CABG, CABG preceded by CEA or CAS, concomitant CEA or CAS at the time of CABG). remain challenging.

Indications for carotid revascularization: The decision to revascularize the carotid artery hinges on the presence or absence of symptoms attributable to ECAS, degree of ECAS and urgency of CABG.

The current multisocietal vascular guidelines recommend that carotid revascularization by CEA or CAS with embolic protection before or concurrent with myocardial revascularization

surgery is reasonable in patients with greater than 80% carotid stenosis who have experienced ipsilateral retinal or hemispheric cerebral ischemic symptoms within 6 months. They also state that in patients with asymptomatic carotid stenosis, even if severe, the safety and efficacy of carotid revascularization before or concurrent with myocardial revascularization are not well established..(Brott, Halperin et al. 2011)

The American College of Cardiology and American Heart Association CABG guidelines state that is reasonable to revascularize ECAS of 50-99% in patients with previous history of stroke or TIA and In those who do not have a prior history of stroke or TIA, they consider it reasonable to revascularize especially in the setting of bilateral ECAS of 70-99% or unilateral ECAS of 70-99% with contralateral occlusion. (Hillis, Smith et al. 2011)

In addition to it is necessary to identify and appropriately treat other factors such as atrial fibrillation, low output cardiac state, aortic arch atheroma, age, diabetes etc which also increase the risk for perioperative stroke.

Strategies for carotid revascularization in patients undergoing CABG:

The 2 revascularization modalities most commonly used are CEA and carotid stenting. Both of these modalities are approved by the Food and Drug Administration (FDA) for carotid revascularization. (FDA 2011)

Carotid endarterectomy: CEA has proven to beneficial in stroke reduction in patients with symptomatic and asymptomatic ECAS.(1991; 1991; 1995; 1996; 1998; Barnett, Taylor et al. 1998; Halliday, Mansfield et al. 2004; Halliday, Harrison et al. 2010)

There are three surgical strategies for carotid revascularization in patients undergoing CABG:

Concomitant CEA-CABG: CEA is performed prior CABG under the same anesthesia.

"Staged CEA- CABG": CEA is performed prior to CABG in different settings. Patient is initially schedule for CEA and then later for CABG,

"Reverse staged": Here CABG is initially performed and then CEA is scheduled at a later date or time.

A meta-analysis of 56 reports comparing these 3 surgical strategies showed higher rates of stroke in patients undergoing reverse staged procedures (10%) as compared to concomitant (6%) and staged procedures (5%) However, staged procedures had the highest rates of perioperative MI (11%[p=0.01]) and death (9%[p=0.02]) compared to concomitant(5% & 6%) and reverse staged procedures (3% and 4%).(Moore, Barnett et al. 1995) Another meta-analysis of 16 studies with over 800 concomitant and 920 staged procedures showed a increased risk of composite endpoint of stroke or death among patients undergoing combined procedure compared to staged procedures (9.5% v 5.7%; relative risk 1.49; 95% confidence interval 1.03-2.15; p = 0.034).(Borger, Fremes et al. 1999) Naylor et al performed a systematic review comparing outcomes following staged or concomitant procedures which included 94 studies with concomitant procedures and 24 studies with staged procedures.(Naylor, Cuffe et al. 2003) 60% of the patients in these studies were asymptomatic. Bilateral 50-99% ECAS or carotid occlusion was present in 30-37% of the patients. Thirty nine % of patient who underwent

http://dx.doi.org/10.5772/55669

concomitant were labeled as having "urgent" surgery, 72% of them were classified as having New York Heart Association grade 3 or 4 and 25% of patients had left main disease.(Naylor, Cuffe et al. 2003) It was noted that mortality was highest among the patients undergoing concomitant (4.6%, 95% CI 4.1-5.2) and death ± stroke rate was also higher compared to other staged procedure (8.7%, 95% CI 7.7-9.8). Reverse staged procedures had the highest risk of ipsilateral stroke (5.8%, 95% CI 0.0-14.3) and any stroke (6.3%, 95% CI 1.0-11.7) but with the lowest risk for peri-operative MI (0.9%, 95% CI 0.5-1.4). Staged procedures had the lowest rate of death ± stroke (6.1%, 95% CI 2.9-9.3) but the highest rate of peri-operative MI (6.5%, 95% CI 3.2-9.7). However, the benefit seen with staged procedures on reduction in stroke and death was no longer significant when peri-operative MI was also included in the combined outcomes. The risk of death/stroke/ MI was 11.5% (95% CI 10.1-12.9) following concomitant procedures versus 10.2% (95% CI 7.4-13.1) after staged procedures. Non of these studies had randomized patients to the different strategies and hence may have selection bias.

Carotid Artery Stenting: Randomized clinical trials have shown that carotid stenting is an effective method of revascularization equivalent to carotid endarterectomy.(Yadav, Wholey et al. 2004; Brott, Hobson et al. 2010) The protected carotid-artery stenting versus endarterectomy in high-risk patients (SAFFIRE) trial proved efficacy of carotid stenting. It consisted of patients at high surgical risk who were randomized to carotid stenting with embolic protection device or carotid endarterectomy. The study proved that carotid stenting was non-inferior to CEA (cumulative incidence, 20.1 percent; absolute difference, -7.9 percentage points; 95 percent confidence interval, -16.4 to 0.7 percentage points; P=0.004 for noninferiority, and P=0.053 for superiority). (Massop, Dave et al. 2009) Sixteen percent of patients in the SAFFIRE trial had severe CAD too. In the Stenting versus Endarterectomy for Treatment of Carotid-Artery Stenosis (CREST) trial, 2502 patients with indication for carotid revascularization were randomized to carotid stenting or CEA regardless of level of surgical risk. The CREST showed that CAS had similar adverse outcomes as CEA proving it to be equivalent to CEA for revascularization (7.2% and 6.8%, respectively; hazard ratio with stenting, 1.11; 95% confidence interval, 0.81 to 1.51; P=0.51).(Brott, Hobson et al. 2010).

Three different strategies can be utilized when carotid stenting is performed in patients undergoing CABG:

1. "Staged": CAS followed by CABG (CABG is done weeks later after CAS)

2. "Same day hybrid": CAS followed by CABG on the same day.

3. Concomitant ("true hybrid"): CAS followed by CABG on the same day in the same OR done immediately after CAS is completed.

In the staged method after carotid stenting, patients are treated with dual antiplatelet therapy with aspirin and clopidogrel for a few weeks (most commonly 4 weeks). Later, clopidogrel is held for 5-7 days prior to CABG. Patients undergoing hybrid procedures (true or same day) are placed on heparin between procedures and later on clopidogrel as soon as possible after CABG.

Mendiz et al reported 30 high surgical risk patients for CEA who underwent synchronous CAS then CABG and/or valve surgery. Among these patients, 1 patient had TIA and no patients suffered stroke or MI.(Mendiz, Fava et al. 2006) Versaci et al reported 101 patients who underwent CABG immediately after CAS. The 30-day composite incidence of disabling stroke, AMI or death was 4%: 2 patients had stroke after CAS. (Versaci, Reimers et al. 2009). Another series of 22 patients who underwent true hybrid procedure showed no deaths or MI and one case of contralateral stroke. There were no cases of major postoperative bleeding or stent thrombosis.(Palombo, Stella et al. 2009) Van der Heyden et al reported 356 patients with asymptomatic ECAS who underwent staged CAS - CABG with a mean interval of 22 days between the 2 procedures. The 30-day post-CABG stroke and death rate was 4.8%, MI was 2% and MI and death was 6.7%.(Van der Heyden, Suttorp et al. 2007) Naylor et al performed a meta-analysis of 11 studies involving 760 CAS plus CABG procedures.(Naylor, Mehta et al. 2009) Majority of the patients in this analysis were asymptomatic (87%) and majority had unilateral ECAS (82%). The study reported a mortality of 5.5% (95% confidence interval, CI: 3.4-7.6), ipsilateral stroke rate of 3.3% (95% CI: 1.6-5.1), all-cause stroke rate of 4.2% (95% CI: 2.4-6.1) and a MI rate of 1.8% (95% CI: 0.5-3.0) at 30-day follow-up. These results are comparable to systematic reviews of staged and concomitant carotid CEA-CABG, and suggest that staged CAS-CABG appears to as effective as staged CEA-CABG.

Decision regarding appropriate procedure and strategy for carotid revascularization in patients with undergoing CABG:

There are no randomized clinical trials comparing CAS and CEA in this patient group. Data from the Nationwide Inpatient Sample consisting of 27,084 patients who underwent carotid stenting before CABG or combined CEA - CABG surgery during the 5 years from 2000 to 2004 reported that 96.7% underwent CEA plus CABG surgery versus 3.3% who had carotid stenting plus CABG. Fewer perioperative strokes were reported among patients undergoing staged carotid stenting - CABG than among those undergoing staged CEA - CABG stroke (2.4% versus 3.9%). In this non-randomized data, patients undergoing staged CEA - CABG surgery faced a 62% greater risk of postoperative stroke than patients undergoing staged CAS-CABG surgery (OR 1.62, 95% CI 1.1 to 2.5; p<0.02).(Timaran, Rosero et al. 2008) There was no difference in the combined risk of stroke and death between the treatment (OR 1.26, 95% CI 0.9 to 1.6; p=NS).(Timaran, Rosero et al. 2008) Another study compared hybrid CAS - CABG procedures (n=56) to concomitant CEA-CABG procedure (n=111). In this study patients undergoing CAS at baseline were more likely to have unstable/severe angina (52% vs 27%, p = 0.002), severe left ventricular dysfunction (20% vs. 9%, p = 0.05), symptomatic carotid disease (46% vs. 23%, p = 0.002), and the need for repeat open heart surgery (32% vs. 9%, p = 0.0002). Severe contra-lateral carotid disease was more prevalent in the concomitant CEA+CABG group (28% vs. 11%, p = 0.01). On 30-day follow-up, CAS group had a significantly lower incidence of stroke or MI (5% vs. 19%, p = 0.02). (Ziada, Yadav et al. 2005) Another study involving 659 patients in whom CEA-CABG, CAS–CABG (staged) or CAS-CABG (hybrid) was performed in 28.1%, 57.4% and 13.5% of patients respectively showed a 30-day compo-

http://dx.doi.org/10.5772/55669

site endpoint of death, MI and stroke of 4.8%, 2.4% and 8.6% respectively (p=0.01). (Ribichini, Tomai et al. 2010)

Timing of carotid revascularization when indicated is chosen based on symptoms status of the carotid and coronary territory, severity of carotid and coronary disease and level of expertise available at the institution.(Venkatachalam and Shishehbor 2011)

Symptomatic carotid artery disease with ECAS >50-99% stenosis:

1. Symptomatic carotid disease and asymptomatic coronary disease or stable angina: In these patients carotid revascularization should be pursued prior to CABG, staged carotid stenting then followed by 4 weeks of dual antiplatelet and then CABG or staged CEA - CABG or concomitant CEA-CABD is usually considered. Selection of patients for carotid stenting or CEA is based co-morbidities, anatomy and local expertise available.

2. Symptomatic carotid disease and symptomatic coronary disease (acute coronary syndromes): In these patients carotid disease should be revascularized initially or concomitantly. Concomitant CEA-CABG or "same day" or "true hybrid" stenting procedures are usually considered. In case need for emergent CABG's, reverse stages CABG-CEA procedures can be considered.

Asymptomatic carotid stenosis (ECAS> 80-99%) is further classified as high risk or low risk groups. High risk group consists of patients with bilateral ECAS > 80-99% or unilateral ECAS >80-99% with contralateral occlusion and asymptomatic ECAS 80-99% with impaired cerebral perfusion reserve. Patients without these features are considered low risk.

1. Asymptomatic ECAS with high risk features and symptomatic coronary disease (acute coronary syndromes): These patients are at high risk for myocardial infarction as well as stroke and hence should be considered for concomitant CEA-CABG or "same day" or "true hybrid" CAS-CABG.

2. Asymptomatic ECAS with high risk features with stable angina: These patients should be considered for staged CAS-CABG.

3. Asymptomatic ECAS with low risk features and stable angina or acute coronary syndromes: These patents should initially undergo coronary revascularization with carotid revascularization (stenting or CEA) at a later date on an elective basis.

5. Conclusion

To date, stroke remains one of the most devastating complications after open heart surgery with serious adverse economic, psychological and clinical implications on healthcare and individuals suffering from it.(Roach, Kanchuger et al. 1996; Hogue, Murphy et al. 1999) Identifying patients at risk of stroke after CABG and applying measures to reduce its occurrence are extremely vital.

Author details

Aditya M. Sharma[1] and Herbert D. Aronow[2]

1 University of Virginia, Charlottesville, VA, USA

2 St. Joseph Mercy Hospital, Ann Arbor MI, USA

References

[1] (1991). "Beneficial effect of carotid endarterectomy in symptomatic patients with high-grade carotid stenosis. North American Symptomatic Carotid Endarterectomy Trial Collaborators." *N Engl J Med* 325(7): 445-453.

[2] (1991). "MRC European Carotid Surgery Trial: interim results for symptomatic patients with severe (70-99%) or with mild (0-29%) carotid stenosis. European Carotid Surgery Trialists' Collaborative Group." *Lancet* 337(8752): 1235-1243.

[3] (1995). "Endarterectomy for asymptomatic carotid artery stenosis. Executive Committee for the Asymptomatic Carotid Atherosclerosis Study." *JAMA* 273(18): 1421-1428.

[4] (1996). "Endarterectomy for moderate symptomatic carotid stenosis: interim results from the MRC European Carotid Surgery Trial." *Lancet* 347(9015): 1591-1593.

[5] (1998). "Randomised trial of endarterectomy for recently symptomatic carotid stenosis: final results of the MRC European Carotid Surgery Trial (ECST)." *Lancet* 351(9113): 1379-1387.

[6] (2002). "Collaborative meta-analysis of randomised trials of antiplatelet therapy for prevention of death, myocardial infarction, and stroke in high risk patients." *BMJ* 324(7329): 71-86.

[7] (2008). "Screening for carotid artery stenosis: recommendation statement." *Am Fam Physician* 77(7): 1006-1010.

[8] Amarenco, P., J. Bogousslavsky, et al. (2006). "High-dose atorvastatin after stroke or transient ischemic attack." *N Engl J Med* 355(6): 549-559.

[9] Amarenco, P., J. Labreuche, et al. (2004). "Statins in stroke prevention and carotid atherosclerosis: systematic review and up-to-date meta-analysis." *Stroke* 35(12): 2902-2909.

[10] Anastasiadis, K., T. D. Karamitsos, et al. (2009). "Preoperative screening and management of carotid artery disease in patients undergoing cardiac surgery." *Perfusion* 24(4): 257-262.

[11] Barnett, H. J., D. W. Taylor, et al. (1998). "Benefit of carotid endarterectomy in patients with symptomatic moderate or severe stenosis. North American Symptomatic Carotid Endarterectomy Trial Collaborators." *N Engl J Med* 339(20): 1415-1425.

[12] Bates, E. R., J. D. Babb, et al. (2007). "ACCF/SCAI/SVMB/SIR/ASITN 2007 clinical expert consensus document on carotid stenting: a report of the American College of Cardiology Foundation Task Force on Clinical Expert Consensus Documents (ACCF/SCAI/SVMB/SIR/ASITN Clinical Expert Consensus Document Committee on Carotid Stenting)." *J Am Coll Cardiol* 49(1): 126-170.

[13] Beique, F., M. Ali, et al. (2006). "Canadian guidelines for training in adult perioperative transesophageal echocardiography. Recommendations of the Cardiovascular Section of the Canadian Anesthesiologists' Society and the Canadian Society of Echocardiography." *Can J Cardiol* 22(12): 1015-1027.

[14] Bhatt, D. L., K. A. Fox, et al. (2006). "Clopidogrel and aspirin versus aspirin alone for the prevention of atherothrombotic events." *N Engl J Med* 354(16): 1706-1717.

[15] Borger, M. A., S. E. Fremes, et al. (1999). "Coronary bypass and carotid endarterectomy: does a combined approach increase risk? A metaanalysis." *Ann Thorac Surg* 68(1): 14-20; discussion 21.

[16] Brott, T. G., J. L. Halperin, et al. (2011). "2011 ASA/ACCF/AHA/AANN/AANS/ACR/ASNR/CNS/SAIP/SCAI/SIR/SNIS/SVM/SVS guideline on the management of patients with extracranial carotid and vertebral artery disease. A report of the American College of Cardiology Foundation/American Heart Association Task Force on Practice Guidelines, and the American Stroke Association, American Association of Neuroscience Nurses, American Association of Neurological Surgeons, American College of Radiology, American Society of Neuroradiology, Congress of Neurological Surgeons, Society of Atherosclerosis Imaging and Prevention, Society for Cardiovascular Angiography and Interventions, Society of Interventional Radiology, Society of NeuroInterventional Surgery, Society for Vascular Medicine, and Society for Vascular Surgery." *Circulation* 124(4): e54-130.

[17] Brott, T. G., J. L. Halperin, et al. (2011). "2011 ASA/ACCF/AHA/AANN/AANS/ACR/ASNR/CNS/SAIP/SCAI/SIR/SNIS/SVM/SVS guideline on the management of patients with extracranial carotid and vertebral artery disease: executive summary. A report of the American College of Cardiology Foundation/American Heart Association Task Force on Practice Guidelines, and the American Stroke Association, American Association of Neuroscience Nurses, American Association of Neurological Surgeons, American College of Radiology, American Society of Neuroradiology, Congress of Neurological Surgeons, Society of Atherosclerosis Imaging and Prevention, Society for Cardiovascular Angiography and Interventions, Society of Interventional Radiology, Society of NeuroInterventional Surgery, Society for Vascular Medicine, and Society for Vascular Surgery." *Circulation* 124(4): 489-532.

[18] Brott, T. G., J. L. Halperin, et al. (2011). "2011 ASA/ACCF/AHA/AANN/AANS/ACR/ASNR/CNS/SAIP/SCAI/SIR/SNIS/SVM/SVS guideline on the management of pa-

tients with extracranial carotid and vertebral artery disease: executive summary. A report of the American College of Cardiology Foundation/American Heart Association Task Force on Practice Guidelines, and the American Stroke Association, American Association of Neuroscience Nurses, American Association of Neurological Surgeons, American College of Radiology, American Society of Neuroradiology, Congress of Neurological Surgeons, Society of Atherosclerosis Imaging and Prevention, Society for Cardiovascular Angiography and Interventions, Society of Interventional Radiology, Society of NeuroInterventional Surgery, Society for Vascular Medicine, and Society for Vascular Surgery." *Circulation* 124(4): 489-532.

[19] Brott, T. G., R. W. Hobson, 2nd, et al. (2010). "Stenting versus endarterectomy for treatment of carotid-artery stenosis." *N Engl J Med* 363(1): 11-23.

[20] Brown, P. P., A. D. Kugelmass, et al. (2008). "The frequency and cost of complications associated with coronary artery bypass grafting surgery: results from the United States Medicare program." *Ann Thorac Surg* 85(6): 1980-1986.

[21] Chobanian, A. V., G. L. Bakris, et al. (2003). "The Seventh Report of the Joint National Committee on Prevention, Detection, Evaluation, and Treatment of High Blood Pressure: the JNC 7 report." *JAMA* 289(19): 2560-2572.

[22] Colhoun, H. M., D. J. Betteridge, et al. (2004). "Primary prevention of cardiovascular disease with atorvastatin in type 2 diabetes in the Collaborative Atorvastatin Diabetes Study (CARDS): multicentre randomised placebo-controlled trial." *Lancet* 364(9435): 685-696.

[23] Diener, H. C., J. Bogousslavsky, et al. (2004). "Aspirin and clopidogrel compared with clopidogrel alone after recent ischaemic stroke or transient ischaemic attack in high-risk patients (MATCH): randomised, double-blind, placebo-controlled trial." *Lancet* 364(9431): 331-337.

[24] Diener, H. C., L. Cunha, et al. (1996). "European Stroke Prevention Study. 2. Dipyridamole and acetylsalicylic acid in the secondary prevention of stroke." *J Neurol Sci* 143(1-2): 1-13.

[25] Eagle, K. A., R. A. Guyton, et al. (1999). "ACC/AHA guidelines for coronary artery bypass graft surgery: executive summary and recommendations : A report of the American College of Cardiology/American Heart Association Task Force on Practice Guidelines (Committee to revise the 1991 guidelines for coronary artery bypass graft surgery)." *Circulation* 100(13): 1464-1480.

[26] FDA. (2011). "http://www.fda.gov/NewsEvents/Newsroom/PressAnnouncements/ucm254430.htm."

[27] Furlan, A. J., C. A. Sila, et al. (1992). "Neurologic complications related to cardiac surgery." *Neurol Clin* 10(1): 145-166.

[28] Gerstein, H. C., M. E. Miller, et al. (2008). "Effects of intensive glucose lowering in type 2 diabetes." *N Engl J Med* 358(24): 2545-2559.

[29] Go, A. S., D. Mozaffarian, et al. (2012). "Heart Disease and Stroke Statistics--2013 Update A Report From the American Heart Association." *Circulation*.

[30] Goldstein, L. B., R. Adams, et al. (2006). "Primary prevention of ischemic stroke: a guideline from the American Heart Association/American Stroke Association Stroke Council: cosponsored by the Atherosclerotic Peripheral Vascular Disease Interdisciplinary Working Group; Cardiovascular Nursing Council; Clinical Cardiology Council; Nutrition, Physical Activity, and Metabolism Council; and the Quality of Care and Outcomes Research Interdisciplinary Working Group: the American Academy of Neurology affirms the value of this guideline." *Stroke* 37(6): 1583-1633.

[31] Gupta, A., J. L. Chazen, et al. (2012). "Cerebrovascular reserve and stroke risk in patients with carotid stenosis or occlusion: a systematic review and meta-analysis." *Stroke* 43(11): 2884-2891.

[32] Halliday, A., M. Harrison, et al. (2010). "10-year stroke prevention after successful carotid endarterectomy for asymptomatic stenosis (ACST-1): a multicentre randomised trial." *Lancet* 376(9746): 1074-1084.

[33] Halliday, A., A. Mansfield, et al. (2004). "Prevention of disabling and fatal strokes by successful carotid endarterectomy in patients without recent neurological symptoms: randomised controlled trial." *Lancet* 363(9420): 1491-1502.

[34] Hillis, L. D., P. K. Smith, et al. (2011). "2011 ACCF/AHA Guideline for Coronary Artery Bypass Graft Surgery: executive summary: a report of the American College of Cardiology Foundation/American Heart Association Task Force on Practice Guidelines." *Circulation* 124(23): 2610-2642.

[35] Hogue, C. W., Jr., S. F. Murphy, et al. (1999). "Risk factors for early or delayed stroke after cardiac surgery." *Circulation* 100(6): 642-647.

[36] Howard, G., L. E. Wagenknecht, et al. (1998). "Cigarette smoking and other risk factors for silent cerebral infarction in the general population." *Stroke* 29(5): 913-917.

[37] Iso, H., D. R. Jacobs, Jr., et al. (1989). "Serum cholesterol levels and six-year mortality from stroke in 350,977 men screened for the multiple risk factor intervention trial." *N Engl J Med* 320(14): 904-910.

[38] Kallikazaros, I., C. Tsioufis, et al. (1999). "Carotid artery disease as a marker for the presence of severe coronary artery disease in patients evaluated for chest pain." *Stroke* 30(5): 1002-1007.

[39] Kurth, T., B. M. Everett, et al. (2007). "Lipid levels and the risk of ischemic stroke in women." *Neurology* 68(8): 556-562.

[40] Lawes, C. M., D. A. Bennett, et al. (2004). "Blood pressure and stroke: an overview of published reviews." *Stroke* 35(4): 1024.

[41] Manninen, H., K. Makinen, et al. (2009). "How often does an incomplete circle of Willis predispose to cerebral ischemia during closure of carotid artery? Postmortem and clinical imaging studies." *Acta Neurochir (Wien)* 151(9): 1099-1105.

[42] Massop, D., R. Dave, et al. (2009). "Stenting and angioplasty with protection in patients at high-risk for endarterectomy: SAPPHIRE Worldwide Registry first 2,001 patients." *Catheter Cardiovasc Interv* 73(2): 129-136.

[43] Mendiz, O., C. Fava, et al. (2006). "Synchronous carotid stenting and cardiac surgery: an initial single-center experience." *Catheter Cardiovasc Interv* 68(3): 424-428.

[44] Mitchell E, M. G., Zwiebel W, Pellerito J (2004). *Introduction to Vascular Ultrasonography*. Philadelphia, Elsevier.

[45] Mohr, J. P., J. L. Thompson, et al. (2001). "A comparison of warfarin and aspirin for the prevention of recurrent ischemic stroke." *N Engl J Med* 345(20): 1444-1451.

[46] Moore, W. S., H. J. Barnett, et al. (1995). "Guidelines for carotid endarterectomy. A multidisciplinary consensus statement from the ad hoc Committee, American Heart Association." *Stroke* 26(1): 188-201.

[47] Naylor, A. R., R. L. Cuffe, et al. (2003). "A systematic review of outcomes following staged and synchronous carotid endarterectomy and coronary artery bypass." *Eur J Vasc Endovasc Surg* 25(5): 380-389.

[48] Naylor, A. R., Z. Mehta, et al. (2009). "A systematic review and meta-analysis of 30-day outcomes following staged carotid artery stenting and coronary bypass." *Eur J Vasc Endovasc Surg* 37(4): 379-387.

[49] Naylor, A. R., Z. Mehta, et al. (2002). "Carotid artery disease and stroke during coronary artery bypass: a critical review of the literature." *Eur J Vasc Endovasc Surg* 23(4): 283-294.

[50] Palombo, G., N. Stella, et al. (2009). "Safety and effectiveness of combining carotid artery stenting with cardiac surgery: preliminary results of a single-center experience." *J Cardiovasc Surg (Torino)* 50(1): 49-54.

[51] Patel, A., S. MacMahon, et al. (2008). "Intensive blood glucose control and vascular outcomes in patients with type 2 diabetes." *N Engl J Med* 358(24): 2560-2572.

[52] Qureshi, A. I., A. V. Alexandrov, et al. (2007). "Guidelines for screening of extracranial carotid artery disease: a statement for healthcare professionals from the multidisciplinary practice guidelines committee of the American Society of Neuroimaging; cosponsored by the Society of Vascular and Interventional Neurology." *J Neuroimaging* 17(1): 19-47.

[53] Qureshi, A. I., A. V. Alexandrov, et al. (2007). "Guidelines for screening of extracranial carotid artery disease: a statement for healthcare professionals from the multidisci-

plinary practice guidelines committee of the American Society of Neuroimaging; cosponsored by the Society of Vascular and Interventional Neurology." *J Neuroimaging* 17(1): 19-47.

[54] Ribichini, F., F. Tomai, et al. (2010). "Clinical outcome after endovascular, surgical or hybrid revascularisation in patients with combined carotid and coronary artery disease: the Finalised Research In ENDovascular Strategies Study Group (FRIENDS)." *EuroIntervention* 6(3): 328-335.

[55] Roach, G. W., M. Kanchuger, et al. (1996). "Adverse cerebral outcomes after coronary bypass surgery. Multicenter Study of Perioperative Ischemia Research Group and the Ischemia Research and Education Foundation Investigators." *N Engl J Med* 335(25): 1857-1863.

[56] Rooke, T. W., A. T. Hirsch, et al. (2012). "2011 ACCF/AHA focused update of the guideline for the management of patients with peripheral artery disease (updating the 2005 guideline): a report of the American College of Cardiology Foundation/American Heart Association Task Force on Practice Guidelines: developed in collaboration with the Society for Cardiovascular Angiography and Interventions, Society of Interventional Radiology, Society for Vascular Medicine, and Society for Vascular Surgery." *Catheter Cardiovasc Interv* 79(4): 501-531.

[57] Sacco, R. L., H. C. Diener, et al. (2008). "Aspirin and extended-release dipyridamole versus clopidogrel for recurrent stroke." *N Engl J Med* 359(12): 1238-1251.

[58] Salasidis, G. C., D. A. Latter, et al. (1995). "Carotid artery duplex scanning in preoperative assessment for coronary artery revascularization: the association between peripheral vascular disease, carotid artery stenosis, and stroke." *J Vasc Surg* 21(1): 154-160; discussion 161-152.

[59] Schwartz, L. B., A. H. Bridgman, et al. (1995). "Asymptomatic carotid artery stenosis and stroke in patients undergoing cardiopulmonary bypass." *J Vasc Surg* 21(1): 146-153.

[60] Shahar, E., L. E. Chambless, et al. (2003). "Plasma lipid profile and incident ischemic stroke: the Atherosclerosis Risk in Communities (ARIC) study." *Stroke* 34(3): 623-631.

[61] Shirani, S., M. A. Boroumand, et al. (2006). "Preoperative carotid artery screening in patients undergoing coronary artery bypass graft surgery." *Arch Med Res* 37(8): 987-990.

[62] Tarakji, K. G., J. F. Sabik, 3rd, et al. (2011). "Temporal onset, risk factors, and outcomes associated with stroke after coronary artery bypass grafting." *JAMA* 305(4): 381-390.

[63] Tell, G. S., G. H. Rutan, et al. (1994). "Correlates of blood pressure in community-dwelling older adults. The Cardiovascular Health Study. Cardiovascular Health Study (CHS) Collaborative Research Group." *Hypertension* 23(1): 59-67.

[64] Timaran, C. H., E. B. Rosero, et al. (2008). "Trends and outcomes of concurrent carotid revascularization and coronary bypass." *J Vasc Surg* 48(2): 355-360; discussion 360-351.

[65] Van der Heyden, J., M. J. Suttorp, et al. (2007). "Staged carotid angioplasty and stenting followed by cardiac surgery in patients with severe asymptomatic carotid artery stenosis: early and long-term results." *Circulation* 116(18): 2036-2042.

[66] van der Meer, I. M., A. Iglesias del Sol, et al. (2003). "Risk factors for progression of atherosclerosis measured at multiple sites in the arterial tree: the Rotterdam Study." *Stroke* 34(10): 2374-2379.

[67] Venkatachalam, S. and M. H. Shishehbor (2011). "Management of carotid disease in patients undergoing coronary artery bypass surgery: is it time to change our approach?" *Curr Opin Cardiol* 26(6): 480-487.

[68] Versaci, F., B. Reimers, et al. (2009). "Simultaneous hybrid revascularization by carotid stenting and coronary artery bypass grafting: the SHARP study." *JACC Cardiovasc Interv* 2(5): 393-401.

[69] Wilson, P. W., J. M. Hoeg, et al. (1997). "Cumulative effects of high cholesterol levels, high blood pressure, and cigarette smoking on carotid stenosis." *N Engl J Med* 337(8): 516-522.

[70] Yadav, J. S., M. H. Wholey, et al. (2004). "Protected carotid-artery stenting versus endarterectomy in high-risk patients." *N Engl J Med* 351(15): 1493-1501.

[71] Ziada, K. M., J. S. Yadav, et al. (2005). "Comparison of results of carotid stenting followed by open heart surgery versus combined carotid endarterectomy and open heart surgery (coronary bypass with or without another procedure)." *Am J Cardiol* 96(4): 519-523.

Chapter 22

Infected Aneurysm and Inflammatory Aorta: Diagnosis and Management

Takao Kato

Additional information is available at the end of the chapter

http://dx.doi.org/10.5772/54415

1. Introduction

Due to the increase of aged patients with atherosclerosis, more attention should be paid to the endothelial damage of great vessels. The damaged endothelium is more susceptible to bacterial infections. The reports or papers of infected aneurysms (mycotic aneurysms) are increasing in Pubmed search (Figure 1), which is consistent with personal experience in daily practice. The reasons for the increase were due to several causes: 1) the increase of aged patients with more risk of atherosclerosis than before, 2) an improvement of CT imaging and MR imaging, 3) more awareness of the disease. We focused the diagnosis and managements of infected aneurysms, and the diseases needed to differentiate from infected aneurysms, such as collagen vascular diseases and periaortitis.

1.1. Diagnosis of infected aneurysms

Risk factors for infected aneurysm include: 1) Endothelial damage caused by atherosclerosis including pre-existing aneurysm [1], 2) Antecedent infection including bacteremia, 3) Arterial injury including iatrogenic mechanisms, such as percutaneous coronary intervention [2]. When the intima is diseased, bacteria can pass through it into deep layers of the aorta and can establish infection. Infective endocarditis (IE) remains to be main cause of infected aneurysm [3], because the risk factors of IE are very similar to those of infected aneurysms, and bacteremia and septic emboli from heart are often common features of IE.

Staphylococcus species (spp) and Salmonella spp are two major bacteria causing infected aneurysm, 28 to 71 percent and 15 to 24 percent of causes, respectively [4,5]. Streptococcus pneumoniae may be the third major, re-emerging, cause of infected aneurysms [6]. The pathology of the diseased site includes acute or chronic inflammation with bacterial

infection, abscesses, and necrosis. The suprarenal abdominal aorta is most commonly involved site.

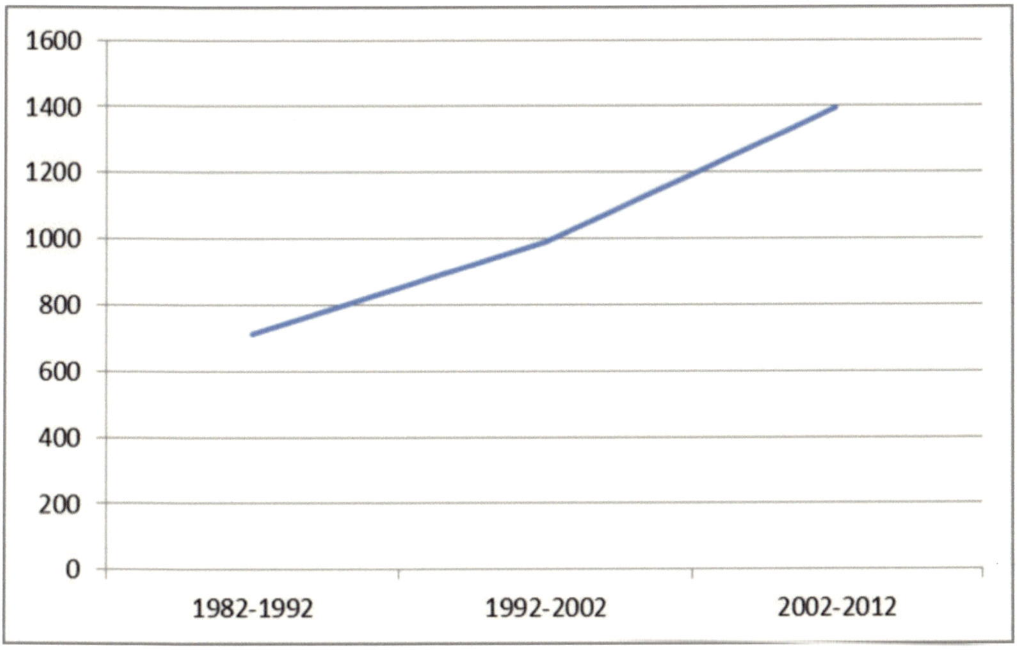

Figure 1. Results of Pubmed search using mycotic aneurysm or infected aneurysm.

Symptoms of an infected aneurysm vary according the lesion diseased. For example, abdominal pain and diarrhea is observed if abdominal aorta is involved, painful pulsatile mass if superficial artery is involved, and chest pain if thoracic aorta is involved. An infected aneurysm involving deep arteries or aorta may cause only fever. It might be followed as fever of unknown origin, and could be diagnosed as an infected aneurysm only after CT imaging is acquired. If the patients were with bacteremia or a persistent high fever and their etiology was not determined, the contrast-enhanced CT imaging would be the choice for searching the diseased lesion, and an asymptomatic infected aneurysm would be one of differential diagnoses.

The next step of diagnosing an infected aneurysm is based on blood cultures and imaging. In all suspicious patients, blood cultures should be examined. About 50-85% of patients may be positive [5,7]. If negative, however, the infected aneurysm cannot be ruled out. Contrast-enhanced CT imaging identified the infected aneurysm. Findings on CT angiography of an infected aneurysm include a disruption of aortic wall calcification, soft tissue inflammation or mass around a vessel, and periaortic fluid or air collection [8,9]. These findings can differentiate from other inflammatory aortic disease. The wall of inflammatory aorta is thickened and periaortic fibrosis sometimes observed in adhesion to surrounding organs. MR imaging is another strong tools. The T2-weighted images or mixed T1/T2-weighted STIR images are

http://dx.doi.org/10.5772/54415

able to visualize the edematous lesion. The diffusion images can detect fluid collection, and gadolinium enhancement indicates the increase of inflammatory connective tissue.

In summary, the important things for the diagnosis of an infected aneurysm are the high suspicion of this disease and obtaining blood cultures and enhanced CT or MR imaging.

1.2. Management of infected aneurysms

Surgical replacement or debridement is the treatment of choice combined with antibiotic therapy [4]. The main aims of surgical procedures are removal of infected tissue and re-vascularization if distal perfusion is limited. Mortality rate without surgery was 85 percent with infected thoracic aneurysm and 96 percent with infected aortic aneurysm [10,11]. Figure 2 shows a gradually enlarged infective aneurysm treated on medication alone despite the control of bacteremia [12]. Among patients who underwent surgery, mortality rates were the highest for patients with infected arch aneurysms (50 %) compared with supra-renal aortic aneurysms (43%), distal descending thoracic aneurysms (33 %), proximal descending thoracic aneurysms (16 %), or infra-renal aortic aneurysms (4 %) [10,13]. Endovascular stenting is reported to be effective in some systematic reviews with low mortality [14,15]. Because the infected focus is not removed by endovascular stenting, the procedures may be palliative, and more persistent or recurrent infections are likely to occur compared to surgical procedures. However, endovascular procedures could be a secondary choice for patients who refuse surgery, those with a very high risk for surgery, and those with a ruptured infected aneurysm.

The initial choice of antibiotic therapy should be based on the culture and susceptibility results. Until the results become available, the combination treatment with vancomycin and a ceftriaxone, a fluoroquinolone, or piperacillin-tazobactam is preferable targeting gram-negative Salmonella and enteric bacteria. The optimal duration of antibiotic therapy is uncertain because of the lack of randomized clinical trials. In general, four to six weeks of parenteral antimicrobial therapy is performed for the treatment of infected aneurysm followed by principles of vascular graft infection or infective endocarditis of prosthesis valve. A longer duration of treatment or additional oral antibiotics may be warranted in the clinical course of persist elevation of C-reactive proteins or recurrence of fever when drug-related fever is excluded.

In summary, the surgical replacement in combination with antibiotics is the treatment of choice, and endovascular procedures may be palliative. The management is followed by principles of vascular graft infection or infective endocarditis of prosthesis valve.

2. Inflammation of aorta: "Aortits"

Large vessel vasculitits such as Takayasu's arteritis and giant cell arteritis, rheumatic and HLA-B27–associated spondyloarthropathies, Behçet's syndrome, and infections such as syphilis, tuberculosis may be the cause of inflammation of aorta, and we must differ-

entiate these from infected aneurysms when blood culture is negative or infected focus remains unclear. Another disease which we must differentiate is IgG4-related diseases (chronic periaortits).

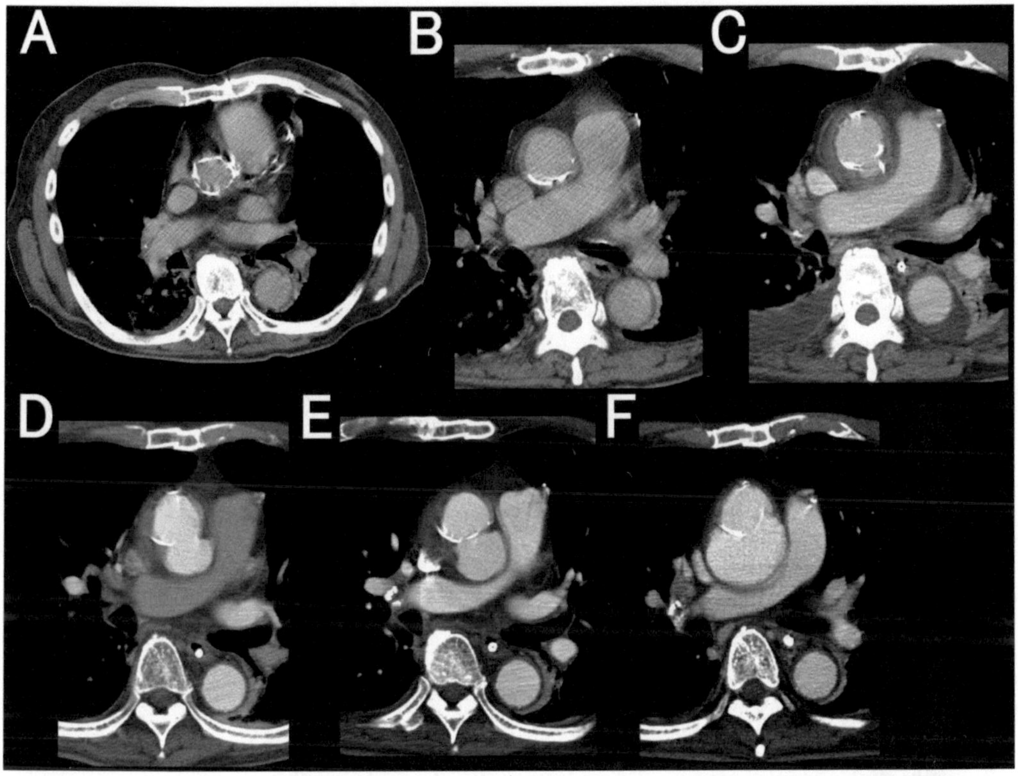

Figure 2. A case of medical treatment of an infected aneurysm. A 75-year-old man with familial hypercholesterolemia, cerebral infarction, and coronary bypass grafting presented with high fever and chest pain. Panel A and B showed a severely calcified ascending aorta. The repeated CE-CT on the 5th day revealed aneurysmal change with protrusion (Panel C), indicating an infected aneurysm. Due to a prohibitive risk of surgery, medical treatment was the choice of him and his family, but the infected aneurysm gradually enlarged despite the control of bacteremia with antibiotics (13th day: Panel D, 24th day: Panel E, and 58th day; Panel F), and he died 2 months after onset.

A detailed history and a careful physical examination are important for the diagnosis and assessment of the extent of vascular lesions. The mean age at onset of Takayasu's arteritis and giant cell arteritis was between 17 and 26 years of age and with 69 years, respectively, primarily in women (about 80 %) [16]. Systemic symptoms are common such as fatigue, weight loss, and low-grade fever are common in these disorders, along with local symptoms, for example, arthralgia, skin lesion (erythema nodosum), and abdominal pains. HLA-B27–associated spondyloarthropathies accompanies with ankylosing spondylitis, reactive arthritis, or inflammatory bowel disease with negative rheumatic factors. Skin and mucosa, ocular system, GI manifestations include abdominal pain, nausea, and diarrhea with or without blood, and/or musculoskeletal and neurological system are involved in Behçet's

http://dx.doi.org/10.5772/54415

syndrome. Allergic features such as atopy, asthma, and modest peripheral eosinophilia, along with tumorous swelling in many organs and elevated serum IgG4 levels above the upper limit of normal(>135 mg/dL) are the characteristics of IgG-4 related diseases [17].

3. Takayasu's arteritis, giant cell arteritis

Takayasu's arteritis, also called pulseless disease, involves the ascending aorta and aortic arch, and carotid and subclavian arteries, causing dilations and obstruction at the stage of healing and recurrences. CT angiography revealed the diseased lesion, thickened arterial wall in acute phase and aneurysmal or stenotic lesion in chronic phase [18]. The ultrasonography and MR angiography are also useful. In acute phase, the high signal of T2-weighted and/or STIR MR images and the increased uptake of ^{18}Fluorodeoxy-glucose indicate the presence of active inflammation [19]. The mainstay of therapy for Takayasu's arteritis is glucocorticoids. Giant cell arteritis (GCA) is a chronic vasculitis of large and medium sized vessels. The following classification criteria were as follows: 1) Age older than 50 years at onset, 2) Localized headache de novo, 3) Tenderness or decreased pulse of the temporal artery, 4) Erythrocyte sedimentation rate (ESR) greater than 50 mm/h, 5) Biopsy-proven necrotizing arteritis with multinucleated giant cells [20].

4. IgG4-related diseases: Chronic periaortits

IgG4 -related disease is a newly recognized syndrome of unknown etiology characterized by fibroinflammatory condition, in which tumefactive lesions, a dense lymphoplasmacytic infiltrate rich in IgG4-positive plasma cells. Various symptoms are observed according to the lesions involved, although patients feel well at the time of diagnosis without fever. Seventy percent of patients have elevated serum IgG4 concentrations [17]. CT imaging features of arterial lesions are characterized by homogeneous wall thickening and enhancement in the late phases after contrast infusion accompanying the increase of connective tissue indicating sclerosing inflammation [21]. This indicates chronic periaortitis, which resembles the infected aneurysm with periaortic abscess (Figure 3). Therefore, the diseases should be differentiated from infected aneurysm by not only the imaging features but also clinical symptoms or negative blood cultures. Glucocorticoids typically the first line of therapy.

5. Conclusions

Due to the increase of aged patients with atherosclerosis, more attention should be paid to the endothelial damage of great vessels and an infected aneurysm should be properly diagnosed and carefully managed.

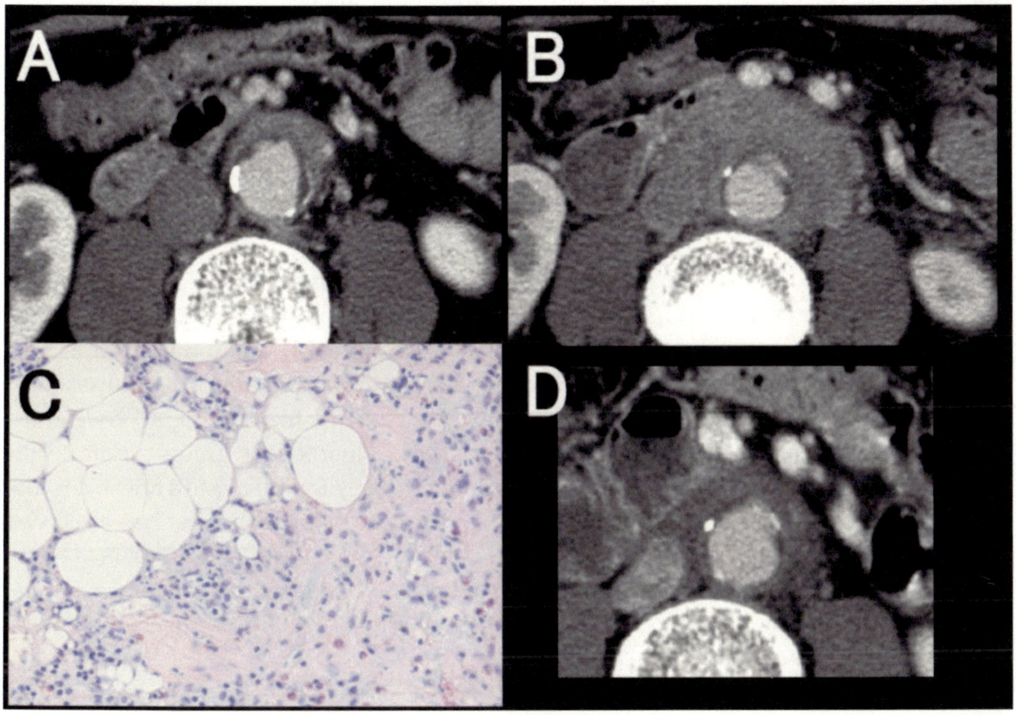

Figure 3. A case of chronic periaortitis with retroperitoneal fibrosis. A 75-year-old man presented with vague discomfort of lower abdomen. Panel A was at presentation. Two months later the symptoms remained unchanged with 8.5mg/dL of C-reactive protein but without fever. Repeated CT was performed (Panel B). Biopsy of the tissue revealed the infiltration of inflammatory cells and no bacteria (Panel C). Panel D was three weeks after the glucocorticoid therapy.

Disclosures

None.

Author details

Takao Kato*

Address all correspondence to: takao-kato@kitano-hp.or.jp

Cardiovascular Center, The Tazuke Kofukai Medical Research Institute, Kitano Hospital, Osaka, Japan

http://dx.doi.org/10.5772/54415

References

[1] Ernst CB, Campbell HC Jr, Daugherty ME, Sachatello CR, Griffen WO Jr. Incidence and significance of intra-operative bacterial cultures during abdominal aortic aneurysmectomy. Ann Surg 1977; 185: 626-33.

[2] Samore MH, Wessolossky MA, Lewis SM, Shubrooks SJ Jr, Karchmer AW. Frequency, risk factors, and outcome for bacteremia after percutaneous transluminal coronary angioplasty. Am J Cardiol 1997; 79:873-7.

[3] Johansen K, Devin J. Mycotic aortic aneurysms. A reappraisal. Arch Surg 1983; 118:583-8.

[4] Moneta GL, Taylor LM Jr, Yeager RA, Edwards JM, Nicoloff AD, McConnell DB, Porter JM. Surgical treatment of infected aortic aneurysm. Am J Surg 1998; 175:396-9.

[5] Johnson JR, Ledgerwood AM, Lucas CE. Mycotic aneurysm. New concepts in therapy. Arch Surg 1983; 118:577-82.

[6] Brouwer RE, van Bockel JH, van Dissel JT. Streptococcus pneumoniae, an emerging pathogen in mycotic aneurysms? Neth J Med 1998; 52:16-21.

[7] Maeda H, Umezawa H, Goshima M, Hattori T, Nakamura T, Umeda T, Shiono M. Primary infected abdominal aortic aneurysm: surgical procedures, early mortality rates, and a survey of the prevalence of infectious organisms over a 30-year period. Surg Today 2011; 41:346-51.

[8] Gomes MN, Choyke PL. Infected aortic aneurysms: CT diagnosis. J Cardiovasc Surg (Torino) 1992; 33:684-9.

[9] Lee WK, Mossop PJ, Little AF, Fitt GJ, Vrazas JI, Hoang JK, Hennessy OF. Infected (mycotic) aneurysms: spectrum of imaging appearances and management. Radiographics 2008; 28:1853-68.

[10] Weis-Müller BT, Rascanu C, Sagban A, Grabitz K, Godehardt E, Sandmann W. Single-center experience with open surgical treatment of 36 infected aneurysms of the thoracic, thoracoabdominal, and abdominal aorta. Ann Vasc Surg 2011; 25:1020-5.

[11] Taylor CF, Lennox AF. Treatment options for primary infected aorta. Ann Vasc Surg 2007; 21:225-7.

[12] Kato T, Kimura M, Inoko M, Nohara R. Infected aneurysm in an atherosclerotic lesion. Intern Med. 2012; 51:983.

[13] Lee CH, Hsieh HC, Ko PJ, Li HJ, Kao TC, Yu SY. In situ versus extra-anatomic reconstruction for primary infected infrarenal abdominal aortic aneurysms. J Vasc Surg 2011; 54:64-70.

[14] Kan CD, Lee HL, Yang YJ. Outcome after endovascular stent graft treatment for mycotic aortic aneurysm: a systematic review. J Vasc Surg 2007; 46:906-12.

[15] Kpodonu J, Williams JP, Ramaiah VG, Diethrich EB. Endovascular management of a descending thoracic mycotic aneurysm: mid-term follow-up. Eur J Cardiothorac Surg 2007; 32:178-9.

[16] Hunder GG, Arend WP, Bloch DA, Calabrese LH, Fauci AS, Fries JF, Leavitt RY, Lie JT, Lightfoot RW Jr, Masi AT, McShane DJ, Michel BA, Mills JA, Stevens MB, Wallace SL, Zvaifler NJ. The American College of Rheumatology 1990 criteria for the classification of vasculitis. Introduction. Arthritis Rheum 1990; 33:1065-7.

[17] Stone JH, Zen Y, Deshpande V. IgG4-related disease.N Engl J Med. 2012; 366:539-51.

[18] Yamada I, Nakagawa T, Himeno Y, Numano F, Shibuya H. Takayasu arteritis: evaluation of the thoracic aorta with CT angiography. Radiology 1998; 209:103-9.

[19] Kissin EY, Merkel PA. Diagnostic imaging in Takayasu arteritis. Curr Opin Rheumatol 2004; 16:31-7.

[20] Hunder GG, Bloch DA, Michel BA, Stevens MB, Arend WP, Calabrese LH, Edworthy SM, Fauci AS, Leavitt RY, Lie JT, et al. The American College of Rheumatology 1990 criteria for the classification of giant cell arteritis. Arthritis Rheum 1990; 33:1122-8.

[21] Inoue D, Zen Y, Abo H, Gabata T, Demachi H, Yoshikawa J, Miyayama S, Nakanuma Y, Matsui O. Immunoglobulin G4-related periaortitis and periarteritis: CT findings in 17 patients. Radiology 2011;251:625-33.

Chapter 23

Endovascular Treatment of Ascending Aorta: The Last Frontier?

Eduardo Keller Saadi, Rui Almeida and
Alexandre do Canto Zago

Additional information is available at the end of the chapter

http://dx.doi.org/10.5772/55149

1. Introduction

The treatment of ascending aorta diseases is usually performed by traditional surgery with median sternotomy and cardiopulmonary bypass. However, in some patients, the operative risk of this approach may be prohibitive. In these instances, endovascular approaches to the ascending aorta may be an alternative.

Endovascular approaches are being increasingly utilized to treat a variety of thoracic aortic diseases including aneurysms, pseudoaneurysms, dissections, penetrating aortic ulcers, traumatic aortic rupture, coarctation and abdominal aortic aneurysms [1].

Ascending aorta has several limitations for the endovascular approach, such as its larger diameter and the presence of the aortic valve and the coronary arteries.

2. Access and technique

The endovascular procedure is usually performed through the femoral arteries [1-3]. Sometimes this access is impossible or not recommended because of small size vessels, obstruction, calcification, dissection or extreme tortuosity.

The feasibility of endovascular treatment depends on many anatomic factors, including the diameter and the disease state of the access vessels [4,5]. Stenosis, calcifications, tortuosity, small size or dissection in both femoral and iliac arteries can make introduction of large sheath hazardous or impossible.

Endoprosthesis deployment in the ascending aorta usually requires large diameter and long sheath. There is always possibility of damaging the aortic valve, since the nose of the commercially available devices is designed for descending and/or abdominal aorta. The vascular prosthesis should be large enough to oversize by 15-20 % the aortic diameter and short in length to fit between the coronary arteries and the brachiocephalic trunk. This length usually measures 8 cm or less. The endovascular technique would have several advantages over the open surgical alternatives if the right tools for the procedure were available. Current thoracic aortic stent-grafts are too long, while abdominal aortic stent-grafts are too short and narrow. Moreover, abdominal aortic delivery systems are too short to traverse the long and tortuous path from the femoral artery to the ascending aorta.

Several different approaches have been presented and published over the last years as an attempt to solve very dramatic situations stretching the limits of the current technology [6-8].

The technique should be carefully planned. Rapid pacing and adenosine are useful to lower blood pressure and allow precise deployment. A rigid (Landerquist or super stiff) and long (260 cm) guidewire is usually placed in the left ventricle to give adequate support near the coronary arteries. This is similar to what we use when performing transcatheter aortic valve implantation (TAVI). One important tip is to perform a "wide J-shape" at the end of the rigid guidewire in order to prevent left ventricule perforation and, consequently, cardiac tamponade or left ventricular pseudoaneurysm.

Similar to other endovascular procedures, besides careful planning, patient selection and technical expertise are crucial to obtain satisfactory results. In this setting multidetector computed tomography (MDCT) plays an important role in selecting the patients suitable for the procedure and allows a careful and detailed step by step preoperative planning.

We have recently published a series of five clinical cases and described the technique in which the axillary artery was used to deliver the endograft for the treatment of different thoracic aortic diseases [9]. We also demonstrated the possibility of concomitant treatment of ascending aorta disease and coronary stent implantation [10,11].

Transcarotid is another alternative access and, recently, transapical approach through a small left thoracotomy has been described.

3. Clinical cases

In this part we will discuss clinical cases of endovascular treatment of ascending aortic diseases showing different approaches and techniques.

3.1. Clinical case 1

A 32-year-old female presenting cardiogenic shock (Figures 1-2).

http://dx.doi.org/10.5772/55149

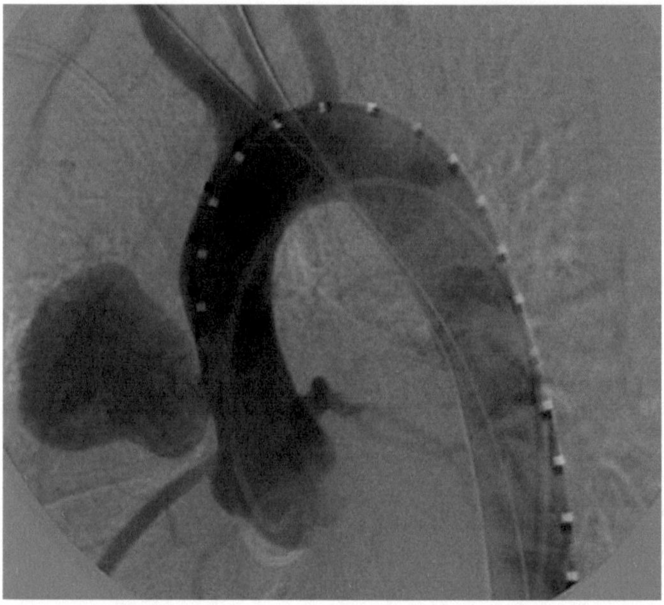

Figure 1. Aortogram showing bovine trunk and a pseudoaneurysm in the anterolateral wall of the ascending aorta 1 cm above the ostium of the right coronary artery.

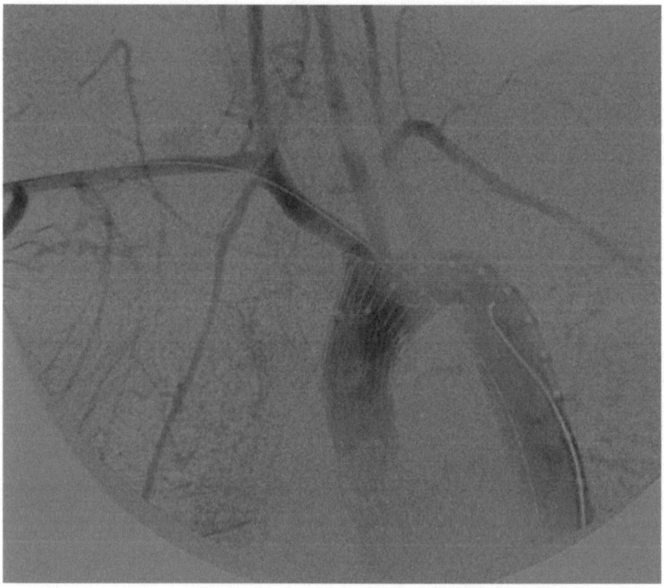

Figure 2. Final aortogram of emergency endovascular correction of a pseudoaneurysm through transfemoral implantation of a Cook endoprosthesis. The shorter device we had available was a 8 cm length endoprosthesis. In order to preserve flow in the brachiocephalic trunk and left carotid artery (bovine trunk) we had to use a chimney (snorkel) technique in this two vessels arch using two Viabahns to preserve flow.

3.2. Clinical case 2

A 57-year-old female underwent coronary artery bypass graft in another hospital with left internal mammary artery to the left anterior descending and saphenous vein graft to the right coronary artery. The patient developed mediastinitis and had 7 reinterventions resulting in acute bleeding through the sternum. She was sent to our hospital in cardiogenic shock and manual compression of the bleeding site in the sternum. Previous computed tomography showed ruptured pseudoaneurysm at the proximal anastomosis of saphenous vein graft to the (Figures 3-6).

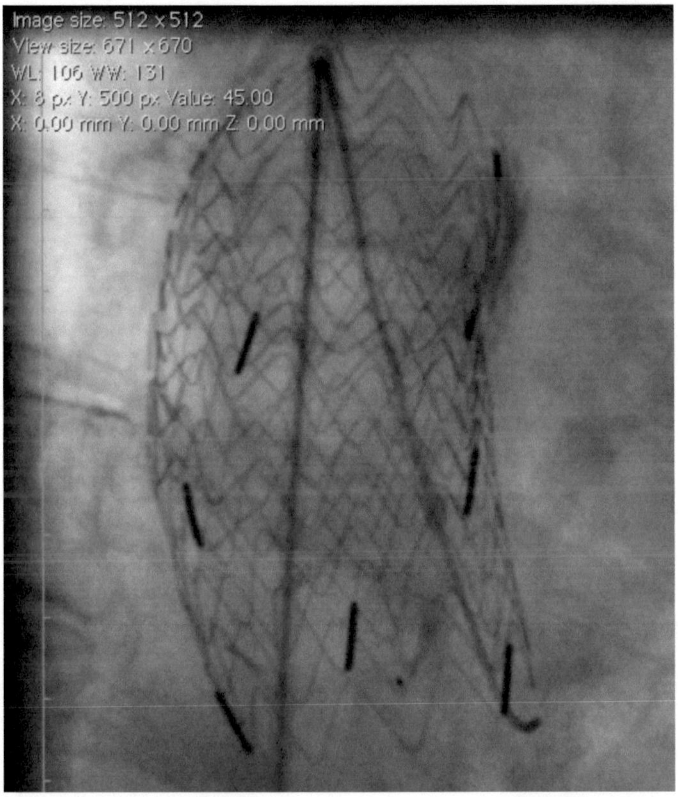

Figure 3. Emergency endovascular deployment of two abdominal extension cuffs (Gore-Tex) in the ascending aorta between the coronary ostium and the brachiocephalic trunk through the left axillary artery. The bleeding stopped immediately and the patient became stable.

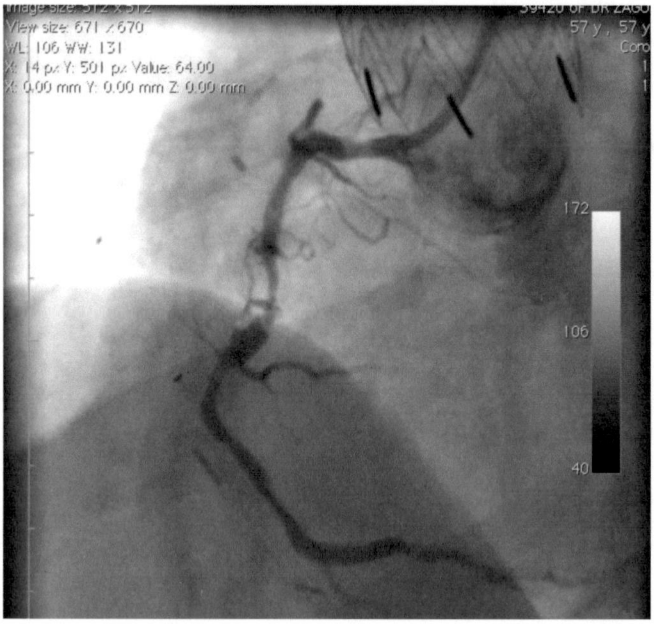

Figure 4. Right coronary angiography demonstrating severe stenosis. Once saphenous vein graft to the right coronary artery had occluded by the endoprosthesis, the native right coronary artery had to be treated.

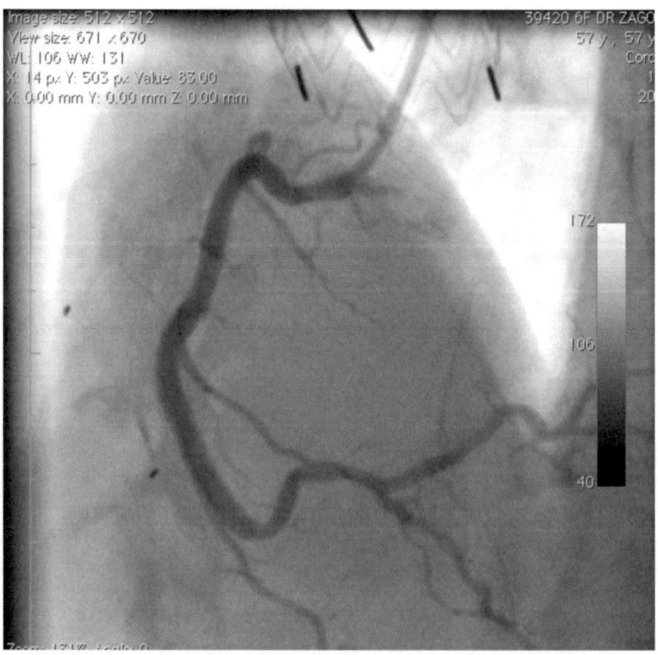

Figure 5. Deployment of three stents in the right coronary artery.

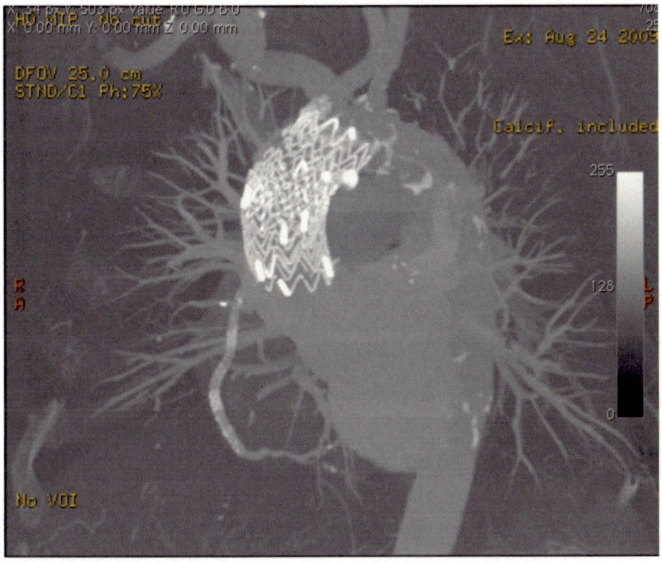

Figure 6. Computed tomography showing the two extension cuffs in the ascending aorta and the three stents in the right coronary artery.

3.3. Clinical case 3

A 74-year-old male with previous coronary artery bypass graft presented with iatrogenic ascending aortic pseudoaneurysm that occurred during angiography. The patient was at very high risk for surgical treatment, therefore an (Figures 7-9).

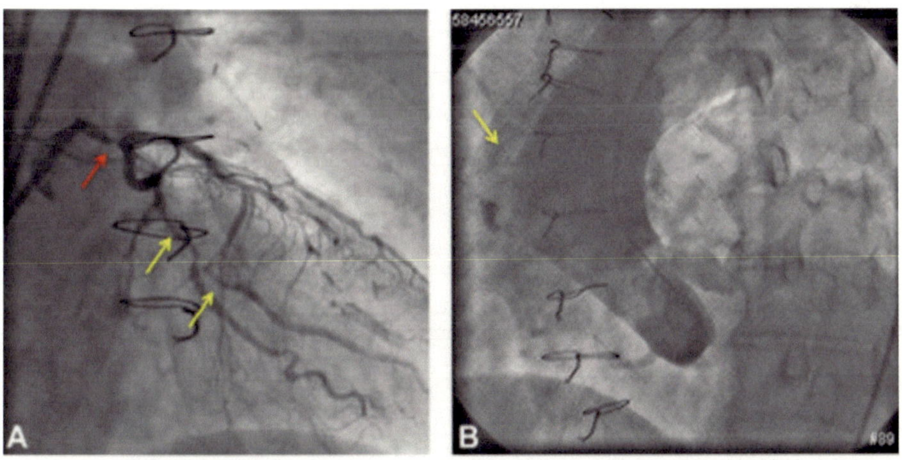

Figure 7. A) Coronary angiogram showing left main bifurcation with severe stenosis and circumflex with severe stenosis extending to large marginal branch. (B) Aortic angiogram demonstrating ascending aorta dilatation and image suggesting dissection at the saphenous vein graft ostium.

http://dx.doi.org/10.5772/55149

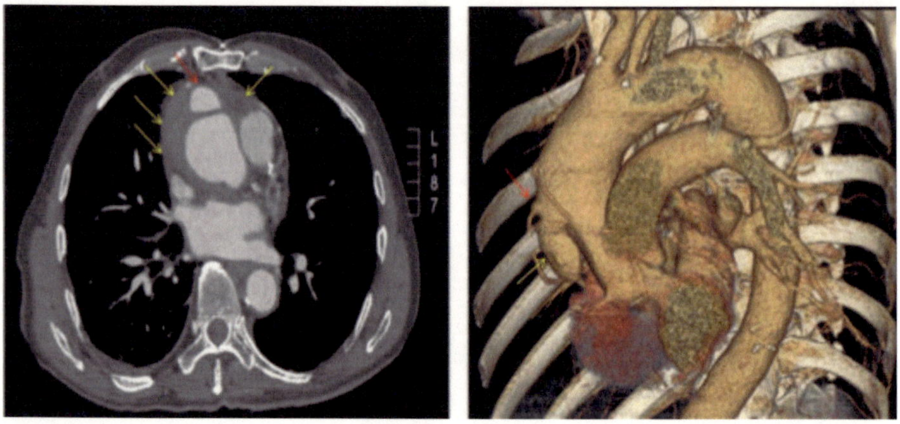

Figure 8. Computerized tomographic angiography showing a 3.4-cm pseudoaneurysm with partial thrombosis in ascending aorta and surrounding intramural hematoma.

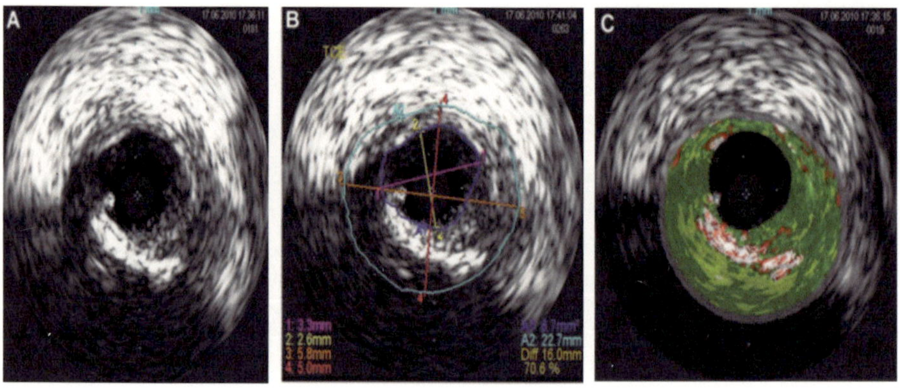

Figure 9. A) Intravascular ultrasound of left main artery evidencing significant stenosis due to calcified plaque. (B) Intravascular ultrasound measurements confirming the presence of a large left main artery and significant plaque burden. (C) Virtual histology showing predominantly fibrous plaque and superficial calcium arch.

Both procedures were successfully performed and the patient was discharged without (Figures 10-12). At 6 months and 1 year clinical follow-up the patient had no symptoms as well as no other adverse cardiovascular events.

4. Target diseases

There are several pathologies of the ascending aorta that can be potentially addressed by the endovascular approach. Pseudoaneurysms or sacular aneurysms in the mid-ascending aorta are adequate for this technique because they usually appear with a sufficient proximal and

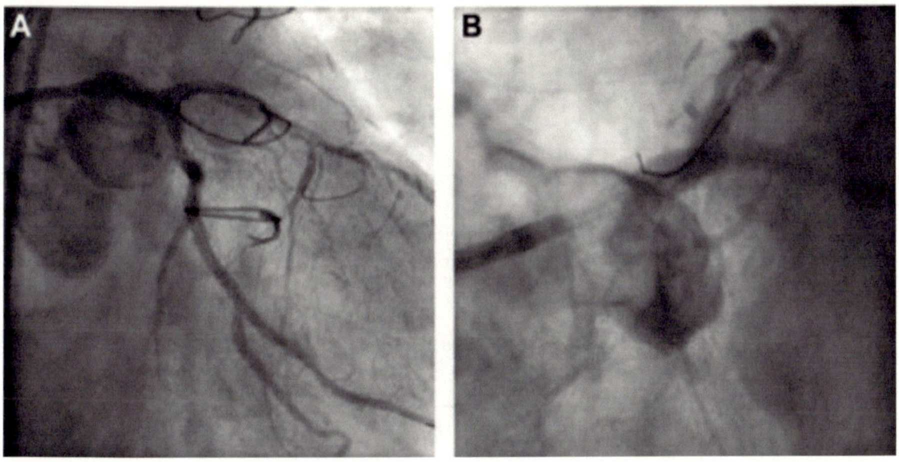

Figure 10. Coronary angiogram showing final result in right anterior oblique projection (A) and spider view (B).

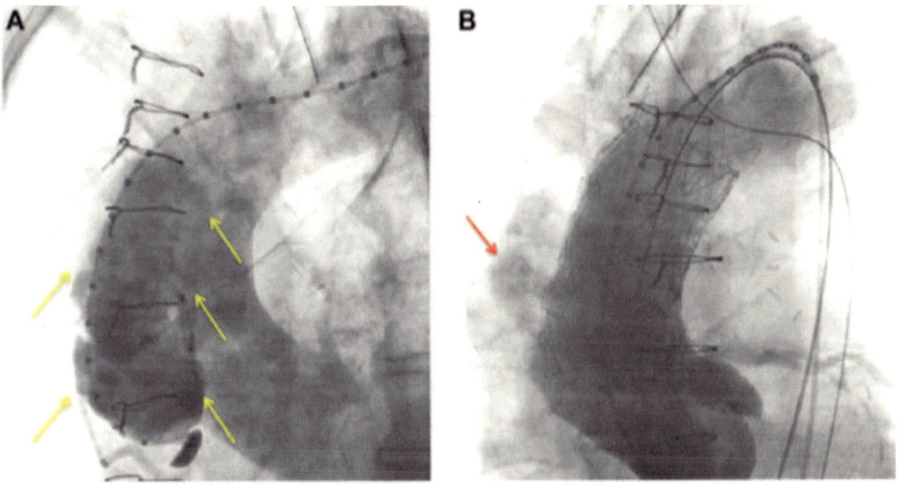

Figure 11. (A) Ascending aorta angiogram before endoprosthesis deployment showing a large pseudoaneurysm (yellow arrow). (B) Ascending aorta angiogram after endoprosthesis deployment evidencing sealed pseudoaneurysm and a type 1 endoleak (red arrow).

distal landing zone. On the other hand, fusiform aneurysms have the limitation of lacking a sufficient landing zone in many cases.

Thoracic endovascular stent grafting has revolutionized the treatment of distal [type B] acute aortic dissection. Endovascular surgeons are now seeking the ways to improve the treatment of type A dissection by offering endovascular techniques to replace conventional surgical therapy. Less invasive endovascular therapy, obviates the need for sternotomy and cardiopulmonary bypass, reduces perioperative morbidity, and offers an alternative solution for

http://dx.doi.org/10.5772/55149

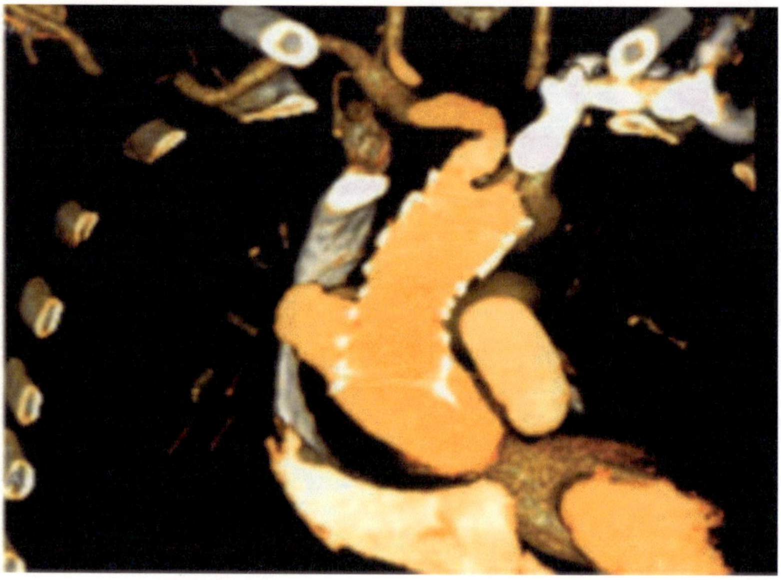

Figure 12. Computerized tomographic angiography showing final result after endoprosthesis deployment.

those patients not eligible for conventional intervention due to co-morbidity or severe complications of the disease.

Thoracic stent grafting in the ascending aorta presents specific challenges and the role of uncovered stents is unclear in this situation. The majority of patients with acute type A aortic dissection has the intimal tear originated in the sinotubular junction. More than 90% of patients with this disease does not have sufficient proximal or distal landing zone required for secure fixation. Therefore, the site of the intimal tear as well as aortic valve insufficiency and aortic diameter >38mm are major factors limiting the use of endovascular therapy for acute type A dissection. Current available stents in use to treat type B aortic dissection do not address anatomical constraints present in type A aortic dissection in the majority of cases, hence the development of new devices is required.

5. Technical limitations

Endovascular approach of the ascending aorta has several limitations and is still in its beginning phase.

The diameter of the ascending aorta is usually larger than the rest of the aorta and the proximity with the aortic valve and the presence of the coronary arteries pose special challenges.

The length of the delivery system, which is designed for the abdominal aorta, does not allow to reach the ascending aorta through the groin.

Finally, the length of the endoprosthesis itself for descending aorta may be too long to be positioned between the coronary ostia and the brachiocephalic trunk.

6. Conclusions

Despite the fantastic progress in this field and the clear advantages of endovascular approaches for the ascending aorta in some clinical situations, one must bear in mind the high level of risk that these procedures entail.

Long-term data are not available to establish the safety and durability of stent-graft repairs. The cases described represent an off-label use of this technology and should be considered with the above mentioned limitations in mind.

The surgeon will need special skills in open aortic surgery and catheter based interventions to be able to plan the procedure carefully, to properly deliver the devices and to manage the potential serious complications [12].

Challenges in endograft design are the development of branched endografts and of pathology-specific endografts [13]. However, the unique composition of the proximal thoracic aorta and the associated mechanical properties have to be taken into account and make this effort by far more complex than initially expected. Moreover, there is a need for reducing the stent-graft devices profile as well as for increasing conformability and trackability.

We believe that future advances with devices specifically designed for the treatment of ascending aorta diseases will allow this technique to be incorporated into routine medical practice.

Author details

Eduardo Keller Saadi[1,2,3], Rui Almeida[4,5,6] and Alexandre do Canto Zago[1,2,7]

1 Federal University of Rio Grande do Sul, Porto Alegre, RS, Brazil

2 Federal University of Rio Grande do Sul Hospital, Porto Alegre, RS, Brazil

3 Mãe de Deus Hospital, Porto Alegre, RS, Brazil

4 West Paraná State University, Cascavel, PR, Brazil

5 Mãe de Deus Hospital, Cascavel, PR, Brazil

6 Cardiovascular Surgery Institute of West Paraná, Cascavel, PR, Brazil

7 Lutheran University Hospital, Porto Alegre, RS, Brazil

References

[1] Melissano, G, Bertoglio, L, Civilini, E, Marone, E. M, Calori, G, Setacci, F, & Chiesa, R. Results of Thoracic Endovascular Grafting in Different Aortic Segments. J Endovasc Ther (2007). , 14, 150-157.

[2] Guidelines for the Diagnosis and Management of Patients with Thoracic Aortic DiseaseA Report of the American College of Cardiology Foundation/American Heart Association Task Force on Practice Guidelines, American Association for Thoracic Surgery, American College of Radiology, American Stroke Association, Society of Cardiovascular Anesthesiologists, Society for Cardiovascular Angiography and Interventions, Society of Interventional Radiology, Society of Thoracic Surgeons, and Society for Vascular Medicine. Circulation (2010). ee369., 266.

[3] Nienaber, C. A, Rousseau, H, Eggebrecht, H, Kische, S, Fattori, R, Rehders, T. C, Kundt, G, Scheinert, D, Czerny, M, Kleinfeldt, T, Zipfel, B, & Labrousse, L. Ince HS for the INSTEAD Trial. Randomized Comparison of Strategies for Type B Aortic Dissection. Circulation (2009). , 120, 2519-2528.

[4] Alric, P, Canaud, L, Branchereau, P, Marty-ané, C, & Berthet, J. P. Preoperative assessment of anatomical suitability for thoracic endovascular aortic repair. Acta Chir Belg (2009). , 109(4), 458-64.

[5] Almeida, R. M, Leal, J. C, Saadi, E. K, & Braile, D. M. Rocha AST, Volpiani J, Centola C, Zago A. Thoracic endovascular aortic repair- a Brazilian experience in 255 patients over a period of 112 months. Interact CardioVasc Thorac Surg (2009). , 524-528.

[6] Uchida, K, Imoto, K, Yanagi, H, Machida, D, Okiyama, M, Yasuda, S, et al. Endovascular Repair of Ascending Aortic Rupture: Effectiveness of a Fenestrated Stent-Graft. J Endovasc Ther (2010). , 17, 395-398.

[7] Lin, P, Kougias, P, Huynh, T, Huh, J, & Coselli, J. S. Endovascular Repair of Ascending Aortic Pseudoaneurysm: Technical Considerations of a Common Carotid Artery Approach Using the Zenith Aortic Cuff Endograft. J Endovasc Ther (2007).

[8] Chuter TAMEndovascular Repair in the Ascending Aorta: Stretching the Limits of Current Technology. J Endovasc Ther (2007). , 14, 799-800.

[9] Saadi, E. K, Dussin, L. H, Moura, L, & Machado, A. S. The axillary artery--a new approach for endovascular treatment of thoracic aortic diseases. Interact Cardiovasc Thorac Surg. (2010). Nov;, 11(5), 617-9.

[10] Zago, A. C, Saadi, E. K, & Zago, A. J. Endovascular approach to treat ascending aortic pseudoaneurysm in a patient with previous CABG and very high surgical risk. Catheter Cardiovasc Interv. (2011). Oct 1;, 78(4), 551-7.

[11] Saadi, E. K. Moura Ld, Zago A, Zago A. Endovascular repair of ascending aorta and coronary stent implantation.Rev Bras Cir Cardiovasc. (2011). Jul-Sep;, 26(3), 477-80.

[12] Saadi, E. K. Is it possible to train an endovascular surgeon? Rev Bras Cir Cardiovasc. (2007). Jan-Mar;22(1):III-IV.

[13] Greenberg, R, Eagleton, M, & Mastracci, T. Branched endografts for thoracoabdominal aneurysms. J Thorac Cardiovasc Surg (2010). S, 171-8.

Chapter 24

The Role of The Angiosome Model in Treatment of Critical Limb Ischemia

Kim Houlind and Johnny Christensen

Additional information is available at the end of the chapter

http://dx.doi.org/10.5772/54418

1. Introduction

Critical limb ischemia (CLI) is the major cause of amputation in the developed world but revascularization offers an opportunity for limb salvage. Revascularization can be performed either by bypass surgery or by endovascular techniques. Peripheral bypass surgery can be performed using artificial grafts, but vein grafts offer better limb salvage and graft patency [1].

When performing revascularization of the lower limb, common clinical practice and recent guidelines include grafting of the" best vessel" which crosses the level of the ankle in order to restore pulsatile flow to the foot [1]. This may lead to either direct perfusion of the ischemic area or – very often – indirect perfusion relying on collaterals surrounding the diseased zone. This strategy is different from the one used e.g. in coronary artery bypass surgery, where the aim is "complete revascularization" i.e. performing bypasses to every diseased vascular territory [2].

The arterial connections between different parts of the foot may quite often not be sufficient to ensure healing and to prevent amputation. For instance, approximately 15% of heel ulcers do not heal despite an open bypass graft to the dorsal pedal artery [3]

An alternative strategy, called the angiosome model, is based on the pioneering work of Taylor and coworkers [4], who, in the eighties, performed detailed dissections with injection of dye in the vessels. They demonstrated the fact that the body consists of "angiosomes" i.e. three-dimensional blocks of tissue perfused and drained by specific arterial and venous bundles. In a later report from the same group, the angiosomes of the leg and foot were described in detail [5]

Perfusion and drainage can occur between angiosomes by means of connecting "choke" vessels, but this perfusion is less effective than direct supply from the specific feed artery of the angiosome. It is worth noting that the choke vessels are diseased in patients with diabetes and atherosclerosis. This angiosome has had profound impact on the developement of strategies for plastic and reconstructive surgery. However, only little attention has been paid to the angiosome model in treatment of critical limb ischemia. According to the angiosome model, the specific feed artery – rather than the "best vessel" – should be favoured for revascularization. The foot and ankle area consist of six angiosomes.

During the last few years, some studies have compared the results of "best vessel" versus "angiosome" directed revascularization. The studies include comparisons of both arterial bypass and percutaneous revascularization based on the two principles

This chapter aims at describing the role of the angiosome model in critical limb ischemia, and to review the current literature.

2. Anatomy

Blood supply to the foot is derived from the three tibial vessels, the Anterior tibial artery, the Posterior tibial artery, and the Peroneal artery. These three arteries give rise to six end-arteries, each supplying an angiosome (Figure 1).

1. The anterior tibial artery supplies the anterior ankle and continues as the dorsalis pedis artery, which supplies the dorsum of the foot. It gives off the lateral tarsal artery and branches into the first dorsal interosseal artery and the arcuate artery supplying the 2-4 interosseal arteries. It has been pointed out that the dorsalis pedis artery is extremely attenuated or absent in 12% of cases [6].

   The posterior tibial artery divides into three main branches:

2. The calcaneal branch, which arborizes into multiple braches, that supply the medial and plantar portion of the heel,
3. the medial plantar artery, supplying the medial, plantar part of the foot. Its boundaries encompass the instep, and, depending on anatomic variability, can include the hallux.
4. the lateral plantar artery which supplies the lateral midfoot as well as the entire plantar forefoot through the 4 plantar metatarsal arteries that emanate from the deep plantar arch. Normally, this angiosome also includes the plantar aspect of the hallux, depending on anatomic variability.

   The peroneal artery bifurcates into

5. the anterior perforating brach, supplying the lateral anterior upper ankle and
6. a calcaneal branch, supplying the lateral and plantar heel. Together with the calcaneal brach of the posterior tibila artery this artery ensures a double blood supply to the plantar aspect of the heel.

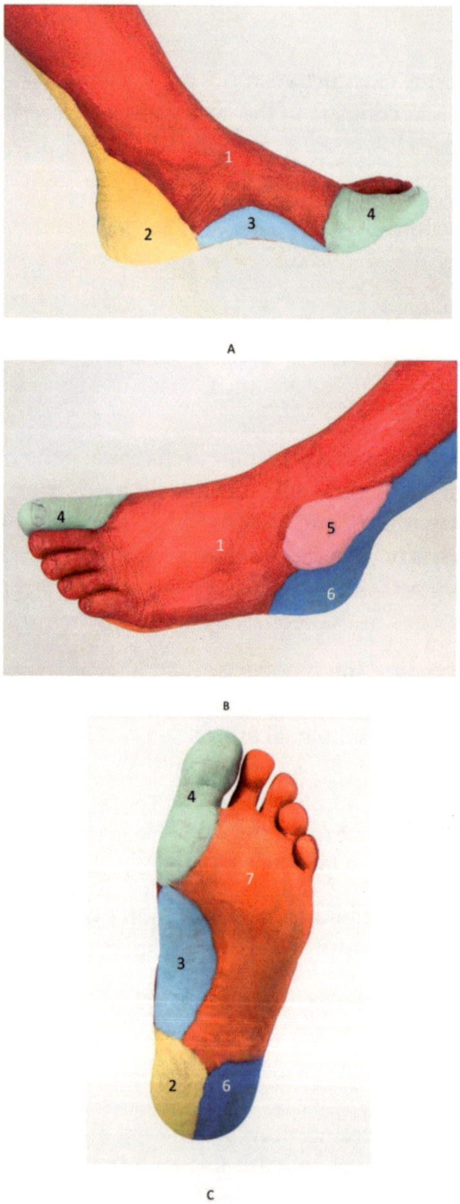

1. Dorsalis pedis angiosome
2. Medial calcaneal artery angiosome
3. Medial plantar artery angiosome
4. The hallux, which may be supplied by the feeding arteries of angiosomes 1, 2, or 6
5. Anterior perforating branch angiosome
6. Lateral calcaneal branch angiosome
7. Lateral plantar artery angiosome

Figure 1. Angiosomes shown on the surface of the foot. A. Medial view, B. Dorso-lateral view, C. Plantar view.

3. Interconnections

A number of interconnections exist between the angiosomes. When present, these interconnections exist *a priori* and – in contrast to the choke vessels described below - do not need a period of ischemia to open. However, as peripheral arterial disease progresses, these connections may be blocked.

The arterial-arterial connections include:

Anterior tibial to peroneal:

The lateral malleolar artery joins with the anterior perforating branch of the peroneal artery just above the ankle joint (Figure 2A).

Anterior tibial to posterior tibial:

The lateral plantar artery forms the deep plantar arch crossing the proximal 2,3, and 4th metatarsals and finally anastomoses directly with the dorsalis pedis artery in the first interspace (Figures 2A and 2B). The superficial and deep medial plantar arteries join at the cruciate anastomosis. Depending on what arteries predominate at or around the cruciate anastomosis, the hallux may be primarily nourished by the lateral plantar artery, medial plantar artery, the first dorsal metatarsal artery or simultaneously by either two or three of these arteries [7].

The medial plantar artery also interconnects with the anterior tibial tree as cutaneous branches connect proximally with medial branches of the dorsalis pedis artery and distally with branches of the first dorsal metatarsal artery.

Peroneal and posterior tibial connections:

Between one and three communicating branches between the peroneal artery and the posterior tibial artery proximal to the ankle joint deep to the Achilles tendon.

On the other hand, no direct arterial-arterial connection exists between the medial and lateral calcaneal arteries, which both supply the plantar aspect of the heel.

4. Choke vessels

Where no "true" arterial-arterial connections are present between neighbouring angiosomes, a network of reduced caliber "choke vessels" form a link. These vessels are normally inadequate to perfuse the area of a distant angiosome but may be provoked to dilate.

This is the theoretical base of the "delay phenomenon" which has been applied in plastic surgery. While the choke vessels between angiosomes in a skin or muscle flap may be sufficient to perfuse an adjacent vascular territory, necrosis will ususally appear in the choke vessel zone defining the next vascular territory. When designing a skin or muscle flap larger than two angiosomes, a two stage procedure might be performed. In the first stage, the perforators of the neighbouring angiosomes are ligated, causing the choke vessels between neighbouring angiosomes to dilate over a period of 4-10 days. After this delay period, a larger flap can be safely elevated [8]. There is good clinical and experimental evidence that this

principle works for the transfer of skin grafts from essentially normal donor sites. These results may, however, not be extrapolated to other situations e.g. in the ischemic foot where distal, aggressive macroangiopathy is associated with microcirculatory changes like thrombosis, neuropathy, local sepsis, arterio-venous shunting and hypercoagulability [9].

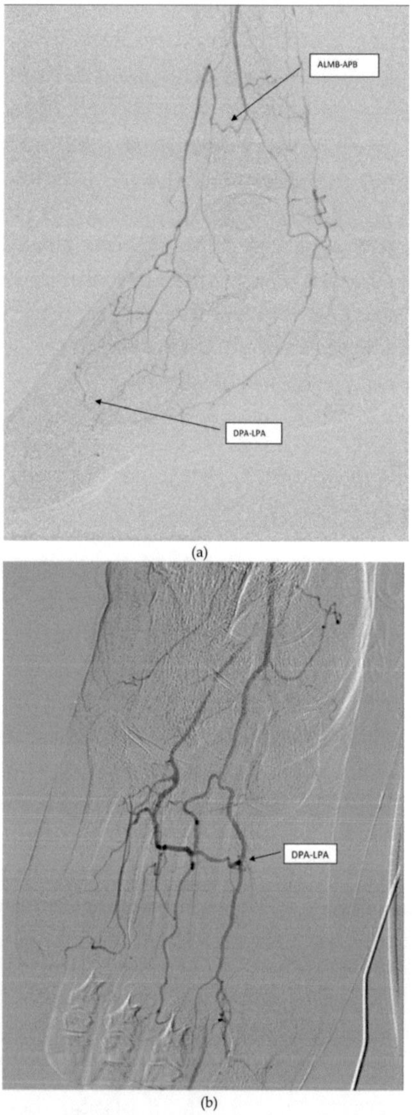

Figure 2. A. Lateral oblique projection of the anterior pedal vessels of a patient with peripheral occlusive arterial disease and patent arterial-arterial connections. ALMB-APB: Connection between the anterior lateral malleolar branch of the anterior tibial artery and the anterior perforating branch of the peroneal artery. DPA-LPA: Perforating branch connecting the dorsal pedal artery with the lateral plantar artery. B. Antero-posterior projection of the perforating branch connecting the dorsal pedal artery with the lateral plantar artery (DPA-LPA).

5. Imaging and assessment

5.1. Angiography

A fundamental prerequisite of providing angiosome-directed revascularization is profound knowledge of the anatomy of the pedal vasculature as well as adequate imaging technique including intraprocedural angiography of both tibial and pedal arteries. Manzi and coworkers have recently reported their experience from more than 2500 antegrade interventional procedures in patients with critical limb ischemia and diabetes [10]. For imaging of the pedal arteries they stress that prolonged filming is often necessary to record delayed enhancement of of pedal vessels from retrograde or collateral circulation and that both standard anteroposterior and lateral oblique projections should be obtained. They have established the following two criteria for correct positioning of the image intensifier: 1) The base of the fifth metatarsal bone must be seen to project outward from the base of the foot in the lateral oblique view and 2) the first proximal metatarsal interspace must be clearly visualized in the anteroposterior view. These two views tend to give a good overview of the pedal arteries and collaterals.

5.2. Doppler ultrasound

Attinger and coworkers have described in detail how to map the arterial-arterial connections using a Doppler device [7].

As an example, the Doppler signal is located from the posterior tibial artery over the tarsal tunnel. If the signal persists when occluding (by digital compression) the artery distally, there is antegrade flow along the posterior tibila artery. If the signal disappears, the flow is retrograde from the anterior tibial artery via the dorsalis pedis and lateral plantar arteries. Similarly, Doppler signal can be obtained from the anterior perforating branch of the peroneal artery in the lateral soft area between the tibia and fibula just above the ankle joint. When the anterior tibial artery is occluded at the takeoff of the lateral malleolar branch, the Doppler signal will persist if there is antegrade flow along the anterior perforating branch of the peroneal artery. If the Doppler signal disappears, filling of the anterior perforating branch must be retrograde from the anterior tibial artery through the lateral malleolar branch. The authors describe how the competence of these connections can have profound significance for the healing potential of an amputation wound.

5.3. Thermography

Nagase and coworkers [11] reported the results of plantar thermography of skin temperature in 129 non-ulcer diabetic patients and 32 normal volunteers. From the pattern of four different plantar angiosomes originally described by Attinger [7], they defined twenty different patterns of temperature distribution. The most common pattern in normal subjects was a "bilateral butterfly pattern" in which the medial arch showed the highest temperature (46.9%) or an even distribution of temperature across the entire planta of the feet (20.3%).

http://dx.doi.org/10.5772/54418

Recordings of the diabetic feet showed a lower proportion of feet with a "bilateral butterfly pattern" (13.9%), higher proportions of even distribution of temperature (39.1%) and a generally more diverse distribution of patterns in the rest. Although interesting, the study did not provide comparisons with angiographic findings that could confirm a correlation between the distribution of skin temperature and the distribution of lesions of feed arteries to the relevant angiosomes.

6. Results from direct versus indirect revascularization

A number of studies have been performed comparing the results of direct revascularization to the relevant angiosome with those of indirect revascularization either through collaterals or choke vessels.

In 2009, Neville and coworkers published a retrospective analysis of 43 patients undergoing bypass surgery for tissue loss due to ischemia [12]. Twenty-two were directly revascularized to the relevant agniosome while 21 were indirectly revascularized. Healing occurred in 91% of the directly revascularized patients and only 62% of the indirectly revascularized patients ($p=0.03$]. Major patient characteristics such as diabetes, tobacco use, and renal failure were evenly distributed between the directly revascularized and indirectly revascularized groups, but wound characteristics and infection were not reported.

On the other hand, Azuma and coworkers [13] reviewed the results of 249 consecutive distal bypasses for critical limb ischemia. 218 limbs were included in the initial analysis which proved significantly lower wound healing rate in the indirect revascularization group than in the direct revascularization group. This was especially the case in a subgroup of patients with end stage renal failure. This finding was, however, compromised by significant baseline differences between the groups especially characterized by a higher proportion of patients with heel ulcers and gangraene in the indirect revascularization group. After applying propensity scored analysis including only 48 pairs of limbs, the healing rate between the two groups did not reach statistical significance ($p=0.185$). The authors concluded that the angiosome concept was not relevant for open surgical treatment of critical limb ischemia in patients without end stage renal failure. This conclusion may be questioned in view of the limited statistical strength of the propensity scored analysis.

Iida and coworkers reviewed the results of endovascular treatment of 203 limbs in 177 consecutive patients with critical limb ischemia, Rutherford 5 or 6 [14]. During up to 4 years follow up, they found significantly higher limb salvage rate in patients with the directly revascularized than indirectly revascularized wounds. Interestingly, the total number of tibial vessels with run off did not influence the limb salvage rate in neither group, indicating that it is not important how much blood can be provided to the foot but rather whether i t reaches the ischemic area. In a later review by the same group [15], including 369 limbs from 329 consecutive patients, including only patients with isolated below-the-knee lesions, patients who had received direct revascularization experienced significantly higher levels of amputation-free survival and freedom from major adverse limb events than patients in

whom only indirect revascularization was possible. In this review the finding was confirmed after propensity matching of groups. In multivariate analysis, elevated levels of c-reactive protein were found to be independent predictors of major amputation in the indirect revascularization group but not in the direct revascularization group. This may imply that indirect revascularization may be inadequate for the healing of infected wounds.

Alexandriescu and collegues have published several reports describing their experience with targeted primary angioplasty of diabetic foot lesions [16-17]. In a series of 124 limbs (98 patients), they were able to achieve direct revascularization in 82% [16]. Limb salvage was 91% at 12 months and 84% at three years follow-up. More recently, they published a historical comparison between their results before and after 2005 when they introduced the angiosome concept in their practice. Despite similar graft patency and technical success, they experienced a significantly better wound healing rate and limb preservation in the group of patients treated according to the angiosome concept [18]. This result is interesting although it is probably biased by the general learning curve of the group.

In a paper published together with Alexandriescu, the vascular surgery department at the University Hospital in Helsinki, Finland recently reported their results from the last three years [19]. In a population including approximately the same number of direct and indirect endovascular revascularizations, they found 74% of the wounds to have healed within one year in the directly revascularized group compared to 46% in the indirectly revascularizd group (p=0.002). The number of patients was, however, not reported.

Two studies, one surgical by Deguchi [20] and one endovascular by Blanes Ortí [21] failed to show any difference in wound healing time or limb salvage between directly or indirectly revascularized patients. Due to small numbers, the statistical strengh of these comparisons is, however, limited.

6.1. The influence of collaterals

The prognostic significance of indirect revascularization via collaterals was studied by Varela in a mixed cohort of venous bypass and endovascular treated patients with ischemic wounds [22]. Defining collaterals visible on perioperative angiograms, either between distal calcaneal peroneal branches and anterior or posterior tibial artery (n=16) or patent pedal arch connecting dorsal and plantar blood supply (n=2), they found a similar wound healing rate for indirect revascularization of the wound area through collaterals as for direct revascularization to the angiosome specific feed artery (92% versus 88% wound healing at 12 months follow-up). When including indirect revascularizations without visible collaterals, only 73% of the wounds had healed after 12 months (p=0.008).

6.2. The significance of venosomes

Anatomically, the venous drainage follows the arterial perfusion of the angiosomes [23] and Alexandriescu used the term venosome, when reporting the results of surgical deep calf vein arterialization. In a series of 26 limbs in 25 diabetic patients with very advanced below the knee occlusive disease, a PTFE bypass was made between an arterial inflow and a deep

calf vein followed by selective embolization of collaterals, directing arterial blood to the relevant venosome. Using this strategy, a 73% three year limb salvage rate was achieved [24].

7. Discussion

The concept of angiosome-directed revascularization is, theoretically, attractive and in accordance with pathophysiological knowledge. It is also in line with experience from coronary bypass surgery, where reperfusion through collaterals does not provide a similar freedom from cardiac events as that provided by complete direct revascularization of all the diseased vascular territoria [2].

It is well established that healing of an ishemic pedal wound is more effectively achieved when pulsatile arterial blood flow is established across the ankle and it seems logical to expect that this effect is larger when the pulsatile flow is provided all the way to the site of the injury.

As suggested by the above mentioned papers, the effect of direct revascularization may especially be relevant in the settings of end stage renal failure, infected wounds, endovascular rather than surgical repair, and in cases where collaterals are absent.

The angiosome concept represents a novel approach to improving the therapy of critical limb ischemia. It may potentially provide the rationale not only for the choice of target artery. It may also influence the indications for endovascular or open repair according to which target artery is accessible by which method.

Although the evidence in favour of an angiosome directed treatment is mounting fast, it is, however, still circumstantial. All of the studies comparing the results of direct and indirect revascularization are retrospective and, thus, biased by heterogeneity in patient selection. More often than not, the angiosome specific artery will also be the most diseased artery and the ability to recanalize this vessel will most probably select the least atherosclerotic patients to the "direct revascularization" group. It is also likely that the advocates of an angiosome-directed revascularization strategy would attempt direct revascularization first and only perform indirect revascularization if this attempt was unsuccessful. Regardless of any retrospective matching of the groups this would lead to patients with extensive distal atherosclerosis to be placed in the indirect revascularization groups, thus biasing the comparisons in favour of the angiosome specific approach. The differences in healing rate and limb salvage between groups may, therefore, merely reflect preoperative differences in the extent of occlusive disease. It is possible that this is what is reflected in the lack of statistically significant differences after propensity scoring in the study by Azuma [13].

As highlighted in the study by Varela, the presence or absence of collaterals merit further investigation [22]. For this purpose, the Doppler method described by Attinger [7] seems to be a good and non-invasive technique.

As evidence stands at the moment, there is some, although limited, evidence that when there is a choice of target artery for revascularization, preference should be given to the ar-

tery directly feeding the wound´s angiosome. Specific analysis, based on prospectively collected data of homogeneous cohorts of patients are needed. Unbiased evidence will only be achievable by performing a prospective, randomized controlled trial with a blinded endpoint assessment.

Author details

Kim Houlind[1] and Johnny Christensen[2]

1 Dept. of Vascular Surgery, Kolding Hospital, Denmark and Institute of Regional Health Services Research, University of Southern Denmark, Denmark

2 Dept. of Radiology, Kolding Hospital, Denmark

References

[1] Norgreen L, Hiatt WR, Dormandy JA, Nehler MR, Harris KA, Fowkes FGR on behalf of the TASC II Working Group. Inter-society Concensus for the management of peripheral arterial disease (TASC II). Eur J Endovasc Surg 2007;33(Suppl 1): S32-55.

[2] Vieira RD, Hueb W, Gersh BJ, Lima EG, Pereira AC, Rezende PC, Garzillo CL, Hueb AC, Favarato D, Soares PR, Ramires JA, Filho RK. The effect of complete revascularization on 10-year Survival of Patients with Stable Multivessel Coronary artery Disease: MASS II Trial. Circulation 2012;126 (11 Suppl 1): S158-63

[3] Berceli SA, Chan AK, Pomposelli FB jr. Gibbons GW, Campbell DR, Akbari CM, Brophy DT, LoGerfo FW. Efficacy of dorsal pedal artery bypass in limb salvage for ischemic heel ulcers. J Vasc Surg 1999;30(3):499-508

[4] Taylor GI, Palmer JH. The vascular territories (angiosomes) of the body: Experimental study and clinical implication. Br J Plast Surg 1987;40:113-

[5] Taylor GI, Pan WR. Angiosomes of the leg: anatomic study and clinical implications. Plast Reconstr Surg 1998;102:599-616

[6] Clemens MW, Attinger CE. Angiosomes and wound care in the diabetic foot. Foot Ankle Clin N Am 2010;15:439-64

[7] Attinger CE, Evans KK, Bulan E, Blume P, Cooper P. Angiosomes of the Foot and Ankle and Clinical Implications for Limb Salvage: Reconstruction, Incisions, and Revascularization. Plast. Reconstr. Surg 2006; 117 (Suppl) 261S-293S

[8] Taylor GI, Corlett RJ, Caddy CM, Zeit RG. An anatomic review of the delay phenomenon: II. Clinical applications. Plast Reconstr Surg:89 (3):408-16

[9] Jörneskog G. Why critical limb ischemia criteria are not applicable to diabetic foot and what the consequences are. Scand J Surg 2012:101;114-18

[10] Manzi M, Cester G, Palena LM, Alek RT, Candeo A, Ferraresi R. Vascular Imaging of the Foot: The first step toward endovascular recanalization. Radiographics 2011;31(6):1623-36

[11] Nagase T, Sanada H, Takehara K, Oe M, Iizaka S, Ohashi Y, Oba M, Kadowaki T, Nakagami G. Variations of planatar thermographic patterns in normal controls and non-ulcer diabetic patients: Novel classification using angiosome concept. Journal of Plastic, reconstructive & aesthetic Surgery 2011; 64: 860-66

[12] Neville RF, attinger CE, Bulan EJ, Ducic I, Thomassen M, Sidaway AN. Revascularization of a Specific Angiosome for Limb salvage: Does the Target artery Matter? Ann Vasc Surg 2009;23:367-373

[13] Azuma N, Uchida H, kokubo T, Koya A, Akasaka N, sasajima T. factors influencing wound healing og critical ischaemic foot after bypass surgery: Is the angiosome important in selecting bypass traget artery. European journal of vascular and endovascular surgery 2012;43:322-328

[14] Iida O, Nanto S, Uematso M, Ikeoka K, Okamoto S, Dohi T, Fujita M, Terasi H, Nagata S. Importance of the angiosome concept for endovascular therapy in patients with critical limb ischemia. Catheterization and cardiovascular Interventions 2010; 75: 830-836

[15] Iida O, Soga Y, Hirano K, Kawasaki D, Suzuki K, Miyashita Y, Terasi H, Uematsu M. Long term reults of direct and indirect endovascular revascularization base don the angiosome concept in patients with critical limb ischemia presenting with isolated below-the knee lesions. J Vasc surg 2012;55:363-70

[16] Alexandriescu V-A, Hubermont G, Philips Y, Guillaumie B, Ngongang C, Vandenbossche P, Azdad K, Ledent G, Horion J. Selective primary angioplasty following an angiosome model of reperfusion in the treatment of Wagner 1-4 diabetic foot lesions: Practice in a multidisciplinary diabetic limb service. J Endovasc Ther 2008;15:580-593

[17] Alexandriescu V, Hubermont G. The challenging topic of diabetic foot revascularization: does the angiosome-guided angioplasty may improve outcome. Journal of Cardiovascular Surgery 2012;53:3-12.

[18] Alexandriescu V, Vincent G, Azdad K, Hubermont G, Ledent G, Ngongang C, Filimon A-M. A reliable approach to diabetic neuroischemic foot wounds: Below-the-knee angiosome-oriented angioplasty. J Endovasc Ther 2011;18:376-387

[19] Alexandriescu V, Söderström M, Venermo M. Angiosome theory: Fact or fiction? Scandinavian Journal of surgery 2012;101:125-31

[20] Deguchi J, Kitaoka T, Yamamoto K, Matsumoto H, Sato. Impact of Angiosome on Treatment of Diabetic Ischemic Foot with Paramalleolar Bypass. J Jpn Coll Angiol 2010;50:687-691

[21] Blanes Orti P, Vázquez R, Minguell P, García V, Manuel-Rimbau Munoz E, Lozarno Vilardell P. Percutaneous revascularization of specific angiosome in critical limb ischaemia. Angiologia 2011;63:11-17

[22] Varela C, Acin F, de Haro J, Bleda S, Esparza L, March JR. The role of foot collateral vessels on ulcer healing and limb salvage after successful endovascular and surgical distal procedures according to the angiosome model. Vasc Endovasc Surg 2010;44:654-660

[23] Taylor G.I, Caddy CM, Waterson PA, Crock JG. The venous territories (venosomes) of the human body. Experimental study and clinical implications. Plast Reconstr Surg 1990;86:185-

[24] Alexandriescu V, Ngongang C, Vincent G, Ledent G, Hubermont G. Deep calf veins arterialization for inferior limb preservation in diabetic patients with extended ischemic wounds, unfit for direct arterial reconstruction; preliminary results according to an angiosome model of perfusion. Cardiovascular revascularization Medicine 2011;12:10-19

Chapter 25

Impact of Renal Dysfunction and Peripheral Arterial Disease on Post-Operative Outcomes After Coronary Artery Bypass Grafting

Muhammad A. Chaudhry, Zainab Omar and Faisal Latif

Additional information is available at the end of the chapter

http://dx.doi.org/10.5772/54417

1. Introduction

In-hospital and long-term outcomes after Coronary artery Bypass grafting (CABG) are impacted by various factors including age, gender and various co-morbidities including chronic obstructive pulmonary disease, hypertension, diabetes Mellitus, dyslipidemia, chronic kidney disease (CKD), Peripheral arterial disease (PAD) and even connective tissue disorders such as systemic lupus erythematosus, and rheumatoid arthritis.

Both CKD and PAD have been considered a major risk factor for morbidity and mortality post-CABG [1]. Therefore, both are always considered as a variable when calculating risk for peri-operative mortality in patients undergoing CABG in the popular EUROSCORE and society of Society of Thoracic Surgeons National Cardiac Surgery Database scoring system [1,2].

We will discuss the degree of importance of these co-morbidities along with the epidemiology, underlying proposed pathogenetic mechanisms, significant associated co-factors, and also highlight the pertinent existing data on these parameters.

2. CKD and its impact on outcomes after CABG

Chronic kidney disease is defined as derangement in renal function for a period of at least six months. It is broadly divided into five stages based on creatinine clearance or glomerular filtration rate (GFR) obtained from either Cockcroft-Gault or modification of diet in renal disease (MDRD) equations [3,4]:

Cockcroft-Gault equation: Creatinine Clearance (ml/min) = [([140 − age] × weight [kg])/72 × serum creatinine (mg/dl)] (× 0.85 for women),

MDRD equation: GFR (mL/min/1.73 m^2) = 175 × (serum creatinine)$^{-1.154}$ × (Age)$^{-0.203}$ × (0.742 if female) × (1.212 if African American) (conventional units)

Creatinine clearance or glomerular filtration rate (GFR) represents renal function. Declining values represent a decline in renal function. Stage 1 refers to glomerular filtration rate (GFR) >90 ml/min and is generally asymptomatic. GFR between 60-90 ml/min is stage 2 CKD. Stage 3 is GFR between 30 and 60 ml/min and is further subdivided into Stage 3A (GFR 45-60 ml/min) and Stage 3B (GFR 30-45 ml/min). Stage 4 is defined by GFR between 15-30 ml/min while GFR <15 ml/min signifies Stage 5 and is considered an indication for renal replacement therapy i.e. dialysis. The most common etiological factors for CKD include diabetes mellitus and hypertension resulting in diabetic nephropathy and hypertensive nephrosclerosis, respectively.

The presence of CKD is considered a major independent predictor for development of coronary artery disease (CAD). An analysis from the atherosclerosis risk in communities (ARIC) study, Manjunath et al demonstrated that in 15,350 subjects with a mean follow up of over 6 years, there was a significant increase in acute coronary syndrome events in patients with stage 3 and 4 CKD (14.2%) compared with 5.5% in patients with stage 1 CKD (HR 1.38 (1.02, 1.87). Additionally, with every 10 ml/min/1.73 m^2 decline in GFR, there was a progressive increase in the incidence of cardiac events [5].

2.1. Proposed pathogenic mechanisms

Many factors contribute in the mechanisms associated in the renal contribution to increased risk of cardiovascular events. We briefly discuss a few here: Impaired renal function is associated with reduced erythropoietin synthesis and consequent anemia, which has been associated with cardiovascular disease [6]. Reduced 1, 25 (OH) vitamin D synthesis is associated with increased parathyroid hormone levels and higher prevalence of vascular calcification and arteriosclerosis [7].

Abnormal calcium phosphate metabolism is a consequence of renal dysfunction and it has a strong association with increased adverse cardiovascular events. Hyperphosphatemia and hypercalcemia are distinctly independent risk factors leading to a greater occurrence of cardiovascular events in patients with CKD and additionally, are also associated with poor surgical outcomes in patients undergoing CABG. Increased calcium-phosphate product greater than 55 and hyperphosphatemia escalates the development of secondary hyperparathyroidism which has been linked to increased osteoclastic activity and enhanced calcium-phosphate precipitation in the vasculature. There is also increase in the number of protein receptors in vessel cell membrane which increases deposition of calcium. In patients with CKD, vitamin D deficiency is also present even in the early stages. Vitamin D levels have a pivotal role in calcium-phosphorus homeostasis, regulation of parathyroid hormone (PTH), and bone metabolism and turnover. Three plausible mechanisms have been suggested in the protective effects of vitamin D against cardiovascular disease mortality are that vitamin D can inhibit various foci of inflam-

http://dx.doi.org/10.5772/54417

mation which is a key pathogenic mechanism in atherosclerosis; vitamin D also has an anti-proliferative effect on myocardial cell hypertrophy and proliferation and prevents remodeling which underlies the pathogenesis of congestive heart failure and vitamin D acts as an inhibitory endocrine regulator for the renin-angiotensin system, which triggers the cascade of hypertension and decompensated heart failure[8]. Thus, with low 1,25 hydroxy cholecalciferol levels, this effect is pronounced causing even further increase in cardiovascular risk.

We will discuss the outcomes of patients with CKD with the two modes of revascularization namely percutaneous and then, surgical. Additionally, we will take into account the impact of various comorbidities such as diabetes, dyslipidemias with respect to lipoprotein levels as well as the role of oxidative stress in this patient population.

Although long-term mortality may improve with surgical revascularization in dialysis patients with coronary artery disease, perioperative mortality continues to remain higher among patients with end-stage renal disease (ESRD) requiring CABG. Various studies have compared the outcomes of percutaneous coronary intervention (PCI) versus CABG and showed that mortality is not different [9-11]. However, these studies were from the 1990s and percutaneous techniques have been refined since then with improved outcomes. Newer studies are required to compare outcomes of percutaneous versus surgical revascularization.

2.2. Outcomes with percutaneous coronary intervention

In hemodialysis dependent patients (CKD stage 5), clinical outcomes of PCI are especially poor. Before the advent of coronary stents 20 years ago, when percutaneous revascularization was performed with balloon angioplasty alone, it was found that patients with ESRD experience a higher rate of coronary restenosis and recurrent angina, when compared to patients without ESRD [12]. In another case control study of twenty patients with ESRD and 20 age and sex matched controls without renal disease, it was shown that the rate of restenosis was 60% in ESRD patients, as compared to 35% in patients without renal disease. Restenosis was found to be dependent on size of vessel dilated and there was increased prothrombotic risk secondary to increased fibrinogen concentrations [13].

Many patients with ESRD experience silent ischemia. The possible mechanism being uremic polyneuropathy and therefore, may not experience typical ischemic symptoms.

In a prospective study of 5327 patients undergoing percutaneous coronary intervention (PCI) with a follow up of over five years, rate of death or myocardial infarction at one year was 1.5% in CKD patients with creatinine clearance >70 ml/min, 3.6% in patients with creatinine clearance between 50-70 ml/min, 7.8% between 30 and 49 ml/min and 18.1% with creatinine clearance less than 30ml/min. This study showed a progressive increase in adverse outcomes with worsening renal function. CKD was a strong predictor of adverse cardiovascular events including death and MI [14].

2.3. CABG in patients with renal dysfunction

Even though conflicting studies exist, a large study has shown that although there is increased risk of mortality in patients with ESRD undergoing CABG when compared to pa-

tients without significant renal disease, it still portends a better outcome in terms of mortality when compared to percutaneous revascularization in this patient population [15].

2.4. Hard endpoints after CABG

It has been shown that the lower the GFR, the worse the mortality after CABG. In a study of 2067 patients, it was found that estimated GFR was a powerful and independent predictor of mortality in multivariate analysis. Estimated average GFR in patients who died was 57.9+/-17.6 mL/min per 1.73 m^2 mg/dl, as compared to 64.7 +/- 13.8 mL/min per 1.73 m^2 in those who survived at an average follow-up for 2.3 years [16].

In a database review of 483,914 CABG patients over a three year period, it was shown that the post-operative mortality rates for stage 2, stage 3, and stage 4 CKD patients were 1.8%, 4.3% and 9.3 % respectively. Also, there was a higher incidence of stroke, need for re-operation, sternal infection, prolonged mechanical ventilation greater than 48 hours and a hospital stay of longer than two weeks [17]. In a prospective study of 15,500 CABG patients over a five year period, it was shown that dialysis dependent patients with CABG had higher risk of in-hospital mortality as compared to non- dialysis dependent CABG patients (12.2% as compared to 3.1%) and also significantly higher risk of mediastinitis (3.6 vs. 1.2%) [18].

One of the largest initial studies on CABG outcomes in ESRD patients 13 years ago was a retrospective study on 82 patients in which patients had a mean follow-up of 3 years. 18.5 % of the patients had left ventricular ejection fraction (LVEF) <0.45 and the aortic cross clamp time was fairly good at 50 ± 3 minutes [10]. Mean number of grafts was 2.3. Sixty-two percent of patients received left internal mammary grafts. In this study, 30-day mortality rate was 14.6%, and the mean survival rate at one, three and five years was 71%, 56% and 39% respectively. Thirty day mortality was 14.6% due to a variety of causes including myocardial infarction, cardiac arrest or cardiac tamponade. This study showed that although there was high peri and post- operative as well as long term mortality in ESRD patients undergoing CABG, there was a significant improvement in functional status as a result of CABG. The use of internal mammary artery grafts was related with less in-hospital mortality as well. Perioperative atrial fibrillation occurred in 12.1 % of patients within the first thirty days. With patients having preoperative Newyork Heart Association (NYHA) class III or class IV symptoms, LVEF less than 45% and age greater than 60 years, there was higher long term mortality. The incidence of post- operative bleeding and sternal infection was 3.6% which was higher when compared to patients not on dialysis.

Patients with CKD have a poor baroreceptor reflex. Therefore, they do not adjust very well in conditions like post-operative hypotension. Therefore, poor cardiac output can be more symptomatic in this group of patients [19].

In a study of 2438 CKD patients undergoing CABG over a three year period, operative mortality was 4.8% in individuals with stage 3 CKD and 7.1% in individuals with stage 4–5 CKD while it was 2.2% in those without significant CKD [20]. CKD was associated with increased post-operative blood transfusion requirement, acute kidney injury superimposed on CKD,

myocardial injury and cardiac arrest. Use of blood transfusions and acute kidney injury were strongly associated with in-hospital death in CKD patients.

2.5. Impact of mode of dialysis on outcomes after CABG

The mode of dialysis is equally important in influencing CABG outcomes, namely peritoneal (PD) and hemo-dialysis (HD). Peritoneal dialysis has been associated with worse outcomes when compared with hemodialysis [21,22]. Following CABG, diaphragmatic splinting, atelectasis and hypoxemia can occur after early post-operative initiation of PD. In a retrospective analysis of 105 patients, among whom 40 were on PD, and 65 on HD and all patients had been on dialysis for at least 2 months prior to CABG, it was demonstrated that the incidence of post- operative dialysate leak and peritonitis was 10% and 12.5% respectively in patients on PD. On the other hand, incidence of arterio-venous access thrombosis was 4.6% in patients on HD. Besides older age, PD was an independent risk factor of high operative mortality (adjusted OR for in hospital mortality in PD patients was 22.58). Actual causes of mortality included sepsis, cardiac arrest, pneumonia and gastrointestinal bleed. Chief infective organisms in septic patients were Staphylococcus aureus (coagulase negative), Pseudomonas aeruginosa, and Enterococcus faecalis [21]. Risk of peritonitis is higher if gastroepiploic artery is harvested for CABG as it requires diaphragmatic incision [22].

2.6. Impact of comorbidities in patients with CKD undergoing CABG

Diabetes and hypertension are the most common causes of CKD and they are also the major risk factors for coronary artery disease, therefore, the incidence of CAD is higher in these patients.

2.6.1. Diabetes

Diabetes is present in almost one third of CKD patients undergoing CABG and is considered a strong predictor of mortality in this patient group [23,24].

Szabo et al showed in a study of 2779 CABG patients that in 19.4% of patients with diabetes, the cross-clamp and cardiopulmonary bypass times as well as the need for inotropic support, transfusion of blood products and progression of renal failure were all higher in patients with CKD. Additionally, the incidence of post-operative stroke was greater in diabetic patients (4.3% vs. 1.7%). Five year survival rate was 84.4% in diabetic group while it was 91.3% in the non- diabetic group [25]. Another study showed that diabetes was an independent major predictor of morbidity and mortality in CABG patients. In 12,198 patients, it was observed that the diabetic group had higher rates of post-operative mortality (3.9% vs. 1.6%) and stroke (2.9% vs. 1.4%). The five and ten year survival rates were 78% and 50% among patients with diabetes as compared to 88 and 71% in the non-diabetic group [26]. Morris et al demonstrated in a study of 5654 patients undergoing CABG that the five year survival rate for diabetic patients was 80% as compared to 91% for non- diabetics [27]. Outcomes of CABG are improved in diabetic patients who undergo grafting of internal mammary arteries, with two being better than one. In a retrospective analysis of 4382 patients undergoing CABG, it was shown at 10 year follow-up that bilateral internal mammary ar-

tery grafting in addition to SVGs in diabetic patients improved survival and decreased need for revascularization compared with single internal mammary artery grafting along with SVGs [28]. The strong correlation between diabetes and cardiovascular outcomes including survival and myocardial infarction is due to the diffusely extensive and rapidly progressive nature of atherosclerotic coronary artery disease (CAD) in this group of patients. Various other factors such as oxidized low-density lipoproteins (LDL), hyperglycemia causing adverse metabolic shifts, deranged fibrinolysis, increased coagulability, and advanced renovascular hypertension resulting in change in vessel architecture also contribute to the progressive nature of CAD in diabetics. There is increased tendency for LDL induced atherosclerotic plaque formation and there is greater predisposition to thrombosis due to increased blood viscosity secondary to high plasma protein levels. There is also platelet and endothelial dysfunction and increased production of thromboxane A2 and von- willebrand factor along with decreased production of prostacyclins which creates a procoagulant state. Coronary vasodilation is impaired as a result of loss of the hyperpolarizing mechanics normally present in endothelial cells. Autonomic neuropathy in diabetes increases cardiac chrontropic workload and subsequently leads to greater oxygen demand even at rest. There is enhanced vascular tone in the coronary atherosclerotic plaque area leading to further reduction in blood flow, producing orthostatic changes which leads to reduction in coronary perfusion pressure and mitigates warning signs of ischemia such as angina [27,29-32].

2.6.2. *Hypertension*

Hypertension has also been associated with worse post CABG outcomes. In a multi centre study of 2417 patients among whom patients were categorized into patients with normal preoperative blood pressure, isolated systolic hypertension (systolic blood pressure >140 mm Hg), diastolic hypertension (diastolic blood pressure >90 mm Hg), or a combination of systolic and diastolic hypertension. It was found that isolated systolic hypertension was associated with a 40% greater risk of adverse outcomes such as stroke, renal failure, congestive heart failure and all cause mortality after CABG. Even after correction for confounding risk factor adjustment, the increased risk of adverse outcomes was significantly more pronounced in hypertensive patients [33].

2.6.3. *Impact of other risk factors*

In a study of 936 hemodialysis patients to elucidate correlation of recognized risk factors in CKD patients, it was found that correlation with diabetes, smoking, African-American race and increasing age of above fifty- five years was strong. It is suspected that non-traditional risk factors like uremic environment and hemodialysis procedure using arteriovenous fistulae and high output state associated with these fistulae also impact the outcomes after CABG adversely [34].

Dyslipidemia with a high LDL is a classic risk factor for development of CAD in the general population. However, it is likely not a major risk factor in patients with advanced renal disease. In a study of 210 dialysis dependent patients compared with 223 control subjects with normal renal function, it was found that high density lipoprotein (HDL) levels were low

while intermediate and very low density lipoprotein (IDL and VLDL) levels as well as triglyceride levels were higher in dialysis patients while there was no significant difference in LDL levels [35]. In part, the role of decreased renal metabolism of lipids leads to a decreased level of LDL is likely the cause.

Atherosclerosis is regarded as an inflammatory process [36]. It has also been shown that in dialysis-dependent patients, oxidative stress is increased resulting in a pro-inflammatory environment. As a result, incidence of cardiovascular events is increased. In a comparison study of 28 healthy subjects and 31 patients with renal disease, it was discovered that glutathione peroxidase and superoxide dismutase activities were increased in patients on HD while total glutathione and glutathione reductase activity is reduced resulting in increased oxidative stress [37].

2.6.4. Impact of renal artery stenosis on CABG

Renal artery stenosis (RAS) can lead to refractory hypertension and gradual deterioration in kidney function. The presence of underlying RAS and its effect on CABG outcomes has been studied and variable results have been obtained. In a study of 798 patients undergoing isolated CABG with 18.7% having renal artery stenosis (>50% stenosis), acute renal failure developed in 10.2% of patients post procedure. The mortality rate was 14% in patients who developed acute renal failure (ARF) post operatively, while it was 0.2% in patients who did not develop ARF. However, presence of RAS was not associated with development of ARF post-operatively [38].

In a series of eighteen patients undergoing CABG who also had varying degrees of RAS with mean serum creatinine of 2.6±2.7 mg/dl, RAS was not associated with adverse outcomes post-operatively [39].

2.7. Post-CABG complications in patients with CKD

Besides relatively increased short-term mortality in patients with CKD undergoing CABG, they also encounter increased morbidity from infections, blood transfusions, and stroke. In a retrospective analysis of 3954 patients where 82.7% patients had creatinine <1.5 mg/dl, and 16% had a serum creatinine level between 1.5 and 3.0 mg/dl, it was demonstrated that patients with a serum creatinine level >1.5 mg/dl had a mortality of 7% compared to 3% in patients with serum creatinine <1.5 mg/dl. Additionally, patients with a higher serum creatinine level had a higher incidence of requiring prolonged mechanical ventilation (15% vs. 8%), risk of stroke (7% vs. 2%), and bleeding complications (8% vs. 3%). Three infectious complications (mediastinitis, graft harvest site infection, and chest wound infections) were not different among these groups, whereas the occurrence of pneumonia and endocarditis was significantly higher in patients with a higher serum creatinine [40].

2.7.1. Prolonged mechanical ventilation

It is believed that the prolonged mechanical ventilation and the need for re-intubation after CABG in patients with renal dysfunction are due to a compromised ability to eliminate fluid

volume, thereby predisposing patients to impaired alveolar gas exchange. Additionally, renal failure would result in decreased metabolism and elimination of sedative, anxiolytic and analgesic drugs leading to impairment of respiratory drive.

A study showed that ventilatory complications such as need for greater than 48 hours of mechanical ventilation and re- intubation is high in patients with significant renal dysfunction undergoing CABG, when compared to patients with normal or mild renal dysfunction [40]. Another study showed a stepwise increase in need for prolonged mechanical ventilation as the renal function deteriorates. In this study, the ventilator dependence rate greater than 24 hours was 8.6%, 14.7%, and 20.2%, as the stage of CKD increased [20].

2.7.2. *Bleeding complications post CABG*

Platelet dysfunction is a consequence of uremia in patients with CKD and they are more prone to bleeding complications requiring blood transfusion. A study showed that significant renal dysfunction (serum creatinine of 1.5 to 3.0 mg/dl) significantly increases bleeding complications such as disseminated intravascular coagulation, gastrointestinal hemorrhage, or thoracic hemorrhage sufficient to require reoperation, or result in cardiac complications such as cardiac arrest and low cardiac output [40].

The association of transfusion with mortality is particularly interesting. CKD impairs erythropoiesis in the bone marrow due to reduced synthesis of erythropoietin, and is associated with pre-operative anemia of chronic disease and also leads to increased risk of bleeding after CABG [41]. Strategies to optimize preoperative hemoglobin and to minimize post-operative transfusion could possibly improve operative outcomes in patients with CKD. Transfusion needs are also increased as a result of uremia induced platelet dysfunction which can cause an increase in bleeding tendency in these patients.

2.7.3. *Other post-CABG complications in CKD*

Interestingly, occurrence of post-operative atrial fibrillation has been shown to increase with worsening renal function as well. In a study, the occurrence of atrial fibrillation was 22.2%. 19.2% and 16.5% in severe, moderate and mild CKD patients respectively [20].

Different studies have demonstrated the increased incidence of stroke in patients with CKD. In an analysis on 2438 patients undergoing CABG, the incidence of stroke was 3%, 2.7% and 1.7% in severe, moderate and mild CKD groups [20].

Infectious complications occur more commonly in patients with CKD undergoing CABG as well. A study showed that deep sternal infection, pneumonia, septicemia, infection involving a leg vein and overall infection rate was higher as the CKD stage increased (9.0%, 5.1%, and 3.5% in severe, moderate and mild CKD respectively) [20].

2.8. Impact of aortic cross clamp time in CABG

Aortic cross clamping time is the period during which an occlusive clamp is placed on the ascending aorta close to the innominate artery as a part of achieving cardioplegia before proceed-

http://dx.doi.org/10.5772/54417

ing with coronary bypass grafting. The mechanism of induction of cardioplegia involves prevention of repolarization of myocardial cell membrane due to the high potassium concentration of the cardioplegic fluid causing inactivation of the sodium channels which initiate the action potential. The hypothermic fluid of cardioplegia induces asystole. When the solution is administered in the aortic root it is termed antegrade and when administered in the coronary sinus, it is called retrograde. Myocardial protection with cardioplegia decreases the energy demands of the heart by arrest of the contractile apparatus. This is considered to be an extension of ischemia tolerance which is considered to minimize the deleterious effects of induced cardiac arrest. However, it still is desirable to keep duration of cardioplegia at a minimum as the aortic cross-clamp time is an important factor in predicting mortality in cardiac surgery and the lesser it is, the better the outcomes. The metabolic processes resulting from cardiac ischemia include sudden cessation of normal aerobic cardiac metabolic events, reduction in creatine phosphate, initiation of anaerobic glycolysis, and build-up of lactate and alpha glycerol phosphate as well as nucleotide metabolites. This is associated with contractile impairment and electrical pathway alterations consistent with typical EKG changes. The myocardial demand for high energy phosphate substrates is increased when the availability of adenosine triphosphate decreases. The predominant mode of energy derivation is switched to anaerobic glycolysis in the ischemic tissue. With early ischemic component, contractile activity and later on ion transport utilizes available adenosine triphosphate but gradually with the increase in ischemic time period, the metabolic demands undergo a compensatory reduction to prevent further ischemic damage. Irreversible injury in cardiac muscle is highlighted by very low levels of adenosine triphosphate, lack of energy production even by anaerobic mode, progressive accumulation of hydrogen ions, adenosine monophosphate, and lactic acid with a consequently high osmotic load, mitochondrial swelling and amorphous densities in matrix, and loss of integrity of the sarcolemmal membrane. The precise mechanism of pathogenesis is still elusive. In animal models, severe ischemia causes irreversible cell injury and death in one hour while with less severe ischemia in the mid and sub-epicardial myocardium, survival is possible up to six hours. Irreversible injury and cell death after six hours is inevitable. The ischemic injury changes reverse to a certain degree after reperfusion but how quickly and completely this transformation occurs is highly variable ranging from minutes to days. Aerobic metabolism is restored early while adenine nucleotide pool and stunning resolve slowly [42].

Systolic dysfunction with reduction in LVEF <0.40 is also an indicator of poor prognosis in CKD patients undergoing CABG. In a comparison study of aortic cross clamp times in patients with normal versus reduced ejection fraction in 27,215 patients in which 99.8 % received antegrade, retrograde or combined cardioplegia, it was found that prolonged aortic cross clamp time was an independent predictor of mortality [43]. It was shown that a combination of reduced LVEF and prolonged aortic cross clamp time especially with CKD compounds the ischemic effects and increases overall risk of perioperative mortality. In this study, the mean aortic cross clamp time was 68± 20 minutes, number of distal grafts was 3.1± 1.4 and 68.7% of patients underwent grafting of the left internal mammary artery. The incidence of pulmonary complications was 12.2% and stroke was 2.27%. Fifty-two percent of the patients had baseline hypertension, 29% had diabetes and 7% were dialysis dependent.

It has been shown that patients undergoing CABG with off pump or beating heart technique experience improved post-operative outcomes and less perioperative mortality. In a study

of 638 patients with acute coronary syndrome undergoing emergency CABG out of which 240 were operated off pump and 398 had standard on-pump CABG. 14.5% of patients were in cardiogenic shock along with serum creatinine greater than 1.8 mg /dl. Follow-up was up to 5 years. The results showed that in the off pump CABG group, in-hospital outcomes were significantly better. With off-pump CABG, skin incision to culprit lesion revascularization time was significantly reduced. There was less requirement for prolonged mechanical ventilation, less need for inotropic support, less incidence of atrial fibrillation, lower stroke rate (2.5 % vs. 6.7%), shorter intensive care unit stay and less sternal wound healing complications (2.5% vs. 3.5%). The overall hospital mortality rate was also reduced (5.7%) as compared to those on cardiopulmonary bypass (8.6%) [44].

2.9. Conclusion

As we have discussed, numerous studies have shown that patients with CKD have worse outcomes including an increased mortality and other complications after undergoing CABG, when compared to patients without CKD. However, an increasing number of patients with ESRD continue to undergo CABG and additionally, these patients are getting more complex a higher presence of comorbidities including diabetes, hypertension and obesity [Figure 1]. However, fortunately, in-hospital mortality rates have declined remarkably from over 31% to 5.4% in patients with ESRD (versus 4.7% to 1.8% among patients without ESRD) [45]. However, the mortality in ESRD patients remains 3-fold higher which indicates the need of continued work to improve outcomes in these patients [Figure 2].

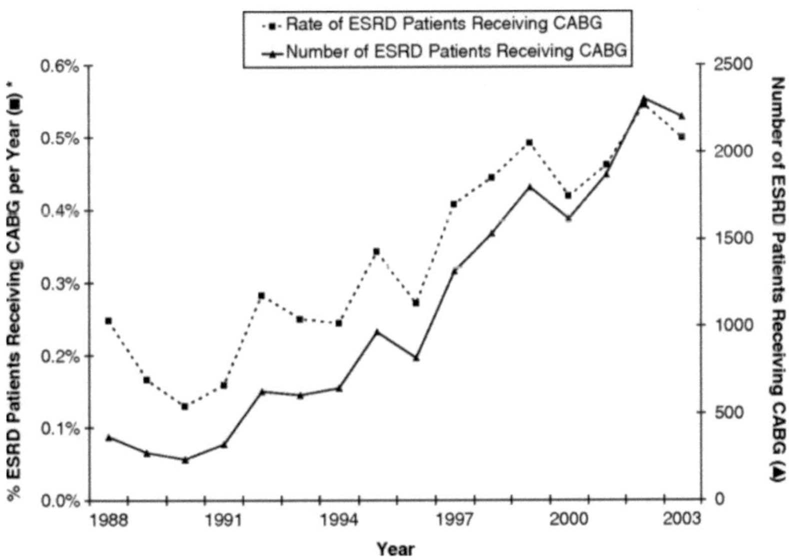

Figure 1. Graph depicting the increasing trend in the number of patients with end-stage renal disease (ESRD) undergoing coronary artery bypass grafting (CABG) over a 15-year period (Data from Parikh DS, Swaminathan M, Archer LE, et al. Perioperative outcomes among patients with end-stage renal disease following coronary artery bypass surgery in the USA. Nephrol. Dial. Transpl 2010; 25(7):2275-2283).

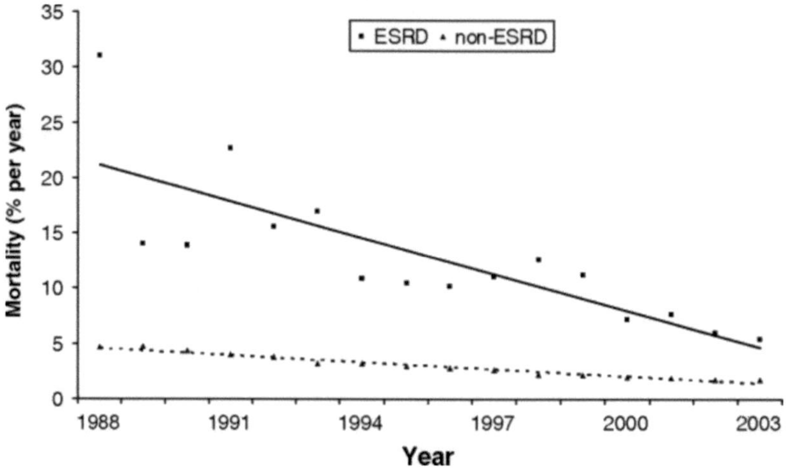

Figure 2. Graph depicting the constantly decreasing trend in mortality of patients with end-stage renal disease (ESRD) undergoing coronary artery bypass grafting (CABG) compared to patients without ESRD, over a 15-year period (Data from Parikh DS, Swaminathan M, Archer LE, et al. Perioperative outcomes among patients with end-stage renal disease following coronary artery bypass surgery in the USA. Nephrol. Dial. Transpl 2010; 25(7):2275-2283)..

Studies have shown that cardiovascular risk modification using ACC/AHA guideline recommended therapies for CAD, such as aspirin, beta blockers, hydroxymethyl coenzyme A (HMG-Co A inhibitors popularly known as statins) and angiotensin converting enzyme (ACE) inhibitors are used less frequently in patients with CKD when compared to patients without CKD [14,46-48]. These medications have been shown to decrease the risk of cardiovascular events across the population at risk. However, it is also true that many of those trials excluded patients with significant renal disease, which therefore poses a questions mark on their efficacy in patients with advanced CKD. Randomized trials to evaluate efficacy of these medications in patients with advanced renal dysfunction are warranted.

3. Peripheral arterial disease and CABG outcomes

The presence of peripheral arterial disease (PAD) plays a significant role in the potential morbidity and mortality of patients undergoing CABG. Coexisting CAD and PAD significantly influences long term survival adversely [49,50]. In the Coronary Artery Surgery Study (CASS), PAD was found to carry a higher risk of mortality even when compared to patients who had previously experienced myocardial infarction and angina [51].PAD is included as a major risk factor when calculating risk of mortality in patients undergoing CABG [1,2]. Non-invasive diagnostic testing for PAD includes segmental pressure measurement, treadmill stress, and Doppler ultrasound with the most significant information provided by the ankle-brachial index (ABI). Normally it is greater than 1.0 while <0.9 is considered abnormal. In patients with critical limb ischemia, the ABI is commonly <0.4. It is suspected that in PAD patients, poor surgical outcomes after CABG could be related to rapid progression of atherosclerotic coronary artery disease and more extensive small vessel

CAD with poor target foci for intervention resulting in higher mortality rates. Also the highly variable rates of CAD progression in patients with and without PAD leads to poor outcomes as well [52].

In comparison with PCI, CABG has been shown to improve mortality significantly more in patients with PAD. Data from 1305 consecutive patients undergoing coronary revascularization (PCI, n = 341; CABG, n = 964) between 1994 and 1996 showed that patients with PAD undergoing CABG had better survival at 3 years when compared to PCI (hazard ratio 0.68; 95% CI 0.46-1.00; p = 0.05) [53].

In a retrospective analysis on 1,164 consecutive patients who underwent CABG (370 with PAD), it was shown that PAD did not impact 30-day mortality. However, multivariable analysis showed that patients with PAD had a significantly worse 9-year survival rate compared to patients without PAD (72.9% vs. 82.8%; adjusted hazard ratio, 1.7; p = 0.004) [54]. Trachiotis et al studied long-term survival in 11,830 CABG patients, 744 of whom had LVEF <0.35. Among all patients, regardless of ventricular function, diabetes was linked with a 59% increase in the relative risk of death [55]. It was shown by Birkmeyer et al that patients undergoing CABG with history of PAD had a 20% five-year mortality rate as compared to 8% for those without known PAD [56,57]. Kaul et al showed that after risk factor adjustment, patients with PAD had mortality rates twice as high as patients without PAD [58]. Loponen et al showed in a multicenter study on 3000 patients that patients with PAD undergoing CABG had a 71% greater in-hospital mortality rate than those without PAD [59].

In a ten year prospective study of 8000 patients with PAD undergoing CABG, it was seen that they had a higher incidence of various intra- and post-operative complications including arrhythmias, stroke, pulmonary complications, low cardiac output state, longer hospital stay, infections, and acute renal failure. These results have been borne out by other studies as well [60-63].

The anatomic diversity of obstructive atherosclerotic disease process is particularly interesting. Patient can have isolated cerebrovascular disease involving carotid arteries, or lower extremity arterial disease or a combination thereof. It has been shown that as the number of involved arterial beds increases, the mortality increases. In a study on 2817 patients undergoing CABG, it was demonstrated that when compared to patients with CAD alone, the mortality was 1.6 times, 2.5 times, and 2.8 times higher for patients with concomitant cerebrovascular disease, lower extremity arterial disease and both cerebrovascular and lower extremity arterial disease, respectively [64]. Another study found that in patients younger than 40 years, the most common pattern of lower extremity arterial disease is aortoiliac disease while in patients older than 40 years, femoro-popliteal disease is predominant and causes intermittent claudication in 65% of these patients [65].

Commonly, patients with iliac disease have hemodynamically significant stenoses, while majority of patients with femoral disease have total occlusions characteristically involving long segments of the superficial femoral artery. Consequently, percutaneous revascularization of the femoral arterial segments is technically difficult as compared to iliac endovascular repair. The risk factors associated with PAD are similar to those for CAD, with diabetes

and smoking being the major ones. Diabetes is a major predictor of outcomes of CABG in patients with PAD. It is associated with more than 50% of major amputations in patients with PAD. In a study of 261 patients by Jonason et al (47 diabetic and 224 non diabetic), at six year follow up, showed an incidence of gangrene in 31% of diabetics as compared to 5% in non-diabetics [66]. Also hypertension, strong family history of premature atherosclerotic vascular disease, and hyperlipidemia are also contributory. Progression to severe ischemia or amputation in symptomatic patients with intermittent claudication occurs at 1.4% per year with poor prognosis in patients with diabetes and smoking [66,67].

The rate of all-cause mortality in patients with large-vessel PAD compared with the normal population is three times greater, while the risk of cardiovascular mortality is six-fold more, with the most common etiology being myocardial infarction or stroke [67]. In an analysis of 900 patients with LVEF of 0.35 or less, among whom 38% were diabetics, all-cause mortality was 26% in diabetics and 24% in non-diabetics ($p>0.05$). However, 4 -year re-hospitalization rates were 85% in diabetics and 69% in non-diabetics ($p = 0.0001$). The incidence of superficial sternal wound infection was 3.3 times higher and of renal failure was 2.2 times greater in diabetic patients as compared to non- diabetics [68].

Finally, a combination of CKD and PAD is even worse for the overall outcomes of patients undergoing CABG. In a prospective study of 36,641 CABG patients over a ten year period, long term survival rates of patient groups stratified as non- diabetic, diabetic with PAD and CKD, and diabetics without PAD and CKD were determined. The follow up was equivalent to 154,140 person-years. Annual mortality rates for non-diabetic and diabetic groups were 3.1 deaths per 100 person-years and 4.4 deaths per 100 person-years, respectively. The annual mortality rate for diabetic subjects with CKD, PAD, or both was significantly higher at 9.4 deaths per 100 person-years. Thus, patients undergoing CABG who are diabetic along with having PAD and CKD are at highest mortality risk over long term follow up of 10 years [69].

3.1. Impact of cerebrovascular disease on outcomes of CABG

Carotid artery stenosis is an important risk factor in determining post CABG outcomes such as stroke and additionally, has a direct impact on perioperative mortality [70,71]. Duplex ultrasonography or contrast-based techniques can be utilized pre-operatively in high risk patients with age greater than 65 years and multiple risk factors such as diabetes mellitus, hypertension, and previous transient ischemic attacks or stroke. In case of severe carotid disease, surgical planning might need to include carotid endarterectomy along with CABG simultaneously versus consideration for endovascular repair of carotid disease pre-operatively.

In a study of 582 patients undergoing CABG, preoperative carotid artery duplex scans were performed to assess the presence of asymptomatic carotid artery stenosis. >50% uni- or bilateral stenosis was present in 22% while >80% uni- or bilateral stenosis was present in 12% of patients. The post-operative hemispheric stroke rate in patients with carotid stenosis >50% was 3.8% as compared to 0.34% in patients without carotid

stenosis (p = 0.0072). Also the risk of hemispheric stroke was 5.3% in patients with unilateral 80% to 99% stenosis, or bilateral 50% to 99% stenosis, or unilateral occlusion with contralateral 50% or greater stenosis. Patients with a unilateral 50% to 79% stenosis did not suffer a stroke in this study [70].

In a study of 3344 patients undergoing CABG who were followed over a three year period to assess the effect of carotid artery stenosis on perioperative stroke and mortality, it was found that the clinical outcomes were directly related to the degree of carotid stenosis. Patients with carotid stenosis <60% had a significantly less risk of suffering perioperative stroke and mortality when compared to patients with >60% stenosis, especially patients with a totally occluded carotid artery [71].

These studies signify carotid artery disease as an important subset of patients with PAD which can adversely affect post CABG outcomes in terms of incidence of stroke and mortality rates.

3.2. Impact of microvascular disease on CABG

Microvascular disease, such as that which occurs in diabetic patients has also been shown to adversely affect outcomes after CABG. These complications generally stem from a cumulative poor glycemic control. In a study on 223 patients with diabetic retinopathy followed 11 years post-CABG, it was found that diabetic retinopathy was a strong independent predictor of overall mortality (relative risk [RR], 4.0), and repeat revascularization (RR, 3.0) [72].

3.3. Use of LIMA and SVG grafts

Use of internal mammary artery (IMA) grafts in patients undergoing CABG have been associated with improved short and long-term survival, increased patency and decreased perioperative mortality. However, in patients with significant PAD, it could be the major source of collateral flow to the lower extremities in patients with aorto-iliac disease. The finding that the mammary artery collateralized the iliac artery led to major treatment changes in all patients undergoing CABG [73]. Therefore, it is advisable to perform angiography of this conduit before referral for CABG in patients with PAD.

In a study on 21,873 patients among whom 87% underwent grafting of left IMA, and were followed for 7 years, there was a significantly decreased risk of mortality in all subgroups. Additionally, the incidence of stroke, repeat intervention, bleeding complications, mediastinitis or sternal dehiscence requiring surgery was less with use of IMA grafts. The adjusted mortality rate was 2.2% vs. 4.9%, and rate of stroke was 1.6% vs. 1.9% in patients undergoing IMA versus no IMA grafting, respectively. Infective mediastinitis or sternal dehiscence was seen in 1.1% of the LIMA group and 1.3% of the non-LIMA group [74].

It has been shown that use of LIMA grafts is even associated with lower in hospital mortality even in patients with a higher number of risk factors such as age greater than 70 years, elevated left ventricular end-diastolic pressure, left ventricular ejection

http://dx.doi.org/10.5772/54417

fraction less than 40%, small body mass index, or clinical presentation in acute or emergency setting. So, there is a proven consistent trend of protective LIMA effect in high risk groups as well [75].

3.4. Impact of PAD on graft failure in CABG

A major cause of short-term mortality post CABG and therefore, poor surgical outcome is graft failure. In 1972, Lesperance et al reported that out of a total of 105 saphenous vein grafts (SVG) used during CABG, 20% had early occlusion [76]. In a review of SVG disease, Motwani and Topol showed an early SVG occlusion rate of 15% and elucidated the diverse etiology of SVG closure [77]. At one month post CABG, the major cause of graft failure is thrombosis. From a month to one year post CABG, intimal hyperplasia is the chief contributor while after one year, atherosclerotic changes have been primarily implicated. They also demonstrated that arterial runoff was the single most important determinant of short-term graft survival. Occluded vessels distal to the SVG anastomosis resulted in thrombosis and graft failures.

The internal diameter of the mid-LAD is approximately1.7 mm, while that of the saphenous vein is 4-5 mm. This difference leads to variable flow rates and slow flow velocity in the SVG as compared to mid-LAD. The sluggish flow causes red blood cell sledging and consequent thrombosis. The internal diameter of the IMA is almost equivalent the mid-LAD, and thus there is decreased risk of graft thrombosis. They also highlighted that LIMA graft in addition to matching favorable dimensions of native LAD, lacks valves, has less endothelial fenestrations, and has a greater resistance to trauma while it is being harvested [78]. Other advantageous physiological characteristics of the IMA include higher flow reserve and shear stress, greater nitric oxide and prostacyclin production leading to vasodilation and inhibition of platelet aggregation, appropriate relaxation response to thrombin, less vasoconstrictor sensitivity and high vasodilator sensitivity along with decreased number of fibroblast growth factor receptors thus reducing plaque formation [78].

In a patent population in whom both radial artery and SVG grafts were used for CABG, it was found that radial artery grafts fared worse than SVGs in patients with PAD [79].

3.5. Off pump CABG and standard CABG

Off pump CABG (OPCAB) is referred to as CABG without use of cardiopulmonary bypass or cardioplegia while on pump CABG is referred to the use of cardiopulmonary bypass and cardioplegia. There have been various studies which generally show benefits of OPCAB as compared to standard CABG. Benefits include less bleeding complications, stroke and renal failure after OPCAB.

In a retrospective analysis of 68,000 patients by Ractz et al, 9000 OPCAB revascularizations were performed with this group comprising many high-risk patients including those with >60 years of age, female gender, low LVEF, previous history of CABG, stroke, PAD, conges-

tive heart failure, calcified aortic disease, and renal failure. It was seen that the standard CABG group as compared to OPCAB group had higher rates of stroke (2.0% vs. 1.6%), higher bleeding complications (2.2% vs. 1.6%), and prolonged hospital stay by one day. At 3-year follow-up, the need for repeat revascularization was also greater in standard CABG versus the OPCAB group [80].

In another retrospective study by Mack et al in which 17401 patients were reviewed and 7283 received OPCAB, it was found that even in patients with PAD among other risk factors, patients undergoing OPCAB had improved mortality when compared to patients undergoing on-pump CABG (1.9% vs. 3.5%). The rate of complications including major bleeding, wound infection, atrial fibrillation, permanent stroke, gastrointestinal and respiratory complications, renal failure, myocardial infarction, and multiorgan failure was higher in standard CABG group [81].

In another study comprising 214 patients at high risk (high EuroSCORE) with >50% of patients with significant PAD, it was found that off-pump CABG was safer and was associated with less early post-operative complications including multi-organ failure [82].

Patients with PAD are likely to have complex atheromatous plaques in the arch of aorta which poses a risk for peri-operative stroke during manipulation for on-pump CABG surgery An analysis of 422 patients demonstrated that there was a significant reduction in post-operative stroke in patients who had OPCAB when compared to patients undergoing on-pump surgery (0.9% vs. 5.7%, p=0.007) [83]. Therefore, for patients with PAD needing CABG, OPCAB would help avoid manipulation of aorta and in turn, decrease post-operative cerebrovascular complications.

Over a period of time, an increasing body of evidence has indicated that OPCAB is better than on-pump CABG, especially in high-risk groups. This includes a significant benefit of OPCAB in patients with PAD as it reduces the risk of postoperative stroke. As it has been shown in the SYNTAX trial, which is the largest contemporary trial comparing PCI versus CABG, showed that the major risk with CABG appears to be the increased risk of stroke from it [84]. OPCAB can, at least reduce that chance which might improve the overall benefit of CABG in patients with advanced CAD.

4. Conclusion

Based on current data, there is sufficient evidence to suggest that diabetes, peripheral arterial disease, CKD, on-pump CABG, increased aortic cross clamp and cardiopulmonary bypass duration, lack of use of IMA graft are strongly associated with poor in hospital, short term and long term outcomes after CABG. Rigorous modification of these risk factors to the maximum possible extent preoperatively can result in further improvement of surgical outcomes following CABG.

http://dx.doi.org/10.5772/54417

Author details

Muhammad A. Chaudhry[1], Zainab Omar[2] and Faisal Latif[3]

*Address all correspondence to: faisal-latif@ouhsc.edu

1 Scripps Green Hospital, La Jolla, California, USA

2 King Edward Medical College, Lahore, Pakistan

3 University of Oklahoma Health Sciences Center, Oklahoma City, Oklahoma, USA

References

[1] Roques F, Nashef SA, Michel P, Gauducheau E, de Vincentiis C, Baudet E, Cortina J, David M, Faichney A, Gabrielle F, Gams E, Harjula A, Jones MT, Pintor PP, Salamon R, Thulin L. Risk factors and outcome in European cardiac surgery: analysis of the EuroSCORE multinational database of 19030 patients. Eur J Cardiothorac Surg. 1999 Jun;15(6):816-22; discussion 822-3.

[2] Edwards FH, Grover FL, Shroyer AL, Schwartz M, Bero J, Clark RE. The Society of Thoracic Surgeons National Cardiac Surgery Database: current risk assessment Ann Thorac Surg 1997;63:903-908.

[3] Cockcroft DW, Gault MH. Prediction of creatinine clearance from serum creatinine. Nephron 1976;16 (1): 31–41.

[4] Levey AS, Bosch JP, Lewis JB, Greene T, Rogers N, Roth D. A more accurate method to estimate glomerular filtration rate from serum creatinine: a new prediction equation. Modification of Diet in Renal Disease Study Group. Annals of Internal Medicine 1999;130 (6): 461–70.

[5] Manjunath G, Tighiouart H, Ibrahim H, MacLeod B, Salem DN, Griffith JL, Coresh J, Levey AS, Sarnak MJ. Level of kidney function as a risk factor for atherosclerotic cardiovascular outcomes in the community. J Am Coll Cardiol. 2003; 41(1):47-55.

[6] Strippoli GF, Craig JC, Manno C, et al. Hemoglobin targets for the anemia of chronic kidney disease: a meta analysis of randomized, controlled trials. J Am Soc Nephrol 2004; 15: 3154-3165.

[7] Cozzolino M, Brancaccio D, Gallieni M, et al. Pathogenesis of vascular calcification in chronic kidney disease. Kidney Int 2005;68: 429-436.

[8] Levin A, Li YC. Vitamin D and its analogues: do they protect against cardiovascular disease in patients with kidney disease? Kidney Int. 2005 Nov; 68(5):1973-81.

[9] Agirbasli M, Weintraub WS, Chang GL, et al.Outcome of coronary revascularization in patients on renal dialysis. Am J Cardiol 2000;86:395-399.

[10] Labrousse L, de Vincentiis C, Madonna F, et al. Early and long term results of coronary artery bypass grafts in patients with dialysis dependent renal failure. Eur J Cardiothorac Surg 1999;15:691-696.

[11] Ivens K, Gradaus F, Heering P, et al. Myocardial revascularization in patients with end-stage renal disease: comparison of percutaneous transluminal coronary angioplasty and coronary artery bypass grafting. Int Urol Nephrol 2001; 32: 717-723.

[12] Kahn JK, Rutherford BD, McConahay DR, et al.Short- and long-term outcome of percutaneous transluminal coronary angioplasty in chronic dialysis patients. Am Heart J 1990;119:484-489.

[13] Schoebel F, Gradaus F, Ivens K, Heering P, Jax TW, Grabensee B, Strauer B, Leschke M. Restenosis after elective coronary balloon angioplasty in patients with end stage renal disease: a case-control study using quantitative coronary angiography. Heart. 1997; 78(4): 337–342.

[14] Latif F, Kleiman NS, Cohen DJ, Pencina MJ, Yen CH, Cutlip DE, Moliterno DJ, Nassif D, Lopez JJ, Saucedo JF; EVENT Investigators. In-hospital and 1-year outcomes among percutaneous coronary intervention patients with chronic kidney disease in the era of drug-eluting stents: a report from the EVENT (Evaluation of Drug Eluting Stents and Ischemic Events) registry. JACC Cardiovasc Interv. 2009;2(1):37-45.

[15] Herzog CA, Ma JZ, Collins AJ. A comparative survival of dialysis patients in the United States after coronary angioplasty, coronary artery stenting, and coronary artery bypass grafting and impact of diabetes. Circulation 2002;106:2207-11.

[16] Hillis GS, Croal BL, Buchan KG, et al. Renal function and outcome from coronary artery bypass grafting: Impact on mortality after a 2.3-year follow up. Circulation 2006; 113:1056-1062.

[17] Cooper WA, O'Brien SM, Thourani VH, et al. Impact of renal dysfunction on outcomes of coronary artery bypass surgery: Results from the Society of Thoracic Surgeons National Adult Cardiac Database. Circulation 2006; 113:1063-1070.

[18] Liu JY, Birkmeyer NJ, Sanders JH, et al. Risks of morbidity and mortality in dialysis patients undergoing coronary artery bypass surgery. Circulation. 2000; 102: 2973–2977.

[19] Zoccali C, Ciccarili M, Maggiori Q. Defective reflex control of heart rate in dialysis patients: evidence for an autonomic afferent lesion. Clin Sci Mol Med 1982;63: 285-292.

[20] Charytan DM, Yang SS, McGurk S, Rawn J. Long and short-term outcomes following coronary artery bypass grafting in patients with and without chronic kidney disease. Nephrol. Dial. Transplant 2010; 25(11): 3654-3663.

[21] Zhong H, David T, Zhang AH, Fang W, Ahmad M, Bargman JM, Oreopoulos DG. Coronary artery bypass grafting in patients on maintenance dialysis: is peritoneal dialysis a risk factor of operative mortality? Int Urol Nephrol. 2009; 41(3):653-62.

[22] Hamada Y, Kawachi K, Nakata T, Takano S, Tsunooka N, Sato M, Watanabe Y, Nakano N, Miyauchi K, Kohtani T. Cardiac surgery in patients with end-stage renal disease. Utility of continuous ambulatory peritoneal dialysis. Jpn J Thorac Cardiovasc Surg. 2001 Feb; 49(2):99-102.

[23] Herlitz J, Wognsen GB, Karlson BW, et al. Mortality, mode of death and risk indicators for death during 5 years after coronary artery bypass grafting among patients with and without a history of diabetes mellitus. Coron Artery Dis. 2000; 11:339–346.

[24] Clough RA, Leavitt BJ, Morton JR, et al. The effect of comorbid illness on mortality outcomes in cardiac surgery. Arch Surg. 2002; 137: 428–432.

[25] Szabo Z, Hakanson E, Svedjeholm R. Early postoperative outcome and medium-term survival in 540 diabetic and 2239 non-diabetic patients undergoing coronary artery bypass grafting. Ann Thorac Surg. 2002; 74: 712–719.

[26] Thourani VH, Weintraub WS, Stein B, et al. Influence of diabetes mellitus on early and late outcome after coronary artery bypass grafting. Ann Thorac Surg. 1999; 67: 1045–1052.

[27] Morris JJ, Smith LR, Jones RH, et al. Influence of Diabetes and Mammary Artery Grafting on Survival after Coronary Bypass. Circulation. 1991; Suppl III: III-275–III-284.

[28] Stevens LM, Carrier M, Perrault LP, Hébert Y, Cartier R, Bouchard D, Fortierand A, Pellerin M. Influence of diabetes and bilateral internal thoracic artery grafts on long-term outcome for multivessel coronary artery bypass grafting.. Eur J Cardiothorac Surg (2005) 27 (2): 281-288.

[29] Salomon NW, Page US, Okies JE, Stephens J, Krause AH, Bigelow JC.Diabetes mellitus and coronary artery bypass. Short-term risk and long-term prognosis. J Thorac Cardiovasc Surg 1983; 85(2):264-271.

[30] Jacoby RM, Nesto RW. Acute myocardial infarction in the diabetic patient: pathophysiology, clinical course and prognosis. J Am Coll Cardiol 1992;20(3):736-744.

[31] OsendeJI, Badimon JJ, Fuster V, Herson P, Rabito P, Vidhun R, Zaman A, Rodriguez OJ, Lev EI, Rauch U, Heflt G, Fallon JT, Crandall JP. Blood thrombogenicity in type 2 diabetes mellitus patients is associated with glycemic control. J Am Coll Cardiol 2001;38(5):1307-1312.

[32] Williams SB, Cusco JA, Roddy MA, Johnstone MT, Creager MA. Impaired nitric oxide-mediated vasodilation in patients with non-insulin-dependent diabetes mellitus. J Am Coll Cardiol 1996; 27(3):567-574.

[33] Isolated Systolic Hypertension Is Associated with Adverse Outcomes from Coronary Artery Bypass Grafting Surgery. Solomon Aronson, Denis Boisvert, William Lapp.A & A May 2002 vol. 94 no. 5 1079-1084.

[34] Cheung AK, Sarnak MJ, Yan G, Dwyer JT, Heyka RJ, Rocco MV, Teehan BP, Levey AS. Atherosclerotic cardiovascular disease risks in chronic hemodialysis patients. Kidney Int. 2000 Jul;58(1):353-62.

[35] Shoji T, Nishizawa Y, Kawagishi T, Tanaka M, Kawasaki K, Tabata T, Inoue T, Morii H. Atherogenic lipoprotein changes in the absence of hyperlipidemia in patients with chronic renal failure treated by hemodialysis. Atherosclerosis. 1997 Jun; 131(2): 229-36.

[36] Ross R. Atherosclerosis-An inflammatory disease. N Engl J Med1999;340:115-26.

[37] Schettler V, Wieland E, Methe H, Schuff-Werner P, Müller GA. Oxidative stress during dialysis: effect on free radical scavenging enzyme (FRSE) activities and glutathione (GSH) concentration in granulocytes. Nephrol. Dial. Transpl 1998; 13(10): 2588-2593.

[38] Conlon PJ, Crowley J, Stack R, Neary JJ, Stafford-Smith M, White WD, Newman MF, Landolfo K. Renal artery stenosis is not associated with the development of acute renal failure following coronary artery bypass grafting. Ren Fail. 2005; 27(1):81-6.

[39] Erentug V, Bozbuga N, Polat A, Tuncer A, Sareyyupoglu B, Kirali K, Akinci E, Yakut C. Coronary bypass procedures in patients with renal artery stenosis. J Card Surg. 2005; 20(4):345-9.

[40] Anderson RJ, O'brien M, MaWhinney S, VillaNueva CB, Moritz TE, Sethi GK, Henderson WG, Hammermeister KE, Grover FL, Shroyer AL. Renal failure predisposes patients to adverse outcome after coronary artery bypass surgery. VA Cooperative Study #5. Kidney Int. 1999 Mar; 55(3):1057-62.

[41] Winkelmayer WC, Levin R, Avorn J. Chronic kidney disease as a risk factor for bleeding complications after coronary artery bypass surgery. Am J Kidney Dis 2003;41: 84-89.

[42] Jennings RB, Reimer KA. The cell biology of acute myocardial ischemia. Annu Rev Med, 1991; 42:225-46.

[43] Doenst T, Borger MA, Weisel RD, Yau TM, Maganti M, Rao V. Relation between aortic cross-clamp time and mortality — not as straightforward as expected. Eur J Cardiothorac Surg 2008; 33(4):660-665.

[44] Rastan AJ, Eckenstein JI, Hentschel B, Funkat AK, Gummert JF, Doll N, Walther T, Falk V, Mohr FW. Emergency Coronary Artery Bypass Graft Surgery for Acute Coronary Syndrome Beating Heart Versus Conventional Cardioplegic Cardiac Arrest Strategies. Circulation. 2006; 114: I-477-485.

[45] Parikh DS, Swaminathan M, Archer LE, Inrig JK, Szczech LA, Shaw AD, Patel UD. Perioperative outcomes among patients with end-stage renal disease following coronary artery bypass surgery in the USA. Nephrol. Dial. Transpl 2010; 25(7):2275-2283.

[46] Wright RS, Reeder GS, Herzog CA, et al. Acute myocardial infarction and renal dysfunction: a high-risk combination. Ann Intern Med. 2002; 137:563–570.

[47] Best PJ, Lennon R, Ting HH, Bell MR, Rihal CS, Holmes DR, Berger PB. The impact of renal insufficiency on clinical outcomes in patients undergoing percutaneous coronary interventions. J Am Coll Cardiol 2002;39(7):1113-9.

[48] Smith SC, Benjamin EJ, Bonow RO, et al. AHA/ACCF Secondary Prevention and Risk Reduction Therapy for Patients With Coronary and Other Atherosclerotic Vascular Disease: 2011 Update: Title and subTitle Break A Guideline From the American Heart Association and American College of Cardiology Foundation Endorsed by the World Heart Federation and the Preventive Cardiovascular Nurses Association. J Am Coll Cardiol. 2011;58(23):2432-2446.

[49] Casser A, Poldermans D, Rihal CS, Gersch BJ. The management of combined coronary artery disease and peripheral vascular disease. European Heart Journal 2010;31(13):1565–1572.

[50] Steg G, Bhatt DL, Wilson PWF, D'Agostino R, Ohman M, Rother J, et al. for the REACH registry investigators one-year cardiovascular event rates in outpatients with atherothrombosis. The Journal of the American Medical Association, 297 (11) (2007), pp. 1197–1206

[51] Eagle KA, Rihal CS, Foster ED, Mickel MC, Gersch BJ for the Coronary Artery Surgery Study (CASS) investigators. Long-term survival in patients with coronary artery disease: importance of peripheral vascular disease. J Am Coll Cardiol 1994;23(5): 1091–1095.

[52] Shub C, Vlietstra RE, Smith HC, Fulton RE, Elveback LR. The unpredictable progression of symptomatic coronary artery disease: a serial clinical-angiographic analysis Mayo Clin Proc 1981; 56:155-160.

[53] O'Rourke DJ, Quinton HB, Piper W, Hernandez F, Morton J, Hettleman B, et al. Survival in patients with peripheral vascular disease after percutaneous coronary intervention and coronary artery bypass graft surgery. The Annals of Thoracic Surgery 2004;78(2): 466–470.

[54] Chu D, Bakaeen FG, Wang XL, Dao TK, LeMaire SA, Coselli JS, Huh J. The Impact of peripheral vascular disease on long-term survival after Coronary Artery Bypass Graft Surgery. Ann Thorac Surg. 2008;86(4):1175-80.

[55] Trachiotis GD, Weintraub WS, Johnston TS, Jones EL, Guyton RA, Craver JM. Coronary artery bypass grafting in patients with advanced left ventricular dysfunction, Ann Thorac Surg 1998;66:1632-1639.

[56] Birkmeyer JD, O'Connor GT, Quinton HB. et al. The effect of peripheral vascular disease on in-hospital mortality rates with coronary artery bypass surgery. J Vasc Surg 1995; 21445- 452.

[57] Birkmeyer JD, Quinton HB, O'Connor NJ. et al. The effect of peripheral vascular disease on long-term mortality after coronary artery bypass surgery. Arch Surg 1996;131316- 321.

[58] Kaul TK, Fields BL, Wyatt DA, Jones CR, Kahn DR. Surgical management in patients with coexistent coronary and cerebrovascular disease: long-term results. Chest 1994; 1061349-1357.

[59] Loponen P, Taskinen P, Laakkonen E. et al. Peripheral vascular disease as predictor of outcome after coronary artery bypass grafting. Scand J Surg 2002;91160- 165.

[60] Criqui MH, Langer RD, Fronek A, et al. Mortality over a period of 10 years in patients with peripheral arterial disease. N Engl J Med. 1992; 326: 381–386.

[61] Minakata K, Konishi Y, Matsumoto M, Aota M, Sugimoto A, Nonaka M, et al. Influence of peripheral vascular occlusive disease on the morbidity and mortality of coronary artery bypass grafting. Japanese Circulation Journal 2000;64(12):905–908.

[62] Collison T, Smith JM, Engel AM. Peripheral vascular disease and outcomes following coronary artery bypass graft surgery. Archives of Surgery 2006;141(12):1214–1218.

[63] Cooper EA, Edelman B, Wilson MK, Bannon PG, Vallely MP. Off-pump Coronary Artery Bypass Grafting in Elderly and High-risk Patients – A Review. Heart Lung and Circulation 2011;20(11):694-703.

[64] Pokorski RJ. Effect Of Peripheral Vascular Disease On Long-Term Mortality After Coronary Artery Bypass Graft Surgery. Journal of Insurance Medicine 1997, 29:192-194.

[65] Krajewski LP, Olin JW. Atherosclerosis of the aorta and lower-extremity arteries. In: Young JR, Olin JW, Bartholomew JR, eds. Peripheral Vascular Diseases. St Louis, Mo: Mosby-Year Book, Inc; 1996:208–233.

[66] Jonason T, Bergstrom R. Cessation of smoking in patients with intermittent claudication: effects on the risk of peripheral vascular complications, myocardial infarction and mortality. Acta Med Scand. 1987;221: 253–260.

[67] DeBakey ME, Glaeser DH. Patterns of atherosclerosis: effect of risk factors on recurrence and survival-analysis of 11,890 cases with more than 25-year follow-up. Am J Cardiol. 2000;85: 1045–1053.

[68] Whang W, Bigger JT. Diabetes and outcomes of coronary artery bypass graft surgery in patients with severe left ventricular dysfunction: results from The CABG Patch Trial database. J Am Coll Cardiol. 2000; 36(4):1166-1172.

[69] Leavitt BJ, Sheppard L, Maloney C, et al. Effect of Diabetes and Associated Conditions on Long-Term Survival After Coronary Artery Bypass Graft Surgery. Circulation. 2004;110(11 Suppl 1):I-I41-4.

[70] Schwartz LB, Bridgman AH, Kieffer RW, Wilcox RA, McCann RL, Tawil MP, Scott SM. Asymptomatic carotid artery stenosis and stroke in patients undergoing cardiopulmonary bypass. J Vasc Surg. 1995; 21(1):146-53.

[71] Tunio AM, Hingorani A, Ascher E. The impact of an occluded internal carotid artery on the mortality and morbidity of patients undergoing coronary artery bypass grafting. Am J Surg. 1999; 178(3):201-5

[72] Ono T, Kobayashi J, Sasako Y, Bando K, Tagusari O, Niwaya K, Imanaka H, Nakatani T, Kitamura S. The impact of diabetic retinopathy on long-term outcome following coronary artery bypass graft surgery. J Am Coll Cardiol. 2002;40(3):428-36.

[73] Ben-Dor I, Waksman R, Satler LF, Bernardo N, Torguson R, Li Y, Gonzalez MA, Maluenda G, Weissman G, Hanna NN, Monath A, Gallino R, Lindsay J, Kent KM, Pichard AD. A further word of caution before using the internal mammary artery for coronary revascularization in patients with severe peripheral vascular disease! Catheter Cardiovasc Interv. 2010 Feb 1;75(2):195-201.

[74] Leavitt BJ, O'Connor GT, Olmstead EM, Morton JR, Maloney CT, Dacey LJ, Hernandez F, Lahey SJ. Use of the Internal Mammary Artery Graft and In-Hospital Mortality and Other Adverse Outcomes Associated With Coronary Artery Bypass Surgery; Circulation. 2001; 103: 507-512.

[75] Cosgrove DM, Loop FD, Lytle BW, et al. Does mammary artery grafting increase surgical risk? Circulation. 1985;72:II-170–II-174.

[76] Lesperance J, Bourassa MG, Biron P, et al. Aorta to coronary artery saphenous vein grafts: preoperative angiographic criteria for successful surgery. Am J Cardiol. 1972;30: 459–465.

[77] Motwani JG, Topol EJ. Aortocoronary saphenous vein graft disease: pathogenesis, predisposition, and prevention. Circulation. 1998; 97:916–931.

[78] O'Connor NJ, Morton JR, Birkmeyer JD, et al. Effect of coronary artery diameter in patients undergoing coronary bypass surgery: the Northern New England Cardiovascular Disease Study Group. Circulation. 1996; 93: 652–655.

[79] Hata M, Yoshitake I, Wakui S, Unosawa S, Kimura H, Hata H, Shiono M. Long-term patency rate for radial artery vs. saphenous vein grafts using same-patient materials. Circ J. 2011;75(6):1373-7.

[80] Racz MJ, Hannan EL, Isom OW, Subramanian VA, Jones RH, Gold JP, Ryan TJ, Hartman A, Culliford AT, Bennett E, Lancey RA, Rose EA. A comparison of short- and long-term outcomes after off-pump and on-pump coronary artery bypass graft surgery with sternotomy. J Am Coll Cardiol. 2004; 43: 557–564.

[81] Mack MJ, Pfister A, Bachand D, Emery R, Magee MJ, Connolly M, Subramanian VA. Comparison of coronary bypass surgery with and without cardiopulmonary bypass in patients with multivessel disease. J Thorac Cardiovasc Surg. 2004; 127: 167–173.

[82] Munos E, Calderon J, Pillois X, Lafitte S, Ouattara A, Labrousse L, Roques X, Barandon L. Beating-heart coronary artery bypass surgery with the help of mini extracorporeal circulation for very high-risk patients. Perfusion. 2011;26(2):123-31.

[83] Karthik S, Musleh G, Grayson AD, Keenan DJM, Pullan DM, Dihmis WC, et al. Coronary surgery in patients with peripheral vascular disease: effect of avoiding cardiopulmonary bypass. The Annals of Thoracic Surgery, 77 (4) (2004), pp. 1245–1249.

[84] Serruys PW, Morice MC, Kappetein AP, et al. for the SYNTAX Investigators. Percutaneous Coronary Intervention versus Coronary-Artery Bypass Grafting for Severe Coronary Artery Disease. N Engl J Med 2009; 360:961-972.

Section 5

Miscellaneous Cardiac Surgical Topics

Chapter 26

Short and Long Term Effects of Psychosocial Factors on the Outcome of Coronary Artery Bypass Surgery

Zsuzsanna Cserép, Andrea Székely and Bela Merkely

Additional information is available at the end of the chapter

http://dx.doi.org/10.5772/54622

1. Introduction

Coronary heart disease (CHD) is the commonest form of heart disease in the developed world, and one of the leading causes of mortality and morbidity in these countries. Over the past decades numerous studies focused on the link between CHD and different psychosocial factors. The prevalence of depression in patients with diagnosed CHD is quoted between 20 and 45%. Elevated anxiety scores have been reported for 20 to 55% [1]. Emotional factors and the experience of chronic stress contribute to the development of atherosclerosis and cardiac events. Emotional factors include affective disorders such as major depression and anxiety disorders as well as hostility and anger. Chronic stressors include factors such as low social support and low socioeconomic status [2]. Similar prevalence ratios have been found for patients undergoing coronary artery bypass graft surgery (CABG). Symptoms of anxiety and unipolar depression are common psychological disturbances among patients undergoing CABG surgery. Numerous prospective cohort studies focus on the short and long term outcome of CABG. Research revealed that not only clinical factors e.g. cardiac status, comorbities and intraoperative factors have impact on the outcome [3]. Comparison of morbidity and mortality rates associated with psychosocial factors to morbidity and mortality rates related to traditional risk factors (smoking, obesity, and physical inactivity) showed priority of psychosocial background [4].

The purpose of this review is to provide a selected summary of key findings in this literature. We summarize some of the classic studies and historical developments important to the field and focus on prospective data on cardiac surgery patients. We review the literature on the important psychosocial domains (depression, anxiety, self rated health, happiness, illness intrusiveness, quality of life, gender differences, social support, negative affectivity, social inhibition, education) that have received much of the research attention, discuss key patho-

physiological mechanisms and pathways by which psychosocial factors may influence the outcome after surgery, and discuss some treatment directions likely to be critical to advancing the field.

2. Depression

2.1. Depression and Coronary Heart Disease (CHD)

Among emotional factors, depression has been most widely studied in recent years. Depressive disorders vary from mild (subclinical) depressive symptoms to classic major depression. According to the Diagnostic and Statistical Manual of Mental Disorders, depression is characterized by low mood and/or anhedonia (lose interest in activities that once were pleasurable) that lasts for two weeks or more and is accompanied by significant functional impairment and somatic complaints (insomnia, excessive sleeping, fatigue, loss of energy, or aches, pains or digestive problems that are resistant to treatment) [2]. Depression is 3 times more common in patients after an acute myocardial infarction than in the general community. In-hospital prevalence of major depression was 15% to 20% of patients with myocardial infarction, and an even more patients showed an elevated level of depressive symptoms [5]. Depression is regarded as an independent risk factor for atherosclerotic deposits in coronary arteries. The pathophysiological background covers hypercortisolaemia related to e.g. insulin resistance, sympathetic vagal dysbalance related to e.g. disturbed regulation of blood pressure, reduced heart rate variability, hypothalamic-pituitary-adrenal axis dysfunction, increased plasma platelet factor 4 (suggesting enhanced platelet activation), impaired vascular function, and increased C-reactive protein and fibrinogen levels (suggesting increased inflammatory response) and an unfavourable lifestyle like cigarette smoking, unhealthy diet, and lack of physical activity, medication adherence, as well as social isolation and chronic life stress [1, 5]. Depressive patients have higher risk of non-compliance with medical treatment regimens, therefore reduced chances of successful modifications of other cardiac risk factors and participation in cardiac rehabilitation, and have greatly reduced quality of life [5]. Major depression and elevated depressive symptoms are associated with worse prognosis in patients with CHD: in the Prospective Epidemiological Study of Myocardial Infarction (PRIME) Study, a multicenter, observational, prospective cohort, in healthy, European, middle-aged men were surveyed for the occurrence of first coronary heart disease and stroke events over 10 years. At baseline a questionnaire was used to define the presence of depressive symptoms. Results suggested that, baseline depressive symptoms are associated with an increased risk of coronary heart disease in the short-term and for stroke in the long-term [6]. Barefoot et al. assessed 1250 patients with documented CHD using the Zung Self-Report Depression Scale at the time of diagnostic coronary angiography and followed patients for up to 19.4 years. Results showed that patients with moderate to severe depression were at 69% greater risk for cardiac death and 78% greater risk for all-cause death [7]. Frasure-Smith et al. assessed gender differences in the impact of depression on 1-year cardiac mortality in patients hospitalized for an acute myocardial infarction. Increased depression scores were

http://dx.doi.org/10.5772/54622

significantly related to cardiac mortality for both genders (the odds ratio for women was 3.29, for men, the odds ratio was 3.05). Data were controlled for other multivariate predictors of mortality (age, Killip class, the interactions of gender by non-Q wave myocardial infarction, gender by left ventricular ejection fraction, and gender by smoking) and showed that depression was independent predictor for either gender [8]. Most studies that have examined the relationship between increasing depression severity and cardiac events have shown a dose-response relationship: in a 5-year-follow-up study post-myocardial infarction patients were recruited and assigned to categories based on the severity of depressive symptoms, ranging from no depressive symptoms to moderate to severe depressive symptoms. During follow-up period, a gradient relationship was observed between the magnitude of depressive symptoms and the frequency of deaths, with increased events occurring even in patients with mild depressive symptoms [9]. In the prospective study of Brown et al. elderly adults with significant depressive symptoms at baseline and without a current diagnosis of CHD at baseline were more likely to experience a cardiac event over a 15-year follow-up period. Depressed patients were 1.5 times more likely to suffer a cardiac event (i.e., acute myocardial infarction or cardiac death), even after controlling for demographics and known cardiovascular risk factors. The elevated depressive symptom severity is a predictor of cardiac events among older women and men as well as older white and black adults [10]. Despite methodological differences (sample sizes, sample characteristics, selection of covariates, etc) from study to study, the data from prospective studies with objective outcome measures and validated questionnaires for depression are remarkably consistent in their results suggesting depression is a risk factor for both the development of and the worsening of CHD [5].

2.2. Depression and CABG

CABG surgery is a common surgical intervention for CHD patients and prevalence of depression before or after CABG surgery is about 20–25% [4]. The presence of elevated levels of depressive symptoms results in a higher risk of mortality and significantly increased overall risk of major cardiac events following cardiac surgery [11]. In the prospective study of Connerney et al. 309 CABG patients were followed for 1 year after surgery. Compared with non depressed patients, depressed patients were more than twice as likely to have a cardiac event within 12 months after surgery but were not at higher risk for mortality within the first year [4]. In a larger sample of 817 CABG patients followed for up to 12 years, Blumenthal et al. assessed the effect of depression on mortality after CABG surgery. Depression was assessed both at baseline and 6 months after surgery. Results indicated that moderate to severe depression on the day before surgery as well as depression that persisted from baseline to 6 months after surgery were associated with 2-fold to 3 fold increased risk of mortality after adjustment for other risk factors [3]. Readmission following cardiac surgery is a significant burden on the healthcare system. In a prospective study, 226 CABG patients completed baseline self-report measures of depression, anxiety and stress and 222 patients completed these measures after surgery on the hospital ward. In multivariable analyses more than two-fold increase in readmission risk was associated with preoperative anxiety and postoperative depression, independent of covariates [12]. When our work group investigated the relation-

ship between depression, anxiety, education, social isolation and mortality 7.5 years after cardiac surgery, we found that there was a significant difference in depression (measured with Beck Depression Inventory (BDI)) between survivors and non survivors preoperatively, after discharge and in both intervals (Figure 1) [13].

First author and title	Number of patients	Methods	Results
Blumenthal JA. Depression as a risk factor for mortality after coronary artery bypass surgery.	817	CABG patients completed the Center for Epidemiological Studies-Depression (CES-D) scale before surgery, 6 months after CABG, and were followed-up for up to 12 years.	Patients with moderate to severe depression at baseline (adjusted hazard ratio [HR] 2.4, [95% CI 1.4-4.0]; p=0.001) and mild or moderate to severe depression that persisted from baseline to 6 months (adjusted HR 2.2, [1.2-4.2]; p=0.015) had higher rates of death than did those with no depression.
Connerney I. Relation between depression after coronary artery bypass surgery and 12-month outcome: a prospective study.	207 men and 102 women	CABG patients screened for depression with a structured psychiatric interview (diagnostic interview schedule) and a questionnaire (Beck depression inventory) before discharge. Outcome: cardiac events included angina or heart failure that needed admission to hospital, myocardial infarction, cardiac arrest, percutaneous transluminal coronary angioplasty, repeat CABG, and cardiac mortality. Non-cardiac events consisted of all other reasons for mortality or readmission.	63 patients (20%) met criteria for major depressive disorder. At 12 months, 17 (27%) of these patients had a cardiac event compared with 25 of 246 (10%) who were not depressed (p<0.0008). In a Cox proportional-hazard model with these five and two other variables of cardiac severity, major depressive disorder (risk ratio 2.3 [95% CI 1.17-4.56]), low ejection fraction (2.3 [1.07-5.03]), and female sex (2.4 [1.24-4.44]) were associated with adverse outcomes. Depression did not predict deaths or admissions for non-cardiac events.
Majed B. Depressive symptoms, a time-dependent risk factor for coronary heart disease and stroke in middle-aged men: the PRIME Study.	9601 men	The occurrence of first coronary heart disease (n=647) and stroke events (n=136) over 10 years among healthy men.	Depressive symptoms at baseline were associated with coronary heart disease in the first 5 years of follow-up (hazard ratio, 1.43; 1.10 1.87) and with stroke in the second 5 years of follow up (hazard ratio, 1.96; 1.21-3.19) after adjustment. The association was even stronger for ischemic stroke (n=108; hazard ratio, 2.48; 1.45-4.25).
Barefoot JC. Depression and long-term mortality risk in patients with coronary artery disease.	1250	Patients with established CAD were assessed for depression with the Zung Self-Rating Depression Scale and followed for subsequent mortality. Follow-up ranged up to 19.4 years.	Depression was associated with increased risk of cardiac death (p = 0.002) and total mortality (p < 0.001) after controlling for initial disease severity and treatment. Patients with moderate to severe depression had a 69% greater odds of cardiac death and a 78% greater odds of mortality from all causes than nondepressed patients. Patients with moderate to severe

			depression had an 84% greater risk 5 to 10 years later and a 72% greater risk after "/> 10 years compared with the nondepressed.
Frasure-Smith N. Gender, depression, and one-year prognosis after myocardial infarction.	613 men 283 women	Beck Depression Inventory (BDI) was used to assess depression symptoms during hospitalization after an acute myocardial infarction.	There were 290 patients (133 women) with at least mild to moderate symptoms of depression; 8.3% of the depressed women died of cardiac causes in contrast to 2.7% of the nondepressed. For depressed men, the rate of cardiac death was 7.0% in contrast to 2.4% of the nondepressed. Increased BDI scores were significantly related to cardiac mortality for both genders [the odds ratio for women was 3.29 (95% confidence interval (CI) = 1.02-10.59); for men, the odds ratio was 3.05 (95% CI = 1.29-7.17)]. Control for other multivariate predictors of mortality in the data set (age, Killip class, the interactions of gender by non-Q wave MI, gender by left ventricular ejection fraction, and gender by smoking) did not change the impact of the BDI for either gender.
Lesperance F. Five-year risk of cardiac mortality in relation to initial severity and one-year changes in depression symptoms after myocardial infarction	896	Beck Depression Inventory was administered to the patients after myocardial infarction during admission and at 1 year. Five-year survival was ascertained using Medicare data	Significant long-term dose-response relationship between depression symptoms during hospitalization and cardiac mortality was observed. Results remained significant after control for multiple measures of cardiac disease severity. Although 1-year scores were also linked to cardiac mortality, most of that impact was explained by baseline scores. Improvement in depression symptoms was associated with less cardiac mortality only for patients with mild depression. Patients with higher initial scores had worse long-term prognosis regardless of symptom changes.
Brown JM. Risk of coronary heart disease events over 15 years among older adults with depressive symptoms	2728	Depressive symptom severity at baseline was assessed by the Center for Epidemiologic Studies Depression Scale among primary care practice patients. Data regarding baseline demographic and clinical variables, as well as laboratory evidence of acute MI, were obtained from an electronic medical record system. All-cause mortality and CHD death were determined from the National Death Index through 2006.	Cox proportional hazards models showed that individuals with elevated depressive symptoms were more likely to experience a CHD event, even after adjustment for demographics and comorbid health conditions (relative risk = 1.46, 95% confidence interval: 1.20-1.77). Depression status was also a significant predictor of all-cause mortality in adjusted models.

Tully PJ. The role of depression and anxiety symptoms in hospital readmissions after cardiac surgery.	226	Hospital readmissions after coronary artery bypass graft surgery were assessed.	When analyzed as continuous variables in multivariable analyses, preoperative anxiety and postoperative depression predicted readmissions independent of medical covariates. In multivariable analyses with dichotomized anxiety, depression and stress, more than two-fold increase in readmission risk was attributable to preoperative anxiety and postoperative depression, independent of covariates.

Table 1. Some important studies about depression and CABG

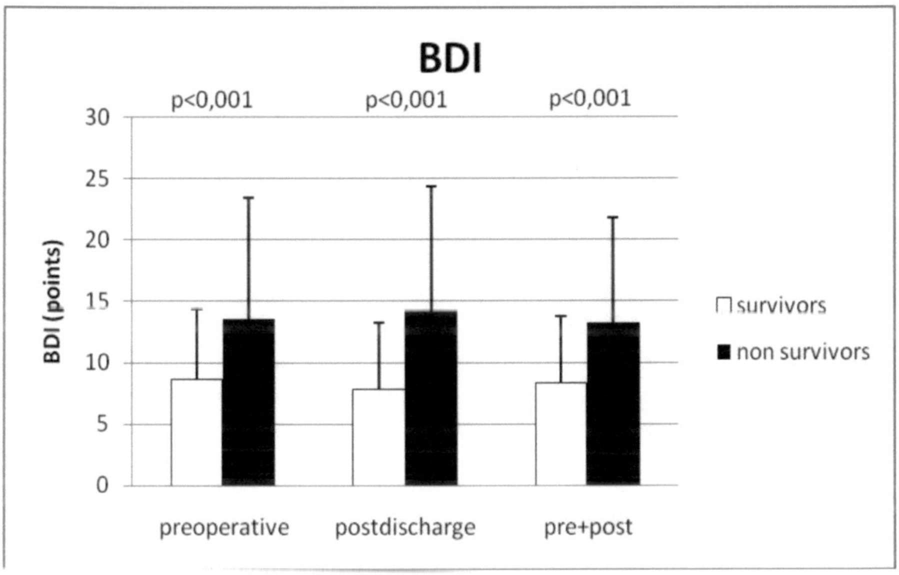

Figure 1. Figure showes significant difference in depression (BDI points) between survivors and non survivors preoperatively, after discharge and in both intervals.

3. Anxiety

3.1. Anxiety and coronary heart disease

Anxiety has been characterized as a future-oriented, negative affective state with a component of fear, resulting from the perception of threat and the individual's perceived inability to predict, control, or obtain the desired results in upcoming situations. Somatic manifestations are tachycardia, hyperventilation, sweating, psychological manifestations are feelings of apprehension, nervousness, restlessness, and may also cause changes in sleeping pattern [13].

http://dx.doi.org/10.5772/54622

Pathophysiological background by which anxiety influences outcome in ischemic heart disease is largely unknown. An increased incidence of ECG QT interval prolongation has been demonstrated among patients with anxiety, which increases the occurrence of ventricular arrhythmia [14]. Patients with anxiety have been shown consistently to have sympathetic nervous system upregulation, with excessive catecholamine production [15]. Furthermore, impaired vagal control, manifest as an impaired baroreflex response and a decrease in heart rate variability has been noted in patients with anxiety. Impairment of the baroreflex response and decreased heart rate variability are each thought to be sensitive markers for abnormalities in autonomic cardiovascular regulation and are independent risk factors for sudden cardiac death [16, 17, 18]. Patients with anxiety and CAD often show an exaggerated systemic response to stress, characterized by an abnormally increased production of catecholamines, which can result in increased myocardial oxygen demand due to elevations in heart rate, blood pressure, and the rate of ventricular contraction [19]. In addition to the biological risks of anxiety, the additive effects of adverse behavioural risk factors (e.g., excessive nicotine and perhaps caffeine) in anxious patients have also be taken into account [20]. Anxiety is very common in patients with myocardial infarction, with an inhospital occurrence rate of 30% to 40% [21]. Studies with coronary patients suggest that anxiety disorders may be associated with greater mortality, particularly sudden cardiac death, and greater cardiovascular morbidity. Higher levels of anxiety have been associated with poorer prognosis and greater recurrence of cardiac events after myocardial infarction [22]. In a cohort study the relative importance of depression, anxiety, anger, and social support in predicting 5-year cardiac-related mortality following a myocardial infarction was investigated. Higher level of anxiety predicted greater cardiac-related mortality in a sample of nearly 900 patients with myocardial infarction, but this effect was non significant following adjustment for disease severity [23]. The first meta-analysis on the association of anxiety and coronary heart disease showed a consistent association between anxiety and impaired prognosis after myocardial infarction, with a 36% increased risk for mortality (cardiac and all-cause) and for cardiac events. Limitation of the result was the pooled odds ratios for cardiac death, because it was based on only four studies [21].

3.2. Anxiety and CABG

Anxiety is especially high for CABG patients while they are on the waiting list with an unknown surgery date [24]. The patients have fear of dying before, rather than during surgery, and this fear influenced strongly their level of anxiety. Anxiety also manifests as an activator of sympathetic and parasympathetic nervous systems and cardiovascular excitation that can exacerbate CAD symptoms. After surgery, while anxiety may decrease to below pre-operative level, the severity of anxiety does not necessarily remit to below sub-clinical levels and may warrant intervention [25]. In the Post-CABG Trial the presence of anxiety symptoms was significantly associated with a higher incidence rate of death or myocardial infarction after a median follow-up time of 4.3 years following CABG. After controlling for the presence of depressive symptoms and other covariates (age, gender, race, treatment assignment and years since CABG surgery), a significant dose-response relationship persisted between anxiety and mortality. The observed dose-response relationship between level of anxiety and risk of death or myocardial infarction underlines the importance of even lower levels of anxiety. The risk

of death or myocardial infarction in those with both depressive and anxiety symptoms was what would be expected from the combination of the independent effects [26]. In a study of our workgroup trait anxiety was associated with increased mortality and cardiovascular morbidity. In our population trait anxiety remained an independent predictor for post-discharge cardiovascular events and 4 year mortality. Moreover, post-discharge 6th month trait anxiety scores were more predictive for cardiovascular events compared to the preoperative values. Although anxiety and depression were positively and highly correlated in these patients, only anxiety was associated with increased mortality and morbidity. In addition trait anxiety was significantly higher in patients hospitalized with arrhythmia, congestive heart failure or myocardial infarction during a 4 year period after cardiac (CABG and valve) surgery [27]. In another study of our workgroup depression, anxiety, education, social isolation and mortality together were investigated 7.5 years after cardiac surgery. Our results have suggested that the assessment of psychosocial factors, particularly anxiety and education may help identify patients at an increased risk for long-term mortality after cardiac surgery (Figure 2.) [13]. Anxiety was also reported to be associated with twofold risk for fatal CHD and more than fourfold risk for sudden death [28]. In a retrospective study 17,885 discharge records of patients after primary CABG surgery were identified. In the sample of rural patients the prevalence of anxiety disorder was 27%. Anxiety was a significant independent predictor of both length of hospital stay and non routine discharge [29]. In a prospective study on cardiac-related readmission within 6 months of CABG postoperative anxiety was identified as both a univariate risk factor and a multivariate risk factor for CHD and surgery-related readmission both with and without adjustment for covariates [30].

First author and title	Number of patients	Methods	Results
Cserep Z. The impact of preoperative anxiety and education level on long-term mortality after cardiac surgery.	180	Anxiety (Spielberger State-Trait Anxiety Inventory, STAI-S/STAI-T), depression (Beck Depression Inventory, BDI) and the number and reason for rehospitalizations were assessed each year in cardiac surgery patients.	During a median follow-up of 7.6 years (25th to 75th percentile, 7.4 to 8.1 years), the mortality rate was 23.6% (95% confidence interval [CI] 17.3-29.9; 42 deaths). In a Cox regression model, the risk factors associated with an increased risk of mortality were a higher EUROSCORE (points; Adjusted Hazard Ratio (AHR):1.30, 95%CI:1.07-1.58)), a higher preoperative STAI-T score (points; AHR:1.06, 95%CI 1.02-1.09), lower education level (school years; AHR:0.86, 95%CI:0.74-0.98), and the occurrence of major adverse cardiac and cerebral events during follow up (AHR:7.24, 95%CI: 2.65-19.7). In the postdischarge model, the same risk factors remained.

Frasure-Smith N. Depression and other psychological risks following myocardial infarction	896	Beck Depression Inventory, state scale of the State-Trait Anxiety Inventory, 20-item version of the General Health Questionnaire, Modified Somatic Perception Questionnaire, Anger Expression Scale, Perceived Social Support Scale, number of close friends and relatives, and visual analog scales of anger and stress were assessed to predict 5-year cardiac-related mortality following a myocardial infarction.	The Beck Depression Inventory (P<0.001), the State-Trait Anxiety Inventory (P =0.04), and the 20-item version of the General Health Questionnaire (P = 0.048) were related to outcome, but only depression remained significant after adjustment for cardiac disease severity (hazards ratio per SD, 1.46; 95% confidence interval, 1.18-1.79) (P<0.001). There was also a covariate-adjusted trend between negative affectivity scores and outcome (P = 0.08). Furthermore, residual depression scores (P =0.001) and negative affectivity scores (P = 0.05) were linked to cardiac-related mortality after adjustment for each other and cardiac covariates.
Koivula M. Fear and anxiety in patients at different time-points in the coronary artery bypass process.	171	CABG patients completed questionnaires while awaiting surgery at home, in hospital the evening before surgery and 3 months later. The Bypass Grafting Fear scale was developed to measure fear. Anxiety was measured using State-Trait-Anxiety Inventory.	The highest levels of fear and anxiety were measured in the waiting period to coronary CABG. Compared with the waiting period, fear and anxiety levels dropped in hospital and 3 months later. Female gender was related to change in fear and anxiety.
Rosenbloom JI. Self-reported anxiety and the risk of clinical events and atherosclerotic progression among patients with Coronary Artery Bypass Grafts (CABG).	1317	CABG patients were randomized to either aggressive or moderate lipid lowering and to either warfarin or placebo. Patients were followed up for clinical end points and coronary angiography was conducted at enrollment and after a median follow-up of 4.3 years. Anxiety symptoms were assessed at enrollment using the state portion of the Spielberger State-Trait Anxiety Inventory (STAI)	STAI score "/> or =40 was positively associated with risk of death or myocardial infarction (MI) (OR 1.55, 95% CI 1.01-2.36, P =0.044). This association was attenuated slightly when depressive symptoms were included in the model, but lost statistical significance (P = 0.11). There was a dose-response relationship between STAI score and risk of death or myocardial infarction. There was no association between self-reported anxiety and atherosclerotic progression of grafts.
Székely A. Anxiety predicts mortality and morbidity after coronary artery and valve surgery--a 4-year follow-up study.	180	Patients who underwent cardiac surgery using cardiopulmonary bypass were prospectively studied and followed up for 4 years. Anxiety (Spielberger State-Trait Anxiety Inventory, STAI-S/STAI-T), depression (Beck Depression Inventory, BDI), living alone, and education level along with clinical risk factors and	Average preoperative STAI-T score was 44.8 +/- 10. Kaplan-Meier analysis showed a significant effect of preoperative STAI-T "/>45 points (p =0.008) on mortality. In multivariate models, postoperative congestive heart failure (OR: 10.8; 95% confidence interval [CI]: 2.9-40.1; p =0 .009) and preoperative

		perioperative characteristics were assessed. Psychological self-report questionnaires were completed preoperatively and 6, 12, 24, 36, and 48 months after discharge. Clinical end-points were mortality and cardiac events requiring hospitalization during follow-up.	STAI-T (score OR: 1.07; 95% CI: 1.01-1.15; p = 0.05) were independently associated with mortality. The occurrence of cardiovascular hospitalization was independently associated with postoperative intensive care unit days (OR: 1.41; 95% CI: 1.01-1.96; p =0.045) and post discharge 6th month STAI-T (OR: 1.06; 95% CI:1.01-1.13; p = .03).
Kawachi I. Symptoms of anxiety and risk of coronary heart disease. The Normative Aging Study.	402 cases of incident coronary heart disease	An anxiety symptoms scale was constructed out of five items from the Cornell Medical Index, which was administered to the cohort at baseline. During 32 years of follow-up incidence of CHD was observed.	Compared with men reporting no symptoms of anxiety, men reporting two or more anxiety symptoms had elevated risks of fatal CHD (age-adjusted odds ratio [OR] = 3.20, 95% confidence interval [CI]: 1.27 to 8.09), and sudden death (age-adjusted OR = 5.73, 95% CI: 1.26 to 26.1). The multivariate OR after adjusting for a range of potential confounding variables was 1.94 (95% CI: 0.70-5.41) for fatal CHD and 4.46 (95% CI: 0.92-21.6) for sudden death. No excess risks were found for nonfatal myocardial infarction or angina.
Dao TK. Gender as a moderator between having an anxiety disorder diagnosis and coronary artery bypass grafting surgery (CABG) outcomes in rural patients.	17,885	Patients who underwent a primary CABG surgery were identified. Independent variables included age, gender, race, median household income based on patient's ZIP code, primary expected payer, the Deyo, Cherkin, and Ciol Comorbidity Index, and an anxiety comorbidity diagnosis. Outcome variables included in-hospital length of stay and patient disposition (routine and nonroutine discharge).	27% of rural patients had a comorbid anxiety diagnosis. Rural patients who had nonroutine discharge were more likely to have comorbid anxiety diagnosis compared to rural patients who had a routine discharge. There was a significant interaction effect between having an anxiety diagnosis and gender on length of hospital stay but not for patient disposition.
Oxlad M. Psychological risk factors for cardiac-related hospital readmission within 6 months of coronary artery bypass graft surgery.	119	Consecutive patients awaiting elective CABG, completed a battery of psychosocial measures in a three-stage repeated-measures design. Relevant medical data were also extracted from patients' medical records 6 months postoperatively to allow for the examination of potential covariates.	Increased postoperative anxiety and increased preoperative depression, were identified as risk factors for cardiac-related readmission independent of the only significant covariate identified, cardiopulmonary bypass time.

Table 2. Some important studies about anxiety and CABG

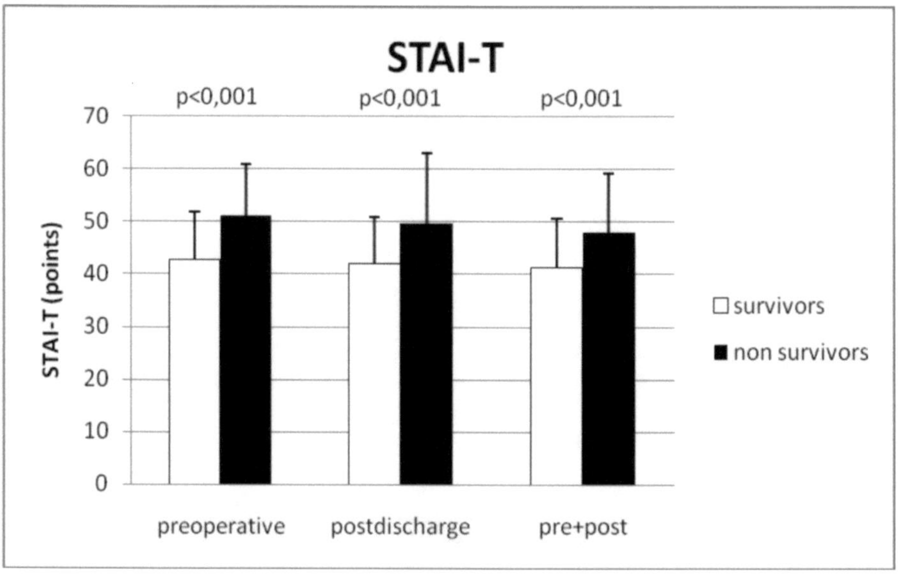

Figure 2. Figure showes significant difference in STAI-T (State-Trait Anxiety Inventory) between survivors and non survivors preoperatively, after discharge and in both intervals.

4. Self rated health

Self-rated health (SRH) is measured with a simple question "How do you rate your health in general?" There are five possible responses: very good, good, fair, poor and very poor [31]. Self rated health has been shown to be a potent predictor of mortality and morbidity, functional decline, disability and utilization of health care even after controlling for several sociodemographic and health indicators The association can be explained by three ways: (1) SRH is a more comprehensive and sensitive measure of health status than the other psychosocial covariates in the analyses; (2) SRH measures individual optimistic or pessimistic disposition, that as such, may be associated with survival; or (3) SRH also measures characteristics other than health status itself, such as family history, health behaviour, and social and psychological resources [32]. In a review SRH was described as an active cognitive process that is independent from formal definitions of health. Self rated health covers bodily sensations that are directly available only to the individuals. These sensations may reflect important physiological dysregulations, such as inflammatory processes. SRH is an individual and subjective conception that is related to death, and builds a connection from the social world and psychological to the biological world. Therefore the answer to the SRH question may summarize the dimensions of health that are most important and determinant to each individual [33]. SRH has been described as one of the most important health outcomes available and recommended as a tool for disease risk screening, as an outcome indicator in the primary care, and standard part of clinical trials [34]. Several studies in different field confirmed the importance of SRH, one of them described that good self health 3 months after PCI predicted good clinical outcome

after 4 years [35]. SRH was reported as an independent predictor of long term mortality in older women after myocardial infarction. Patients dissatisfied with their general health status were at more than six times higher risk of mortality than the satisfied ones [36]. There are only few data available on the link between CABG and SRH. Oxlad et al. investigated consecutive elective CABG patients on self-report measures including optimism, illness representations, self-rated health, social support, coping methods, depression, anxiety and post-traumatic stress disorder. Poor pre-operative psychological functioning was the strongest psychological risk factor for adverse psychological functioning six months post-operatively [37].

5. Happiness

Negative emotional states (e.g., depression, anxiety) are proven risk factors for cardiovascular disease; however, much less is known about the association between positive emotional states (e.g., happiness and optimism) and cardiovascular health. Steptoe et al. have suggested that positive emotions may have direct and beneficial effects on physiological processes including those involving the neuroendocrine, inflammatory, immunological and cardiovascular systems [38]. The association between positive psychological well-being and mortality could be mediated in part via behavioural pathways. For example positive dispositions are related to predictors of prolonged survival, such as not smoking, exercising regularly, reduced alcohol consumption, and better sleep quality. Psychologically balanced persons might have increased adherence to medical regimens because inverse associations between adherence and depression have been described. However, the protective effect of positive emotions on mortality in healthy population studies persisted even after fully controlling for behavioural covariates, suggesting that other pathways may also be involved. Direct physiological pathways might also contribute to associations. Positive psychological well-being could alter people's disease susceptibility via the attenuation of sympathetic nervous system activity and the enhancement of parasympathetic activation. Positive affects may reduce stress-induced elevations of inflammatory and coagulation factors, such as fibrinogen and interleukin-6, which are crucial in cardiovascular disease, and reduce vulnerability to infectious illness. Positive psychological well-being was associated with reduced cardiovascular mortality in healthy population studies, with a near significant effect in patients with established cardiovascular disease [39]. In one of prospective epidemiological cohort studies participants with greater emotional vitality were at markedly reduced risk for CHD, and this effect remained significant after controlling for medical and psychosocial factors [40]. Optimism was associated with recovery from CABG surgery within 6 months [41]. Post hoc analysis of previous data showed that among depressed post-CABG patients, optimists responded to depression treatment at higher rates. Independent of depression, optimists were less likely to be rehospitalized by 8 months after CABG [42].

6. Illness intrusiveness

One of the important determinants of quality of life is taking part in psychologically meaningful activity. Illnesses, mostly chronic ones interfere with valued activities. Illness intrusive-

ness is a determinant of quality of life in patients with chronic disease. Illness intrusiveness covers the disease- and treatment-induced disruptions to lifestyles, activities, and interests [43]. There is only one available study about the relationship of illness intrusiveness and CABG: our work group investigated psychosocial factors like illness intrusiveness, depression, anxiety, sleeping disorders and found an independent association with the occurrence of major adverse cardiac and cerebrovascular events (MACCE) after adjustment of biomedical factors and perioperative variables following cardiac surgery. Additionally, severity of illness intrusiveness, sleeping problems and social inhibition increased in the MACCE positive patients during the three-year period; these tendencies were not observed in the event-free group [44].

7. Quality of life

With aging of the population and sophisticated health care technologies the number of patients with chronic diseases has extremely increased. As a result, improving the daily functioning and quality of life of the chronically ill has become an important goal of medical and surgical interventions. Therefore assessing the quality of life has been brought into the limelight [45]. On the other hand, predictive value of quality of life on survival and other outcomes of cardiac surgery has been also studied. In a prospective study of 6305 patients who underwent isolated coronary artery bypass the overall functional health-related quality of life improved after recovery from cardiac surgery. Reduced long-term survival following cardiac surgery even after adjustment for known risk factors associated with survival after cardiac surgery was associated with lower functional health related quality of life beyond the posthospital recovery phase. The degree of functional recovery was directly related to subsequent survival [46]. In a prospective cohort study the preoperative quality of life was an independent predictor of 6-month mortality following CABG even after adjusting for traditional risk factors. The magnitude of the effect (39% increase in risk for a small difference in quality of life score) was clinically important, and it is a non-invasive, easily available tool for clinicians [47].

8. Gender differences

The increased operative mortality and morbidity of women compared with men undergoing CABG surgery results from differences in methodology, low number of women in studies reporting negative findings, many studies, both positive and negative, did not take into account preoperative differences in health status between the sexes. Women more frequently have factors associated with increased short- and long-term mortality, such as less common use of internal mammary artery grafts. According to the reported analyses, they are older, less educated, have more severe angina and congestive heart failure, lower functional status, and higher level of depressive symptoms. At time of referral, women are at more advanced disease stage than men; however, despite being more symptomatic, women have less extensive coronary artery disease than men as determined by coronary angiography results [48]. This

large number of differences makes the comparison difficult, and studies are not corrected for so many potential imbalances that may influence sex differences in outcome. Additional large prospective studies with substantial numbers of women are needed to evaluate gender-related differences in autonomic responses to myocardial infarction, complications related to cardiopulmonary bypass, susceptibility to abnormalities in coagulation, and other biological factors that might account for discrepant outcomes in men versus women undergoing CABG. Furthermore, specific pharmacologic and therapeutic considerations, such as the role of estrogen replacement therapy, need to be clarified [49]. Compared to conducted studies in this topic the POST CABG Biobehavioral Study enrolled the highest number of women (n = 269) and physical, social, and emotional functioning were investigated after CABG surgery. Both male and female patients improved in physical, social, and emotional functioning after CABG, and recovery over time was similar in men and women. However, women's health-related quality-of-life scale scores remained less favourable than men's women did show less benefit with regard to the symptoms of shortness of breath and tiredness through 1 year after surgery [50]. In another prospective cohort study on quality of life women did not reach the same degree of improvement after 1 year as men, even after adjusting for pre-existing risk factors. Women were at greater risk for subjective cognitive difficulties, increased anxiety and decreased ability to perform tasks for daily living, diminished work-related activities, and reduced exercise capacity [51].

9. Social support

Socially isolated persons are single and/or have small social network. Social isolation is associated with poor outcome in established CAD, while high levels of social support is known to promote psychologic and physical well being [52]. Social support can be divided into two broad categories: social networks, which describe the size, structure, and frequency of contact with the network of people surrounding an individual; and functional support, which may be further divided into received social support, which highlights the type and amount of resources provided by the social network, and perceived social support, which focuses on the subjective satisfaction with available support or the perception that support would be available if needed [2]. The underlying mechanisms remain to be identified. Several factors may confound the effect of isolation such as disease severity, or its associations with demographic measures, because socially isolated patients are generally older and of lower socioeconomic status, which are known to reduce survival. Another possible mechanism is the influence of disease progression via its effect on psychosocial functioning. Psychological distress in CAD patients is more severe in patients with lack of adequate social support. Description of the demographic and psychosocial characteristics of those with few social contacts might aid our understanding of the link between isolation and mortality [52]. Previous studies showed the pivotal role of family ties in preserving cardiovascular health [53, 54]. A strong and consistent inverse gradient was reported between the magnitude of social support and adverse clinical outcomes among both initially healthy subjects and those with known CAD [55]. In our study on cardiac surgery patients (180 patients) 17% of patients admitted living alone, however when

asking about marital status 35% admitted being single. We showed in our study that social isolation was associated with higher mortality after cardiac surgery [27]. Without social network and family support patients face longer hospital stay after CABG. Loneliness increases mortality: in a prospective study 1290 CABG patients were investigated. After controlling for various preoperative factors known to be independently associated with mortality loneliness was found to be associated with mortality, both at 30 days (relative risk 2.61) and at 5 years (relative risk 1.78) after the operation [52]. Kopp et al. found that marital status and spouse support was closely associated with men's mortality. Premature death was significantly lower among married men or men in relationship compared to single men and those who were satisfied with spouse support compared to those who were not [56]. Orth-Gomer et al. reported that following myocardial infarction, women with concomitant marital stress had 2.9-fold increased risk of recurrent cardiac events during a five-year follow-up compared to those with less marital stress after adjustment for age, estrogen status, education level, smoking, diagnosis at index event, diabetes mellitus, systolic blood pressure, smoking, triglyceride level, high-density lipoprotein cholesterol level, and left ventricular dysfunction [57]. In accordance with this finding, higher prevalence of subclinical atherosclerosis, and accelerated progression over time, among healthy women reporting marital dissatisfaction was reported, assuming that marital stress is atherogenic [58].

10. Negative affectivity and social inhibition

Type D personality unifies psychosocial factors related to high cardiovascular risk in one model. Particularly negative affectivity (NA) and social inhibition (SI) are relevant in this context. NA refers to the stable tendency to experience negative emotions across time/ situations. Persons with high-NA experience more feelings of dysphoria, anxiety, and irritability; have a negative view of self; and are looking for signs of impending trouble. NA overlaps with neuroticism and trait anxiety; includes subjective feelings of tension, worry, anxiety, anger, and sadness. SI patients tend to inhibit the expression of emotions/behaviours in social interactions to avoid disapproval by others. They feel inhibited, tense, and insecure when with others. Individuals who are high in both NA and SI have a distressed or Type D personality, given their vulnerability to chronic distress [59]. Type D patients are at increased risk for a wide range of adverse health outcomes, mortality and morbidity, in various cardio-vascular populations, including those with ischemic heart disease [60], coronary intervention [61], cardiac arrhythmias [62], peripheral arterial disease [63]. Global left ventricular dysfunction and type D personality were independent predictors of long-term cardiac events in patients with a reduced ejection fraction after myocardial infarction [64]. Type D personality independently predicted mortality and early allograft rejection after heart transplantation [65]. In our 5-year follow-up, there was no link between the occurrence of major cardiac and cerebral event and NA and SI after CABG [44]. Additionally, severity of illness intrusiveness, sleeping problems and SI increased in the MACCE positive patients during the three-year period Unfavourable effect of Type D is linked to physiological hyperreactivity, immune activation, and inadequate response to cardiac treatment [59].

First author and title	Number of patients	Methods	Results
Cserép Z. Psychosocial factors and major adverse cardiac and cerebrovascular events after cardiac surgery.	180	Depression [Beck depression inventory (BDI)], anxiety [state anxiety subscale in Spielberger State-Trait Anxiety Inventory (STAI-S) and trait anxiety subscale in Spielberger State-Trait Anxiety Inventory (STAI-T)] were investigated annually, social support, negative affectivity, social inhibition (SI), illness intrusiveness, self-rated health and sleeping disorders were investigated by standardized tests at the second and fifth year after cardiac surgery. The end-point was the major adverse cardiac and cerebrovascular event (MACCE) including death.	At the end of the second year after adjustment for medical and perioperative factors worse self-rated health [adjusted hazard ratio (AHR): 0.67, P=0.006], sleeping disorders (AHR: 1.14, P=0.001), higher illness intrusiveness (AHR: 1.03, P=0.018), higher BDI (AHR: 1.12, P=0.001), STAI-S (AHR: 1.09, P=0.001) and higher STAI-T scores (AHR: 1.08, P=0.002) showed higher risk for MACCE. Significant individual elevation in scores of sleeping disorders, illness intrusiveness and SI were observed over the three-year period in the MACCE group.
Denollet J. Personality as independent predictor of long-term mortality in patients with coronary heart disease.	268 men and 35 women	Patients with angiographically documented CHD, who were taking part in an outpatient rehabilitation programme. All patients completed personality questionnaire at entry to the programme. Survival status was followed up for mean 7-9 years. The main endpoint was death from all causes.	The rate of death was higher for type-D patients than for those without type-D (23 [27%]/85 vs 15 [7%]/218; p < 0.00001). The association between type-D personality and mortality was still evident more than 5 years after the coronary event and was found in both men and women.Type-D was an independent predictor of both cardiac and non-cardiac mortality after controlling for medial variables.
Pedersen SS. Type D personality predicts death or myocardial infarction after bare metal stent or sirolimus-eluting stent implantation: a Rapamycin-Eluting Stent Evaluated At Rotterdam Cardiology Hospital (RESEARCH) registry sub-study.	875	Patients completed the Type D Personality Scale (DS14) six months after PCI. The end point was a composite of death and MI.	Type D patients were at a cumulative increased risk of adverse outcome compared with non-Type D patients: 5.6% versus 1.3% (p < 0.002). Type D personality (odds ratio [OR] 5.31; 95% confidence interval [CI] 2.06 to 13.66) remained an independent predictor of adverse outcome adjusting for all other variables.

Pedersen SS. Type D personality is associated with increased anxiety and depressive symptoms in patients with an implantable cardioverter defibrillator and their partners.	221	Patients with implantable cardioverter defibrillator and their partners completed the Hospital Anxiety and Depression Sca le, the Type D Personality Scale, and the Perceived Social Support Scale.	In patients, Type D personality was independently related to anxiety (OR: 7.03; 95% CI: 2.32-21.32) and depressive symptoms (OR: 7.40; 95% CI: 2.49-21.94) adjusting for all other variables. In partners, Type D personality was independently associatedwith increased sym ptoms of anxiety (OR: 8.77; 95% CI: 3.19-24.14) and depression (OR: 4.40; 95% CI: 1.76-11.01).
Aquarius AE. Role of disease status and Type D personality in outcomes in patients with peripheral arterial disease.	150	Patients with peripheral arterial disease were assessed with the Type D Scale-14, World Health Organization Quality of Life Assessment Instrument-100, and Perceived Stress Scale-10 Item assessed type D personality, QOL, and perceived stress	Type D patients reported significantly poorer quality of life than non-type D patients across peripheral arterial disease and healthy subgroups ($p < 0.0001$). After controlling for disease status (presence or absence of peripheral arterial disease), type D personality remained associated with increased risk for impaired quality of life (odds ratio [OR] 7.35, 95% confidence interval [CI] 3.39 to 15.96, $p < 0.0001$) and perceived stress (OR 6.45, 95% CI 3.42 to 12.18, $p < 0.0001$).
Denollet J. Personality, disease severity, and the risk of long-term cardiac events in patients with a decreased ejection fraction after myocardial infarction.	87	Patients with myocardial infarction with a decreased left ventricular ejection fraction (LVEF).	Patients with Type D personality were more likely to experience an event over time compared with non-type D patients (P=0.00005). Cox proportional hazards analysis yielded LVEF of < or =30% (relative risk, 3.0; 95% confidence interval, 1.2 to 7.7; P=.02) and type D (relative risk, 4.7; 95% confidence interval, 1.9 to 11.8; P=0.001) as independent predictors.
Denollet J. Unfavorable outcome of heart transplantation in recipients with type D personality	51	Patients with transplanted heart were identified to have or not to have Type D personality by using the DS14 scale.	Type D recipients had a 10-fold higher mortality rate after hospital discharge (5 of 15, or 33%) as compared with non-Type D recipients (1 of 34, or 3%) ($p = 0.013$, adjusting for age and gender). Among surviving recipients, the rate of Grade "/> or =3A rejection for both groups was 40% vs 27%, respectively ($p = 0.45$). The risk of unfavorable outcomes (death, Grade "/> or =3A rejection, or number rejection-free days < or =14) was greater in Type D recipients (12 of 15, or 80%) than in

	non-Type Ds (13 of 34, or 38%), adjusting for other risk factors (odds ratio: 6.75; 95% confidence interval: 1.47 to 30.97) (p = 0.014).

Table 3. Some important studies about negative affectivity and socal inhibition in cardiology

11. Education

Previous research showed that educational level is an important health determinant, with gender-related differences and ethnic and cultural variations. Low educated men and women, in particular with required schooling only, have usually low income and thus lower socio-economic status may be expected. The lower education level of older persons leads to greater burden for medical services and lower awareness of how to lead a healthy lifestyle, and lower adherence to medication and utilisation of preventive measures. In general, women take part more often in screening programs, are more interested in health prevention and visit their general practitioners more often. Their activity may also relate to a higher rate of diagnosis of depression and anxiety disorders. Besides biological factors including oestradiol, psychosocial factors, culture and education may be responsible for the prevalence of these mental disorders among women [66]. Less education was showed an important risk factor for late-life depression [67]. In survey in South America women's higher education was associated with lower risk for diabetes and hypertension and lower BMI in all areas but more strongly in urban areas. There was no association or even an adverse association between education and these risk factors among men in less urban areas [68]. Controversially, men with low level of education were related to higher BMI, prevalence of diabetes and smoking. Less-educated women had higher blood pressure and BMI and low education in both sexes was associated with twofold increased incidence of stroke and CHD [69]. In an Austrian study both men and women with lower educational levels were associated with unhealthy behaviours, overweight and higher cardiovascular risk. There was in inverse relationship in both men and women between overweight and obesity and educational level. The odds of daily smoking, eating a diet rich in meat and doing no regular vigorous exercise decreased with increasing educational level. Among women, the odds of suffering from diabetes or from hypertension decreased gradually with increasing educational level. There was no clear association between educational level and the risk of diabetes or hypertension in men. Depression among women with only required schooling was frequent, but showed no relationship with education in men [66]. Low education and income are important determinants of all-cause mortality and cardiovascular mortality [70] among patients with myocardial infarction. Low income and education are related to a higher risk profile and poorer treatment [71]. In accordance, in our study, a higher level of education was associated with a longer survival time after CABG. Those patients who had an academic degree had a mean survival time of 8.01 years, patients with 9 to 12 years of education had a mean survival time of 7.73 years and the group with 8 years or less of education had a mean survival time of 7.03 years. There were significant differences among patients with 8 years or less of education and patients with 8 to 12 years of education and patients with an

academic degree in the survival analysis. Patients with less education had a worse life expectancy. There was no significant difference between patients with 9 to 12 years of education and those with an academic degree [13]. Patients with a high level of education are likely to have a higher income and therefore can afford the more expensive "healthy" diet and sport activities [70]. In a recent study, however, the risk for major cardiac event after primary percutaneous coronary intervention depended only on employment status and income, but not education level [72]. More prospective studies are needed to establish the relationship.

12. Interventions

The American Heart Association has recommended routine screening by self- reporting measures to rapid identification of likely depressed CAD patients. The Patient Health Questionnaire is one such depression assessing measurement, focuses on two requisite symptoms for a depression or major depressive episode diagnosis, i.e., (1) little interest or pleasure in doing things, (2) feeling down, depressed, or hopeless. Patients with positive screening results should be evaluated by a professional qualified in the diagnosis and management of depression [5].

12.1. Antidepressants

There are currently several empirically validated treatments for depression. A national survey of cardiovascular physicians reported nearly 50% of respondents treat the symptoms of depression once identified in patients with CAD [73]. The Selective serotonin re-uptake inhibitors (SSRI) are currently considered the safest to use with CAD patients, in contrast to the tricyclics, which may have pro-arrhythmic and cardio-toxic effects. The SSRI have been hypothesized as safe among cardiac patients due to the serotonin transporter affinity and attenuation of platelet functioning. The SADHART trial compared the effects of sertraline and placebo for 24 weeks in major depressive patients with unstable angina or recent MI. The SSRI treatment did not adversely affect cardiac function and was considered to be safe for most patients [74]. However, in the ENRICHD trial, improvements in depression were rather modest. Patients with at least 1 prior episode of depression or more severe depression showed consistent improvement in depression relative to control, suggesting that treatment with SSRIs is a good option for this subset of depressed CAD patients. The ENRICHD trial also found that antidepressant treatment improved prognosis for myocardial infarction patients, they were at decreased risk for death and reinfarction compared with those who did not take antidepressants [75]. In a systematic review [76] only 2 studies had follow-up periods that were long enough to assess cardiac outcomes [76, 77]. None of them found evidence of an effect of depression treatment. Two studies reported that selective serotonin reuptake inhibitors did not affect cardiac function [74, 79]. Possible side effects of SSRIs for CABG surgery patients include increased bleeding, but have not been consistently supported [80]. One study suggested an increased long-term mortality and rehospitalization after CABG surgery attributable to SSRIs [81]. Another study indicated greater renal morbidity and ventilation times, but not greater mortality or bleeding risk [82]. In two recent systematic reviews of randomized, controlled trials in CAD patients both established SSRI vs. placebo there was no difference in

mortality and differential findings were reported on hospital readmissions. One found reduced odds [83], whereas another review did not when applying stringent criteria for properly randomized studies [84]. There is no trial about the role of anxiolytic drugs before or after CABG with or without concomitant depressive symptoms.

12.2. Psychosocial Interventions

Psychosocial interventions (psychotherapy, support, stress reduction) have been used as treatments for depression in CAD patients. The aim of these interventions is to reduce psychological distress, which in theory would ultimately improve clinical outcomes. Patients with depression often do not participate or complete cardiac rehabilitation programs after CABG and thus may form a barrier to improvements in cardiac functioning [85]. From another aspect, isolated patients may be difficult to enroll in interventions because they do feel that they have a problem. Without the experience of need, motivation to change may be low [86]. Numerous behavioural and psychological randomized controlled trial (RCT) interventions have been reported and cognitive behavioural therapy or collaborative care constitutes Class IIa evidence (i.e., it is reasonable to administer treatment, additional studies with focused objectives are needed) [85]. In one of RCT studies on brief, tailored cognitive behavioural therapy targeting preoperative depression and anxiety researchers found that intervention improved depressive and anxiety symptoms, as well as quality of life. Moreover, it reduced in-hospital length of stay [87]. In a Canadian study eight weeks prior to CABG, the treatment group received exercise training twice per week, education and reinforcement, and monthly nurse-initiated telephone calls. After surgery, participation in a cardiac rehabilitation program was offered to all patients. The intervention was not associated with differences in pre-surgery anxiety versus usual care, however length of stay differed significantly between groups. Patients who received the preoperative intervention spent 1 less day in the hospital overall and less time in the intensive care. During the waiting period, patients in the intervention group had a better quality of life than controls. Improved quality of life continued up to 6 months after surgery. Mortality rates did not differ [88]. In a prospective randomized controlled trial the effects of a home-based intervention program on anxiety and depression 6 months after CABG were assessed. Anxiety and depression symptoms were measured before surgery, 6 weeks after surgery, and 6 months after surgery. On 6-week and 6-month follow-ups, significant improvements in anxiety and depression symptoms were found in both groups. There was no significant difference between patients receiving interventions and not [89]. Freedland et al. compared cognitive behaviour or supportive stress management vs usual care and found significant three month depression remission rates in the treatment arms. Cognitive behaviour therapy had greater and more durable effects than supportive stress management on depression and several secondary psychological outcomes [90]. The limitation of psychosocial RCTs among CABG populations is that those patients experiencing significant postoperative morbidity are likely to be excluded from trial inclusion. Therefore, less is known about long term outcomes for patients who experience stroke, deep sternal wound infection, sternal dehiscence, renal failure requiring dialysis and extended length of time on mechanical ventilation, or intensive care during their hospital stay. These moribund patients are at higher risks for developing or exacerbating psychological distress. Moreover, treatment of affective

http://dx.doi.org/10.5772/54622

disorders is important in any context, there is not sufficient evidence whether interventions among cardiac patients can promote and maintain health related behaviour change [25]. Exercise is commonly recommended to promote both primary and secondary CAD prevention, but evidence suggests that exercise may also modify psychosocial risk factors, including depression. Cross sectional studies of both patients and healthy cohorts have consistently demonstrated lower depression rates among those who are most active [55]. A randomized controlled comparison between antidepressant medication versus exercise was performed in depressed patients. After 16 weeks, there was a significant reduction in depression in all groups, confirming the same effect of exercise and sertraline hydrochloride in reducing depressive symptoms. However, a lower rate of relapse was observed in the exercise group after six months [91].

13. Conclusion and future directions

Coronary artery bypass graft surgery (CABG) is a confirmed procedure to relive angina pectoris and reduce the risk from life-threatening ischaemic heart disease, besides reducing the likelihood of future heart attacks and prolonging life-expectancy. Another goal is to improve health-related quality of life and psychological well-being. After successful surgery the majority of patients can have an improved everyday life, with increased performance in physical, social and sexual functioning and decreased levels of depression, anxiety, fatigue and sleep. In some cases quality of life for patients can be disappointing, and attention has increasingly been paid to psychological difficulties following CABG surgery [92]. Psychological problems such as depression and anxiety are widely reported soon after CABG surgery and remain evident for around one-fifth of patients one year after surgery. Poor psychological adjustment following surgery can increase the likelihood of new coronary events, further hospitalisations and even death. According to a recent study 30% of patients have reduced health related quality of life without being clinically anxious or depressed they present with fear of activity, fear of excitement, give up enjoyed hobbies / activities. Evidence suggests that self-perceived health related quality of life, depressive symptoms and anxiety together influence the short and long term recovery following coronary bypass surgery [93]. There is also a higher risk for morbidity and mortality among the lonely and the socially isolated, they are likely to have prolonged postoperative recovery and hospital stay. Lower education and poor social background are associated with higher mortality rates related to CHD and prolonged hospital stay after CABG [93, 94]. Further research on the interaction between these disorders and social factors may improve our understandings and uncover promising ways for intervention. Most studies to date focus on depression, the role of other factors alone or investigated together warrants further research.

In conclusion, compared with community samples the prevalence of depression and anxiety disorders are significantly higher and they confer greater morbidity risks, though the behavioural and biological mechanisms are poorly understood. Researchers and clinicians hope psychosocial intervention might decrease or cease the deleterious impact of depression and anxiety on morbidity and mortality.

Author details

Zsuzsanna Cserép[1], Andrea Székely[1,2] and Bela Merkely[3]

*Address all correspondence to: szekelya@kardio.hu

1 Department of Anesthesiology and Intensive Care, Semmelweis University, Budapest, Hungary and Uzsoki Street Hospital of the Budapest Municipality, Budapest, Hungary

2 Intensive Care, Gottsegen György Hungarian Institute of Cardiology, Budapest, Hungary

3 Department of Cardiology, Semmelweis University, Budapest, Hungary

References

[1] Krannich JH, Weyers P, Lueger S, Herzog M, Bohrer T, Elert O. Presence of depression and anxiety before and after coronary artery bypass graft surgery and their relationship to age. BMC Psychiatry. 2007;7:47.

[2] Rozanski A, Blumenthal JA, Davidson KW, Saab PG, Kubzansky L. The epidemiology, pathophysiology, and management of psychosocial risk factors in cardiac practice: the emerging field of behavioral cardiology. J Am Coll Cardiol. 2005;45:637-51.

[3] Blumenthal JA, Lett HS, Babyak MA, White W, Smith PK, Mark DB, et al; NORG Investigators. Depression as a risk factor for mortality after coronary artery bypass surgery. Lancet, 2003;362:604-9.

[4] Connerney I, Shapiro PA, McLaughlin JS, Bagiella E, Sloan RP. Relation between depression after coronary artery bypass surgery and 12-month outcome: a prospective study. Lancet. 2001;358:1766-71.

[5] Lichtman JH, Bigger JT Jr, Blumenthal JA, Frasure-Smith N, Kaufmann PG, Lespérance F, et al; American Heart Association Prevention Committee of the Council on Cardiovascular Nursing; American Heart Association Council on Clinical Cardiology; American Heart Association Council on Epidemiology and Prevention; American Heart Association Interdisciplinary Council on Quality of Care and Outcomes Research; American Psychiatric Association. Depression and coronary heart disease: recommendations for screening, referral, and treatment: a science advisory from the American Heart Association Prevention Committee of the Council on Cardiovascular Nursing, Council on Clinical Cardiology, Council on Epidemiology and Prevention, and Interdisciplinary Council on Quality of Care and Outcomes Research: endorsed by the American Psychiatric Association. Circulation. 2008;118:1768-75.

[6] Majed B, Arveiler D, Bingham A, Ferrieres J, Ruidavets JB, Montaye M, et al; PRIME Study Group. Depressive symptoms, a time-dependent risk factor for coronary heart disease and stroke in middle-aged men: the PRIME Study. Stroke. 2012;43:1761-7.

[7] Barefoot JC, Helms MJ, Mark DB, Blumenthal JA, Califf RM, Haney TL, et al. Depression and long-term mortality risk in patients with coronary artery disease. Am J Cardiol. 1996;78:613–7.

[8] Frasure-Smith N, Lesperance F, Juneau M, Talajic M, Bourassa MG. Gender, depression, and one-year prognosis after myocardial infarction. Psychosom Med. 1999;61:26–37.

[9] Lesperance F, Frasure-Smith N, Talajic M, Bourassa MG. Five-year risk of cardiac mortality in relation to initial severity and one-year changes in depression symptoms after myocardial infarction. Circulation. 2002;105:1049 –53.

[10] Brown JM, Stewart JC, Stump TE, Callahan CM. Risk of coronary heart disease events over 15 years among older adults with depressive symptoms. Am J Geriatr Psychiatry. 2011;19:721-9.

[11] Mahoney JJ, Voelkel EA, Bannister JA, Gopaldas RR, Dao TK. Psychiatric Factors Which Impact Coronary Heart Disease and Influence Outcomes Post-Coronary Artery Bypass Grafting Surgery. Rijeka: In Tech; 2012. http://www.intechopen.com/books/howtoreference/front-lines-of-thoracic-surgery/psychiatric-factors-which-impact-coronary-heart-disease-chd-and-influence-outcomes-post-coronary-art (accessed 11 October 2012).

[12] Tully PJ, Baker RA, Turnbull D, Winefield H. The role of depression and anxiety symptoms in hospital readmissions after cardiac surgery. J Behav Med. 2008;31:281-90.

[13] Cserep Z, Losoncz E, Balog P, Szili-Török T, Husz A, Juhász B, et al. The impact of preoperative anxiety and education level on long-term mortality after cardiac surgery. J Cardiothorac Surg. 2012;7(1):86.

[14] Fava M, Abraham M, Pava J, Shuster J, Rosenbaum J. Cardiovascular risk factors in depression: the role of anxiety and anger. Psychosomatics. 1996;37:31-37.

[15] Esler M, Turbott J, Schwarz R, Leonard P, Bobik A, Skews H, et al. The peripheral kinetics of norepinephrine in depressive illness. Arch Gen Psychiatry. 1982;39:285-300.

[16] Watkins LL, Grossman P, Krishnan R, Sherwood A. Anxiety and vagal control of heart risk. Psychosom Med. 1998;60:498-502.

[17] Kawachi I, Sparrow D, Vokonas PS, Weiss ST. Decreased heart rate variability in men with phobic anxiety (data from the Normative Aging Study). Am J Cardiol. 1995;75:882-885.

[18] van Boven AJ, Jukema JW, Haaksma J, Zwinderman AH, Crijns HJ, Lie KI. Depressed heart rate variability is associated with events in patients with stable coronary artery disease and preserved left ventricular function. REGRESS Study Group. Am Heart J. 1998;135:571-576.

[19] Krantz D, Helmers K, Bairey CN, Nebel L, Hedges S, Rozanski A. Cardiovascular reactivity and mental stress-induced myocardial ischemia in patients with coronary artery disease. Psychosom Med. 1991;53:1-12.

[20] Carney RM, Freedland KE, Rich MW, Jaffe AS. Depression as a risk factor for cardiac events in established coronary heart disease: a review of possible mechanisms. Ann Behav Med. 1995;17:142-149.

[21] Roest AM, Martens EJ, Denollet J, de Jonge P. Prognostic association of anxiety post myocardial infarction with mortality and new cardiac events: a meta-analysis. Psychosom Med. 2010;72:563-9.

[22] Everson-Rose SA, Lewis TT. Psychosocial factors and cardiovascular diseases. Annu Rev Public Health. 2005;26:469-500.

[23] Frasure-Smith N, Lesperance F. Depression and other psychological risks following myocardial infarction. Arch. Gen. Psychiatry 2003; 60:627–36.

[24] Koivula M, Tarkka MT, Tarkka M, Laippala P, Paunonen-Ilmonen M. Fear and anxiety in patients at different time-points in the coronary artery bypass process. Int J Nurs Stud. 2002;39:811-22.

[25] Tully PJ, Baker RA. Depression, anxiety, and cardiac morbidity outcomes after coronary artery bypass surgery: a contemporary and practical review. J Geriatr Cardiol. 2012;9:197-208.

[26] Rosenbloom JI, Wellenius GA, Mukamal KJ, Mittleman MA. Self-reported anxiety and the risk of clinical events and atherosclerotic progression among patients with Coronary Artery Bypass Grafts (CABG). Am Heart J. 2009;158:867-73.

[27] Székely A, Balog P, Benkö E, Breuer T, Székely J, Kertai MD, et al. Anxiety predicts mortality and morbidity after coronary artery and valve surgery--a 4-year follow-up study. Psychosom Med. 2007;69(7):625-31.

[28] Kawachi I, Sparrow D, Vokonas PS, Weiss ST. Symptoms of anxiety and risk of coronary heart disease. The Normative Aging Study. Circulation. 1994; 90:2225-9.

[29] Dao TK, Voelkel E, Presley S, Doss B, Huddleston C, Gopaldas R. Gender as a moderator between having an anxiety disorder diagnosis and coronary artery bypass grafting surgery (CABG) outcomes in rural patients. J Rural Health. 2012;28:260-7.

[30] Oxlad M, Stubberfield J, Stuklis R, Edwards J, Wade TD. Psychological risk factors for cardiac-related hospital readmission within 6 months of coronary artery bypass graft surgery. J Psychosom Res. 2006;61:775-81.

[31] Kopp MS, Skrabski Á, Réthelyi J, Kawachi I, Adler N. Self Rated Health, Subjective Social Status and Middle Aged Mortality in a Changing Society. Behav Med. 2004;30:65-70.

[32] Jylhä M, Volpato S, Guralnik JM. Self-rated health showed a graded association with frequently used biomarkers in a large population sample. J Clin Epidemiol. 2006;59:465-71.

[33] Jylhä M. What is self-rated health and why does it predict mortality? Towards a unified conceptual model. Soc Sci Med. 2009;69:307-16.

[34] Arnadottir SA, Gunnarsdottir ED, Stenlund H, Lundin-Olsson L. Determinants of self-rated health in old age: a population-based, cross-sectional study using the International Classification of Functioning. BMC Public Health. 2011;11:670.

[35] Schroeder S, Baumbach A, Herdeg C, Oberhoff M, Buchholz O, Kuettner A, et al. Self-rated health and clinical status after PTCA: results of a 4-year follow-up in 500 patients. Eur J Intern Med. 2001;12:101-106.

[36] Norekvål TM, Fridlund B, Rokne B, Segadal L, Wentzel-Larsen T, Nordrehaug JE. Patient-reported outcomes as predictors of 10-year survival in women after acute myocardial infarction. Health Qual Life Outcomes. 2010;8:140.

[37] Oxlad M, Wade TD. Longitudinal risk factors for adverse psychological functioning six months after coronary artery bypass graft surgery. J Health Psychol. 2008;13:79-92.

[38] Steptoe A, Wardle J, Marmot M. Positive affect and health-related neuroendocrine, cardiovascular, and inflammatory processes. Proc Natl Acad Sci USA. 2005;102:6508-12.

[39] Steptoe A, Dockray S, Wardle J. Positive affect and psychobiological processes relevant to health. J Pers. 2009;77:1747-76.

[40] Kubzansky LD, Thurston RC. Emotional vitality and incident coronary heart disease: benefits of healthy psychological functioning. Arch Gen Psychiatry. 2007;64:1393-401.

[41] Scheier MF, Matthews KA, Owens JF, Schulz R, Bridges MW, Magovern GJ, et al. Optimism and rehospitalization after coronary artery bypass graft surgery. Arch Intern Med. 1999;159:829–35.

[42] Tindle H, Belnap BH, Houck PR, Mazumdar S, Scheier MF, Matthews KA, et al. Optimism, response to treatment of depression, and rehospitalization after coronary artery bypass graft surgery. Psychosom Med. 2012;74:200-7.

[43] Devins GM. Using the illness intrusiveness ratings scale to understand health-related quality of life in chronic disease. J Psychosom Res. 2010;68:591-602.

[44] Cserép Z, Balog P, Székely J, Treszl A, Kopp MS, Thayer JF, et al. Psychosocial factors and major adverse cardiac and cerebrovascular events after cardiac surgery. Interact Cardiovasc Thorac Surg. 2010;11:567-72.

[45] Czajkowski SM. Health-related quality of life outcomes in clinical research: NHLBI policy and perspectives. Ann Thorac Surg. 1998;66:1486-7.

[46] Koch CG, Li L, Lauer M, Sabik J, Starr NJ, Blackstone EH. Effect of functional health-related quality of life on long-term survival after cardiac surgery. Circulation. 2007;115:692-9.

[47] Rumsfeld JS, MaWhinney S, McCarthy M Jr, Shroyer AL, VillaNueva CB, O'Brien M, et al. Health-related quality of life as a predictor of mortality following coronary artery bypass graft surgery. Participants of the Department of Veterans Affairs Cooperative Study Group on Processes, Structures, and Outcomes of Care in Cardiac Surgery. JAMA. 1999;281:1298-303.

[48] Vaccarino V. Women and outcomes of coronary artery bypass surgery: do we have an answer? Am Heart J. 2003;146:935-7.

[49] Koch CG, Nussmeier NA. Gender and cardiac surgery. Anesthesiol Clin North America. 2003;21:675-89.

[50] Lindquist R, Dupuis G, Terrin ML, Hoogwerf B, Czajkowski S, Herd JA, et al; POST CABG Biobehavioral Study Investigators. Comparison of health-related quality-of-life outcomes of men and women after coronary artery bypass surgery through 1 year: findings from the POST CABG Biobehavioral Study. Am Heart J. 2003;146:1038-44.

[51] Phillips Bute B, Mathew J, Blumenthal JA, Welsh-Bohmer K, White WD, Mark D, et al. Female gender is associated with impaired quality of life 1 year after coronary artery bypass surgery. Psychosom Med. 2003;65:944-51.

[52] Herlitz J, Wiklund I, Caidahl K, Hartford M, Haglid M, Karlsson BW, et al. The feeling of loneliness prior to coronary artery bypass grafting might be a predictor of short-and long-term postoperative mortality. Eur J Vasc Endovasc Surg. 1998;16:120-5.

[53] Balog P, Janszky I, Leineweber C, Blom M, Wamala SP, Orth-Gomér K. Depressive symptoms in relation to marital and work stress in women with and without coronary heart disease. The Stockholm Female Coronary Risk Study. Journal of Psychosomatic Research. 2003;54:113-9.

[54] Balog P, Mészáros E. Házastársi stressz, depressziós tünetek és a cardiovascularis vulnerabilitás - nőknél. LAM. 2005;8:685-92.

[55] Rozanski A, Blumenthal JA, Kaplan J. Impact of psychological factors on the pathogenesis of cardiovascular disease and implications for therapy. Circulation. 1999;99:2192–217.

[56] Kopp MS, Skrabski A, Székely A, Stauder A, Williams R. Chronic stress and social changes: socioeconomic determination of chronic stress. Ann N Y Acad Sci. 2007;1113:325-38.

[57] Orth-Gomer K, Wamala SP, Horsten M, Schenck-Gustafsson K, Schneiderman N, Mittleman MA. Marital stress worsens prognosis in women with coronary heart disease: the Stockholm Female Coronary Risk Study. JAMA 2000;284:3008 –14.

[58] Gallo LC, Troxel WM, Kuller LH, Sutton-Tyrrell K, Edmundowicz D, Matthews KA. Marital status, marital quality, and atherosclerotic burden in postmenopausal women. Psychosom Med 2003;65:952– 62.

[59] Denollet J. DS14: standard assessment of negative affectivity, social inhibition, and Type D personality. Psychosom Med. 2005;67:89-97.

[60] Denollet J, Sys SU, Stroobant N, Rombouts H, Gillebert TC, Brutsaert DL. Personality as independent predictor of long-term mortality in patients with coronary heart disease. Lancet. 1996;347:417–21.

[61] Pedersen SS, Lemos PA, van Vooren PR, Liu TK, Daemen J, Erdman RA, et al. Type D personality predicts death or myocardial infarction after bare metal stent or sirolimus-eluting stent implantation: a Rapamycin-Eluting Stent Evaluated At Rotterdam Cardiology Hospital (RESEARCH) registry sub-study. J Am Coll Cardiol. 2004;44:997– 1001.

[62] Pedersen SS, van Domburg RT, Theuns DA, Jordaens L, Erdman RA. Type D personality is associated with increased anxiety and depressive symptoms in patients with an implantable cardioverter defibrillator and their partners. Psychosom Med. 2004;66:714– 9.

[63] Aquarius AE, Denollet J, Hamming JF, De Vries J. Role of disease status and Type D personality in outcomes in patients with peripheral arterial disease. Am J Cardiol. 2005;96:996–1001.

[64] Denollet J, Brutsaert DL. Personality, disease severity, and the risk of long-term cardiac events in patients with a decreased ejection fraction after myocardial infarction. Circulation. 1998;97:167-73.

[65] Denollet J, Holmes RV, Vrints CJ, Conraads VM. Unfavorable outcome of heart transplantation in recipients with type D personality. J Heart Lung Transplant. 2007;26:152-8.

[66] Kautzky-Willer A, Dorner T, Jensby A, Rieder A. Women show a closer association between educational level and hypertension or diabetes mellitus than males: a secondary analysis from the Austrian HIS. BMC Public Health. 2012;12:392.

[67] Chang-Quan H, Zheng-Rong W, Yong-Hong L, Yi-Zhou X, Qing-Xiu L. Review Education and risk for late life depression: a meta-analysis of published literature. Int J Psychiatry Med. 2010; 40:109-24.

[68] Fleischer NL, Diez Roux AV, Alazraqui M, Spinelli H, De Maio F. Socioeconomic gradients in chronic disease risk factors in middle-income countries: evidence of effect modification by urbanicity in Argentina. Am J Public Health. 2011;101:294-301.

[69] Veronesi G, Ferrario MM, Chambless LE, Sega R, Mancia G, Corrao G, et al. Gender differences in the association between education and the incidence of cardiovascular events in Northern Italy. Eur J Public Health. 2011;21:762-7.

[70] Kopp M, Skrabski A, Szántó Z, Siegrist J. Psychosocial determinants of premature cardiovascular mortality differences within Hungary. J Epidemiol Community Health. 2006;60:782–88.

[71] Gerber Y, Goldbourt U, Drory Y, Israel Study Group on First Acute Myocardial Infarction: Interaction between income and education in predicting long-term survival after acute myocardial infarction. Eur J Cardiovasc Prev Rehabil. 2008;15:526–32.

[72] Jakobsen L, Niemann T, Thorsgaard N, Thuesen L, Lassen JF, Jensen LO, et al. Dimensions of Socioeconomic Status and Clinical Outcome After Primary Percutaneous Coronary Intervention. Circ Cardiovasc Interv. 2012 Oct http://circinterventions.ahajournals.org/content/early/2012/10/02/CIRCINTERVENTIONS.112.968271.long (accessed 11 October 2012.)

[73] Feinstein RE, Blumenfield M, Orlowski B, Frishman WH, Ovanessian S. A national survey of cardiovascular physicians' beliefs and clinical care practices when diagnosing and treating depression in patients with cardiovascular disease. Cardiol Rev. 2006;14(4):164-9.

[74] Glassman AH, O'Connor CM, Califf RM, Swedberg K, Schwartz P, Bigger JT, et al, SADHEART Group. Sertraline treatment of major depression in patients with acute MI or unstable angina. JAMA. 2002;288:701–9.

[75] Writing committee for the ENRICHD investigators. Effects of treating depression and low social support on clinical events after myocardial infarction: The enhancing recovery in coronary heart disease patients (ENRICHD) randomized trial. JAMA. 2003;289:3106–16.

[76] Thombs BD, de Jonge P, Coyne JC, Whooley MA, Frasure-Smith N, Mitchell AJ, et al. Depression screening and patient outcomes in cardiovascular care: a systematic review. JAMA. 2008;300:2161-71.

[77] Berkman LF, Blumenthal J, Burg M, Carney RM, Catellier D, Cowan MJ, et al; Enhancing Recovery in Coronary Heart Disease Patients Investigators (ENRICHD). Effects of treating depression and low perceived social support on clinical events after myocardial infarction: the Enhancing Recovery in Coronary Heart Disease patients (ENRICHD) randomized trial. JAMA. 2003;289:3106-3116.

[78] van Melle JP, de Jonge P, Honig A, Schene AH, Kuyper AM, Crijns HJ, et al; MIND-IT investigators. Effects of antidepressant treatment following myocardial infarction. Br J Psychiatry. 2007;190:460-66.

[79] Strik JJ, Honig A, Lousberg R, Lousberg AH, Cheriex EC, Tuynman-Qua HG, et al. Efficacy and safety of fluoxetine in the treatment of patients with major depression after first myocardial infarction: findings from a double-blind, placebo-controlled trial. Psychosom Med. 2000;62:783-89.

[80] Lett HS, Blumenthal JA, Babyak MA, Sherwood A, Strauman T, Robins C, et al. Depression as a risk factor for coronary artery disease: evidence, mechanisms, and treatment. Psychosom Med. 2004;66:305-15.

[81] Xiong GL, Jiang W, Clare R, Shaw LK, Smith PK, Mahaffey KW, et al. Prognosis of patients taking selective serotonin reuptake inhibitors before coronary artery bypass grafting. Am J Cardiol. 2006;98:42-7.

[82] Tully PJ, Cardinal T, Bennetts JS, Baker RA. Selective serotonin reuptake inhibitors, venlafaxine and duloxetine are associated with in hospital morbidity but not bleeding or late mortality after coronary artery bypass graft surgery. Heart Lung Circ. 2012; 21:206-14.

[83] Baumeister H, Hutter N, Bengel J. Review Psychological and pharmacological interventions for depression in patients with coronary artery disease. Cochrane Database Syst Rev. 2011; (9):CD008012.

[84] Pizzi C, Rutjes AW, Costa GM, Fontana F, Mezzetti A, Manzoli L. Meta-analysis of selective serotonin reuptake inhibitors in patients with depression and coronary heart disease. Am J Cardiol. 2011; 107:972-9.

[85] Hillis LD, Smith PK, Anderson JL, Bittl JA, Bridges CR, Byrne JG, et al. 2011 ACCF/AHA Guideline for Coronary Artery Bypass Graft Surgery: Executive Summary A Report of the American College of Cardiology Foundation/American Heart Association Task Force on Practice Guidelines Developed in Collaboration With the American Association for Thoracic Surgery, Society of Cardiovascular Anesthesiologists, and Society of Thoracic Surgeons. J Am Coll Cardiol. 2011;58:2584–614.

[86] Brummett BH, Barefoot JC, Siegler IC, Clapp-Channing NE, Lytle BL, Bosworth HB, et al. Characteristics of socially isolated patients with coronary artery disease who are at elevated risk for mortality. Psychosom Med. 2001;63:267-72.

[87] Dao TK, Youssef NA, Armsworth M, Wear E, Papathopoulos KN, Gopaldas R. Randomized controlled trial of brief cognitive behavioral intervention for depression and anxiety symptoms preoperatively in patients undergoing coronary artery bypass graft surgery. J Thorac Cardiovasc Surg. 2011;142:e109-15.

[88] Arthur HM, Daniels C, McKelvie R, Hirsh J, Rush B. Effect of a preoperative intervention on preoperative and postoperative outcomes in low-risk patients awaiting

elective coronary artery bypass graft surgery. A randomized, controlled trial. Ann Intern Med. 2000;133:253-62.

[89] Lie I, Arnesen H, Sandvik L, Hamilton G, Bunch EH. Effects of a home-based intervention program on anxiety and depression 6 months after coronary artery bypass grafting: a randomized controlled trial. J Psychosom Res. 2007;62:411-8.

[90] Freedland KE, Skala JA, Carney RM, Rubin EH, Lustman PJ, Dávila-Román VG, et al. Treatment of depression after coronary artery bypass surgery: a randomized controlled trial. Arch Gen Psychiatry. 2009;66:387-96.

[91] Babyak M, Blumenthal JA, Herman S, Khatri P, Doraiswamy M, Moore K, et al. Exercise treatment for major depression: maintenance of therapeutic benefit at 10 months. Psychosom Med. 2000;62:633– 8.

[92] McKenzie LH, Simpson J, Stewart M. A systematic review of pre-operative predictors of post-operative depression and anxiety in individuals who have undergone coronary artery bypass graft surgery. Psychol Health Med. 2010;15:74-93.

[93] Cserép Z, Losoncz E, Malik A, Székely A, Balog P, Kopp M. Psychosocial factors determining life expectancy of patients undergoing open heart surgery. Orv Hetil. 2008;149:1549-54.

[94] Johnston G, Goss JR, Malmgren JA, Spertus JA. Health Status and Social Risk Correlates of Extended Length of Stay Following CABG Surgery. Ann Thorac Surg. 2004;77:557-62.

Chapter 27

Current Challenges in the Treatment of Deep Sternal Wound Infection Following Cardiac Surgery

Martin Šimek, Martin Molitor, Martin Kaláb,
Patrick Tobbia and Vladimír Lonský

Additional information is available at the end of the chapter

http://dx.doi.org/10.5772/55310

1. Introduction

Median sternotomy due to its technical simplicity and excellent exposure of the heart, great vessels and pulmonary hila is the most common incision performed in cardiothoracic surgery worldwide [1]. Originally described by Julian more than 100 years ago and re-induced by Milton in 1957, median sternotomy replaced gradually thoracotomy or bilateral transverse sternothoracotomy (clamshell incision) for routine access to the heart [2,3]. Even though median sternotomy is still considered to be the gold standard, efforts remain ongoing to use less invasive methods such as partial sternotomy or small thoracotomy to influence the risk of wound healing complications, patient's satisfaction and better quality of life [4].

2. Incidence and risk factors of Deep Sternal Wound Infection (DSWI)

Infection involving the sternal bones and/or retrosternal space is a serious complication of median sternotomy. Although, DSWI can be described from many perspectives, the definition according to the Center for Disease Control and Prevention (CDC), is used for distinguishing DSWI from others types of sternal wound infections (SWIs), and is respected by most authors (Table 1) [5]. Looking through the incidence of DSWI ranging between 0.3 to 3.2%, no considerable changes have been observed in the incidence of DSWI over the last 30 years [6-22]. It could be perceived that the numerous advances in cardiac surgery, post-operative care and employment of preventive measurements may have played a role in reducing the incidence of DSWI in the last 10 years. Today surgically treated patients' cohorts are different than patients operated on 20 years ago in terms of advanced age, co-morbidities, and surgical

complexity. In other words, the relatively steady status of DSWI incidence over the last three decades might be considered a satisfactory result [23]. Recently Matros et al showed from a large single institution experience with 21,000 sternotomies a reduction in the incidence of DSWI from 1.57 to 0.88% in the last 15 years. They concluded that the rate of DSWI was significantly diminished particularly in the diabetic population, from 3.2% to 1.0%, related to tight glycemic control [19].

Diagnosis of DSWI requires at least one of the following criteria:
(1) anorganism is isolated from culture of mediastinal tissue or fluid
(2) evidence of mediastinitis is seen during operation or byhistopathological examination
(3) one of the following, fever("/>38° C), chest pain, or sternal instability, is present
and there is either purulent drainage from the mediastinum
or an organism isolated from blood culture or culture of drainage of the mediastinal area

Table 1. Center for Disease Control and Prevention (CDC) criteria of DSWI (modified from Mangan et al[5])

The identification of risk factors for the development of DSWI is crucial in the effort to reduce the risk of infection [6-22]. Although more than two dozen factors were obtained for uni-, and multivariable analyses, only obesity and diabetes mellitus were constantly proven in published studies [6-18,21,22]. Obesity is a strong risk factor for development of DSWI. Even though BMI does not correlate closely with body fat, there is a step-wise relationship between BMI and the risk of major surgical infection in cardiac surgery [7,15,24]. It is caused not only through technical obesity-related problems, but also through less effective penetration of antibiotics into the fat tissue [24]. Undoubtedly, diabetics are at a higher risk of developing DSWI, making the role of perioperative glycemic control crucial. Unsatisfactory preoperative glycemic control is considered to be an important risk factor for development of DSWI [25,26]. Internal mammary artery (IMA) harvesting, particularly in the pedicled fashion, has been found to have a higher incidence of DSWI in a CABG cohort compared with valvular procedures [7,8]. Furthermore, this risk becomes stronger when both IMA are used for revascularization or in the diabetic population, but this effect might be attenuated when both IMA are taken down in a skeletonized fashion, even in diabetics [10,27,28]. Chronic obstructive pulmonary disease (COPD) or smoking increases the risk of infectious complications, prolonged post-operative ventilation, and jeopardizes sternal stability from excessive coughing [6,12,15]. Data addressing the impact of early tracheostomy on DSWI incidence is conflicting [29-31]. Historically, a strong relationship between early tracheostomy and DSWI has not been confirmed; but tracheostomy is known to reduce the need for mechanical ventilation and thereby may limit risk of pulmonary infection and ICU stay [32]. Furthermore, re-exploration for bleeding has been analyzed as an independent risk factor for DSWI in several studies [11,12]. The components of this risk factor include the risk of iatrogenic bacteriological wound contamination within the inherent re-exposure, the deleterious effect of anemia and/or concomitant hemodynamic instability, and the amount of given allogenic blood transfusion units [10,33]. Other

http://dx.doi.org/10.5772/55310

factors traditionally associated with an increased risk of DSWI are inconsistently seen in analyses of retrospective studies including advanced age, emergency surgery, hemodynamic instability, low ejection fraction, duration of surgery and CPB time, and renal failure [6-22]. Incidence and risk factors based on multivariable analysis from larger retrospective studies are summarized in Table 2.

Authors	Patients´ enrollement	No. of patients	DSWI incidence	Independent risk factors
Loop FD et al [6]	1985-1987	6504	1.1%	Obesity, BIMA+diabetes, time of operation,
Milano CA et al [7]	1987-1995	6459	1.3%	Obesity, CHF, re-do surgery, CPB time
Braxton et al [8]	1992-1996	15406	1.25%	Obesity, low EF, COPD
Eklund et al [9]	1990-1999	10713	1.1%	Obesity, BMI
The Parisian Mediastinitis Study Group [10]	1996	1830	NA	Obesity, BIMA, hemodynamic instability, re-do surgery
Hollenbeak et al [11]	1996-1998	1519	2.7%	Obesity, renal inssuficieny, re-exploration
Filsouri et al [12]	1998-2005	5798	1.80%	Obesity, MI, diabetes, COPD, CPB time, re-exploration, prolonged ventilation
Tang et al [13]	1990-2003	30102	0.77%	Age, diabetes, stroke, CHF, BIMA +diabetes/CHF
Toumpoulis et al [14]	1992-2002	3760	1.1%	Diabetes,dialysis, hemodynamic instability, BIMA
Risnes et al [15]	1989-2000	18532	0.6%	Age, male gender, obesity, COPD, diabetes
Crabtree et al [16]	1996-2003	4004	2.2%	Obesity, diabetes,"/>2 transfusion units
Fowler et al [17]	2002-2003	331429	NA	Obesity, diabetes, MI, urgent surgery
Sjoegren et al [18]	1999-2004	4781	0.95%	Diabetes, obesity, low EF, renal failure
Matros et al [19]	1991-2006	21000	1.35%	Prolonged CPB time
De Feo et al [20]	1979-2009	22366	0.89%	NA
Upton et al [21]	1998-2003	5176	1.2%	Diabetes, urgent surgery, low EF
Sachithanandan et al [22]	2001-2005	4586	1.65%	Diabetes, smoking, age, prolonged ventilation

NA - not adrressed
BIMA - bilateral IMA harvesting
EF - ejection fraction
COPD - chronic obstructive pulmonary disease
CHF - congestive heart failure
MI - myocardial infaction

Table 2. Analyses of incidence and risk factors of DSWI

3. Microbiology of DSWI and routes of infection

Staphylococci, either S. aureus (SA) or coagulase-negative Staphylococcus (CONS) represent the most causative organism of DSWI, accounting for 60 to 80% of cases [34]. The proportion of individual strains of Staphylococcus and their methicillin-sensitivity varies between countries and institutions, reflecting their long-term hygienic and antibiotic policies [35]. Although surgical site infections are typically perceived to be an exogenous problem related to exposure to healthcare workers, the most causative pathogens are endogenous from patient's own skin or mucosal flora [36,37]. Nasal carriage of SA has been identified as a potential risk factor for DSWI [38], and genetically identical SA from nasal flora have been cultivated from sternotomy wounds [39]. Unlike SA which caused a more aggressive presentation, CONS infection accompanied with bacteremia as observed in 50-60% of cases [34, 40] had a rather indolent course, clinically manifested later, and was more prone to recurrence [41, 42]. DSWI is diagnosed in 40-70% of patients post-discharge, thus post-discharge surveillance of up to 90 days is recommended [43]. Gram negative strains contribute less commonly in the pathogenesis of DSWI and mostly translocate from other host site infections, such as pneumonia, urinary or abdominal infections [34]. Finally, no significant difference in mortality was observed between DSWI infections caused by CoNS, when compared to SA, or Gram-negative pathogens [34]. Mekontso-Dessap et al suggested that DSWI caused by methicillin-resistant SA (MRSA) may have worse actuarial survival than sensitive strains (MSSA) in terms of 1 month, 1-year, and 3- year survival (60.0%±12.6%, 52.5%±-3.4%, and 26.3%±19.7% versus 84.6% ±7.1%, 79.0%±8.6%, and 79.0%±-8.65, p=0.04), and a regression analysis revealed MRSA as an independent risk factor for overall mortality [44].

4. Outcomes and cost of DSWI

Unsurprisingly, DSWI negatively affected outcomes in cardiac surgery. Even with the adoption of modern treatment strategies, the reported in-hospital mortality for DSWI varies from 1.1 to 19% [6-9,11,16,45]. Although the mortality rate is similar to data reported from the 1980s, it appears that implementation of negative pressure wound therapy (NPWT) may improve long-term survival of patients [18,20,46]. Regardless of treatment strategy, in-hospital stay of DSWI patients is at least two weeks longer compared to patients with an uncomplicated post-operative course [6,10,11]. DSWI-related morbidity was repeatedly reported in relation to prolonged mechanical ventilation, renal impairment, atrial and ventricular arrhythmias, cerebrovascular accidents, need for hemodynamic support, and healing-related complications [20,47]. The cause of death in the early post-operative period is mostly multiple organ failure initiated by sepsis or specific DSWI-related complications such as serious bleeding [6-8,16,18, 20]. Predictors of a poor outcome in DSWI patients that have been reported include length of intensive care unit (ICU) stay, late indication for surgical revision, bacteremia, hemodynamic instability, and prolonged mechanical ventilation [47,48]. Loop et al presented the worse survival data of DSWI in patients operated on during the 1980s in comparison with a standard CABG population within a 3-year follow-up after surgery [6]. Survival analyses published in

http://dx.doi.org/10.5772/55310

the last decade consistently confirm long-term complications of patients with mid-, and long term survival rates who were successfully treated for DSWI (Table 3) [8,11,12,14,15,18,22,46]. Specific reasons for worsening of long-term survival are not yet clear. Risnes et al reported significantly higher cardiac-related deaths in the post-DSWI group (34.6 vs. 21.4%, p<0.006) and poorer survival for males ten years after surgery [15]. In contrast with this data, Sjoegren et al and Bailot et al showed unimpaired long-term survival of DSWI patients in comparison with patients who had uncomplicated surgery once NPWT was used [18,46].

Authors	Patients´ enrollement	Survival analysis
Loop FD et al [6]	1985-1987	3-year survival of 62.5% compared to 69.0% survival for patients with positive cultures. Overall, the 3-year survival was 75%, which is significantly below previously reported 5-year and even 10-year survival for isolated coronary bypass patients
Braxton et al [8]	1992-1996	The adjusted survival rates at 30 days, 1 year, and 4 years were 93%, 78%, and 65% among patients with mediastinitis and 97%, 95%, and 89% without mediastinitis, respectively (p<0.001)
Hollenbeak et al [11]	1996-1998	DSWI patient had a 1-year survival of 78% vs. 99% for non-infected CABG patients, p=0.0001
Filsouri et al [12]	1998-2005	Survival rates at 1,3, and 5 years were 72.4%, 64.3% and 55.8% for patients with DSWI compared with 93.8%, 88% and 82% for the control (p<0.001)
Toumpoulis et al [14]	1992-2002	Freedom from all cause mortality in patients in whom DSWI developed at 1 year, 5 years, and 10 years after the operation was 66.2%, 50.8%, and 40.6% respectively, compared with 87.2%, 72.8%, and 54.3% in patients without DSWI (p=0.0007)
Risnes et al [15]	1989-2000	The 10-year, long-term survival for patients with mediastinitis was 49.5%, compared with 71.0% in non-mediastinitis patients (p<0.01)
Sjoegren et al [18]	1999-2004	The actuarial survival at 1 year, 3 years, and 5 years was 92.9% , 89.2%, and 89.2% for patients with mediastinitis and 96.5%, 92.1%, and 86.9 for those without mediastinitis(p=0. 578)
Sachithanandan et al [22]	2001-2005	Unadjusted freedom from all-cause mortality in patients with DSWI at 1 year, 2 years, and 3 years after surgery was 78.6 ± 4.8% (95% CI 69–88.2%), 75.6 ± 5.0% (95% CI 65.6–85.6%) and 69.4 ± 5.8% (95% CI 57.8–81%) respectively compared with 92.8 ± –0.4% (95% CI 92.4–93.2%), 90.7 ± 0.5% (95% CI 90.2–91.2%) and 87.7 ± 0.6% (95% CI 87.1–88.3%) for patients without DSWI (p < 0.001)
Bailot et [46]	1992-2007	Survival in patients with DSWI showed freedom from all-cause mortality at 1, 5 and 10 years to be, respectively, 91.8%, 80.4% and 61.3% compared with 94.0%, 85.5% and 70.2%, respectively, for patients (p = 0.01). Adjusted survival for patients with DSWI treated with NPWT was 92.8%, 89.8% and 88.0%, respectively, at 1, 2 and 3 years, compared with 83.0%, 76.4% and 61.3%, respectively, for patients with DSWI treated conventionaly(p = 0.02)

Table 3. Analyses of compared mid-term and long-term survival of patients with DSWI with non-DSWI patients

Patients who develop DSWI are 2.5 to 3 times more expensive to manage compared with patients who have an uncomplicated post-operative course [6,11]. The first calculation of cost originated from the Loop et al paper, published in the late 1980´s, and found a 2.8 times increase in cost [6]. Patients who died of DSWI consequences consumed 60,500 USD more, making the total cost of these patients approximately 80,000 USD compared with 11,000 USD an uncomplicated CABG patient cost, as showed by Hollenbeak et al [11]. Recent data from Germany showed a doubling in cost (36,261 vs. 13,356 EUR, $p<0.001$) for DSWI patients [49], while Ennker et al calculated a 9,000 EUR increase in cost on average for any DSWI case [50]. The majority of the increased cost is spent on repeat surgical and ICU service, and extension of in-hospital stay [11,51,52]. In looking for cost-effectiveness of treatment strategies, NPWT does not seem to be a more expensive treatment in comparison with the conventional therapy for DSWI, as calculated in the Swedish healthcare system by Mokhari et al [52]. Atkins et al reported lower NPWT costs than Medicare charges for conventional therapy (152,000 vs. 300,000 USD) of DSWI [53].

5. Strategies preventing DSWI

As mentioned previously, diabetes mellitus is a strong independent risk factor for development of DSWI, and concomitant obesity doubles the risk of further infection [24]. Unfortunately, both risk factors are difficult to modify. Zerr et al showed that a continuous insulin infusion started immediately after surgery to maintain a serum glucose level of 150-200mg/dl (8-11 mmol/l) led to a significant decrease in the incidence of DSWI in diabetics (2.4% to 1.5%, $p < 0.02$) compared with subcutaneously administered insulin [54]. A tight glycemic control protocol appears beneficial from the Portland group experience, nevertheless, decreasing serum glucose below 100mg/dl (6 mmol/l) did not bring any additional impact on DSWI rate, and was associated with a higher risk of stroke or death [55].

It has been demonstrated many times that antibiotic prophylaxis effectively prevents sternal wound infection [56]. As Staphylococcal stains are a major causative pathogen, beta-lactam antiobiotics are recommended for prophylaxis, particularly first or second generation cephalosporins [57]. The use of glycopeptides, which are highly effective against MRSA, has not been linked with a reduction in sternal wound infection rates compared to standard prophylaxis, with one study suggesting higher SSI´s rate (3.7 vs. 1.3%, $p<0.05$) when vancomycin prophylaxis was chosen [58]. Local application of a gentamicin soaked-collagen sponge between the sternal lamella was suggested to reduce all SWI´s, particularly DSWI. Friberg et al reported a significant reduction in SWI´s (3.7 vs. 9%, $p<0.001$), and also DSWI (1.5 vs. 3.3%, $p<0.003$) [59,60], however, further randomized controlled trials and meta-analyses did not confirm a benefit of using a gentamicin sponge for DSWI prevention as well as a recently published meta-analysis [61,62]. Although SA caused DSWI might be reduced by locally applied gentamicin, primarily gentamicin-resistant strains such a CONS may overgrow [62].

Another prophylactic issue is patient decontamination before surgery. As Staphylococci colonization is seen in a majority of DSWI, skin and nasopharyngeal decontamination became

popular [38,39]. The use of chlorhexidine for skin care before surgery showed a significant reduction in the microbial count including SA [63]. In comparison to general surgery where reduction of SSI´s due to skin decontamination was confirmed [64], data for cardiac surgery is lacking, nevertheless, protocols involving chlorhexidine or a different skin cleanser are already widely accepted. Locally applied ointment containing mupirocin is 80 to 90% effective in eradicating all types of SA from the nasopharyngeal mucosa [65]. Cimochowski et al reported about the efficacy of this practice on reducing DSWI rates from 2.7% to 0.9% [66]. A randomized controlled trial published by Konvalinka et al did not confirm a reduced DSWI rate from the use of nasal mupirocin ointment (0.8 vs. 0.8%) [67].

The surgical technique in performing median sternotomy and its closure certainly influences the risk of DSWI. Careful handling of skin and pre-sternal soft tissue, mid-lined sternal incision and avoidance of bone wax are essential, in addition to keeping scrub protocol, checking for glove injury, changing gloves after sternotomy and after sternal wiring, and leaving the closed wound primarily covered for at least 48 hours [68].

It has been proposed that the method of IMA harvesting affects the incidence of DSWI, particularly when both IMA (BIMA´s) are demanded for revascularization [7,8,10,27,28]. A recent meta-analysis published by Saso et al showed a reduced risk of SWI´s once IMA or BIMA´s were harvested in a skeletonized fashion compared with a pedicled graft. The risk was reduced both in the non-diabetic (2.96% vs. 11.7%) and diabetic populations (2.4% vs. 14.2%) [69]. Besides harvesting methods of BIMA´s in diabetics, as was mentioned above, tight long-term glycemic control influenced the risk of DSWI. A hemoglobin A1c (HbA1c) ≥7% had a higher incidence of DSWI compared with patients who had a HbA1c <7% (5.0% vs. 1.4%, P = 0.014). A 31% increased risk of DSWI (OR = 1.31, 95% CI 1.16-1.49, P < 0.001) was seen by Halkos et al [26]. Even through diabetic patients may have a comparable risk of developing DSWI when IMA in skeletonized fashion is taken down, the BIMA´s harvesting need is to be considered carefully because additional risk factors such an obesity and COPD are commonly presented in this cohort [24,70].

The crucial point in preventing DSWI is achievement of stable sternal approximation. Standard sternal wire cerclage, if performed well, is fast, easy and effective [71]. Facing poor sternal quality, sternal fracture, or increased traction forces in obese or COPD patients, some modifications of this technique were proposed. Parasternal wire reinforcement, described originally by Robicsek and modified by Sharma, proved to reduce the risk of sternal wound complications [72,73]. Friberg et al reported that the use of more than 6 or 7 simple wires may also reduce DSWI rates (0.4% vs. 4.2%, p=0.001) [74]. Recently, a large multicenter prospective study conducted by Schimmer et al comparing the Robicsek technique with standard cerclage failed to reduce the risk of SWI and sternal dehiscence [75]. Primary plating, mirroring the experience in maxillofacial surgery, was proposed for patients at high risk of sternal non-union [76]. Plates could be anchored only into the sternal bone (SternaLock system™,Biomet Microfixation Inc, Jacksonville, US) or into the ribs (Titanium Sternal Fixation system™, Syntes, Switzeland). Raman et al reported better chest bone healing after primary plating than rewiring at 6-month follow up (70 vs. 24%, p=0.003) and lower pain scores, with no difference in SWI rates [77]. Others systems are used for sternal approximation including, thermoreactive nitinol clips

(Flexigrip™, Praesidia SRL, Bologna, Italy), titanium locked staples (Sternal Talon™, KLS Martin Group, US), and Poly-Ether-Ether-Ketone tapes (Sternal ZipFix system™, Syntes, Switzeland), all designed for parasteral fixation. Negri et al reported a significant reduction of mechanical dehiscence (2.8% vs. 0.2%, p=0.002), but the same risk of DSWI (1.2% vs. 2.4%) when thermoactive clips were compared with standard wire cerclage [78]. Snyder et al reported 5 years of experience with the SternaLock system™ for primary plating in high risk patients. Superiority of plate over wires was seen in the incidence of early presentation (<30 days) of SWI (0% vs. 12%, p<0.06) and shorter in-hospital stay (7 vs. 8 days, p=0.02) [79]. A pilot study published by Bennett-Guerrero et al showed insignificantly higher spirometry volume in the SternalTalon™ arm (67% ± 32%) versus the wire arm (58% ± 24%). Use of the Talon was associated with decreased use of opiates (21.3 ± 11.8 vs. 25.4 ± 21.6 mg, P = 0.44), duration of mechanical ventilation (0.5 vs. 1.0 days, P = 0.24) and hospital length of stay (4.5 ± 3.2 vs. 5.3 ± 4.0 days, P = 0.40) [80].

A promising method to reduce SSI seems to be the application of NPWT on surgically closed sternal wounds. A commercially available system (Prevena® Incision Management System, KCI, St. Antonio, USA) is used, with skin preservation through a semipermeable membrane that has contact with foam, and one proposal pump system with reservoir is added [81]. Limited clinical experience has shown a decreased risk of wound hematoma, seroma and SSI [82]. Other positive effects from wound application of NPWT might include promotion of microvascular flow and decreased tissue edema and myofibroblast activation [83]. Colli and Atkins et al reported no wound healing complications in patients at high risk for sternal wound infections after cardiac surgery, but both studies were retrospective and done on smaller cohort of patients, 10 and 57, respectively [84,85].

6. Treatment strategies for DSWI

Even though treatment of DSWI has considerably evolved, a generally accepted treatment strategy remains controversial. Robicsek postulated three valid principles addressing this issue: first, that the infectious process should be brought under control within the shortest possible time, secondly, that adequate debridement and drainage of the infected area should occur, and third that sternal stability should be assured [86]. Until the 1960s, patients suffering from DSWI were treated conservatively with antibiotic therapy, limited drainage, or exposure of the sternotomy wound until closure with granulation tissue occurred [87]. Mortality rates then reached over 50% and survivors' quality of life was limited due to significant morbidity [87]. In 1964, Shumacker and Mandelbaum reported their experience with single-stage technique of wound debridement, primary sternal re-wiring and continuous antibiotic irrigation [88]. Their original method was consequently modified in terms of the type of antibiotic or antiseptic solution used including its amount, or the setting of indwelling drains for irrigation and suction [89-90]. Closed chest drainage became widely used with reported mortality from DSWI ranging from 4.8% to 28%, with an associated risk of primary therapy failure ranging from 12.5% to 48% [89,90-92]. Lee et al proposed in 1976 the use of an omental flap for covering infected sternotomy wounds [93]. Vital greater omentum was turned into the

http://dx.doi.org/10.5772/55310

chest cavity following sternal debridement. It was suggested that well-vascularized omentum fulfills dead spaces, ensures high antibiotic levels, and yielded angiogenic and absorptive capacity [13,93]. Jurkiewicz et al first reported the use of muscle flaps, preferably the pectoralis flap, and radical sternal debridement in the treatment of DSWI in 1980 [94]. Consequently, 20-years of experience in the Emory group with 409 patients showed 8.1% in-hospital mortality and 5.1% primary therapy failure. 87.1% of procedures were done in single-stage fashion; the pectoralis major was used in 76.6%, rectus abdominis in 19.4%, and omentum in 2.2% [95]. This approach has received many modifications regarding the timing of wound closure, choice of flap, and type of advancement, with reported mortality ranging from 0% to 19% [96,97]. Comparing the omental to the pectoralis flap, Milano et al reported that the omental flap had lower mortality (4.8% vs. 10.5%, $p<0.05$), early wound related complications (9.5% vs. 27.7%,$p<0.001$), and in-hospital stay (10.7 vs. 18.8%, $p<0.05$) [98]. El Oakley and Wright suggested classification of DSWI based on the time of presentation, presence of risk factors such as obesity, diabetes or immunosuppressive therapy, and number of failed therapeutic attempts in 1996 (Table 3) [99]. The identification of five subtypes of DSWI seemed to be a relevant tool for choice of therapeutic method and patient prognosis. Adjusted to the El Oakley and Wright classification, closed chest irrigation has comparable mortality data for type I and II DSWI compared with radical sternal resection and concomitant flap, but with lower flap-related associated morbidity [100-102]. Ringelman et al noted that at 48 month follow-up, 51% of patients had pain or discomfort, 44% had numbness, 42% complained of sternal instability, and 33% claimed to have shoulder weakness, when pectoral flap was used for reconstruction [103]. Closed chest irrigation carries a higher rate of therapy failure when used for type III, and particularly type IV and V El Oakley and Wright classification [104-107]. Thus, these patients might have benefit from more radical sternal debridement and employment of well-vascularized tissue to replenish residual defects. Flap-related morbidity may be addressed with less invasive techniques such as a laparoscopic greater omentum harvesting [108]. Atkins et al recently reported on the influence of sternal repair choice (pectoral, omental flap, or secondary closure) on long-term survival [109].

There is limited data evaluating hyperbaric oxygen (HBO) therapy in the treatment of SWI, despite theoretical advantages, availability of HTO close to the cardiac surgical unit impedes its routine use [110]. Siondalski et al reported successful healing of 55 DSWI patients with no mortality, nevertheless therapy required 20-40 HBO sessions after surgical revision. HTO was taken as an adjunct therapy to perform radical debridement and muscle flap [111].

Class	Description of DSWI
Type I	Mediastinitis presenting within 2 weeks after operation in the absence of risk factors
Type II	Mediastinitis presenting at 2 to 6 weeks after operation in the absence of risk factors
Type IIIA	Mediastinitis type I in the presence of one or more risk factors
Type IIIB	Mediastinitis type II in the presence of one or more risk factors
Type IVA	Mediastinitis type I, II, or III after one failed therapeutic trial

Class	Description of DSWI
Type IVB	Mediastinitis type I, II, or III after more than one failed therapeutic trial
Type V	Mediastinitis presenting for the first time more than 6 weeks after operation
Accepted risk factors: diabetes, obesity, immunosupressive therapy intake	

Table 4. El Oakley and Wright classification of DSWI (modified from El Oakley et[99])

In 1997, Obdeijin et al described the first application of NPWT for treatment of DSWI in 3 consecutive patients [112]. They found that physical therapy contracted the wound, provided sufficient chest stability, and allowed patients to be extubated. Catarino et al reported the first retrospective comparison between NPWT and closed chest irrigation in 2000. In comparing 9 versus 10 patients, they found superiority of NPWT in length of in-hospital stay (15 vs. 40.5 days, p=0.02) and therapy failure (0 vs. 5, p=0.03) [113]. Furthermore, Gustafsson et al and Fleck et al, from the two most active European centers (Lund and Vienna), reported similar in-hospital and 30-day or 90-day mortality of DSWI patients, with 60% of all cases having class III according to El Oakley and Wright [114,115]. Consequently, the Lund group reported survival data from 1,3, and 5 year follow-up which showed comparable survival (92.9%, 89%, 89%) with patients without DSWI after CABG (96%, 92%, 86%) and showed potential survival benefit of NPWT therapy unlike data known from conventional therapy [18]. Recently published data from a larger group of patients showed 1.1-5.4% mortality at 30 days and 8-15% 1 year mortality with a 2 to 6% risk of primary therapy failure [116-119]. The mean length of application of NPWT was 8 to 14 days with a mean number of 4 to 6 dressing changes [116-119]. The amount of dressing used by centers has only minor variability in first-line application protocol, with the only differences reported being the materials used for interface dressing and the timing of wound closure [116-119]. It was suggested that low C-reactive protein level (<50 mg/l) might be a good indicator for timing of wound closure [120]. Since the introduction of NPWT, its comparison with conventional therapy, closed chest irrigation or sternal resection and flap have been studied. So far, we have data only from retrospective comparative studies, with the compared arms being heterogeneous in number of patients, time periods and type of DSWI based on El Oakley classification. It was suggested that NPWT positively influenced the risk of primary therapy failure and survival of patients at short and long-term follow-up [18,46,121-138]. Outcomes of NPWT are DSWI causative pathogen independent, even comparing therapeutic response to MRSA and MSSA caused DSWI [139]. From multivariable analyses, obesity, renal failure and sepsis were calculated as independent risk factors of NPWT failure [128,129]. Results of comparative studies and published meta-analyses are shown in Table 5.

Authors	Follow-up	Patients ´cohort	Endpoints	Results
Catarino et al [113]	Retrospective	11 pts NPWT vs. 9 pts closed irrigation	In-hospital stay, primary therapy failure	NPWT linked with shorter in-hospital stay (15 vs. 40.5 days, p=0.02) and lower therapy failure (0 vs. 5%, p=0.03) than closed irrigation

http://dx.doi.org/10.5772/55310

Authors	Follow-up	Patients ´cohort	Endpoints	Results
Berg et al [121]	Retrospective	31 pts NPWT vs. 29 pts closed irrigation	Primary therapy failure, in-hospital stay and mortality	NPWT group had a lower risk of therapy failure (52 vs. 16%, p<0.05) and in-hospital stay (22 vs. 26 days, p<0.05), with comparable in-hospital mortality (6,9 vs. 6,6%, NS) to closed irrigation
Doss et al [122]	Retrospective	22 pts NPWT vs. 22 closed irrigation	Primary therapy failure, in-hospital stay and mortality	NPWT group had shorter overall length of therapy (17.2±5.8 vs. 22.9±10.8 days, p=0.01) and in-hospital stay (27.9±6.6 vs. 33.0±11.0 dnů, p=0.03), with comparable mortality (5 vs. 5%, NS) to closed irrigation
Song et al [123]	Retrospective	17 pts NPWT vs. 18 pts open packing	Primary therapy failure, number of dressing changes, in-hospital stay and mortality	NPWT associated with shorter length of therapy (6.2 vs. 8.5 days, p<0,05), lower number of dresssing changes (3±2.5 vs. 17±8.6 , p<0.01), and comparable in-hospital mortality (11 vs. 6%, NS)
Luckraz et al [124]	Retrospective	27 pts NPWT vs. 13 pts closed irrigation	Primary therapy failure, in-hospital mortality, and cost of therapy	NPWT linked with lower therapeutic failure rate (15 vs. 30.7%, p<0.05), in-hospital mortality (7.5% vs. 18.5%, p<0.05) and overall cost of therapy (16 400 vs. 20 000 USD) compared with closed irrigation
Fuchs et al [125]	Retrospective	35 pts NPWT vs. 33 pts open packing	Lenght to achieve sterile woud, length of therapy, in-hospital stay, and 1-year survival	NPWT led to faster bacterial decontamination of wounds (16 vs. 26 days, p<0.01), shorter length of therapy (21 vs. 28 days, p<0.01) and in-hospital stay (25 vs. 34 days, p<0.01) and better 1-year survival (97.1 vs. 74.7%, p<0,05) compared with open packing
Sjoegren at el [126]	Retrospective	61 pts NPWT vs. 40 closed irrigation/ open packing	Therapy failure, 1- and 5-year mortality	NPWT had lower risk of therapy failure (0 vs. 15%,p<0.01), 90 day mortality (0 vs. 15%, p<0,01), and 1- and 5-year survival (93 vs. 82%, 83 vs. 59%, p<0.05) against conventional therapy
Immer et al [127]	Retrospective	38 pts NPWT vs. 17 sternectomy and flap	In-hospital stay and in-hospital mortallity, quality of life	NPWT led to shorter in-hospital stay (51.5±20.8 vs. 70.7±28.8 dnů, p<0.05), non-significantly lower in-hospital mortality (5.3 vs 11.8, NS) and better quality of life based on questionnaire SF-36 compared with sternectomy and flap

Authors	Follow-up	Patients ´cohort	Endpoints	Results
Segers [128]	Retrospective	29 pts NPWT vs. 34 pts closed irrigation	Therapy failure, in-hospital, and 1-year mortality	NPWT decreased primary therapy failure (27.6 vs. 58.9%, p<0.05), with comparable 30 day (3,5 vs. 2,9%, NS)and 1-year mortality (31.0 vs. 23.5%, NS) to closed irrigation
Bailot et al [46]	Retrospektive conventional and prospective for NPWT	125 pts NPWT vs. 24 pts. open packing	In-hospital mortality and 1-,5-, and 10 years survival	Lower mortality in NPWT group (4.8 vs. 14.1%, p=0.01), but insignificantly better 1,5, and 10 year survival(92.8 vs. 83.0%, 89.8 vs. 76.4%, 88.0 vs. 61.3%, NS)
Petzina et al [129]	Retrospective	69 pts NPWT vs. 49 closed irrigation	Primary therapy failure, in-hospital stay and mortality	NPWT associated with lower therapeutic failure (2.9% vs.18.3% p<0.05) and in-hospital mortality (5.8% vs. 24.5% p<0.05), but comparable in-hospital stay (38 vs. 41 days, NS) with closed irrigation
Simek et al [130]	Retrospective for conventional and propective pro NPWT	38 pts withNPWT vs. 28 pts closed irrigation	Primary therapy failure, in-hospital stay, in-hospital, and 1 year mortality	NPWT had lower failure of primary therapy (5.8 vs. 39.2%, p<0.05), ICU stay (209.6±33.3 vs. 516.1±449.5 hours, p<0.01),and in-hospital (5.8 vs. 21.4%, p<0.05) and 1-year mortality (14.7 vs 39.2%, p<0.05), but comparable in-hospital stay (40.2±16.3 vs. 48.8±29.2, NS) with closed irrigation.
De Feo et al [131]	Retrospective	74 pts NPWT vs. 83 pts closed irrigation	Primary therapy failure, in-hospital stay and mortality	NPWT group with lower risk of therapy failure (1.4 vs. 16.9%, p<0.001), shorter in-hospital stay (23.3±9 vs. 3.0.5±3, p<0,05), and lower in-hospital mortality (1.4 vs. 3,6 %, p<0,.05) compared with closed irrigation
Assman et al [132]	Retrospective	82 pts NPWT vs. 38 closed irrigation	In-hospital stay and mortality	NPWT patients had shorter in-hospital stay (45.6 ± 18.5 vs. 55.2 ± 23.6 dnů, p<0.05), and lower in-hospital mortality (14.6 vs. 32.4 %, p<0.05)
Vos et al [133]	Retrospective	89 pts NPWT vs. 24 open packing	In-ICU and hospital stay and mortality	NPWT led to shorter ICU stay (6.8±14.4 vs. 18.5±21.0 dnů, p<0.01), in-hospital stay (74.4±61.2 vs. 69.1±62.7 days, p<0.01), and lower in-hospital mortality (12.4 vs. 41.7%, p<0.01)
Deniz et al [134]	Retrospective	47 pts NPWT vs. 43 pts closed irrigation	Primary therapy failure, in-hospital stay and 1-, 3 years mortality	NPWT had insignificantly lower rate of primary therapy failure (2.1% vs. 4.7%, NS) and shorter in-hospital stay (18±9 vs. 24±10 days, NS), 90 days mortality significantly lower (8.5 vs. 23.2%, p<0.05) and better 1-, and 3-year

http://dx.doi.org/10.5772/55310

Authors	Follow-up	Patients ´cohort	Endpoints	Results
				survival (91.5% vs.76.7%, p<0,05, 87.2 vs. 69.8%, P<0.05)
Fleck et al [135]	Retrospective	326 pts NPWT vs. 198 closed irrigation/ open packing	Primary therapy failure, in-hospital mortality	NPWT was associated with lower primary therapy failure (8.5% vs. 34% p<0.001), and in-hospital mortality (3.6% vs. 10%, p<0.05)
Sjoegren at el [18]	Meta-analysis	12 papers focused on comparison of NPWT with conventional therapy	Primary therapy failure, in-hospital stay and mortality	NPWT associated with lower primary therapy failure, shorter in-hospital stay, and lower in-hospital and 1-year mortality
Raja et al [136]	Meta-analysis	13 papers focused on comparison of NPWT with conventional therapy	Primary therapy failure, in-hospital stay and mortality	NPWT seemed to be effective at high-risk DSWI patients, but weak evidence for routine first-line application in DSWI
Schimmer et al [137]	Meta-analysis	15 papers focused on comparison of NPWT with conventional therapy	Primary therapy failure, in-hospital stay and mortality, evaluation of German hearts centers protocols	NPWT is associated with lower therapeutic failure, and in-hospital mortality. Routinely applied as first-line treatment in 35% of German heart centers
Damiani G et al [138]	Meta-analysis	6 papers focused on comparison of NPWT with conventional therapy and chest reconstruction options	Primary therapy failure, in-hospital stay and mortality	NPWT prone to have shorter in-hospital stay and lower mortality

Table 5. Analyses and Meta-analyse of comparison NPWT with conventional therapy

Addressing specific complications of DSWI, it is seen that NPWT does not increase the risk of late infection recurrence. Reported rates of chronic fistulas after conventional therapy and NPWT were comparable between 8-12% [18,130,134,140,41], and long-term survival of these patients is negatively affected [140,142]. CONS was identified as a pathogen with a higher risk

of recurrence; its low virulence, ability to create biofilm on metallic materials and inherent low sensitivity against prophylactically administrated antibiotics limit its eradication [41,143].

With the rise in use of NPWT came an increased number of reported serious bleeding complications [144,145]. The risk of heart injury, particularly the right ventricle, bypass grafts or great vessels is well known from conventionally treated patients. Infectious erosion, displacement of heart structures towards sternal margins, or tractions of fibrosis adhesion were identified as potential mechanism of injury [146]. The incidence of these complications by conventional therapy was found to be between 2-14.8% [147-149], with data from a larger group of NPWT treated patients showing 2 to 5%, thus NPWT does not seem to increase the incidence of serious complications [116,118,127,130,146,150]. Mortality from these complications varies between 25 to 70%, with emergency surgery as well as proper covering of mediastinal structures with interface dressing being crucial for management [146-148,150]. Several layers of paraffin gauze or silicone mesh are usually put below sternal margins on the heart and grafts. Development towards more suitable material, particularly rigid barrier for mediastinal protection is in progress, including mediastinal protection and preserved drainage ability of therapy [151].

7. Reconstruction of sternal bone defect after DSWI in cardiac surgery

Wire re-cerclage was a commonly used method for addressing sternal approximation in patients with sternal dehiscence after DSWI [72,86,102]. The quality of residual sternal bone or its loss makes re-cerclage troublesome or even risky for achieving sternal stability. The occurrence of extensive adhesions below the sternum in DSWI patients increases the risk of damage to the right ventricle and bypass grafts when peri-, trans- and parasternal wiring techniques are used [72,99,100]. Today, stable osteosynthesis of the sternum, particularly using transverse plates, has become a method of treatment of post-DSWI sternal dehiscence [76]. Voss at el reported an institutional experience with Titanium Sternal Fixation system™ plates for sternal non-union in 15 patients, in which four patients had more than two previous attempts to stabilize the chest with some modification of wire re-cerclage, and four patients were treated for DSWI with NPWT prior to plating. All patients were successfully stabilized and healed, with one patient from the DSWI group experiencing a late infection recurrence and one dying from a complication not related to plating [152]. Larger experience with the same plate system has been reported by Baillot et al in a group of 92 patients after DSWI [46]. They achieved chest stabilization in all cases, with 9 patients (9.8%) undergoing further procedure for late infection recurrence including removal of the plate with no impact on sternal stability [153]. Chest stability after a healed DSWI improves respiratory function, augments wound healing processes, shortens in-hospital stay, and improves patient quality [46,72,80]. Plating seems to be an effective method of chest wall stabilization, but may fail in cases of massive loss of chest bone tissue. In these cases, the bone residue does not allow sufficient anchoring for the plates or there is a large bone tissue gap. Shear forces may loosen screws and threaten stability. Persistent pain and respiratory discomfort were also reported in this case [154]. A conventional surgical approach to manage the large residual bone defect leaves the

sternotomy wound unstable and employs the greater omentum or a muscle flap to fulfill any dead spaces [93,95,99,103]. This approach resulted in sternal instability and flap-related morbidity even when wounds were well-healed [154]. Some case reports have included the use of an autologous bone iliac crest graft or allogenous fibula graft to supply residual bone defects after DSWI [155,156]. Marulli reported the first use of an allogenous sternocostal bone graft for sternal reconstruction after chondrosarcoma removal [157]. Consequently, Dell'amore et al described four patients who were managed with the same technique with no wound healing complications and preserved chest wall stability [158]. The same authors proposed this technique for major post-DSWI defects, and [159] Kalab et al described the possibility of using an allogenous calva bone graft to address this issue. Allogenous bony grafts being fixed with transverse plates in mentioned cases [158-160]. Bone allograft usage for transplantation is under law restriction of local governments and European Association of Tissue Banks [161,162].

8. Options in soft tissue defects reconstruction after DSWI in cardiac surgery

There are a broad range of possibilities for managing sternal soft tissue defects caused by DSWI. In the case of minor defects, a direct suture with tissue undermining can be effective. In wide dehiscence, some type of flap transfer is needed and excessive bone and soft tissue loss are dependent on close co-operation between the cardiac and reconstructive surgeons. There are two crucial conditions influencing the reconstructive strategy. The first condition is the size of the defect, while the second is the vascular network, which would optimally remain uncompromised after primary surgery or previously failed reconstructions. Although various flaps and their modifications have been proposed, none have been found to be a reconstructive option for all defects [97,163,164], therefore Greig et al suggested a simple classification system to address the choice of flap based on the size and location of the post-sternotomy defect (Table 6) [165]. It is not possible, however, to follow this classification system because various factors and conditions influencing the result must be taken into the account.

Wound type	Site of sternal wound	Recommended flap for reconstruction
Type A	Upper half sternum	Pectoralis major
Type B	Lower half sternum	Combined pectoralis major and rectus abdominis bipedicled flap
Type C	Whole sternum	Combined pectoralis major and rectus abdominis bipedicled flap

Table 6. Classification of sternal wounds according to anatomical site (modified from Greig et al [165])

In 1976, Lee et al were the first to report on the use of a pedicled greater omentum to fulfill the large defect after total sternectomy [93]. In 1980, Jurkiewicz et al introduced the bilateral pectoralis turnover flap for the same indication. Although various muscle flaps, along with their modifications have been reported, there is still debate about using muscular versus

cutaneous or fasciocutaneous flaps to cover difficult defects. It has been presumed that muscular flaps carry richer vascular networks, thus bringing a better blood supply to the defect, along with a higher antibiotic concentration. Recent studies, however, did not support this hypothesis and suggested that muscle flaps have no particular advantage over fasciocutaneous flaps in terms of improving vascularity and eradicating infection [166,167]. Nevertheless, there is still a reasonable argument for muscular flaps as additional muscle brings enough tissue for planed reconstruction.

8.1. The pectoralis major flap

The pectoralis major provides many qualities that make it a suitable flap choice for covering sternal defects including close proximity to the sternotomy, triple blood supply (the thoracoacromial artery, perforating branches of the internal thoracic artery and the lateral thoracic artery), and versatility of the flap as either the thoracoacromial or internal thoracic artery vascular axis may be used separately to nourish the flap [168]. Netcher et al did not show an adverse influence of the pectoral muscle transposition on pulmonary function [169], moreover, pain and loss of strength appeared to be related more to sternal instability rather than to the muscle transposition. Additionally, Cohen et al reported an improvement of spirometric parameters (forced vital capacity and standardized forced expiratory volume in 1 second) before and after pectoral flap transfer, thus supporting the crucial role of the flap in chest stabilization [170].

8.1.1. Pectoral muscle advancement flap

The pectoral muscle advancement flap is based on the thoracoacromial pedicle and is considered to be the best muscular reconstructive option in this area due to its technical simplicity, versatility, and low risk of flap loss (<3%). There is, however, some risk of skin island necrosis or partial necrosis (≈30%) [171, 172]. Dissection and elevation of the flap begins along the median line of the costal grid until reaching the relatively avascular plane under the muscle. Undermining then proceeds by blunt dissection laterally as necessary to achieve approximation of the bilateral flaps at the median line without tension. The thoracoacromial vascular pedicle is visible at the dorsal plane of the muscle. The humeral and clavicular insertion of the muscle can be released if needed. If the distal portion of the sternum is exposed, dissection continues distally under the anterior sheet of the rectus abdominis which then becomes part of the flap [164]. Though the flap is elevated mostly in a myocutaneous fashion [73,163,164,173,174], Brutus et al reported on the use of a pectoral muscle flap released from skin for covering the entire sternal defect [175]. Completely dissected and freed from all of its origins, the pectoral muscle was advanced medially on the skeletonized vascular pedicle to cover the full length of the sternal defect. Separating the skin from the muscle can jeopardize the cutaneous blood supply and increase risk of skin necrosis. This technique included the release of humeral insertion from a short skin counter incision [175].

If the defect is wide, it may be difficult to achieve tension-free suturing in the midline. A modification of the advancement flap with a skin relaxing incision has been reported [176]. Majure et al proposed shifting the skin island over the pectoralis muscle in the V-Y manner to

cover the entire sternotomy defect, but this method requires secondary skin grafting from an island donor site [177]. This technique was adopted and modified by Molitor et al [178]. The skin island is dissected, while the underlying muscle fascia and pectoralis major are elevated and completely released from their insertions to the humerus, sternocostal junctions and abdominal muscles. The thoracoacromial vessels are visualized and the clavicular insertion of the muscle is released to achieve comfortable advancement of the flap to the defect. The secondary defect in the lateral thoracic wall is then sutured in the V-Y manner and no skin graft is needed [178].

Finally, the pectoralis major musculocuteneous flap can be mobilized in a rotational manner when the skin-muscle flap is elevated based on the thoracoacromial pedicle and is rotated to the defect [179].

8.1.2. Pectoral muscle turnover flap

This flap is based on perforators of the internal mammary artery. Once the skin is elevated off of the anterior pectoralis fascia, the distal rib, proximal clavicular origin and humeral insertion of the muscle are divided. Then, the thoracoacromial pedicle is dissected and ligated, and the pectoralis major is elevated from lateral to medial until the perforating vessels from the internal thoracic artery are identified, and the muscle is then turned into the defect. To gain additional width of the narrowing humeral portion of the flap, fascial release incisions along the direction of the muscle fibers can be done. By this maneuver an average increase in flap width of 5.8 cm can be obtained [181]. Usually bilateral turnover muscle flaps are used [94,95]. The disadvantages of this flap include limitations in the distal parts of the sternum, need for wide skin undermining, dependence on an intact internal mammary artery, and an unfavorable aesthetic consequence including a missing anterior axillary line and parasternal subcutaneous tissue bulkiness [95].

8.2. The rectus abdominis flap

This flap was first used in cardiac surgery by Jurkiewicz in the case of a pectoral turnover flap failing to cover the entire defect [94,95]. To cover the sternal defect, the rectus abdominis flap is used exclusively as a pedicled flap based on the superior epigastric artery [182]. Because this artery is the terminal branch of the internal thoracic artery, the flap cannot be used if the ipsilateral internal thoracic artery was used for bypass grafting. The functional consequences of using the rectus abdominis to reconstruct sternal defects were assessed by Netscher et al [169]. They found no significant differences in abdominal wall function between the groups of patients in whom the rectus muscle was used for reconstruction and the group without sternal wound complications. There is a higher associated risk of hernia (11%) or fascial weakness (42%) as was reported [103,183]. The rectus abdominis flap may be used as a muscular flap [94,184) or as a myocutaneous island flap [171,185].

8.2.1. Rectus abdominis muscular flap

The rectus abdominis muscular flap may be dissected without the use of a skin island. The skin incision continues distally to the desired point according to the necessary flap length. The

skin is undermined over the rectus fascia to expose the muscle. Then, the rectus anterior sheet is divided and the muscle is dissected and mobilized. The distal pedicle inferior epigastric vessels are ligated and divided. The muscle is then turned to the defect. The exposed muscle and pedicle is covered either by skin suture or grafting [95].

8.2.2. Rectus abdominis musculocutaneous flap

The myocutaneous flap can have a skin island oriented vertically along the used muscle (VRAM-vertical rectus abdominis muscle flap), or horizontally, as well as perpendicular to the muscle distal to the umbilicus (TRAM-transverse rectus abdominis muscle flap). The transverse orientation permits harvest of a larger skin paddle. Dissection of the VRAM starts with marking the skin island over the used muscle. The skin component should be placed medially near the umbilicus to include important periumbilical perforators. The skin island is cut and the skin overlying the muscle is undermined above the muscle fascia. Then, the rectus sheet is divided bilaterally at the edges of the muscle and the muscle is dissected and mobilized. The distal pedicle inferior epigastric vessels are ligated and divided. The flap is then turned to the defect. The TRAM is marked transversely under the umbilicus and skin island which can involve the entire area between the umbilicus and symphysis bilaterally. The flap is dissected in the similar way as the VRAM flap, but the mobilization of the skin island continues away from the muscle pedicle crossing the midline to the contralateral side [171,185]. Care must be taken to avoid pedicle compression passed through the subcutaneous tunnel to the sternal defect.

8.3. Combined pectoral muscle — Rectus abdominis muscle flap

For full length sternal defects, a combined pectoralis major and rectus abdominis flap (Pec-Rec flap) was proposed [186]. The flap is predominantly created on the left side, but can occasionally be bilateral. The skin overlying the pectoral muscle is elevated up to the mid-axillary line laterally and from the clavicle to the inferior costal line in a vertical direction. The pectoral muscle is elevated while preserving the thoracoacromial vessels. The muscle is detached from its humeral insertion and medially from one third of the clavicle. Dissection of the flap continues distally while elevating the thoracoepigastric fascial attachments from the chest wall between the pectoralis major and the rectus abdominis. Distal to the fascia, the anterior sheet of the rectus abdominis is incised medially and laterally and the muscle is mobilized from the posterior fascia. The muscular connections of the rectus abdominis to the distal ribs are detached as the last step of flap harvesting. The superior epigastric artery can be preserved or it can be divided close to the muscle if necessary for better medial transposition of the flap [186].

8.4. The latissimus dorsi muscle flap

The latissimus dorsi flap is based on a thoracodorsal artery that has not been jeopardized by previous cardiac surgery. Moreover, a large flap can be harvested (the main surface area of muscle is 105 cm^2 for women and 192 cm^2 for men) [187]. The main disadvantages of this flap include the need for a lateral decubital position during flap harvesting that can endanger patients with large sternal bone defect and sternal instability and shoulder functional limitation followed latissimus dorsi muscle harvesting. Patients who are dependent on their

shoulder girdle strength, such as paralytic patients in a wheelchair or walker dependent patients, may endorse strength difficulties after muscle harvesting as well as tennis and golf players or those whose profession involves overhead tasks [187]. Up to 50% of patients may complain of localized numbness at the harvesting area [172].

Usually the muscle from the non-dominant side is used. The arc of rotation and position of the skin island is assessed and marked. The skin component is predominantly oriented perpendicular to the muscle fibers near the vertebral column, but a longitudinal course from the medial axillary line to the medial caudal dorsum is also possible. The flap is dissected using the whole muscle up to the pedicle. Thoracodorsal vessels are skeletonized and humeral muscle insertion is divided, allowing an additional 4-10 cm of flap advancement. Then the flap is transposed to the defect through a subcutaneous tunnel superficial to the pectoralis major [188,189].

8.5. Breast flap

Obese female patients with large breasts are at higher risk of sternal dehiscence due to the infero-lateral tension of the breasts, especially on the distal third of the sternotomy [72].This instability results from the greater protrusion of the lower thorax and abdomen during respiration, greater dimensions of the lower versus the upper thorax, the concentration of forces from the attachment of the ribs, and the reduced thickness of the lower sternum [72]. Therefore a special bandage, supporting bra, or other garment is used to release the tension resulting from large breasts. The technique of covering the sternal dehiscence with a bilateral pectoral muscle advancement flap with simultaneous breast reduction has been reported [190-192]. Large breasts carry an enormous amount of relatively well vascularized tissue that can potentially be used to cover the sternal defect [193,194]. The vascular supply of the breast is basically the same as the pectoral muscle. There is, however, a unique vascular network inside the breast gland, known as Würinger´s septum. Uygur et al reported a method of covering a large distal sternum defect with bilateral fasciocutaneous V-Y flaps from the breasts [193]. These flaps were anatomically based on the Würinger´s septum [193,195]. Another method has been suggested by Hamdi et al [196]. They performed a septum-based therapeutic mammoplasty on two patients. The principle of this technique is to reduce breast mass with harvesting of a large fasciocutaneous flap from the inferomedial part of the breast

Another possibility for utilizing the breasts to cover the sternal defect is a Cyclops´ flap. In this technique the whole breast is transposed to the central or even contralateral chest defect, so that the areola is centralized. The breast flap in this case is based on the lateral and central vascular pedicles of the breast [197,198].

8.6. Omentum

The greater omentum is a well-vascularized tissue with plentiful lymphatic drainage and angiogenic activity [93,98,199]. Its size can be up to 36x46 cm and is reliable to cover large defects. It is difficult, however, to predict the flap size preoperatively because the greater omentum volume has no direct correlation with the patient's habitus [200]. The omentum can be transposed to the defect in various ways such as, pedicled on both gastroepiploic arteries

for defects in the distal part of sternotomy wound or mobilized on either of the gastroepiploic vessels to cover full-length sternotomy defects [201-203]. Passing the omental flap subcutaneously from the upper portion of the laparotomy bears up to a 21% risk of late herniation [202], thus, a better solution seems to create the transdiaphragmatical tunnel just right of the falciform ligament [204]. The risk of abdominal cavity infection is rare [205], but the traction on the gastroepiploic artery can cause motility disturbances of the stomach and duodenum [206], and one case of fatal cecum volvulus have been reported [207]. Laparoscopic harvesting seems to be promising in reduction of access complications and pain [108,208,209].

8.7. Microsurgical flaps

Microsurgical free flaps can be used to cover sternal defects in particular situations. This technique, due to its duration and technical complexity, should serve as a last treatment option. The use of the tensor fascia lata myocutaneous flap, rectus abdominis myocutaneous flap and deep inferior epigastric artery fasciocutaneous flap for this indication have been reported [210]. As a donor vessel, the thoracoacromial, internal thoracic or cervical vessels can be used. The cephalic vein attached to the thoracoacromial or cervical arteries, can be used for lengthening the donor vessel (arterio-venous loop) [210,211].

8.8. Specifics of care after flap surgery in cardiac surgery

There are special requirements for care after flap surgery. In general, it is important to protect the blood circulation within the flap, maintaining both general and local hemodynamics. Vascular spasm must be prevented by using vasodilator drugs if possible. The elevated and transposed flap usually loses most of its physiological blood and lymphatic network and is dependent only on a small part of it, so varying degrees of edema are usually present. Large swelling of the tissue compresses the capillaries and decreases the blood flow in the flap, increasing the tension on the suture. Corticosteroids are used to prevent swelling for several days in most flap surgeries unless serious contraindications are present. The flap must be kept from topical pressure, particularly in places of passing vascular pedicle and in peripheral parts of the flap because of limited vascular competence. Undoubtedly, changes in body position influence the blood supply of the flap. Furthermore, stretching of the arms causes increased tension on the medial sternal suture. In the case of the pectoral and latissimus dorsi flap, the use of muscles of the shoulder girdle should be avoided. When using the rectus abdominis flap, the abdominal wall must be relaxed and supported with bandages for several weeks to prevent hernia formation. Finally, nutritional support with enteral feeding is essential for successful healing.

9. University hospital Olomouc management of DSWI after cardiac surgery

9.1. Adopted treatment strategy for DSWI

We retrospectively analyzed our experience with treatment strategies of DSWI since February 2002, when our department was established. A total of 100 patients fulfilling CDC criteria [5]

http://dx.doi.org/10.5772/55310

for DSWI were enrolled until September 2011 with an overall incidence of DSWI of 1.36%. The results of 28 patients (March 2002-June 2004) primarily treated with closed chest irrigation using diluted iodine solution were compared with 76 patients (September 2004 to September 2009) treated with NPWT (VAC ATS™, KCI, St. Antonio, USA). A standardized protocol for first-line application of NPWT is depicted in Figure 1. Six patients from the interim period (June to September 2004) when closed irrigation and NPWT were combined were excluded from the analysis. Both groups had comparable demographic and perioperative characteristics, however, the NPWT arm had an insignificant trend towards advanced age, higher logistic EUROSCORE, more complex primary cardiac surgery. No difference in the rate of causative agent was found, with SA and CONS identified in almost 70% of cases. Escherichia coli (5.8%) and Pseudomonas species (7.2%) as leading Gram negative strains were cultivated. The time to presentation of DSWI was insignificant between groups (17.5±15.0 vs. 13.8±16.3, $p=0.55$) as well as readmission for late clinical presentation of DSWI (38.6% vs. 50%, $p=0.12$). Although the overall length of DSWI therapy was comparable (14.3±11.9 vs. 14.9±7.9 days, $p=0.82$), NPWT required more dressing changes (5.4±2.3 vs. 1.8±1.2, $p<0.001$), but was associated with substantially lower failure of primary therapy (5.1 vs. 39.2%, $p<0.01$) with closed chest irrigation. In-ICU stay was significantly shorter in the NPWT group (209.6±331.3 vs. 516.1±449.5 hours, $p<0.001$), nevertheless, shortened in-hospital stay (40.2±16.3 vs. 48.8±29.2 days, $p=0.16$) was insignificant in this group. Addressing mortality, 30-day and 1-year mortality was considerably lower in the NPWT arm (3.9 vs. 21.4%, $p<0.05$, 15.8 vs. 39.2%, $p<0.05$, respectively). A Kaplan-Meier 1 year-survival analysis is shown in Figure 2. The risk of major bleeding complications was comparable between groups, with 2 patients (3.6%) from the closed chest irrigation group having erosion of venous bypass graft and right ventricle (RV), and 3 patients (3.9%) from the NPWT group, including 1 debridement-related and 2 spontaneous injuries of the RV. Employment of local and advancement flaps for covering of residual defects was higher in the NPWT groups (65.7 vs. 17.8%, $p<0.01$). Our experience showed that NPWT is effective in the treatment of DSWI, compared with closed chest irrigation, leading to lower failure of primary therapy, ICU stay, and better short- and mid-survival of patients. We did not prove NPWT influenced length of in-hospital stay or risk of major bleeding, however, residual defects required more complex approach to assure sternal stability and covering defects [119,130].

9.2. Sternal stabilization and management of residual bone defects

Non-complicated sternal dehiscence following DSWI that is not associated with considerable bone loss can be stabilized with transverse titanium plates (Titanium Sternal Fixation system™, Synthes, Switzerland) at our department. Plates are applied on the anterior surface of the ribcage to achieve sufficient stability of the chest wall while minimizing the risk of an iatrogenic injury to the heart. From January 2008 to September 2012 we performed 31 sternal wall reconstructions using the Titanium Sternal Fixation system™. In four cases, osteosynthesis was applied to treat a sterile mechanical dehiscence of the median sternotomy, while 27 other chest osteosyntheses were performed after DSWI when wound bed decontamination was achieved with NPWT. In the postoperative period, 2 patients (7.4%) needed to be operatively revised due to bleeding from pectoral flap advancement; in 3 cases (11.1%) the plates needed

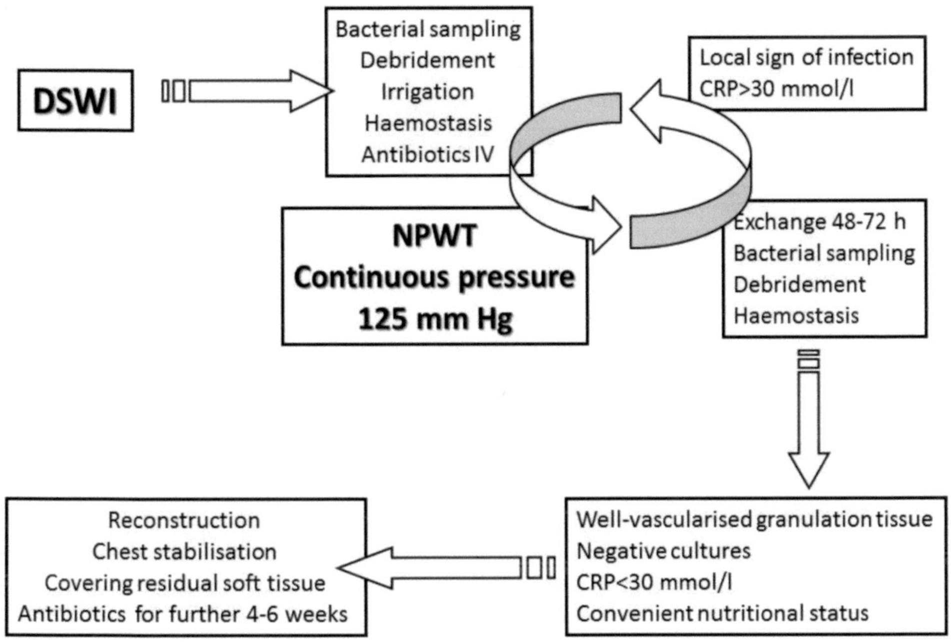

Figure 1. The first-line application protocol of NPWT for treatment of DSWI

to be removed for soft tissue healing complications post-reconstruction. Nevertheless, removal could be postponed until satisfactory healing of the sternal bones was achieved. One patient (3.7%) had to be drained for iatrogenic pneumothorax. We also retrospectively analyzed 21 patients with post-DSWI sternal dehiscence from January 2005 to January 2010, comparing 11 patients with re-cerclage wiring and 10 patients with titanium plate osteosynthesis. DSWI was managed with the same protocol of NPWT prior to reconstruction mentioned above [119]. Plating was accompanied by a lower risk of therapy failure (1% vs. 1.85%), shorter in-hospital stay (22 vs. 59%), and reduction in costs ((€8,243 vs. €33,365) (unpublished data).

In cases of minor sternal bone loss, we use an autologous bone graft harvested from the patient ´s own iliac crest. The graft is preferably prepared as bi-cortical. There is a limit to the extent of bone tissue that can be solved through this method. Fixation of the bone graft and chest stabilization is done in the manner described above. From 2009 to 2012 we used this method in 2 patients. In both cases the wounds healed successfully and the sternal wall regained full stability. Both sternal defects represented partial loss of bone tissue from 6 to 8 cm in length.

Based on this experience, we decided to apply a novel approach for the treatment of massive bone loss after DSWI, by supplying the bone defect with an allogenous bone graft. It allows

http://dx.doi.org/10.5772/55310

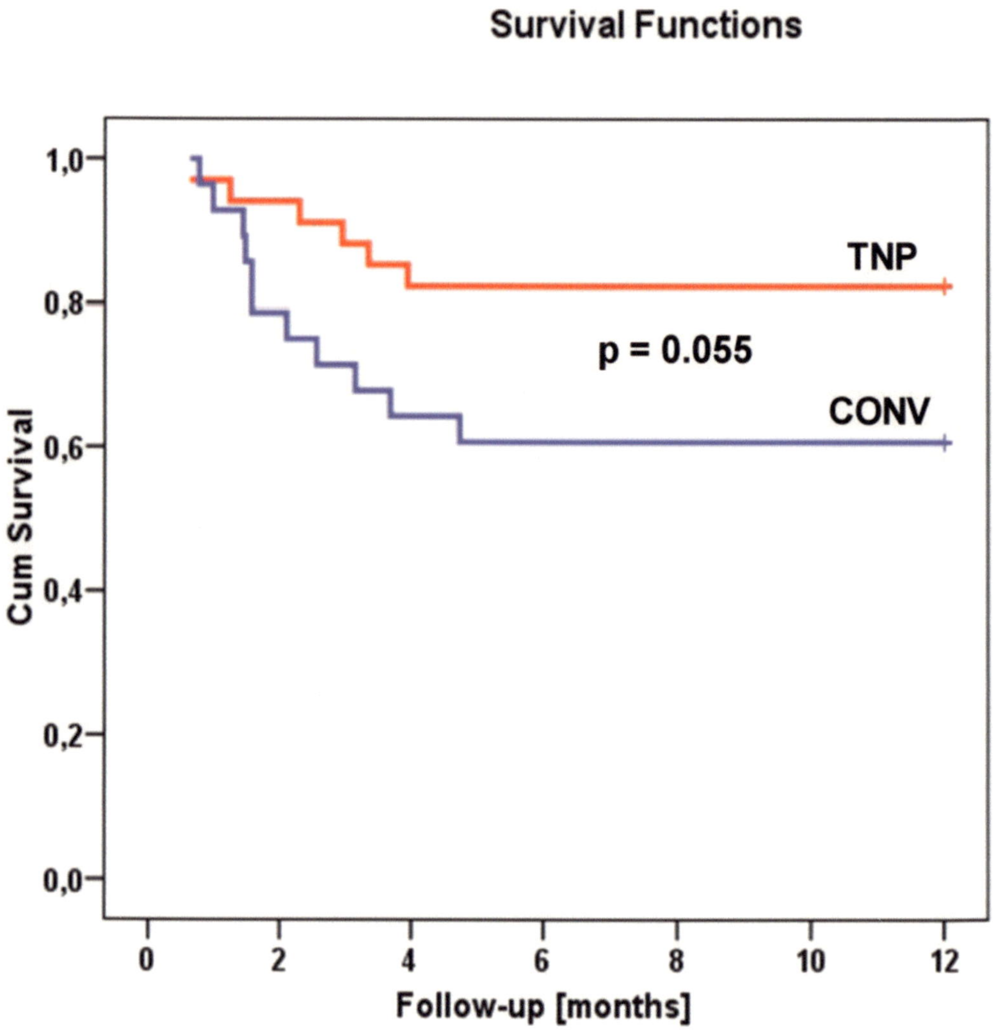

Figure 2. 1-year Kaplan-Meier survival analysis comparing NPWT with conventional therapy (CONV)

treating large sternal defects in the same way as a total or near-total sternectomy and fixed properly with titanium plate system ensures chest cage stability. An allogenous bone transplant doesn´t contain any vital bone marrow cells, which eliminates difficulties in immunogenetic acceptance of the graft by a patient; it represents a biological tissue transfer, which even under conditions of maximum precautions represents a minor risk for transmission of viral or bacterial infections. An allogenous graft must meet legislative criteria from the Czech Republic and the European Association of Tissue Banks [161,162]. Prior to graft harvesting, each donor is cross-checked for registration within the National Registry for organ donation refusal. All deceased donors treated for infectious disease, sepsis, malignant tumors, or systemic and autoimmune diseases at the time of death are withdrawn from the donor list. Donor blood serum samples are tested for antibodies and HIV types 1 and 2, hepatitis B surface

antigen (HbsAg), hepatitis C antibodies (anti-HCV), and HTLV I and II antibodies. Harvest of a sternal bone graft is performed under strictly sterile conditions by a team from the National Tissue Center in Brno. The graft is harvested under sterile conditions and stored in the freezer at −80°C. Prior to its clinical use, the graft is thawed at 4-6°C for 12 hours, soaked with a 1% gentamicin solution, prepared for its final shape, and stored in the freezer again at −80°C. If bacterial sampling is negative, the graft is thawed for 12 hours before transplantation, and submerged in a bath with 1% neomycin solution immediately before surgery.

Inherent surgical technique is modified by a more aggressive debridement of residual chest bone or ribs (1-2 cm safety line). Afterwards, the bone graft is adjusted to the size of the bone defect and fixed with plates anchored by self-cutting or self-drilling cortical screws. An uneven surface and tiny bone deficiency can be filled in with a spongy bone which is prepared from another graft provided by the tissue bank (femoral or tibial graft source). Residual soft tissue defect is covered with monolateral or bilateral pectoral muscle flap transfer. Within the postoperative period, it is strongly recommended to avoid excessive coughing or any rough mechanical strain on the sternal wall. Intravenous antibiotics are administered for at least three weeks after the reconstruction. Between January 2010 and September 2012, we performed six reconstructions of the sternal wall using an allogenous bone graft. We used a cadaveric sternum in four cases (Figure 3), and due to a lack of allografts, we had to use a calva bone in one patient (Figure 4) and a split femoral diaphysis in one patient. Successful healing after the reconstruction was achieved in five cases (83%), while one patient required additional treatment for partial skin necrosis. One obese female experienced flap failure and died from multiple organ failure. Follow-up of the other patients at 3, 6 and 12 months after reconstruction proved stability of the chest wall. A radio-isotope scan using technetium as a tracer of autologous leukocytes (Technetium-HMPAO) carried out at 3, 6 and 12 months after the reconstruction showed a high level of healing activity within the area of the allogenous bone implant, and further chest wall stability with allograft union was confirmed through 3D-CT evaluation done 5 to 7 months after the reconstruction (unpublished data).

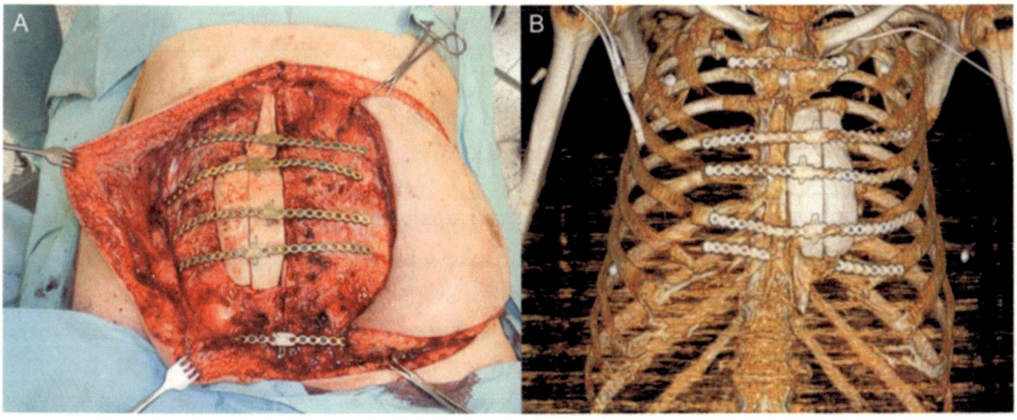

Figure 3. Cadaveric sternal allograft and its use for large residual bone defect

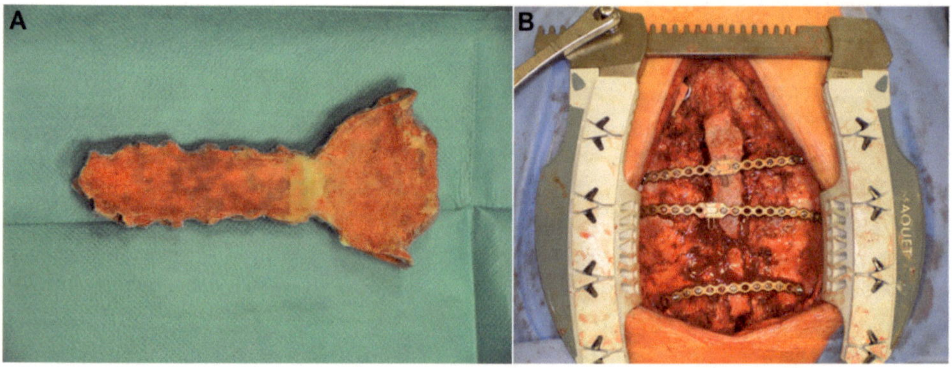

Figure 4. Cadaveric calva bone allograft in large bone defect repair and CT reconstruction showing the bone re-union

9.3. Reconstruction of residual soft tissue defects

In a group of 76 consecutive patients primarily treated with NPWT for DSWI from September 2004 to September 2011, 19 residual defects (25%) were closed by direct suture, and 57 patients (75%) underwent flap transfer to achieve reliable tension-free suture. All but 2 patients (2.7 %) underwent sternal stabilization with re-cerclage (61.8%) or transverse plates with or without bone graft (35.5%). Local fasciocutaneous advancement was used in 12 patients (21.1%), bilateral pectoralis advancement flap in 35 patients (61.2%), monolateral pectoralis flap with V-Y skin island in 7 patients (12.3%), bipedicled pectoral and rectus abdominis flap in 1 patient (1.7%), and vertical rectus abdominis flap in 2 patients (3.5%). We faced 2 flap failures (3.5%) and one whole monolateral pectoralis flap with V-Y skin island was lost due to vascular pedicle thrombosis, with 50% of the mass of the VRAM flap needing to be removed for flap necrosis. Minor healing complications requiring further local wound care were noted in 15 cases (26.3%). While the bilateral pectoralis advancement flap is a technique used by cardiac surgeons, other flaps used for covering larger residual soft tissue defects are utilized by plastic surgeon. The pectoral major flap with V-Y skin island is the first choice (Figure 5). When the defect is wide and deep, or in a female patient with large breasts, the VRAM pedicled flap is considered. If these two options fail or are not accessible, the latissimus dorsi pedicled flap is the next choice, and as a last resort, the microsurgical transfer is taken into account.

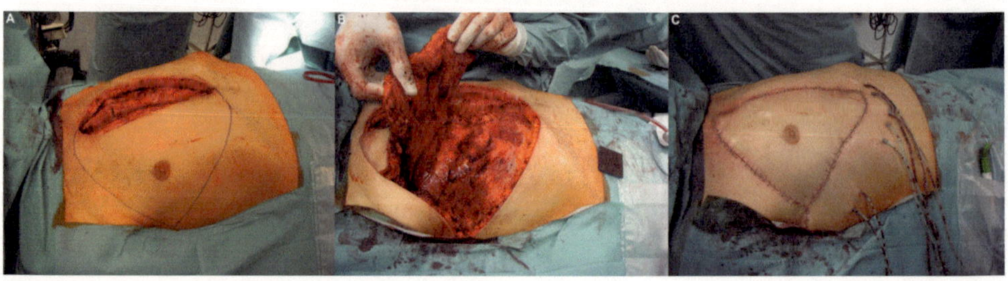

Figure 5. Technique of unilateral pectoral muscle flap advancement with V-Y skin island

10. Conclusion

DSWI remains a potentially fatal complication of cardiac surgery. Even though risk factors for development of DSWI have been identified, few are modifiable. Tight perioperative glycemic control, proper surgical technique, skeletonization of IMA grafts particularly in diabetics, and primary stable sternal approximation for high risk patients including diabetics, obese, immunosuppressed or those with COPD seem to reduce the risk of DSWI. Thanks to the unique combination of closed and open chest treatment, NPWT positively influences the survival of DSWI patients even at long-term follow-up in comparison with conventional therapy. Transverse titanium plates alone or with auto- or allograft bone allows chest cage stability irrespective to the bone mass loss. Better quality of life and lower extent of soft tissue defect might be promising for these patients who faced sternal instability and considerable flap-related morbidity some/few years ago. Plastic surgeons should be included in team planning post-DSWI sternotomy wound closure, not only called when previous closure attempt failed or residual defect seems to be extent.

Author details

Martin Šimek[1*], Martin Molitor[1], Martin Kaláb[2], Patrick Tobbia[3] and Vladimír Lonský[1]

*Address all correspondence to: martin.simek@c-mail.cz

1 Department of Cardiac Surgery, University Hospital Olomouc, Olomouc, Czech Republic

2 Department of Plastic Surgery, University Hospital Bulovka, Prague, Czech Republic

3 Department of Medicine, Cone Health, University of North Carolina, Greensboro, NC, USA

References

[1] Dalton, M. L, Connally, S. R, & Sealy, W. C. Julian's reintroduction of Milton's operation. Ann Thorac Surg (1992). , 53, 532-533.

[2] Milton, H. Mediastinal surgery. Lancet (1897). , 1, 872-5.

[3] Julian, O. C, Lopez-belio, M, Dye, W. S, Javid, H, & Grove, W. J. The median sternal incision in intracardiac surgery with extracorporeal circulation: a general evaluation of its use in heart surgery. Surgery (1957). , 42, 753-61.

[4] Balaguer, J. M, Umakanthan, R, Leacche, M, & Byrne, J. G. Minimally invasive cardiac surgery. Curr Probl Surg. (2012). , 49, 529-49.

[5] Mangram, A. J, Horan, T. C, Pearson, M. L, Silver, L. C, & Jarvis, W. R. The hospital infection control practise advisory committee. Guidelines for prevention of surgical site infection. Infect Control Hosp Epidemiol (2002). , 20, 247-78.

[6] Loop, F. D, Lytle, B. W, Cosgrove, D. M, et al. Maxwell Chamberlain memorial paper. Sternal wound complications after isolated coronary artery bypass grafting: early and late mortality, morbidity, and cost of care. Ann Thorac Surg (1990). , 49, 179-87.

[7] Milano, C. A, Kesler, K, Archibald, N, Sexton, D. J, & Jones, R. H. Mediastinitis after coronary artery bypass graft surgery. Risk factors and long-term survival. Circulation (1995). , 92, 2245-51.

[8] Braxton, J. H. Marrin CAS, McGrath PD, et al. Mediastinitis and long-term survival after coronary artery bypass graft surgery. Ann Thorac Surg (2000). , 70, 2004-7.

[9] Eklund, A. M, Lyytikainen, O, Klemets, P, et al. Mediastinitis after more than 10,000 cardiac surgical procedures. Ann Thorac Surg (2006). , 82, 1784-9.

[10] The Parisian Mediastinitis Study GroupRisk factors for deep sternal wound infection after sternotomy: a prospective, multicenter study. The Journal of Thoracic and Cardiovascular Surgery (1996). , 111, 1200-1207.

[11] Hollenbeak, C. S, Murphy, D. M, Koenig, S, Woodward, R. S, Dunagan, W. C, & Fraser, V. J. The clinical and economic impact of deep chest surgical site infections following coronary artery bypass graft surgery. Chest (2000). , 118, 397-402.

[12] Filsoufi, F, Castillo, J. G, Rahmanian, P. B, et al. Epidemiology of deep sternal wound infection in cardiac surgery. J Cardiothorac Vasc Anesth (2009). , 23, 488-94.

[13] Tang GHL, Maganti M, Weisel RD, Borger MA. Prevention and management of deep sternal wound infection. Semin Thorac Cardiovasc Surg (2004). , 16, 62-9.

[14] Toumpoulis, I. K, & Anagnostopoulos, C. E. Derose JJ Jr, Swistel DG. The impact of deep sternal wound infection on long-term survival after coronary artery bypass grafting. Chest (2005). , 127, 464-71.

[15] Risnes, I, Abdelnoor, M, Almdahl, S. M, & Svennevig, J. L. Mediastinitis after coronary artery bypass grafting risk factors and long-term survival. Ann Thorac Surg (2010). , 89, 1502-10.

[16] Crabtree, T. D, Codd, J. E, Fraser, V. J, Bailey, M. S, & Olsen, M. A. Damiano RJ Jr. Multivariate analysis of risk factors for deep and superficial sternal infection after coronary artery bypass grafting at a tertiary care medical center. Semin Thorac Cardiovasc Surg. (2004). , 2004, 16-53.

[17] Fowler VG JrO'Brien SM, Muhlbaier LH, Corey GR, Ferguson TB, Peterson ED. Clinical predictors of major infections after cardiac surgery. Circulation. 200;112(9 Suppl):I, 358-65.

[18] Sjögren, J, Malmsjö, M, Gustafsson, R, & Ingemansson, R. Poststernotomy mediastinitis: a review of conventional surgical treatments, vacuum-assisted closure therapy and presentation of the Lund University Hospital mediastinitis algorithm.Eur J Cardiothorac Surg (2006). , 30, 898-905.

[19] Matros, E, Aranki, S. F, Bayer, L. R, et al. Reduction in incidence of deep sternal wound infections: random or real? J Thorac Cardiovasc Surg (2010). , 139, 680-5.

[20] De Feo, M, Vicchio, M, Santè, P, Cerasuolo, F, & Nappi, G. Evolution in the treatment of mediastinitis: single-center experience. Asian Cardiovasc Thorac Ann. (2011). , 19, 39-43.

[21] Upton, A, Roberts, S. A, Milsom, P, & Morris, A. J. Staphylococcal post- sternotomy mediastinitis: five year audit. ANZ J Surg. (2005). , 75, 198-203.

[22] Sachithanandan, A, Nanjaiah, P, Nightingale, P, et al. Deep sternal wound infection requiring revision surgery: impact on mid-term survival following cardiac surgery. Eur J Cardiothorac Surg (2008). , 33, 673-8.

[23] Pritisanac, A, Gulbins, H, Rosendahl, U, & Ennker, J. Outcome of heart surgery procedures in octogenarians: is age really not an issue? Expert Rev Cardiovasc Ther (2007).

[24] Prabhakar, G, Haan, C. K, Peterson, E. D, Coombs, L. P, Cruzzavala, J. L, & Murray, C. F. The risks of moderate and extreme obesity for coronary artery bypass grafting outcomes: A study from the Society of Thoracic Surgeons' database. Ann Thorac Surg (2002). , 74, 1125-31.

[25] Furnary, A. P, Zerr, K. J, Grunkemeier, G. L, & Starr, A. Continuous intravenous insulin infusion reduces the incidence of deep sternal wound infection in diabetic patients after cardiac surgical procedures. Ann Thorac Surg (1999). , 67, 352-60.

[26] Halkos, M. E, Puskas, J. D, Lattouf, O. M, et al. Elevated preoperative hemoglobin A1c level is predictive of adverse events after coronary artery bypass surgery. J Thorac Cardiovasc Surg (2008). , 136, 631-40.

[27] Toumpoulis, I. K, Theakos, N, & Dunning, J. Does bilateral internal thoracic artery harvest increase the risk of mediastinitis? Interact Cardiovasc Thorac Surg (2007). , 6, 787-91.

[28] De Paulis, R, De Notaris, S, Scaffa, R, et al. The effect of bilateral internal thoracic artery harvesting on superficial and deep sternal infection: the role of skeletonization. J Thorac Cardiovasc Surg (2005). , 129, 536-43.

[29] Curtis, J. J, Clark, N. C, Mckenney, C. A, et al. Tracheostomy: a risk factor for mediastinitis after cardiac operation. Annals of Thoracic Surgery (2001). , 72, 731-734.

[30] Rahmanian, P. B, Adams, D. H, Castillo, J. G, et al. Tracheostomy is not a risk factor for deep sternal wound infection after cardiac surgery. Annals of Thoracic Surgery (2007)., 84, 1984-1991.

[31] Hubner, N, Rees, W, Seufert, K, et al. Percutaneous dilatational tracheostomy done early after cardiac surgery-outcome and incidence of mediastinitis. The Thoracic and Cardiovascular Surgeon (1998)., 46, 89-92.

[32] Diehl, J. L, El Atrous, S, Touchard, D, et al. Changes in the work of breathing induced by tracheotomy in ventilator-dependent patients. American Journal of Respiratory and Critical Care Medicine (1999)., 159, 383-388.

[33] Banbury, M. K, Brizzio, M. E, Rajeswaran, J, et al. Transfusion increases the risk of postoperative infection after cardiovascular surgery. Journal of the American College of Surgeons (2006)., 202, 131-138.

[34] Gardlund, B, Bitkover, C, & Vaage, J. Postoperative mediastinitis in cardiac surgery microbiology and pathogenesis. Eur J Cardiothorac Surg (2002)., 21, 825-30.

[35] Mekontso-dessap, A, Kirsch, M, Brun-buisson, C, & Loisance, D. Poststernotomy mediastinitis due to Staphylococcus aureus: comparison of methicillin-resistent and methicillin-susceptible cases. Clin Infect Dis (2001)., 32, 877-83.

[36] San Juan R, Chaves F, López Gude MJ, Díaz-Pedroche C, Otero J, Cortina Romero JM, Rufilanchas JJ, Aguado JM.Staphylococcus aureus poststernotomy mediastinitis: description of two distinct acquisition pathways with different potential preventive approaches. J Thorac Cardiovasc Surg. (2007)., 134, 670-6.

[37] Jakob, H. G, Borneff-lipp, M, Bach, A, et al. The endogenous pathway is a major route for deep sternal wound infection. European Journal of Cardio-Thoracic Surgery (2000)., 17, 154-160.

[38] Kluytmans, J. A, Mouton, J. W, Ijzerman, E. P, et al. Nasal carriage of Staphylococcus aureus as a major risk factor for wound infections after cardiac surgery. The Journal of Infectious Diseases (1995)., 171, 216-219.

[39] Von Eiff, C, Becker, K, Machka, K, Stammer, H, & Peters, G. Nasal carriage as a source of Staphylococcus aureus bacteremia. Study Group. N Engl J Med (2001)., 344, 11-16.

[40] San Juan R, Aguado JM, López MJ, et al. Accuracy of blood culture for early diagnosis of mediastinitis in febrile patients after cardiac surgery. Eur J Clin Microbiol Infect Dis. (2005)., 2005, 24-182.

[41] Tegnell, A, Aren, C, & Ohman, L. Coagulase-negative staphylococi and sternal infections after cardiac operation. Ann Thorac Surg (2000)., 69, 1104-9.

[42] Mekontso Dessap A, Vivier E, Girou E, Brun-Buisson C, Kirsch M.Effect of time to onset on clinical features and prognosis of post-sternotomy mediastinitis. Clin Microbiol Infect (2011)., 17, 292-9.

[43] Jonkers, D, Elenbaas, T, Terporten, P, et al. Prevalence of 90 days postoperative wound infections after cardiac surgery. European Journal of Cardio-Thoracic Surgery (2003)., 23, 97-102.

[44] Mekontso-dessap, A, Kirsch, M, Brun-buisson, C, & Loisance, D. Poststernotomy mediastinitis due to Staphylococcus aureus: comparison of methicillin-resistant and methicillin-susceptible cases. Clin Infect Dis. (2001)., 32, 877-83.

[45] Mauermann, W. J, & Sampathkumar, P. Sternal wound infection. Best Practice & Research Clinical Anaesthesiology (2008)., 22, 423-436.

[46] Baillot, R, Cloutier, D, Montalin, L, et al. Impact of deep sternal wound infection management with vacuum-assisted closure therapy followed by sternal osteosynthesis: a 15-year review of 23,499 sternotomies. Eur J Cardiothorac Surg (2010)., 37, 880-7.

[47] Speir, A. M, Kasirajan, V, Barnett, S. D, & Fonner, E. Jr. Additive costs of postoperative complications for isolated coronary artery bypass grafting patients in Virginia. Ann Thorac Surg (2009)., 88, 40-6.

[48] De Feo, M, Renzulli, A, Ismeno, G, & Gregorio, R. Della Corte A, Utili R, et al. Variables predicting adverse outcome in patients with deep sternal wound infection. *Ann Thorac Surg* (2001)., 71, 324-331.

[49] Graf, K, Ott, E, Vonberg, R. P, Kuehn, C, Haverich, A, & Chaberny, I. F. Economic aspects of deep sternal wound infections. Eur J Cardiothorac Surg (2010)., 37, 893-6.

[50] Ennker, I. C, Kojcici, B, Ennker, J, Vogt, P, & Melichercik, J. Examination of the opportunity costs and turnover situation in patients with deep sternal infections. Zentralbl Chir (2012)., 137, 257-61.

[51] Moidl, R, Fleck, T, Giovanoli, P, Grabenwöger, M, & Wolner, E. Cost effectiveness of V.A.C. therapy after post-sternotomy mediastinitis. Zentralbl Chir (2006). S, 189-90.

[52] Mokhtari, A, Sjögren, J, Nilsson, J, Gustafsson, R, Malmsjö, M, & Ingemansson, R. The cost of vacuum-assisted closure therapy in treatment of deep sternal wound infection. Scand Cardiovasc J (2008)., 42, 85-89.

[53] Atkins, Z. B, & Wolfe, G. Sternal Wound Complications Following Cardiac Surgery. In: Cuneyt N. (ed). Special topics in cardiac surgery. Rijeka, InTech;, 284-308.

[54] Lazar, H. L, Chipkin, S. R, Fitzgerald, C. A, Bao, Y, Cabral, H, & Apstein, C. S. Tight glycemiccontrol in diabetic coronary artery bypass graft patients improves perioperativeoutcomes and decreases recurrent ischemic events. Circulation (2004)., 109, 1497-502.

[55] Gandhi, G. Y, Nuttall, G. A, Abel, M. D, Mullany, C. J, Schaff, H. V, Brien, O, Johnson, P. C, Williams, M. G, Cutshall, A. R, Mundy, S. M, Rizza, L. M, & Mcmahon, R. A. MM. Intensive intraoperative insulin therapy versus conventional glucose management during cardiac surgery: a randomized trial. Ann Intern Med. 200;, 146, 233-43.

[56] Bratzler, D. W, Houck, P. M, Richards, C, Steele, L, et al. Use of antimicrobial prophylaxis for major surgery: baseline results from the National Surgical Infection Prevention Project. Arch Surg. (2005). , 140, 174-82.

[57] Finkelstein, R, Rabino, G, Mashiah, T, et al. Vancomycin versus cefazolin prophylaxis for cardiac surgery in the setting of a high prevalence of methicillin-resistant staphylococcal infections. The Journal of Thoracicand Cardiovascular Surgery (2002). , 123, 326-332.

[58] Bolon, M. K, Morlote, M, Weber, S. G, et al. Glycopeptides are no more effective than beta-lactam agents for prevention of surgical site infection after cardiac surgery: a meta-analysis. Clinical Infectious Diseases (2004). , 38, 1357-1363.

[59] Friberg, O, Svedjeholm, R, Soderquist, B, Granfeldt, H, Vikerfors, T, & Kallman, J. Local gentamicin reduces sternal wound infections after cardiac surgery: a randomized controlled trial. Ann Thorac Surg (2005). , 79, 153-61.

[60] Friberg, O, Dahlin, L. G, Källman, J, Kihlström, E, Söderquist, B, & Svedjeholm, R. Collagen-gentamicin implant for prevention of sternal wound infection; long-term follow-up of effectiveness.Interact Cardiovasc Thorac Surg. (2009). , 9, 454-8.

[61] Bennett-guerrero, E. Ferguson TB Jr, Lin M, Garg J, Mark DB, Scavo VA Jr et al. SWIPE-1 Trial Group. Effect of an implantable gentamicin-collagen sponge on sternal wound infections following cardiac surgery: a randomized trial. J Am Med Assoc (2010). , 304, 755-62.

[62] Mavros, M. N, Mitsikostas, P. K, Alexiou, V. G, Peppas, G, & Falagas, M. E. Gentamicin collagen sponges for the prevention of sternal wound infection: A meta-analysis of randomized controlled trials. J Thorac Cardiovasc Surg. (2012). , 144, 1235-40.

[63] Kaiser, A. B, Kernodle, D. S, Barg, N. L, et al. Influence of preoperative showers on staphylococcal skin colonization: a comparative trial of antiseptic skin cleansers. Annals of Thoracic Surgery (1988). , 45, 35-38.

[64] Byrne DNA, Cuschieri A. The value of whole body disinfection in the prevention of post-operative wound infection in clean and potentially contaminated surgery. Surgical Research Communications (1992). , 12, 43-52.

[65] Perl, T. M, & Golub, J. E. New approaches to reduce Staphylococcus aureus nosocomial infection rates:treating S. aureus nasal carriage. Annals of Pharmacotherapy (1998). S, 7-16.

[66] Cimochowski, G. E, Harostock, M. D, Brown, R, et al. Intranasal mupirocin reduces sternal wound infection after open heart surgery in diabetics and nondiabetics. Annals of Thoracic Surgery (2001). , 71, 1572-1578.

[67] Konvalinka, A, Errett, L, & Fong, I. W. Impact of treating Staphylococcus aureus nasal carriers on wound infections in cardiac surgery. J Hosp Infect. (2006). , 64, 162-8.

[68] Graf, K, Sohr, D, Haverich, A, Kühn, C, Gastmeier, P, & Chaberny, I. F. Decrease of deep sternal surgical site infection rates after cardiac surgery by a comprehensive infection control program. Interact Cardiovasc Thorac Surg. (2009). , 9, 282-6.

[69] Saso, S, James, D, Vecht, J. A, Kidher, E, Kokotsakis, J, Malinovski, V, Rao, C, Darzi, A, Anderson, J. R, & Athanasiou, T. Effect of skeletonization of the internal thoracic artery for coronary revascularization on the incidence of sternal wound infection. Ann Thorac Surg (2010). , 89, 661-70.

[70] Hirose, H, Amano, A, Takanashi, S, & Takahashi, A. Skeletonized bilateral internal mammary artery grafting for patients with diabetes. Interact Cardiovasc Thorac Surg (2003). , 2, 287-92.

[71] Baskett RJF, MacDougall CE, Ross DB. Is mediastinitis a preventable complication? A 10-year review. Ann Thorac Surg (1999). , 67, 462-5.

[72] Robicsek, F, Daugherty, H. K, & Cook, J. W. The prevention and treatment of sternum separartion following open-heart surgery J Thorac Cardiovasc Surg (1977). , 73, 267-268.

[73] Sharma, R, Puri, D, Panigrahi, B. P, & Virdi, I. S. A modified parasternal wire technique for prevention and treatment of sternal dehiscence Ann Thorac Surg (2004). , 77, 210-213.

[74] Friberg, Ö, Dahlin, L. G, Söderquist, B, Källman, J, & Svedjeholm, R. Influence of more than six sternal fixation wires on the incidence of deep sternal wound infection Thorac Cardiovasc Surg (2006). , 54, 468-473.

[75] Schimmer, C, Reents, W, Berneder, S, et al. Prevention of sternal dehiscence and infection in high-risk patients: a prospective randomized multicenter trial. Ann Thorac Surg (2008). , 86, 1897-904.

[76] Plass, A, Emmert, M. Y, Pilsl, M, Salzberg, S. P, Genoni, M, Falk, V, & Grunenfelder, J. Sternal plate closure: indications, surgical procedure and follow-up. Thorac Cardiovasc Surg (2011). , 59, 30-3.

[77] Raman, J, Lehmann, S, Zehr, K, et al. Sternal Closure With Rigid Plate Fixation Versus Wire Closure: A Randomized Controlled Multicenter Trial. Ann Thorac Surg. (2012). doi:pii:S0003-4975(12)01863-2. 0.1016/j.athoracsur.2012.07.085. [Epub ahead of print]

[78] Negri, A, Manfredi, J, Terrini, A, Rodella, G, Bisleri, G, El Quarra, S, & Muneretto, C. Prospective evaluation of a new sternal closure method with thermoreactive clips. Eur J Cardiothorac Surg (2002). , 22, 571-5.

[79] Snyder, C. W, Graham, L. A, Byers, R. E, & Holman, W. L. Primary sternal plating to prevent sternal wound complications after cardiac surgery: early experience and patterns of failure. Interact CardioVasc Thorac Surg (2009). , 9, 763-766.

[80] Bennett-guerrero, E, Phillips-bute, B, Waweru, P. M, Gaca, J. G, Spann, J. C, & Milano, C. A. Pilot study of sternal plating for primary closure of the sternum in cardiac surgical patients. Innovations. (2011). , 6, 382-8.

[81] http://www.kci1.com/KCI1/prevena

[82] Stannard, J. P, Atkins, B. Z, Malley, O, Singh, D, Bernstein, H, Fahey, B, Masden, M, & Attinger, D. CE. Use of negative pressure therapy on closed surgical incisions: a case series. Ostomy Wound Management (2009). , 55, 58-66.

[83] Wackenfors, A, Sjögren, J, Gustafsson, R, Algotsson, L, Ingemansson, R, & Malmsjö, M. Effects of vacuum-assisted closure therapy on inguinal wound edge microvascular blood flow. Wound Repair Regen (2004). , 12, 600-6.

[84] Colli, A. First experience with a new negative pressure incision management system on surgical incisions after cardiac surgery in high risk patients. Journal of Cardiothoracic Surgery (2011).

[85] Atkins, B. Z, Wooten, M. K, Kistler, J, Hurley, K, & Hughes, G. C. Wolfe WG: Does negative pressure wound therapy have a role in preventing poststernotomy wound complications? Surg Innov (2009).

[86] Robicsek, F. Postoperative Sterno-mediastinitis. Am Surg (2000). , 66, 184-192.

[87] Sarr, M. G, Gott, V. L, & Townsend, T. R. Mediastinal infection after cardiac surgery. Ann Thorac Surg (1984).

[88] Shumacker, H. B, & Mandelbaum, I. Continuous antibiotic irrigation in the treatment of infection. Arch Surg (1963).

[89] Merrill, W. H, Akhter, S. A, Wolf, R. K, & Schneeberger, E. W. Flege JB Jr. Simplified treatment of postoperative mediastinitis..Ann Thorac Surg. (2004). , 78, 608-12.

[90] .Poncelet, A. J, Lengele, B, Delaere, B, et al. Algorithm for primary closure in sternal wound infection. a single institution 10-year experience. Eur J Cardiothorac Surg. (2008). , 33, 232-8.

[91] Kirsch, M, Mekontso-dessap, A, Houël, R, Giroud, E, Hillion, M. L, & Loisance, D. Y. Closed drainage using redon catheters for poststernotomy mediastinitis: results and risk factors for adverse outcome.. Ann Thorac Surg. (2001). , 71, 1580-6.

[92] Levi, N, & Olsen, P. S. Primary closure of deep sternal wound infection following open heart surgery: a safe operation? J Cardiovasc Surg (Torino). (2000). Apr;, 41(2), 241-5.

[93] Lee, A. B, Schimert, G, Shaktin, S, et al. Total excision of the sternum and thoracic pedicle transposition of the greater omentum; useful stratagems in managing severe mediastinal infection following open heart surgery. Surgery (1976). , 80, 433-6.

[94] Jurkiewicz, M. J, Bostwick, J, Hester, T. R, et al. Infected median sternotomy wound: successful treatment by muscle flaps. Ann Surg (1980).

[95] Jones, G, Jurkiewicz, M. J, et al. Management of the infected median sternotomy wound with muscle flaps. Ann Surg (1997). , 225, 766-78.

[96] Brandt, C, & Alvarez, J. M. First-line treatment of deep sternal infection by a plastic surgical approach: superior results compared with conventional cardiac surgical orthodoxy. Plast Reconstr Surg. (2002). , 109, 2231-7.

[97] Wong CHK, Senewiratne S, Garlick G, Mullany D. Two-stage management of sternal wound infection using bilateral pectoralis major advancement flap. Eur J Cardiothorac Surg (2006). , 30, 148-152.

[98] Milano, C. A, Georgiade, G, Muhlbaier, L. H, Smith, P. K, & Wolfe, W. G. Comparison of omental and pectoralis flaps for poststernotomy mediastinitis. Ann Thorac Surg (1999). , 67, 377-81.

[99] El Oakley, R. M, & Wright, J. E. Postoperative mediastinitis: classification and management. Ann Thorac Surg (1996). , 61, 1030-6.

[100] Molina, E. Primary closure for infected dehiscence of the sternum. Ann Thorac Surg (1993). , 55, 459-63.

[101] Scully, H. F, Leclerc, Y, Martin, R. D, et al. Comparison between antibiotic irrigation and mobilization of pectoral muscle flaps in treatment of deep sternal infection. J Thorac Cardiovasc Surg (1985). , 90, 523-31.

[102] Rand, R. P, Cochran, R. P, Aziz, S, Hofer, B. O, Allen, M. D, Verrier, E. D, et al. Prospective trial of catheter irrigation and muscle flaps for sternal wound infection. *Ann Thorac Surg* (1998). , 65, 1046-1049.

[103] Ringelman, P. R, Vander, K. C, Cameron, D, Bumgartner, W. A, & Manson, P. N. Long-term results of flap reconstruction in median sternotomy wound infection. Plast Reconstr Surg (1994). , 93, 1208-14.

[104] Pairolero, P. C, & Arnold, P. C. Management of recalcitrant median sternotomy wounds. J Thorac Cardiovasc Surg (1984). , 88, 357-64.

[105] Levi, N, & Olsen, P. S. Primary closure of deep sternal wound infection following open heart surgery: a safe operation? J Cardiovasc Surg (Torino). (2000). , 41, 241-5.

[106] Nahai, F, Rand, R. P, Hester, T. R, et al. Primary treatment of the infected sternotomy wound with muscle flaps: a review of 211 consecutive cases. Plast Reconstr Surg (1989)., 84, 434-441.

[107] Kutsal, A, Ibrisim, E, Catav, Z, et al. Mediastinitis after open heart surgery. Analysis of risk factors and management. J Cardiovasc Surg (Torino) (1991)., 32, 38-41.

[108] Van Wingerden, J. J, Coret, M. E, Van Nieuwenhoven, C. A, & Totté, E. R. The laparoscopically harvested omental flap for deep sternal wound infection. Eur J Cardiothorac Surg (2010)., 37, 87-92.

[109] Atkins, B. Z, Onaitis, M. W, Hutcheson, K. A, Kaye, K, Petersen, R. P, & Wolfe, W. G. Does method of sternal repair influence long-term outcome of postoperative mediastinitis? Am J Surg. (2011)., 202, 565-7.

[110] Christian, M. The role of hyperbaric oxygen therapy in the treatment of sternal wound infectionEur J Cardiothorac Surg (2006)., 30, 153-159.

[111] Siondalski, P, Keita, L, Sicko, Z, Zelechowski, P, Jaworski, L, & Rogowski, J. Surgical treatment and adjunct hyperbaric therapy to improve healing of wound infection complications after sterno-mediastinitis. Pneumonol Alergol Pol (2003)., 71, 12-16.

[112] Obdeijn, M. C, De Lange, M. Y, Lichtendahl, D. H, & De Boer, W. J. Vacuum-assisted closure in the treatment of poststernotomy mediastinitis. Ann Thorac Surg (1999)., 68, 2358-60.

[113] Catarino, P. A, Chamberlain, M. H, Wright, N. C, Black, E, Campbell, K, Robson, D, & Pillai, R. G. High-pressure suction drainage via a polyurethane foam in the management of poststernotomy mediastinitis. Ann Thorac Surg (2000)., 70, 1891-5.

[114] Gustafsson, R. I, Sjögren, J, & Ingemansson, R. Deep sternal wound infection: a sternal-sparing technique with vacuum-assisted closure therapy. Ann Thorac Surg. (2003)., 76, 2048-53.

[115] Fleck, T. M, Fleck, M, Moidl, R, et al. The vacuum-assisted closure system for the treatment of deep sternal wound infections after cardiac surgery. Ann Thorac Surg (2002)., 74, 1596-600.

[116] Sjögren, J, Gustafsson, R, Nilsson, J, Lindstedt, S, Nozohoor, S, & Ingemansson, R. Negative-pressure wound therapy following cardiac surgery: bleeding complications and 30-day mortality in 176 patients with deep sternal wound infection. Interact Cardiovasc Thorac Surg (2011)., 12, 117-20.

[117] Fleck, T, Moidl, R, Giovanoli, P, et al. A conclusion from the first 125 patients treated with the vacuum assisted closure system for postoperative sternal wound infection. Interact Cardiovasc Thorac Surg. (2006)., 5, 145-8.

[118] Ennker, I. C, Malkoc, A, Pietrowski, D, Vogt, P. M, Ennker, J, & Albert, A. The concept of negative pressure wound therapy (NPWT) after poststernotomy mediastinitis--a single center experience with 54 patients. J Cardiothorac Surg. (2009). Jan 12;4:5.

[119] Šimek, M, Kaláb, M, Molitor, M, et al. Topical negative pressure in the treatment of deep sternal infection following cardiac surgery: 5-year results of first-line application protocol. The EWMA Journal (2011). , 11, 38-41.

[120] Gustafsson, R, Johnsson, P, Algotsson, L, Blomquist, S, & Ingemansson, R. Vacuum-assisted closure therapy guided by C-reactive protein level in patients with deep sternal wound infection. J Thorac Cardiovasc Surg (2002). , 123, 895-900.

[121] Berg, H. F. Brands WGB, Geldrop van TR, Kluytmans-VandenBergh MFQ, Kluytmans JAJW. Comparison between closed drainage techniques for the treatment of postoperative mediastinitis. Ann Thorac Surg (2000). , 70, 924-929.

[122] Doss, M, Martens, S, Wood, J. P, Wolff, J. D, & Baier, C. Moritz. Vacuum-assisted suction drainage versus conventional treatment in the management of poststernotomy osteomyelitis Eur J Cardiothorac Surg (2002). , 22, 934-938.

[123] Song, D. H, Wu, L. C, Lohman, R. F, Gottlieb, L. J, & Franczyk, M. Vacuum-assisted closure for the treatment of sternal wounds: the bridge between debridement and definitive closure. Plast Reconstr Surg (2003). , 111, 92-97.

[124] Luckraz, H, Murphy, F, Bryant, S, Charman, S, & Ritchie, A. Vacuum-assisted closure as a treatment modality for infections after cardiac surgery J Thorac Cardiovasc Surg (2003). , 125, 301-305.

[125] Fuchs, U, Zittermann, A, Stuetten, B, Groening, A, Minami, K, & Koefer, R. Clinical outcome of patients with deep sternal infection managed by vacuum-assisted closure compared to conventional therapy with open packing: A retrospective analysis. Ann Thorac Surg (2005). , 79, 526-31.

[126] Sjögren, J, Gustafsson, R, Nilsson, J, Malmsjö, M, & Ingemansson, R. Clinical outcome after poststernotomy mediastinitis: vacuum-assisted closure versus conventional treatment. Ann Thorac Surg. (2005). , 79, 2049-55.

[127] Immer, F. F, Durrer, M, Mühlemann, K. S, Erni, D, Gahl, B, & Carrel, T. P. Deep sternal wound infection after cardiac surgery: modality of treatment and outcome. Ann Thorac Surg. (2005). , 80, 957-61.

[128] Segers, P, De Jong, A. P, & Kloek, J. J. de Mol BAJM. Poststernotomy mediastinitis: comparison of two treatment modalities. Interact Cardiovasc Thorac Surg (2005). , 4, 555-560.

[129] Petzina, R, Hoffmann, J, Navasardyan, A, et al. Negative pressure wound therapy for post-sternotomy mediastinitis reduces mortality rate and sternal re-infection rate compared to conventional treatment.Eur J Cardiothorac Surg (2010). , 38, 110-3.

[130] Simek, M, Hajek, R, Fluger, I, et al. Superiority of topical negative pressure over closed irrigation therapy of deep sternal wound infection in cardiac surgery. J Cardiovasc Surg (Torino) (2012). , 53, 113-20.

[131] De Feo, M. Della Corte A, Vicchio M, Pirozzi F, Nappi G, Cotrufo M. Is post-sternotomy mediastinitis still devastating after the advent of negative-pressure wound therapy? Tex Heart Inst J (2011). , 38, 375-80.

[132] Assmann, A, Boeken, U, Feindt, P, Schurr, P, Akhyari, P, & Lichtenberg, A. Vacuum-assisted wound closure is superior to primary rewiring in patients with deep sternal woundinfection. Thorac Cardiovasc Surg (2011). , 59, 25-9.

[133] Vos, R. J, Yilmaz, A, Sonker, U, Kelder, J. C, & Kloppenburg, G. T. Vacuum-assisted closure of post-sternotomy mediastinitis as compared to open packing. Interact Cardiovasc Thorac Surg. (2012). , 14, 17-21.

[134] Deniz, H, Gokaslan, G, Arslanoglu, Y, Ozcaliskan, O, Guzel, G, Yasim, A, & Ustunsoy, H. Treatment outcomes of postoperative mediastinitis in cardiac surgery; negative pressure wound therapy versus conventional treatment. J Cardiothorac Surg (2012).

[135] Fleck, T, & Fleck, M. Negative pressure wound therapy for the treatment of sternal wound infections after cardiac surgery. Int Wound J (2012). doi:j.X.2012.01079.x. [Epub ahead of print], 1742-481.

[136] Raja, S. G, & Berg, G. A. Should vacuum-assisted closure therapy be routinely used for management of deep sternal wound infection after cardiac surgery?Interact CardioVasc Thorac Surg (2007). , 6-523.

[137] Schimmer, C, Sommer, S. P, Bensch, M, Elert, O, & Leyh, R. Management of poststernotomy mediastinitis: experience and results of different therapy modalities.Thorac Cardiovasc Surg. (2008). , 56, 200-4.

[138] Damiani, G, Pinnarelli, L, Sommella, L, Tocco, M. P, Marvulli, M, Magrini, P, & Ricciardi, W. Vacuum-assisted closure therapy for patients with infected sternal wounds: a meta-analysis of current evidence. J Plast Reconstr Aesthet Surg (2011). , 64, 1119-23.

[139] De Feo, M, Vicchio, M, Nappi, G, & Cotrufo, M. Role of vacuum in methicillin-resistant deep sternal wound infection.Asian Cardiovasc Thorac Ann. (2010). , 18, 360-3.

[140] Al-ebrahim, K. E. Sternocutaneous fistulas after cardiac surgery. Ann Thorac Surg (2010). , 89, 1705-6.

[141] Gaudreau, G, Costache, V, Houde, C, Cloutier, D, Montalin, L, Voisine, P, & Baillot, R. Recurrent sternal infection following treatment with negative pressure wound therapy and titanium transverse plate fixation. Eur J Cardiothorac Surg. (2010). , 37, 888-92.

[142] Steingrímsson, S, Gustafsson, R, Gudbjartsson, T, Mokhtari, A, Ingemansson, R, & Sjögren, J. Sternocutaneous fistulas after cardiac surgery: incidence and late outcome during a ten-year follow-up. Ann Thorac Surg (2009). , 88, 1910-5.

[143] Darouiche, R. O. Treatment of infections associated with surgical implants.N Engl J Med (2004). , 350, 1422-9.

[144] Bu-omar, Y, Naik, M. J, Catarino, P. A, & Ratnatunga, C. Right ventricular rupture during use of high-pressure suction drainage in the management of poststernotomy mediastinitis. Ann Thorac Surg. (2003).

[145] Bapat, V, Muttardi, N, Young, C, Venn, G, & Roxburgh, J. Experience with Vacuum-assisted closure of sternal wound infections following cardiac surgery and evaluation of chronic complications associated with its use. J Card Surg. (2008). , 23, 227-33.

[146] Van Wingerden, J. J, Segers, P, & Jekel, L. Major bleeding during negative pressure wound/V.A.C.®--therapy for postsurgical deep sternal wound infection--a critical appraisal. J Cardiothorac Surg. 201;6:121.

[147] Hayward, R. H, Korompai, F. L, & Knight, W. L. The open sternotomy wound and risk of acute hemorrhage. J Thorac Cardiovasc Surg (1992). , 103, 1228-30.

[148] Khoynezhad, A, Abbas, G, Palazzo, R. S, & Graver, L. M. Spontaneous right ventricular disruption following treatment of sternal infection. J Card Surg (2004). , 19, 74-8.

[149] Niclauss, L, Delay, D, & Stumpe, F. Right ventricular rupture due to recurrent mediastinal infection with a closed chest. Interact Cardiovasc Thorac Surg (2010). , 10, 470-2.

[150] Petzina, R, Malmsjö, M, Stamm, C, & Hetzer, R. Major complications during negative pressure wound therapy in poststernotomy mediastinitis after cardiac surgery. J Thorac Cardiovasc Surg.(2010). , 140, 1133-6.

[151] Malmsjö, M, Petzina, R, Ugander, M, Engblom, H, Torbrand, C, Mokhtari, A, Hetzer, R, Arheden, H, & Ingemansson, R. Preventing heart injury during negative pressure wound therapy in cardiac surgery: assessment using real-time magnetic resonance imaging. J Thorac Cardiovasc Surg (2009). , 138, 712-7.

[152] Voss, B, Bauernschmitt, R, Will, A, et al. Sternal reconstruction with titanium plates in complicated sternal dehiscence. Eur J Cardiothorac Surg (2008). , 34, 139-145.

[153] Gaudreau, G, Costache, V, Houde, C, Cloutier, D, Montalin, L, Voisine, P, & Baillot, R. Recurrent sternal infection following treatment with negative pressure wound therapy and titanium transverse plate fixation. Eur J Cardiothorac Surg (2010). , 37, 888-92.

[154] Voss, B, Bauernschmitt, R, Brockmann, G, et al. Osteosynthetic thoracic stabilization after complete resection of sternum. Eur J Cardiothorac Surg (2007). , 32, 391-393.

[155] Piotrowski, J. A, Fischer, M, Klaes, W, & Splittgerber, F. Autologous bone transplant after sternal resection. J Cardiovasc Surg (Torino) (1996). , 37, 179-81.

[156] Nahabedian, M. Y, Riley, L. H, Greene, P. S, et al. Sternal stabilization using allograft fibula following cardiac transplantation. Plastic Reconstr Surg (2001). , 108, 1284-8.

[157] Marulli, G, Hamad, A. M, Cogliati, E, Breda, C, Zuin, A, & Rea, F. Allograft sternochondral replacement after resection of large sternal chondrosarcoma. J Thorac Cardiovasc Surg (2010). e, 69-70.

[158] Dell'amore A, Cassanelli N, Dolci G, Stella F.An alternative technique for anterior chest wall reconstruction: the sternal allograft transplantation. Interact Cardiovasc ThoracInteract Cardiovasc Thorac Surg. (2012). , 15, 944-7.

[159] Dell'Amore A, Dolci G, Cassanelli N, Bini A, Stella F.A massive post-sternotomy sternal defect treated by allograft sternal transplantation. J Card Surg (2012). , 27, 557-9.

[160] Kalab, M, Molitor, M, Kubesova, B, & Lonsky, V. Use of allogenous bone graft and osteosynthetic stabilization in treatment of massive post-sternotomy defects. Eur J Cardiothorac Surg. (2012). Jun;41(6):e, 182-4.

[161] Collection of Laws of The Czech RepublicAct (2008). Collegium on Human Tissues and Cells. Prague, 2008.(296)

[162] European Association of Tissue BanksGeneral Standards for Tissue Banking. ÖBIG-Transplant, Vienna, (1995).

[163] Perkins, D. J, Hunt, J. A, Pennington, D. G, & Stern, H. S. Secondary sternal repair following median sternotomy using interosseous absorbable sutures and pectoralis major myocutaneous advancement flaps. British J Plast Surg (1996). , 49, 214-219.

[164] Brito, J. D, Assumpcao, C. R, Murad, H, & Jazbik, A. P. Sa MPL, Bastos ES, Giambroni Filho R, Silva RS. One-stage management of infected sternotomy wounds using bilateral pectoralis major myocutaneous advancement flap. Rev Bras Cir Cardiovasc (2009). , 24, 58-63.

[165] Greig AVH, Geh JLC, Khanduja V, Shibu M.Choice of flap for the management of deep sternal wound infection- an anatomical classification. J Plast Reconstr Aesth Surg. (2007). , 60, 372-378.

[166] Salgado, C. J, Mardini, S, Mamali, A. A, Ortiz, J, Gonzales, R, & Chen, H. C. Muscle versus nonmuscle flaps in the reconstructon of chronic osteomyelitis defects. Plast Reconstr Surg, (2006). , 118, 1401-1411.

[167] Yazar, S, Lin, Y. T, Ulusal, A. E, & Wei, F. C. Outcome comparison between free muscle and free fasciocutaneous flaps for reconstruction of distal third and ankle traumatic opetn tibial fractures. Plast Reconstr Surg, (2006). , 117, 2468-2475.

[168] Serafin, D. The Pectoralis Major Muscle Flap. In Serafin D. Atlas of Microsurgical Composite Tissue Tranplantation. W.B.Saunders company, London, (1996). , 1996, 161-174.

[169] Netscher, D. T, Eladoumikdachi, F, Mchugh, P. M, Thornby, J, & Soltero, E. Sternal wound debridement and muscle flap reconstruction: functional implications. Annals of Plast Surg (2003). , 51, 115-122.

[170] Cohen, M, Yaniv, Y, Weiss, J, Greif, J, Gur, E, Wertheym, E, & Shafir, R. Median sternotomy wound complication: the effect of reconstruction on lung function. Annals Plast Surg (1997). , 39, 36-43.

[171] Arnold, P. G, & Pairolero, P. C. Chest-wall reconstruction. An account of 500 consecutive patients. Plast Reconstr Surg (1996). , 98, 804-810.

[172] Skoracki, R. J, & Chang, D. W. Reconstruction of the chestwall and thorax. J Surg Oncol (2006). , 94, 455-465.

[173] Ascherman, J. A, Patel, S. M, Malhotra, S. M, & Smith, C. R. Management of sternla wounds with bilateral pectoralis major myocutaneous advancement flaps in 114 consecutively treated patients: refinements in technique and outcomes analysis. Plast Reconstr Surg (2004). , 114, 676-83.

[174] Hugo, N. E, Sultan, M. R, Ascherman, J. A, Patsis, M. C, Smith, C. R, & Rose, E. A. Single-stage management of 74 consecutive sternla wound complications with pectoralis major myocutaneous advancement flaps. Plast Reconstr Surg (1994). , 93, 1433-1441.

[175] Brutus, J. P, Nikolis, A, Perreault, I, & Harris, P. G. The unilateralpectoralis major island flap, an efficient and straightforward procedure for reconstruction of full length sternal defects after postoperative mediastinal wound infection. Brit J Plast Surg (2004). , 57, 803-805.

[176] Chou, E, Tai, Y, Chen, H, & Chen, K. Simple and reliable way in sternum wound coverage-tripedicle pectoralis major musculocutaneous flap. Microsurgery. (2008). , 28, 441-6.

[177] Majure, J. A, Albin, R. E, Donnell, O, & Arganese, R. S. TJ. Reconstruction of the infected median sternotomy wound. Ann Thorac Surg (1986). , 42, 9-12.

[178] Molitor, M, Simek, M, Lonský, V, Kaláb, M, Veselý, J, & Zálešák, B. Pectoral muscle flap with v-y skin paddle for covering sternal defects. Ann Thorac Surg. (2012). e, 131-3.

[179] Hallock, G. G. The breast musculocutaneous flap for complete coverage of the median sternotomy wound. Plast Reconstr Surg (2003). , 112, 199-203.

[180] Nahai, F, Morales, L, Bone, D. K, & Botswick, J. Pectoralis Major Muscle Turnover Flaps for Closure of the infected Sternotomy Wound with Preservation of Form and Function. Plast Reconstr Surg (1982). , 70, 471-474.

[181] Spiess, A. M, Balakrishnan, C. H, & Gursel, E. Fascial release of the pectoralis major:a technique used in pectoralis major muscle closure of the mediastinum in cases of mediastinitis. Plast Reconstr Surg. (2007). , 119, 573-7.

[182] Serafin, D. The Pectoralis Major Muscle Flap. In Serafin D. Atlas of Microsurgical Composite Tissue Tranplantation. W.B.Saunders company, London, (1996). , 1996, 221-247.

[183] Skoracki, R. J, & Chang, D. W. Reconstruction of the chestwall and thorax. J Surg Oncol. (2006). Review., 94, 455-65.

[184] Acinapura, A. J, Godfrey, N, Romita, M, Cunningham, J, Adams, P. X, Jacobowitz, I. S, Rose, D. M, & Nealon, T. Surgical management of infected median sternotomy:Closed irrigation vs muscle flaps. J Cardiovasc. Surg (1985). , 26, 443-446.

[185] Ford, T. D. Rectus abdominis myocutaneous flap used to close a median sternotomy chest defect. S Afr Med J (1985). , 68, 115-116.

[186] Solomon, M. P, & Granick, M. S. Bipedicle muscle flaps in sternal wound repair. Plast Reconstr Surg. (1998). , 101, 356-6.

[187] Laitung JKG, Peck F. Shoulder function following the loss of the latissimus dorsi muscle. British J Plast Surg (1985). , 38, 375-379.

[188] Dejesus, R. A, Paletta, J. D, & Dabb, R. W. Reconstruction of the median sternotomy sound dehiscence using the latissimus dorsi myocutaneous flap. J Cardiovasc Surg (2001). , 42, 359-564.

[189] Fansa, H, Handstein, S, & Schneider, W. Treatment of infected median sternotomy wounds with a myocutaneous latissimus dorsi muscle flap. Scand Cardiovasc J (1998). , 32, 33-39.

[190] Roshan, A, Kotwal, A, & Riaz, M. Stanley PRW. Sternal wound dehiscence complicated by macromastia: report of two cases with discussion of literature. J Plast Reconstr Aesth Surg (2009). ee364., 362.

[191] Copeland, M, Senkowski, C, Ergin, A, et al. Macromastia as a factor in sternal wound dehiscence following cardiac surgery:management combining chest wall reconstruction and reduction mammaplasty. J Card Surg (1992). , 7, 275-278.

[192] Fontaine, S, Devos, S, & Goldschmidt, D. Reduction mammoplasty combined with pectoralis major muscle flaps for median sternotomy wound closure. Br J Plats Surg (1996). , 49, 220-222.

[193] Uygur, F, Sever, C, Ulkur, E, & Celikoz, B. Reconstruction of large post-sternotomy wound with bilateral V-Y fasciocutaneous advancement flaps. Ann Thorac Surg (2008)., 86, 1012-1015.

[194] Roshan, A, Kotwal, A, & Riaz, M. Stanley PRW. Sternal wound dehiscence complicated by macromastia: report of two cases with discussion of literature. J Plast Reconstr Aesth Surg (2009). ee364., 362.

[195] Würinger, E, Mader, N, Posch, E, & Holle, J. Nerve and vessel supplying ligamentous suspension of the mammary gland. Plast Reconstr Surg (1998)., 101, 1486-1493.

[196] Hamdi, M, & Dancey, A. The septum-based therapeutic mammaplasty technique for management of sternal defects. Plast Reconstr Surg (2010)., 569-573.

[197] Hughes, K. C, Henry, M. J, Turner, J, & Manders, E. K. Design of the cyclops flap for chest-wall reconstruction. Plast Reconstr Surg (1997)., 100, 1146-51.

[198] Aydin, A, Güven, E, Keklik, B, Basaran, K, & Özkan, B. Reconstruction of the Chest Wall Defects with Mammary Dermoglandular Advancement Flaps in Female Complicated Cases. Trakya Univ Tip Fak Derg (2009)., 26, 130-133.

[199] Yasuura, K, Okamoto, H, Morita, S, Ogawa, Y, Sawazaki, M, Seki, A, Masumoto, H, Matsuura, A, Maseki, T, & Torii, S. Results of omental flap transposition for deep sternal wound infection after cardiovascular surgery. Annals of Surg (1998)., 227, 455-459.

[200] Mathisen, D. J, Grillo, H. C, Vlahakes, G. J, et al. The omentum in the management of complicated cardiothoracic probleme. J Thorac Cardiovasc Surg (1988)., 95, 677-684.

[201] Weinzweig, N, & Hetman, R. Transposition of the greater omentum for recalcitrant median sternotomy wound infection. Annals Plast. Surg (1995)., 34, 471-477.

[202] Alday, E. S, & Golsdmith, H. S. Surgical technique for ometal lenghtening based on arterial anatomy. Surg Gynecol Obstet (1972).

[203] Das, S. K. The size of the human omentum and methods of lenghtening it for transposition. Br J Plast Surg (1976)., 29, 170-174.

[204] Weinzweig, N, & Hetman, R. Transposition of the greater omentum for recalcitrant median sternotomy wound infection. Annals Plast. Surg (1995)., 34, 471-477.

[205] Pearl, S. N, & Dibbell, D. G. Reconstruction after median sternotomy infection. Surg Gynecol Obstet (1984)., 159, 47-52.

[206] Colen, L. B, Huntsman, W. T, & Morain, W. D. The integrated approach to suppurative mediastinitis: rewiring the sternum over transposed omentum. Plast Reconstr Surg (1989)., 84, 936-943.

[207] Hakelius, L. Fatal complication after use of the greater omentum for reconstruction of the chest wall. Plast Reconstr Surg (1978).

http://dx.doi.org/10.5772/55310

[208] Acarturk, T. O, Swartz, W. M, Luketich, J, et al. Laparoscopically harvested omental flap for chest wall and intrathoracic reconstruction. Ann Plast Surg (2004). , 53, 210-216.

[209] Barragan, B. A, Hallodorsson, A. O, Wachtel, M. S, & Frezza, E. E. Laparoscopic greater omentum harvesting with split-thickness skin grafting for sternal wound dehiscence. The American Surgeon (2006). , 72, 829-832.

[210] Reichenberger, M. A, Harenberg, P. S, Pelzer, M, Gazyakan, E, Ryssel, G, Hermann, G, & Engel, H. Arteriovenous loops in microsurgical free tissue transfer in reconstruction of central sternal defects. J Thorac Cardiovasc Surg (2010). , 140, 1283-1287.

[211] Engel, H, Pelzer, M, Sauerbier, M, Hermann, G, & Heitmann, C. An innovative treatment concept for free flap reconstruction of komplex central chest wall defects- the cephalic-thoraco-acromial (CTA) loop. Microsurgery (2007). , 27, 481-486.